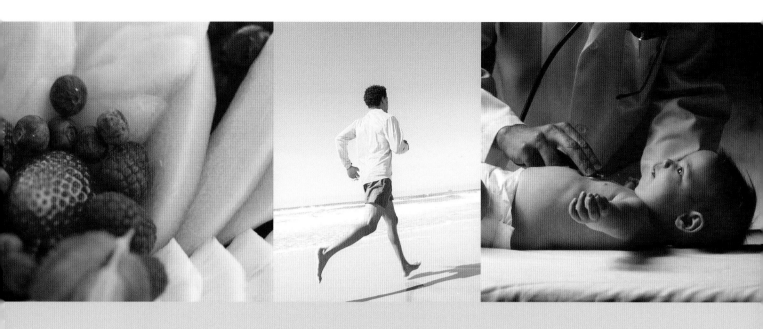

The Duke Encyclopedia of
New Medicine

This edition first published in 2006 by
Rodale International Ltd
7–10 Chandos Street
London W1G 9AD
www.rodalebooks.co.uk

© 2006 Rodale Books International
Text © 2006 Duke University

Produced for Rodale Books International
by
Hydra Packaging, 129 Main Street, Irvington, NY 10533, USA

Cover photographs: Getty Images

Printed and bound in China
using acid-free paper from sustainable sources.

1 3 5 7 9 8 6 4 2

A CIP record for this book is available from the British Library

ISBN-10: 1-4050-9572–5
ISBN-13: 978-1-4050-9572-3

This edition distributed to the book trade by Pan Macmillan Ltd

Notice
This book is intended as a reference volume. The information here is designed to help you make
informed decisions about your health. It is not intended as a substitute for any treatment that may have been prescribed
by your doctor. If you suspect that you have a medical problem, we urge you to seek competent medical help.
Mention of specific companies, organizations or authorities in this book does not imply endorsement by
the publisher, nor does mention of specific companies, organizations or authorities in the book imply that they
endorse the book. Websites and telephone numbers given in this book were accurate at the time the book went to press.

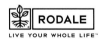

We inspire and enable people to improve their lives and the world around them

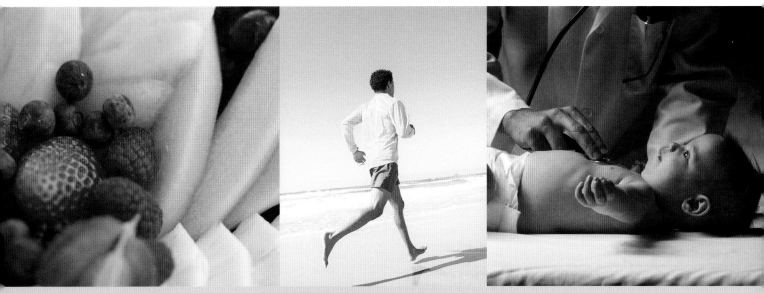

The Duke Encyclopedia of
New Medicine

Conventional and Alternative Medicine for All Ages

Foreword by David Servan-Schreiber, MD, PhD.

 Duke Center for Integrative Medicine
DUKE UNIVERSITY HEALTH SYSTEM

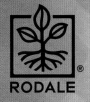
RODALE

Duke Center for Integrative Medicine
DUKE UNIVERSITY HEALTH SYSTEM

The Future of Medicine, Delivered Today

Duke University Health System is a world-class healthcare network, dedicated to providing outstanding patient care, educating tomorrow's healthcare leaders, and discovering new and innovative ways to treat disease through biomedical research. We offer our patients skilful medicine and a thoughtful approach to treatment through a continuum of health services from primary care and antenatal care to hospice. Duke University Medical Center – the hub of the health system – is consistently ranked among the top ten healthcare organizations in the United States.

The Duke Center for Integrative Medicine

The Duke Center for Integrative Medicine (DCIM) is a leader in providing innovative approaches to

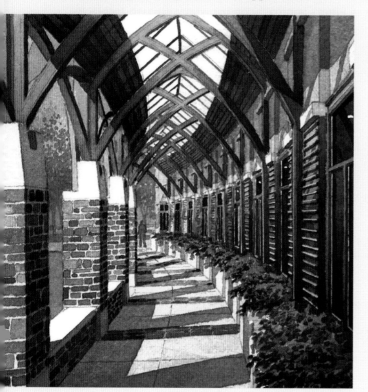

health and healing. Our medical professionals and healing arts practitioners combine the knowledge of modern science with the wisdom of ancient traditions for a 'whole-person' approach to healthcare.

Dedicated exclusively to integrative healthcare, our facility is the first of its kind. Located on the beautifully wooded, 26-acre Duke Center for Living Campus, the 27,000-plus square foot building includes warm and comfortable therapeutic treatment rooms, workshop spaces and gardens where clients can experience an entirely different approach to healthcare. Here, clients can design personal health plans in partnership with skilled medical professionals and take advantage of the best practice of medicine from both conventional and complementary/alternative systems.

The DCIM is a founding member of The Consortium of Academic Health Centers for Integrative Medicine, an association of United States and Canadian universities that have a high level of commitment to integrative healthcare.

Maximizing Your Health and Healing

Whether you are suffering from an illness or simply want to enhance your current state of wellness, you will find that DCIM's primary goal is to maximize your ability to reach optimal vitality and health. We understand that a powerful connection links the mind, body, spirit and community to health and disease. We believe that the human mind and body have essential capacities for self-repair that can be supported and enhanced by appropriate conventional as well as complementary/alternative (CAM) therapies.

The Personalized Health Plan

Our goal is to assist you in creating and following your own Personalized Health Plan. Our team helps

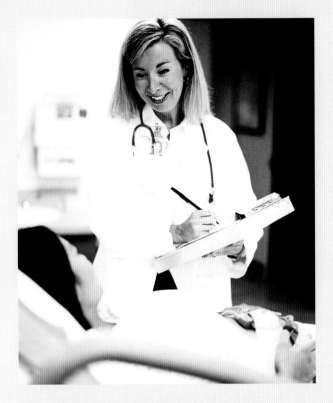

partner or coach to help you create the life you desire. Much like a 'personal trainer' for the whole self, a coach can help you make needed behavioural changes through a structured, supportive partnership of insight, clarity and personal discovery.

Programmes Designed around Your Lifestyle

We understand the challenge of your daily responsibilities and offer flexible, multi-day immersion and educational programmes to fit round your schedule alongside your unique personal health goals. We can also tailor integrative medicine group programmes of up to 60 people for your business, professional group or association.

The Forefront of Integrative Medicine Research

We actively measure the impact of our models of care on patient wellness. Early results from research on our mindfulness-based treatment for eating disorders show it to be a promising means of regulating eating behaviour. Another study examined the effect of the personal health planning model, a keystone of the Center's approach, on patients with high risk factors for developing heart disease. Participants measurably improved their food choices and exercise patterns and reduced their chances of having a cardiovascular incident, such as a heart attack or stroke, over the next ten years.

Agents of Change

At Duke Center for Integrative Medicine, we are agents of change. We are dedicated to the transformation of healthcare from a disease-oriented, doctor-and-technology-centred model into a health-oriented, patient-centred approach that understands and empowers the integration of body, mind, spirit and community in healthcare.

We believe that what is now called 'integrative medicine' will simply become the standard practice of medicine in the future.

To learn more about the Duke Center for Integrative Medicine, visit us online at **www.dcim.org**.

you to assess your current state of health and risk factors for disease, and then works with you to achieve clarity around your health goals and your readiness to change. We then help you to create a comprehensive personal health plan, to experience putting your plan into action in our immersion programme, and then partner with you for maximum effectiveness in taking it home.

The plan includes recommendations from both conventional and complementary/alternative practices, such as conventional medications, herbal supplements, preventative and diagnostic medical screenings, and examinations, Oriental medicine and acupuncture, physical therapy, mind/body therapy, nutritional therapy, movement and exercise assessments.

Individualized Health Coaching

The Duke Center for Integrative Medicine offers each client a health coach: a person who partners with you to make your goals a reality. This provides you with the opportunity to collaborate with an experienced

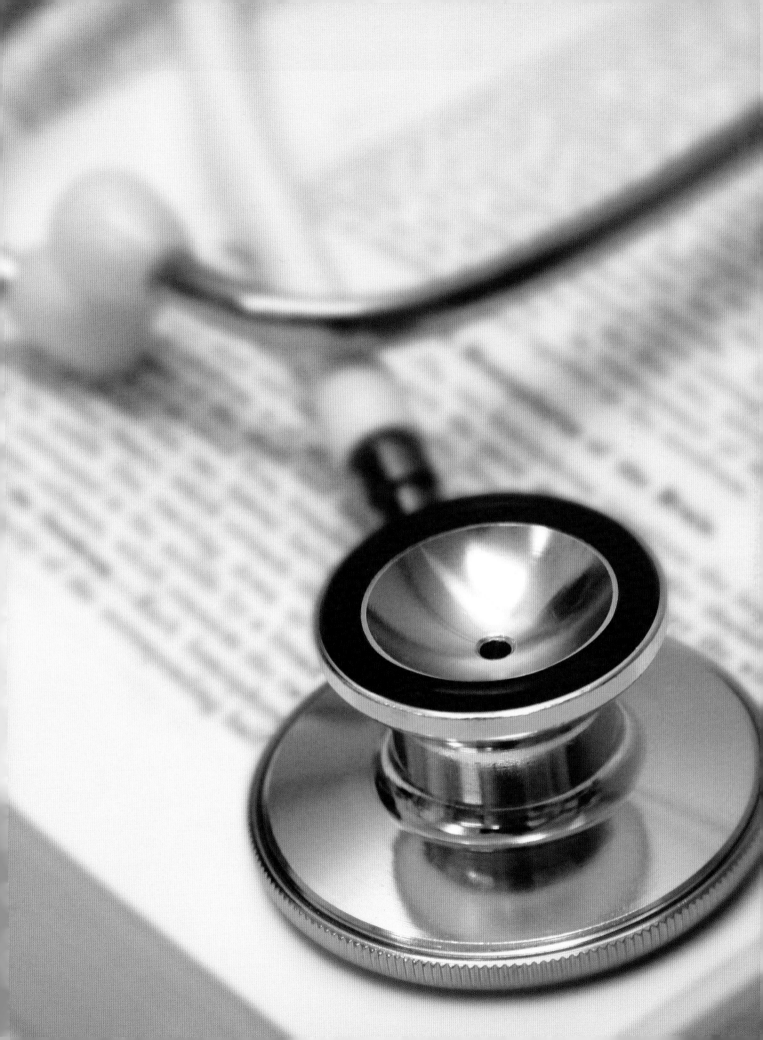

The Duke Center for Integrative Medicine Team

CHIEF MEDICAL EDITORS

Richard Liebowitz, M.D., MHS
Executive Medical Director
Duke Center for Living
Department of Medicine

Linda Smith, PA-C
Director of Programmes
Duke Center for Integrative Medicine
Department of Medicine

MEDICAL CONTRIBUTORS

Tracy W. Gaudet, M.D.
Director
Duke Center for Integrative Medicine
Department of Obstetrics and Gynaecology

Ruth Quillian Wolever, Ph.D.
Health Psychologist and Clinic Director
Duke Center for Integrative Medicine
Department of Psychiatry and Behavioural Sciences

Jeffrey Brantley, M.D.
Director
Mindfulness-Based Stress Reduction Programme
Duke Center for Integrative Medicine
Department of Psychiatry and Behavioural Sciences

Sam Moon, M.D., M.P.H.
Director of Education
Duke Center for Integrative Medicine
Department of Community and Family Medicine

Shelley W. Wroth, M.D.
Department of Obstetrics and Gynaecology
Duke University Medical Center

Greg Hottinger, M.P.H., RD
Nutritionist
Duke Center for Integrative Medicine

Jon Seskevich, R.N., B.S.N, B.A, C.H.T.P.
Nurse Clinician
Duke University Medical Center

Christy K. Mack
Reiki Master
Co-Founder and Director, Bravewell Collaborative

EXTERNAL CONTRIBUTORS

Susan Gilbert, Senior Writer
Award-winning medical journalist and author

Nelly Edmondson Gupta, MA, Contributing Writer
Award-winning medical journalist and magazine
editor

Sheena Meredith MB, BS, MPhil
Contributing Writer
Medical writer, editor and consultant in healthcare
communications

Diana Reese, Contributing Writer
Medical writer specializing in health and medicine

Laura Wallace, MA, Contributing Writer
Writer and editor specializing in health matters

David Servan-Schreiber, MD, PhD
European Medical Consultant
Dr. Servan-Schreiber is Clinical Professor of Psychia-
try, University of Pittsburgh, Lecturer School of Medi-
cine of Lyon, France, and co-founder of the Center for
Integrative Medicine of the University of Pittsburgh.
He is one of the original founders of Doctors Without
Borders-USA, and author of *Healing Without Freud or
Prosac* (Rodale, 2004).

HYDRA PACKAGING

Senior Editor: Myrsini Stephanides
Senior Designer: Brian MacMullen

Editors: Beth Adelman, Franchesca Ho Sang,
Dr Dennis Kuo, Brad Plummer
Designers: Marian Purcell, La Tricia Watford,
Shamona Stokes, Rachel Maloney, Gus Yoo

Editorial Director: Lori Baird
Art Director: Edwin Kuo

Production: Wayne Ellis, Sarah Reilly

Illustrators: Stan Coffman, Kevin Newman,
Rachel Maloney
Photo Researchers: Jeanne Leslie, Ben DeWalt
Indexer: Linda B. Burton

President: Sean Moore
Publishing Director: Karen Prince

RODALE BOOKS INTERNATIONAL

Managing Editor: Miranda Smith
Senior Editor: Dawn Bates
Art Editors: Jo Connor, Vivienne Brar
Production: Sara Granger
DTP: Keith Bambury

Foreword

Some things in medicine have always been unacceptable. That a person with early breast cancer may be steered away from highly effective surgery or chemotherapy for the promise of an ineffective 'alternative' treatment is unacceptable. However, excesses in the other direction have now become equally unreasonable.

Today, I still know of people with depression, who are told that their best treatment option is medication for the rest of their life. Yet, high quality studies have shown that thirty minutes of physical exercise three times a week is equally effective, with none of the side-effects. I also know of people who, after a course of surgery and chemotherapy for colon cancer, have asked their oncologist about measures they could take to keep it from coming back. Often, they are advised to have regular examinations to help catch the cancer at an early stage. Yet, modern studies show that simple nutritional interventions can greatly reduce the incidence of colon cancer. Similar stories can be told about recurrent ear infections in children, people recovering from a heart attack or people dealing with diabetes.

In the 21st century, modern science has shown that our health depends largely on things we can do for ourselves, and no longer only on a doctor's prescriptions for medication. Each of us need to know how to restore balance to our bodies naturally and also how to harness the best of what conventional medicine has to offer.

Ten years ago, as a conventionally trained doctor and scientist, I learned this powerful lesson while on a mission with Doctors Without Borders. I was working with Tibetan refugees in

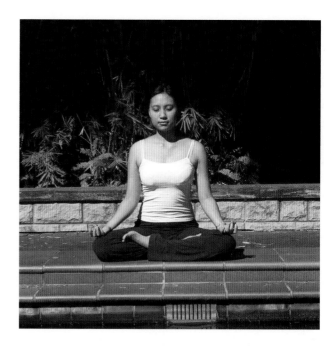

Northern India. The large Tibetan community of Dharamsala – where the Dalai Lama set up his government – benefited from two equally strong health systems. One was a conventional Western system with a hospital, pharmacies and doctors trained in the large cities of India, western Europe and the United Sates. The other was a system of traditional Tibetan Medicine with its own medical school, myriads of practitioners and even a manufacturing plant for herbal remedies. In that system, the only interventions involved meditation, acupuncture, nutritional advice and herbal supplements. At the time, I firmly believed – as I had been taught – that all of these had to be mere placebos. So, when I talked with my counterparts at the Tibetan Ministry of Health, or with well-travelled high Lamas who were interested in improving the health status of the community, I was curious to know their answer to what seemed to be a difficult question: "As a Tibetan who is very familiar with Western civilization, when you get sick yourself, which medicine do you turn to?" To my surprise, they looked at me as if this was almost silly. Their answer was both extremely simple and illuminating: "Obviously, if you have an acute disease, such as pneumonia, a heart attack or appendicitis, you go see a Western doctor. Their treatments are very effective and fast for a medical crisis. But," they continued, "if you have a chronic problem, Western treatments are not enough. You need to work on your body's natural ability to restore its own health, and for this you need the help of a medicine that works on the terrain, not just the illness. This is what Tibetan medicine does. It's slower, but it's also softer and works at a deeper level, by supporting your own natural healing mechanisms."

This was so simple and yet so profound. In 2005, the World Health Organization published a report announcing that the leading causes of illness in the world were now chronic diseases: heart conditions, strokes, cancer, diabetes, depression, etc. Obviously, today we need a new medicine – one that takes advantage of all the advances of modern science in terms of detecting diseases early, understanding their genetic underpinnings, or using precise and focused surgical interventions. However, we also need a medicine that understands natural mechanisms of healing that are part of each one of us, and that knows how to put them to use to help us prevent illness or recover from it when we are sick.

In the last 20 years, pioneering studies have demonstrated the benefits of many natural approaches of treatment. These include studies of nutrition, yoga, meditation, acupuncture, specific supplements or herbal remedies. Duke University was one of the first prestigious medical schools to embrace these treatments as part of a new medicine. The Center for Integrative Medicine at Duke University has focused on natural treatments that have been proved to work and that help give back to each patient some of the natural power and control that had often been lost in the old model of medicine. The success of the Center has been such that it is now contributing to the redefinition of the medical school curriculum in one of the most prestigious medical institutions in the world.

This book, *The Duke Encyclopedia of New Medicine*, is based on the extensive experience of some of the leading doctors and practitioners who have helped advance a practice of medicine that integrates the best of conventional and natural treatments. The book is also rigorously faithful to the scientific evidence that exists for each treatment that is discussed. Reviewing it page by page, I was intrigued by how different this medicine was from the one I had learned about in medical school. It is so much more intelligent, and so much more generous, having learned to make each person more informed and more capable of finding their own capacity to heal.

David SS

David Servan-Schrieiber, MD, PhD

Contents

Part I
Catalogue of
Health
Conditions

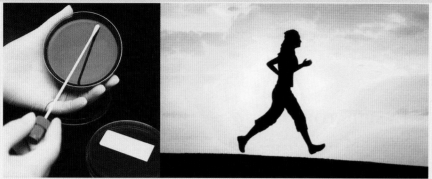

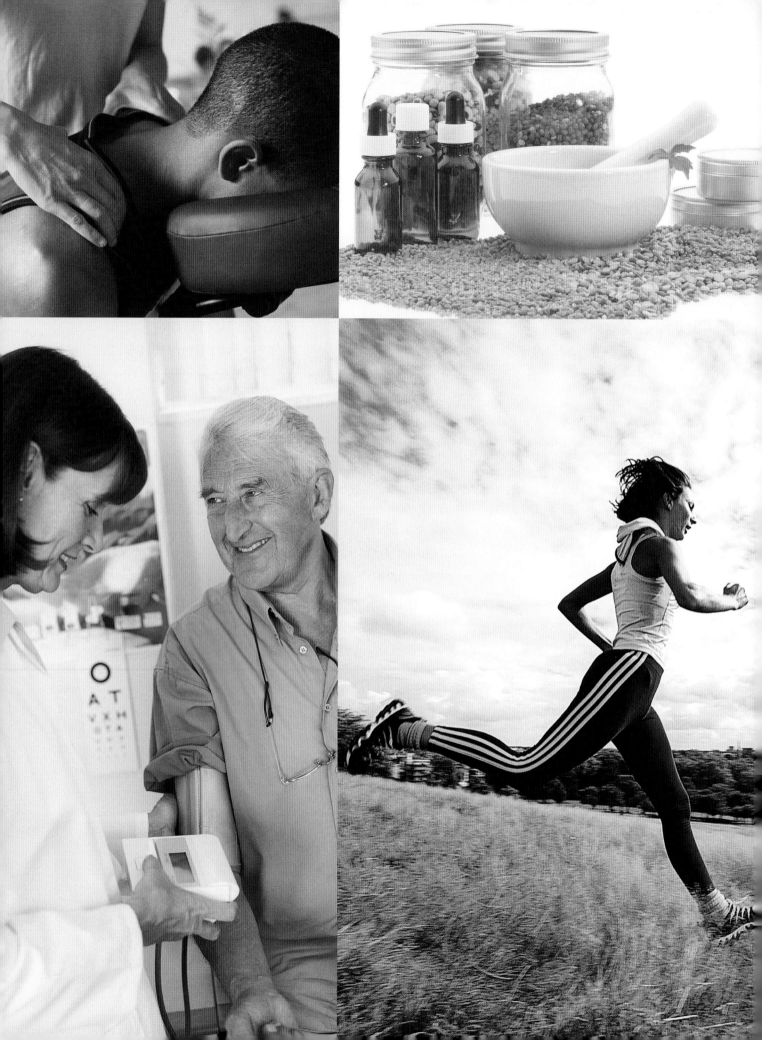

INTRODUCTION

"This is the great error of our day in the treatment of the human being that physicians separate the soul from the body."

This lament could easily describe the state of health care today – with all too much emphasis placed on the diseased parts of the body, and all too little on the whole person. But in fact the quote is from Plato more than 2,000 years ago. Then, as now, a major flaw in the practice of medicine has been an overemphasis on the physical symptoms and too little consideration of the individual's mind and soul.

An Integrative Approach

The emphasis is changing. Around the world, there has been a huge cultural shift in the way people view healthcare. This shift has given rise to integrative medicine, a new paradigm of medical care that considers all factors affecting health, wellness and disease, including the psychosocial and spiritual dimensions of a person's life. The goal of integrative medicine is whole-person care. It is a transformational model of healthcare for the 21st century. It is the future of medicine.

Integrative medicine is 'integrative' in several respects. It joins patients and their health providers in a partnership. Rather than being passive recipients of doctors' orders, patients are active participants in their healthcare and changing health needs. Empowered by information about their options for disease prevention and treatment, patients explore the pros and cons of those options with their health providers to arrive at the plan that is best for them. Integrative health plans are built on mutual trust and respect between patient and practitioner, with the understanding that each individual has a significant, innate capacity for healing that can be supported and enhanced, regardless of the person's initial health condition.

In addition, integrative medicine combines therapeutic interventions from conventional, as well as complementary and alternative disciplines. It integrates state-of-the-art conventional, or allopathic, diagnostic tests and treatments with careful selections from the range of other therapies, including Oriental medicine and acupuncture, herbal medicine, and mind–body interventions such as yoga and meditation, the benefits of which have been widely documented. Whenever possible, integrative medicine favours the evidence-based use of low-tech, low-cost interventions.

Duke University is a world leader in the practice of integrative medicine. The Duke Center for Integrative Medicine, founded in 2000, offers public and professional education programmes, conducts research and practises integrative medicine with individual patient consultation services. In the autumn of 2006, it opened its new facility, the first integrative medicine centre designed to create a healing environment, in which patients and practitioners alike can experience this new approach to health. This centre is committed to addressing the whole person, offering the best of all approaches to healthcare, creating a plan for optimizing an individual's health, immersing them in that actual experience and partnering with them in implementing their plan across time. We at Duke believe that there is a powerful interrelationship between the mind, body, spirit and community in the establishment of both health and disease. Feeling under enormous stress, for example, increases an individual's risk of many conditions such as depression, memory impairment and heart disease. But learning effective mind–body techniques and having strong social ties can buffer the impact of stress and its harmful health effects.

This encyclopedia is a comprehensive resource on integrative medicine. Part I is a catalogue of health conditions – what they are, their causes and the approaches that can be used to prevent and treat them. Part II is a guide to complementary and alternative therapies, with the latest scientific evidence on which treatments are effective for particular health conditions. To help you navigate through Part I and put all of this information into practice, we devised the Wheel of Health (pp.24–5). This is the framework that we use with our patients at the Duke University Center for Integrative Medicine. We have also created a Scale of Evidence (p.23), which provides a guide to the relative benefits and risks for the complementary and alternatives in Part II.

We believe the framework for optimal health rests on three basic strategies, which are represented as three concentric circles in the Wheel of Health. First, at the centre of the wheel, is mindfulness – learning to live in the present moment and, as such, being aware of your own health and being connected to your body, mind and spirit. You are your greatest health resource. But you can only make your best decisions when you are aware of the state of your physical, mental and spiritual health. Next, in the inner circle, are the strategies you can use to improve or maintain your health. These are movement and exercise, nutrition, the physical environment, relationships, personal development and spirituality, and the mind–body connection. The outer circle includes the strategies that involve working with healthcare professionals: preventative medicine, pharmaceuticals and supplements, conventional treatments and complementary/alternative therapies.

What follows is a description of each component of the wheel. You can turn to pages 24–5 for a visual breakdown of the wheel components.

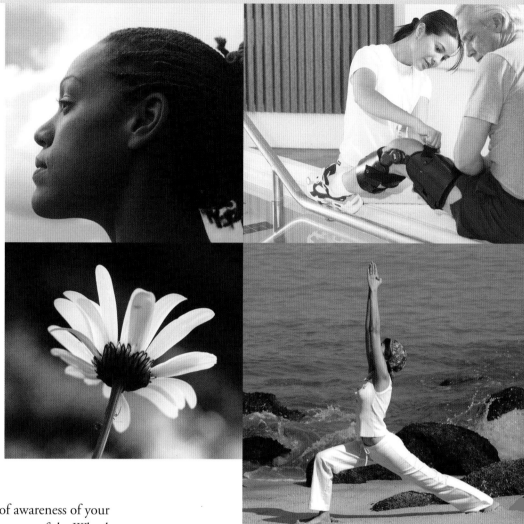

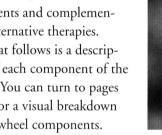

Mindfulness

Mindfulness is a developed sense of awareness of your body, mind and spirit. It is in the centre of the Wheel of Health because all of the other domains of health depend on it. When you are mindful, you are focused on the present – not thinking about the past or planning for the future. To be proactive about your health, you need to learn to be aware of the state of your health, to tune in to your physical, mental and social well-being. Another crucial trait of mindfulness is that it is non-judgmental – you acknowledge a thought or a feeling without criticizing yourself for having it.

Being mindful enables you to notice symptoms early, when they are at the level of a whisper instead of a scream. Recognizing symptoms early is a key to diagnosing health problems early, when they are most readily treatable. Mindfulness is an agent of positive change in your life. It informs the choices you make in the other domains of your health. For example, being aware of a high level of stress in your life allows you to make it a priority to address this risk factor and take steps to reduce it.

Mind–Body Connection

The mind is one of the most powerful tools you have for healing and health. Your state of mind has a huge impact on how your body reacts to stress – whether it reacts in health-harming ways or in health-protective ways. It is estimated that about 70 percent of medical visits are either directly or indirectly related to stress.

Stress is a physical or an emotional factor that causes bodily or mental tension. But here is the key: it is your perception of an event that determines whether or not your body experiences it as stressful. While many events are inherently stressful, you can use the mind to significantly impact the body's response to the stressors. This mind–body connection is key in that it opens the door for protecting your body and mind from the significant health risks of stress.

Stress causes many physiological changes in your body as it activates a number of different hormones.

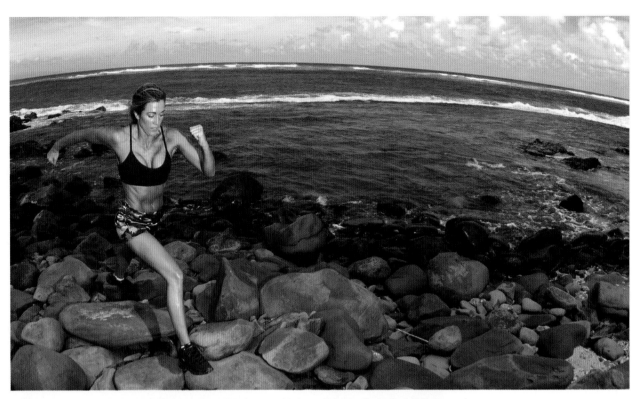

Taking exercise for only twenty minutes a day will help to avoid many diseases, including diabetes and heart disease. It will also help to control weight, which is a major factor in combating health problems.

These changes raise your heart rate, increase your blood pressure and blood sugar, and have major effects on your immune system. While these responses may be helpful in the short term, chronic stress clearly contributes to health problems, including high blood pressure, heart disease, diabetes and cancer.

The opposite of the stress response is the relaxation response. There are many ways to decrease the stress and to activate the relaxation response. Approaches include breathing techniques, meditation, progressive muscle relaxation and guided imagery. Awareness of the ways you can decrease your experience of stress is a key to optimizing your health.

Movement and Exercise

Our bodies are designed to be in motion. And yet, many people barely move at all; this is increasingly true, even of children. Many diseases that are in epidemic proportions, such as diabetes and heart disease, are directly related to the lack of adequate movement and exercise. There is no drug or vitamin that has as many health benefits as exercise. Fortunately, you need not go back to the days before cars and other modern conveniences to remedy this situation.

Twenty minutes of physical activity a day helps to prevent a large number of common diseases. So why do so few of us exercise? Part of the reason is that we have forgotten the joy that comes with moving our bodies. To get back on track, begin paying attention to the kinds of movements your body loves, and build from there. Start with small goals, which will allow your body and mind to get on board instead of rebel. You'll soon realize it can be fun – you will feel better, have more energy, your work will be more efficient and you will feel less stressed.

Find activities that appeal to you and stick with them. To get the most out of your exercise plan, be mindful of your target heart rate and adjust the intensity of your workout to your needs. In addition, incorporate stretching and weight-bearing exercises into your regimen.

Nutrition

When it comes to your health, you certainly are what you eat. A healthy diet supplies you with all the nutrients you need and helps reduce your risk of certain illnesses. A poor diet may leave you vulnerable to substances that can compromise your health. It is not only what you eat, but also where you get your food, how you prepare it and how much you consume that influence its effect on your health.

Do you know which types of fats you consume? Some fats, such as omega-3 fatty acids, help protect against heart disease and other illnesses, whereas other fats increase the risk of illnesses. Tropical oils, such as palm and coconut oil, can markedly increase the level of cholesterol in your blood. The same is true of trans fatty acids, manufactured fats used in processed foods that may increase the risk of certain diseases. Protein is an important component of your diet, but some protein sources are good for your heart and others are not. What is the real story about carbohydrates? Some, such as whole-grains, are very good for you and others, especially processed snack foods, are bad for your health.

These are just a few of the many aspects of nutrition that can have a significant impact on your health. Other considerations are how you prepare your food – proper cleaning is necessary to reduce pesticide residues and other contaminants – and how much you eat. Overeating is one of the main causes of excess weight, and being overweight increases the risk of many illnesses, including heart disease and some forms of cancer. Simply becoming mindful of why you eat – distinguishing between physiological hunger

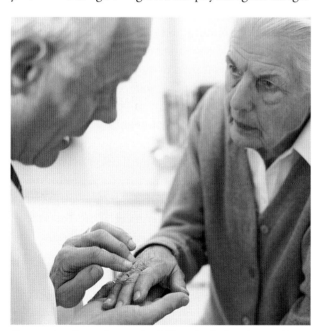

Movement and exercise, good nutrition, physical environment and relationships are very important if remaining in good health to a ripe old age is to be achieved.

and snacking as a result of boredom or anxiety, for example – can be the first step in making significant health improvements.

Physical Environment

Your environment – the spaces where you live and work, as well as the landscape around those spaces – can have profound effects on all aspects of your health. Indoor and outdoor pollutants – fuel emissions, lead paint, secondhand smoke, radon, mercury in fish and the like – can harm your health. Ongoing exposure to loud noise, or 'noise pollution', can also exact a toll on your health in the forms of hearing loss, stress and insomnia. Other environmental hazards include biological agents such as viruses and bacteria, excessive sun exposure, and, to sensitive individuals, allergens. Research suggests that health may also be affected by light, colour, smells and even clutter. All aspects of the physical environment can influence your well-being and your sense of living in a healthy and healing place. Being mindful of your environment goes beyond eliminating toxic or negative aspects. It involves being proactive and creating a healing environment in which to live and work. Pay attention to all of your senses and create environments that nurture them.

Relationships

Human beings are, by nature, social creatures. Research suggests that social support is *the most important psychological buffer of disease*. The level of positive social connection and support in your life exerts a powerful influence over the development, progression and recovery from many diseases.

Inadequate amounts of social support have been linked to an increased risk of dying prematurely from heart attacks, stroke, autoimmune diseases and cancer. It is not only the number of friends and acquaintances you have, but the quality of your relationships with them that matter. For example, research suggests that children who have a poor relationship with their parents are more likely to develop cancer later in life than are children who have a positive, loving relationship with their parents.

Do you have people you can really count on for help and support? Someone you can say anything to? How do you feel about the quality of the important

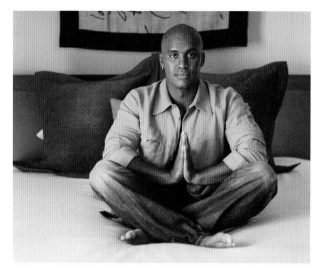

Meditation is a relaxing activity and can help an individual experience spiritual growth. This, in turn, is likely to have a positive effect on health and quality of life.

relationships in your life – those with your parents, children, spouse, siblings, and closest friends? Being aware of the importance of these questions and their answers is the first step to broadening and strengthening the relationships in your life. One way to do this is to pay attention to how well you communicate, both as a listener and a speaker. Spend more time and energy with people who fuel you, and less with people who drain you.

Personal Development and Spirituality

Spirituality, or the capacity to seek purpose and meaning in something larger than yourself, can have a profound effect on health. People around the world derive spiritual guidance and sustenance from religion, but spirituality is not the same as religion. Spirituality can be derived from faith, love, forgiveness, meditation, prayer, nature or the arts – anything that allows a person to transcend everyday experiences and see beyond them.

Research suggests many benefits from spirituality, and the body of literature continues to grow. People who consider themselves spiritual rate their quality of life higher than people who do not consider themselves to be especially spiritual. Those who attend religious services live longer than those who do not.

Whatever the ultimate source of your spirituality, it connects with your soul – the core of who you are. It is the engine of your dreams, goals and personal development. Are there things in your life that give you a sense of joy and motivation? Do you feel fulfilled at home and at work? Do you feel capable of rising above events in your life and maintaining a sense of purpose? These are some of the questions that can help put you in touch with your spirituality and focus on the things that matter most to you. The resilience of the human spirit is tremendous, and nurturing it can be invaluable, particularly in times when your body and mind are faced with health challenges.

Preventative Medicine

Prevention is always preferred to treating a disease. There are many effective ways to prevent disease. Immunizations can shield you from several illnesses. Routine screening tests can alert you to health problems before you would otherwise be aware of them. Avoiding substances such as tobacco and drugs of abuse that are known to cause serious illnesses can dramatically reduce your risk of developing them.

There are many tests that can identify your risk of disease and give you information that can help protect you from illness. Other tests can identify diseases in their early stages, before they cause symptoms and when they are most easily treated. A number of medical groups around the world have made recommendations for routine screening based on age and sex.

Are your immunizations up to date? Do you know when you should have a mammogram? Do you smoke and, if so, have you tried to quit? Have you had a cholesterol screening? Have you seen the dentist lately?

Pharmaceuticals and Supplements

Even when you do 'all the right things', there may be times when you will need medication to treat or prevent an illness. Medication may be prescribed by your health provider and provided by a pharmacist. It may be an over-the-counter medication. You may take a vitamin or supplement to help prevent disease and improve health. Glucosamine, for example, is clearly recognized to decrease both the pain and progression of osteoarthritis of the knee, and folic acid can help prevent certain types of birth defects. Selenium and flax have the potential to lower the risk of certain types of cancer. Omega-3s from fish improve survival after a heart attack.

Before you take any pharmaceuticals or supplements, it is important to learn about them – why you need them, how they can help you and what their side-effects are. Each of them has the potential to help as well as to harm. Certain medications can interact with each other, or with particular supplements, to cause adverse reactions. You can reduce this risk by informing your medical provider of all pharmaceuticals and supplements that you use.

Other information can help you make informed choices about pharmaceuticals and supplements in partnership with your healthcare provider. If your doctor prescribes a drug, make sure you take it as directed – stopping a medicine too soon or taking too-small a dose can reduce its effectiveness. Increasing the dose without checking with your medical provider can be dangerous. And the interactions between over-the-counter supplements and prescribed pharmaceuticals can be significant.

CAM Therapies

If you have a medical condition, following a treatment plan is critical. It is also very important to recognize that there may be more than one medical system to explore. Conventional Western medicine is highly effective with many acute medical problems, such as infection and trauma. But it is less successful in adequately relieving the symptoms of many chronic health problems. Alternative approaches, such as massage, osteopathy, acupuncture and hypnosis, can often help where conventional medicine cannot. The key lies in the appropriate integration of all effective therapies. There are definitely fraudulent and harmful practices being promoted under the banner of CAM. And there are very effective approaches which every patient should be aware of and consider in their health plan.

Integrative medicine combines the best of conventional and complementary and alternative therapies. If you are interested in using an alternative medicine system, it is important to discuss this with your medical provider. It is also important to educate yourself about the evidence supporting the use of any treatment or procedure, be it conventional or alternative. For more information on CAM treatments, refer to the Part II Introduction on pages 434–5.

SCALE OF EVIDENCE

Every treatment decision in medicine strives to achieve a balance between risk and benefits. Chemotherapy, for example, has significant side-effects, but also prolongs survival of people with certain types of cancer, and in some cases can save their lives.

Many complementary/alternative treatments do not have strong studies to support claims of their benefits. (For information on how reasearch for CAM treatments is conducted, refer to pp.434–5.) When deciding on a course of treatment, it is important to integrate the best of all systems, weighing benefits and risks for a complete whole/person approach. Keep in mind that there may be significant risk in selecting an alternative treatment for which there may be limited evidence for effectiveness over a more conventional treatment with significant evidence of benefit. This decision is often best made in discussion with a healthcare professional, especially one who is well versed in integrative medicine including both conventional and alternative approaches.

For each of the complementary/alternative treatments discussed in Part II, we have provided our estimate of how well benefits of the treatment have been established (the green scale, ranging from 1 – minimal to no evidence of benefit, to 3 – strong evidence of benefit). With the red scale, we have provided our estimate of how much risk or danger may be involved in using the treatment – for example: meditation involves minimal risk, whereas ozone therapy can lead to serious side-effects such as anaemia. Some natural supplements such as kava-kava have been associated with liver failure and death and cannot be recommended in most circumstances.

The Wheel of Health

The Wheel of Health symbolizes Duke University's unique approach to integrative medicine. Three concentric circles represent the three elements of optimal health. Each of the conditions and diseases in Part I includes easily recognizable icons that represent the self-care concepts introduced in the Wheel of Health. As you navigate through the ency-clopedia, you can refer back to this introduction for a thorough explanation of the framework of the Wheel – the interrelatedness of mind, body and spirit in the treatment and prevention of disease, and more-over, in an individual's ability to expe-rience optimum vitality and wellness.

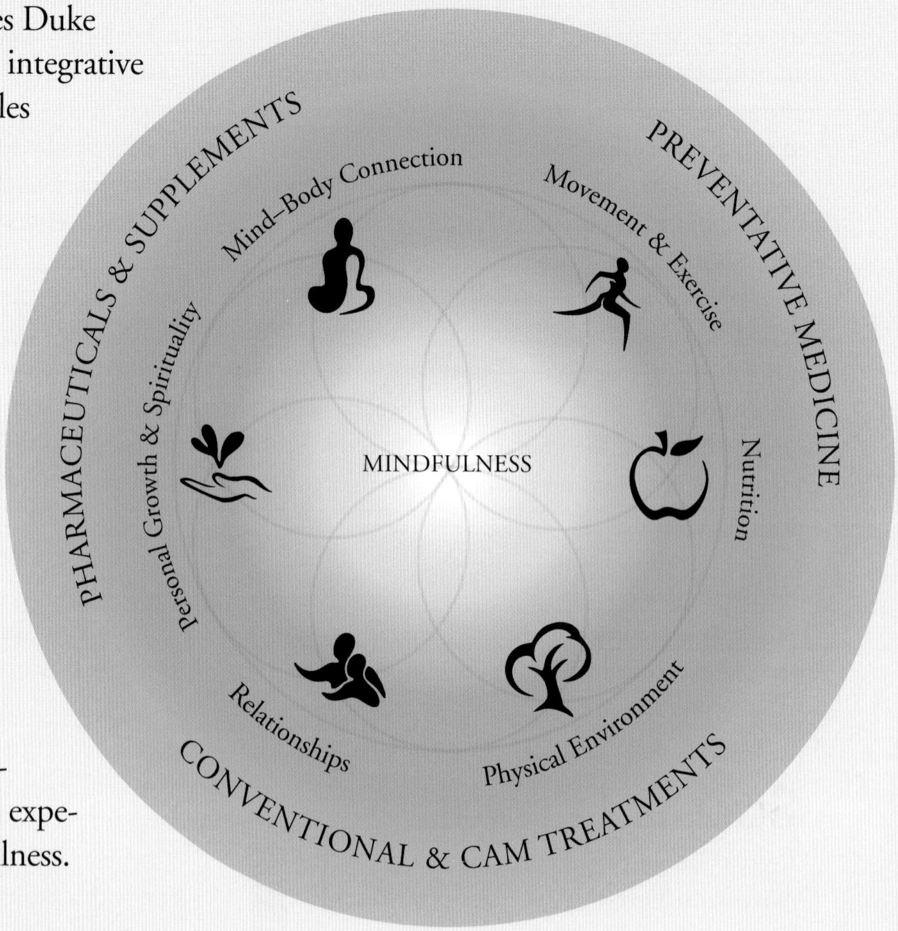

PHARMACEUTICALS & SUPPLEMENTS
PREVENTATIVE MEDICINE
CONVENTIONAL & CAM TREATMENTS

Mind–Body Connection
Movement & Exercise
Personal Growth & Spirituality
Nutrition
MINDFULNESS
Relationships
Physical Environment

Colour and its Meaning

Mindfulness is a pivotal concept that embodies awareness of physical, mental, social and spiritual well-being. Self-awareness enables individuals to recognize symptoms as they emerge, when they are most readily treatable.

Self-Care Individuals are encouraged to explore how the dynamic interplay of the self-care concept resonates in all aspects of health and wellness, and to develop proactive strategies to improve or maintain their health.

Professional Care Recognizing symptoms early is key to diagnosing health problems when they are most treatable, and awareness of the need for professional care is an integral component of the integrative approach to medicine.

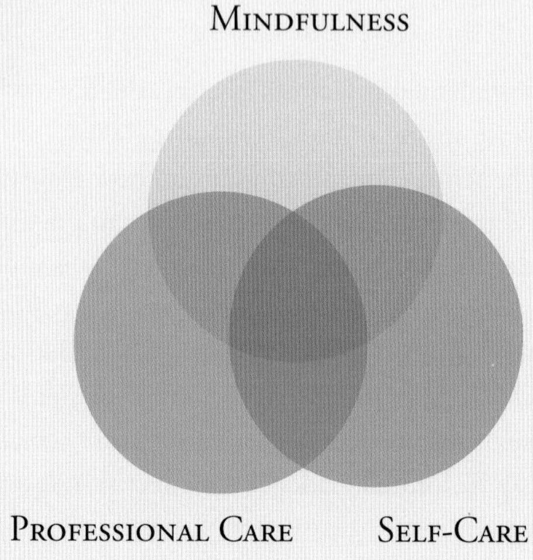

MINDFULNESS

PROFESSIONAL CARE   SELF-CARE

Movement & Exercise

Very few people really exercise, despite the fact that the human body is designed to be in motion. This inertia has serious consequences for our health. A mere 20 minutes of physical activity a day will help to prevent a very large number of common diseases, including heart disease and diabetes. If you start exercising in your chosen way gently and build gradually, you will find yourself enjoying your achievement. What is more, you will feel better, have more energy, your work will be more efficient and you will feel less stressed.

Nutrition

You are what you eat. A healthy diet will both feed you and protect you from many illnesses, while a poorly balanced diet will make you vulnerable to substances that compromise your health. You need to consider not only what you eat, but also where you get it, how it is prepared and how much you eat. Choose foods that will protect, for example those containing omega-3 fatty acids, rather than those that put you more at risk. You should listen to your body, distinguishing between real hunger and snacking because of boredom or anxiety.

Physical Environment

Every aspect of your physical environment can influence your well-being. And the awareness of your environment goes beyond the elimination of any toxic or negative aspects, such as fuel emissions, harmful substances in food or biological agents including viruses and bacteria. It involves being proactive and creating a healing environment in which to live and work. Consider how your health may be affected by noise, light, colour and odours. By paying attention to all of your senses you can create environments that nurture them.

Relationships

Positive social relationships and support are key to well-being.
If you communicate well with those about you, listening as well as speaking, you will benefit from the positive and powerful influence that this gives you over the development, progression and recovery from many diseases. If communication is bad, this can be very harmful, even in some cases, fatal. The quality of relationships is very important, as well, and you should be selective, spending more time with people who give you energy, and less with those that drain you.

Personal Growth & Spirituality

Spirituality is the capacity to seek purpose and meaning in life in something larger than yourself. Spirituality allows people to transcend everyday life and see beyond themselves. Self-awareness of this kind can have very positive beneficial effects on health and well-being. You need to look deep into yourself, searching out the core of who you are. This will help you focus on what matters most to you, and give you strength to cope with times when your body and mind are faced with challenges to your health.

Mind–Body Connection

Your state of mind has a tremendous impact on how your body responds to stress – whether it reacts in ways that harm your health or ways that protect. Awareness of how to decrease stress is the key to optimizing health and well-being. Although life is full of events that are inherently stressful, you can use your mind to significantly impact your body's response to such events. Breathing techniques, meditation, progressive muscle relaxation and guided imagery can be used to activate the body's relaxation response and so reduce stress.

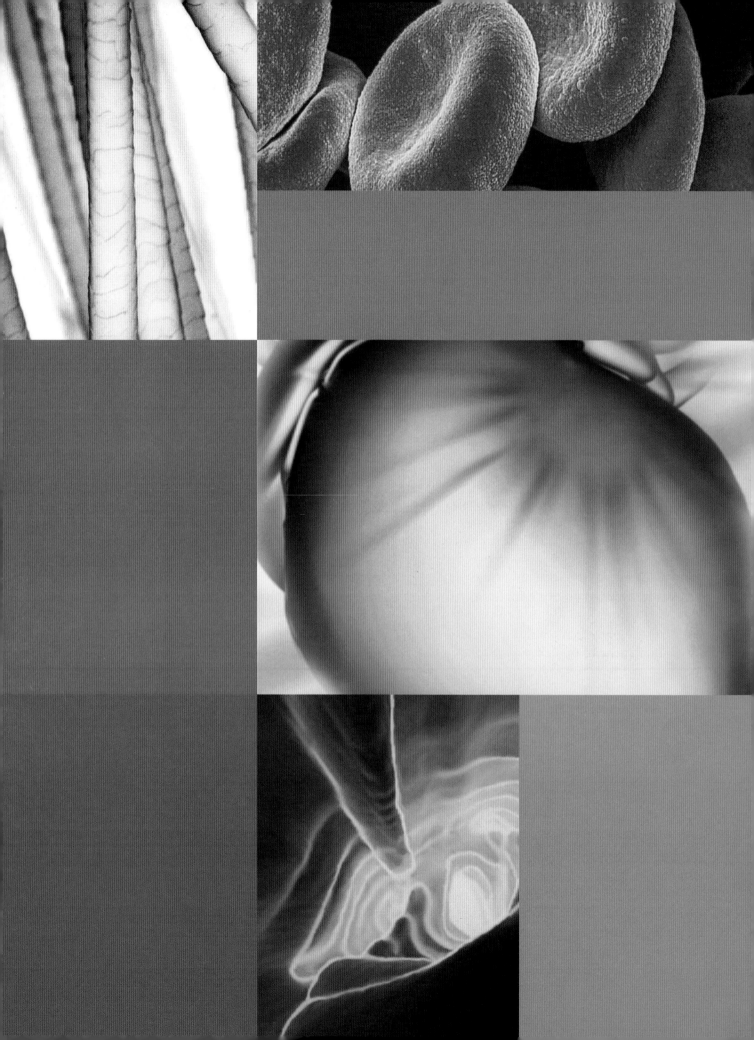

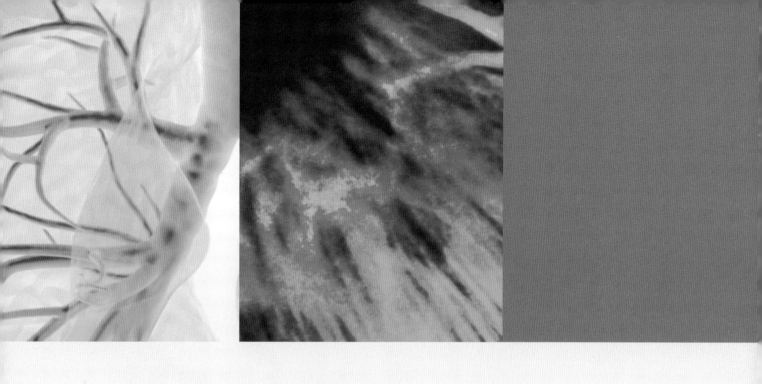

PART I

Catalogue of Health Conditions

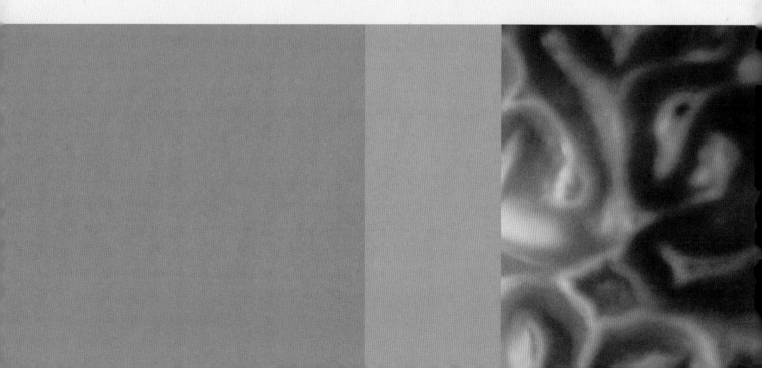

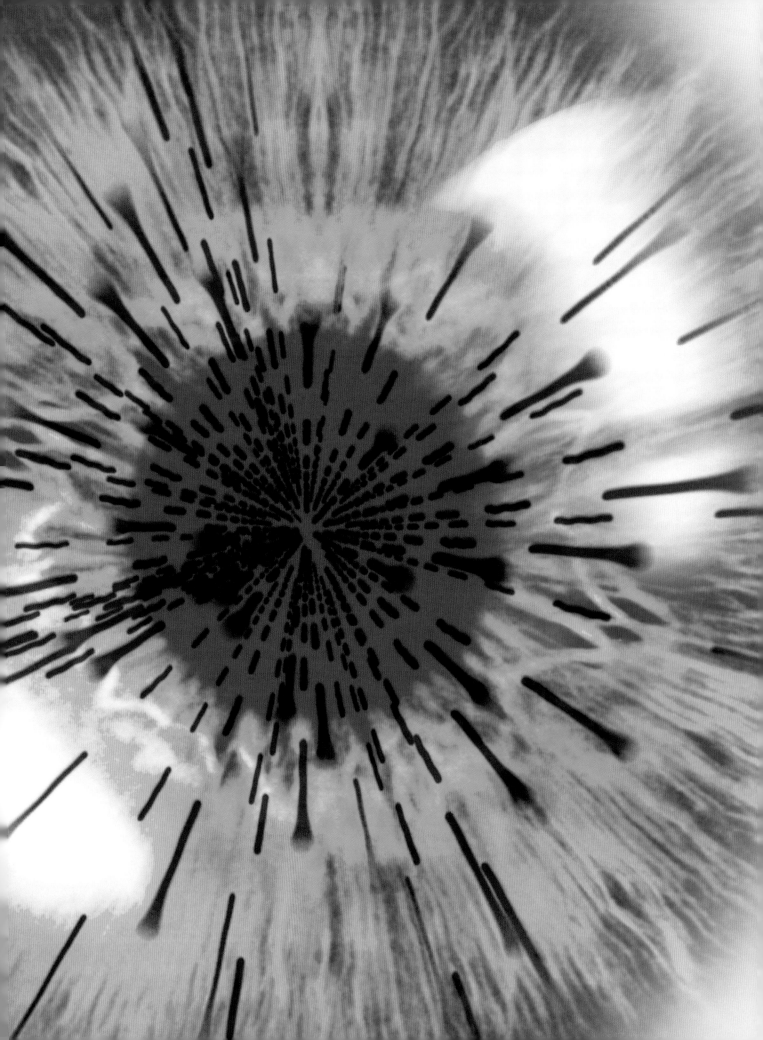

1 | EYES

The eyes are the body's most highly developed sensory organs. In fact, eyesight accounts for a far greater proportion of the brain than hearing, touch, and smell combined. But, despite the complexity of this organ, most of us take vision for granted.

The majority of conditions that affect the eyes are not life-threatening. However, many, such as blepharitis, conjunctivitis and dry eye, can cause considerable discomfort that greatly diminishes quality of life. Diseases such as glaucoma, macular degeneration and – very rarely – eye cancer, can cause blindness.

Although most conditions affecting the eyes may not be preventable, a healthy diet high in fish, nuts and vegetables may lower the risk of diseases such as macular degeneration. Avoiding eye injuries and protecting the eyes from overexposure to the sun are the best ways to guard against most disorders.

Conjunctivitis

Conjunctivitis, also known as pink eye, is an inflammation of the conjunctiva, which are the clear mucous membranes surrounding the white of the eye and the insides of the eyelids. Symptoms are redness or pinkness of the white part of the eye, itching, watery discharge, crusts around the eyelashes and a scratchy feeling when you blink.

CAUSES

Conjunctivitis can be caused by bacteria or a virus, or by environmental factors such as an allergy to eye makeup, pollen or other allergens. Viral conjunctivitis often occurs following a cold or other upper respiratory infection, with adenoviruses being the most common culprits. Bacterial conjunctivitis is very contagious and is easily spread when people rub their eyes with their fingers. It is especially common among children in schools and day care centres, because infected children cannot be relied on to wash their hands after touching their eyes. Neonatal ophthalmia is a form of conjunctivitis that can affect babies during childbirth if their mothers have contracted herpes, chlamydia or gonorrhoea. This form of conjunctivitis can spread throughout the eye and cause blindness unless it is treated promptly.

PREVENTION

Good personal hygiene can significantly reduce the risk of contracting or spreading conjunctivitis. Do not touch your eyes with your hands and instruct children to also avoid doing so. Wash hands frequently. Avoid sharing towels, washcloths and eye makeup, all of which can spread the infection. Prevent allergic conjunctivitis by avoiding substances that have caused it in the past, such as particular brands of mascara or contact lens cleaning solution.

Newborn conjunctivitis can be prevented with good prenatal and neonatal care. Pregnant women should be tested for sexually transmitted diseases (pp.392–3), and treated if necessary. Treating newborns with antibiotic eye drops, which is routine in many countries, can also prevent the disease.

DIAGNOSIS

If you have symptoms of conjunctivitis, go to an eye doctor. Conjunctivitis is diagnosed based on the appearance of the eye. The doctor might take a sample of discharge for testing to see if the cause is bacterial. Since conjunctivitis does not affect the portions of the eye involved in sight, any change in vision needs to be evaluated for other causes.

TREATMENTS

Relieve symptoms by wiping away discharge with a moist cotton ball or tissue. Be sure to wash your hands before and after treating your eyes to avoid spreading the infection to the other eye and to other people in the household.

• MEDICATION Bacterial conjunctivitis must be treated with antibiotic ointment or eye drops to eliminate the infection. Viral conjunctivitis does not respond to antibiotics, but the body's immune system can usually get rid of the infection within a week. Often antibiotics are prescribed to prevent a secondary bacterial infection. Allergic conjunctivitis can be treated with antihistamine eye drops.

• HERBAL MEDICINE Qatoor ramad (QR) is an ophthalmic formulation used in Unani medicine, an ancient herbal medicine system that originated in Afghanistan. Qatoor ramad is effective in treating conjunctivitis and does not cause significant side-effects.

See also: *Allergies, pp.50–1 • STD, pp.392–3 • Pregnancy, pp.398–400*

WHO IS AT RISK?

The risk factors include:
- Upper respiratory infections
- Allergies
- Regular exposure to infected children

Blepharitis

This inflammation of the eyelids can cause considerable discomfort. The margins of the eyelids become red, itchy and inflamed. Crusted mucus forms around the eyelashes and can cause lesions in the skin of the eyelids. The eyes themselves may become red and sensitive to light. Other symptoms include excessive tearing, a distorted appearance of the eyelids and blurred vision. Sometimes blepharitis leads to conjunctivitis of the eyelid (p.30), an infection that causes itching, discharge and redness.

WHO IS AT RISK?

The risk factors include:
- Dandruff
- Rosacea
- Poor hygiene
- Excessive oil production by the glands in the eyelids

CAUSES

The inflammation of blepharitis is not always caused by infection. However, when it affects the margins of the eyelids, the cause may be an infection (usually by *Staphylococcal* bacteria), dandruff, or both. Blepharitis of the inner eyelid can also be caused by dandruff, or by problems with the meibomian glands, which secrete oil in the eyelid. Rosacea (pp.99–101), a skin disorder, is another possible cause.

PREVENTION

Reduce the occurrence and recurrence of blepharitis by keeping the skin around the eyelash follicles clean. Clearing away oil and debris can help prevent the colonization of bacteria that feed on them. Wash around the eyes each morning to eliminate mucus and oil that may have accumulated overnight.

A more elaborate hygiene regimen is required for people who are prone to blepharitis. After washing the hands, mix warm water with a small amount of either a commercial eyelid scrub or non-irritating shampoo. Moisten a washcloth and, with one eye closed, gently rub the washcloth across the eyelashes from one end of the eye to the other. Use a different washcloth to clean the other eye.

DIAGNOSIS

If you think you have blepharitis, see an eye doctor. It is important to determine if antibiotics are needed, or if the irritation is being caused by an even more serious eye condition.

TREATMENTS

Treatment involves keeping the eyelids clean and controlling other conditions. If a bacterial infection is present, antibiotics may be needed.

• MEDICATION Antibiotic eye drops or ointment may be prescribed to eliminate the bacteria. Topical or oral antibiotics are sometimes prescribed if rosacea is also present. To control dandruff, a medicated shampoo may be necessary.

• HYDROTHERAPY Warm compresses on the eyelids several times a day can relieve discomfort and help get rid of blepharitis by loosening debris around the eyelash follicles. After washing the hands, moisten a clean washcloth with warm water. Close the eyes and put the washcloth over them for about five minutes. Next, do an eyelid scrub, as described in Prevention. Apply the compresses and eyelid scrub daily, as directed by a healthcare provider.

See also: *Conjunctivitis, p.30 • Rosacea, pp.99–101 • Hydrotherapy, pp.482–3*

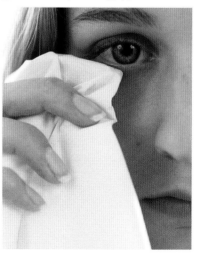

Because belpharitis tends to recur, a regular eyelid hygiene regimen is recommended for those diagnosed with the condition.

Stye

A stye (also known as hordeolum) is a localized infection of the root of the eyelashes involving the hair follicles of the eyelashes or the meibomian glands (small sebaceous glands that lie under the conjunctiva of the eyelids). A person can have more than one stye at the same time. At first, a stye is red and painful due to a build-up of fluid.

A stye can also cause watering, sensitivity to light and the sensation that there is foreign matter in the eye. After several days, a stye usually releases its fluid and within a week or so it heals on its own. A stye that does not heal may develop into a chalazion, a mass of grainy tissue that forms when the sebaceous (oil) gland in the eyelid becomes inflamed and then blocked.

CAUSES

More than 90 percent of cases of stye are caused by *Staphylococcus* bacteria that migrate from the skin of the eyelid into an eyelash follicle.

PREVENTION

Good hygiene can reduce the risk of developing styes. Wash the hands before touching the eyelids. Clean excess oils and discharge from eyelids to help prevent

WHO IS AT RISK?

The risk factors include:

- Chronic blepharitis
- Previous styes
- Diabetes
- Debilitating illness
- Seborrheic dermatitis (dandruff)
- High serum lipids

infection. If you have blepharitis (p.31), an eyelid infection that can lead to styes, consult a doctor.

DIAGNOSIS

A doctor can diagnose a stye based on its appearance.

TREATMENTS

Do not attempt to squeeze a stye. Let it drain on its own.

- MEDICATION If the stye does not disappear, or if it recurs, there may be an underlying infection that must be controlled with an antibiotic cream or ointment.

- HYDROTHERAPY Warm compresses are the first line of treatment. Moisten a washcloth with warm water and apply it to the eyelid for ten minutes, four times a day, until the stye drains.

- LANCING If the stye is large, the doctor may recommend lancing it to drain the fluid and eliminate the infection.

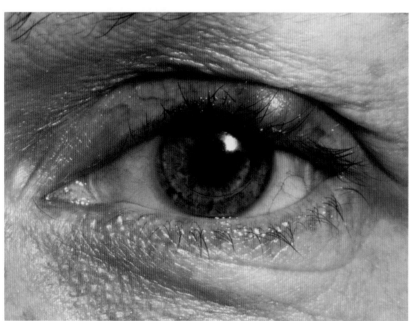

A stye appears on the eyelid as a red bump, similar to a pimple or a boil, and is often filled with pus. Styes are caused by infection of the oil gland at the root of the eyelash, often by staphylococcus bacteria, that migrate from the skin of the eyelid into an eyelash follicle.

See also: *Blepharitis, p.31 • Hydrotherapy, pp.482–3*

Dry Eye

Normally, a film of tears consisting of oil, water and mucus coats the eyeball. But when the lacrimal glands (which produce tears) do not secrete enough fluid or the tears that are produced are abnormal and evaporate too quickly, the result is a condition called dry eye, or keratoconjunctivitis sicca. Both eyes are usually affected by dry eye. It can be very uncomfortable, causing pain, burning, scratchiness, itching and blurred vision. It also makes the eyes feel tired even after only short periods of reading.

CAUSES

Ageing is the most common cause of dry eye. Other contributing agents are smoking, exposure to secondhand smoke and environmental factors such as exposure to sun, wind, and indoor air that is overly dry. Cold and allergy medication, as well as many prescription medicines, can dry out the mucous membranes in the eyes. Dry eye can also result from eye injuries and disorders that interfere with the eye's functioning, as well as from autoimmune disorders such as rheumatoid arthritis (pp.136–9) and lupus (pp.324-5), where the immune system may attack the lacrimal glands.

PREVENTION

Dry eye cannot be prevented, but there are several ways to reduce its severity. The most important is to avoid smoking and exposure to secondhand smoke. Limit exposure to the sun and shield the eyes from wind. During the winter, use a humidifier to add moisture to dry indoor air. If you use a hair dryer, turn your face away from the air. Finally, protect your eyes with goggles when engaged in activities that carry a risk of eye injuries, such as skiing, hockey and carpentry.

DIAGNOSIS

If you think you have dry eye, see your doctor. The condition is diagnosed based on the symptoms and several tests. The Schirmer test gauges the amount of tears the eyes produce. Strips of blotting paper are placed beneath the lower eyelids for five minutes, then a doctor measures the quantity of tears absorbed by the paper. The doctor can also use eye drops to measure how long it takes for tears to evaporate and to identify dry spots on the cornea.

TREATMENTS

Dry eye is treated with a combination of medication and changes to lifestyle and environment.

• MEDICATION Eye drops that help replace the tear film around the cornea can relieve mild cases of dry eye. If necessary, a lubricating ointment can help to reduce the scratchy sensation.

• SILICONE PLUGS If medication does not provide relief, tiny silicone plugs can be fitted into the tear ducts to prevent tears from draining out of the eyes. The plugs are removable.

• CAUTERY A doctor uses a hot wire to seal off the tear ducts to prevent the tears from draining.

• ACUPUNCTURE This may be a useful adjunct to conventional treatment. Although it does not increase the amount of tears that remain in the eyes, some people tolerate the condition better with acupuncture treatments.

• PHYSICAL ENVIRONMENT Making a point to blink frequently can help relieve dry eyes by spreading the tears across the surface of the eyes. The strategies listed under Prevention can also help relieve any discomfort.

See also: *Arthritis, pp.136–9 • Lupus, pp.324–5 • Acupuncture, pp.464–5*

WHO IS AT RISK?

The risk factors include:
• Ageing
• Smoking
• Cold and allergy medications
• Prolonged exposure to dry air
• Eye injuries
• Autoimmune diseases

Cataracts

The lens of the eye, the organ behind the iris that enables the eye to focus, is normally clear. But in an eye with cataracts, it is clouded and opaque. There are many causes of cataracts, but the majority relate to changes in the eye that come about with age. One change is that the lens takes on a brownish yellow tint. This change alone does not usually cause pronounced vision impairment, however. The main reason the lens becomes clouded with cataracts is that with age, protein fibres in the eye tend to clump together.

The condition is painless, but over a period of years vision becomes progressively more blurred. Seeing at night or in dim light becomes especially difficult. Colours appear faded and images may be distorted. Other problems include more pronounced nearsightedness, sensitivity to glare, the appearance of halos around lights, double vision and multiple images in one eye. Cataracts will usually affect both eyes, but one eye will probably be worse than the other.

CAUSES

The main cause of cataracts is ageing. However, when cataracts are due to ageing alone, the condition is usually mild and does not interfere significantly with vision. A number of the factors can lead to the development of cataracts or make cataracts more severe. Diabetes, Down's syndrome and galactosaemia (an abnormal accumulation of the sugar galactose, a constituent of the milk sugar lactose) increase the risk of cataracts.

Other causes include prolonged use of corticosteroid medications, concussion (p.174), eye injury, exposure to certain poisonous substances (such as naphthalene, used in mothballs), smoking, heavy alcohol consumption, and extensive exposure to sunlight and other forms of radiation.

Cataracts can also be congenital, or present at birth. Certain infections in the mother during pregnancy, such as rubella, toxoplasmosis and herpes simplex, can increase the risk of a baby developing congenital cataracts.

PREVENTION

Several approaches may help reduce the risk of developing cataracts, delay the onset of the condition, or reduce the overall severity in how they affect vision. These include getting regular eye examinations – at least every two years, and more often if you are noticing changes in vision. Early detection and treatment of cataracts can minimize damage to the eyes.

WHO IS AT RISK?

The risk factors include:

- Age
- Eye injury
- Concussion
- Diabetes
- Down's syndrome
- Galactosaemia
- Extensive exposure to sunlight or other forms of radiation
- Toxic chemical exposure
- Smoking
- Heavy drinking
- Long-term use of corticosteroid medication
- Infections during pregnancy (can cause congenital cataracts)

Keeping blood sugar under control may help prevent the development of cataracts as the result of diabetes. Good antenatal care can reduce the risk of infections that can cause congenital cataracts.

• PHYSICAL ENVIRONMENT Reduce exposure to sunlight by wearing sunglasses and a wide-brimmed hat when outdoors during midday. Do not smoke and avoid secondhand smoke.

• NUTRITION Eating foods that are rich in antioxidants may protect against cataracts. Antioxidants destroy free radicals – destructive molecules that are believed to accelerate the ageing process and promote several degenerative diseases, including cataracts.

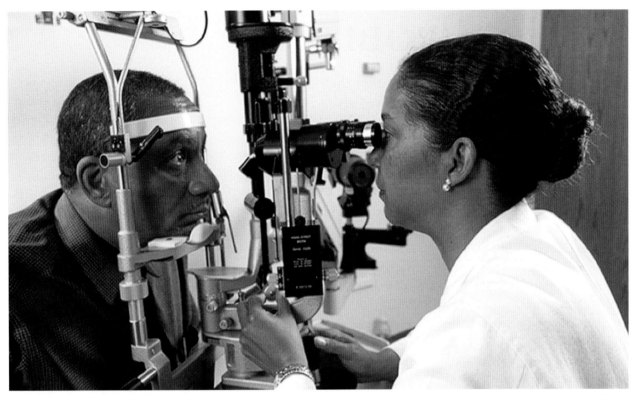

Cataracts occur when the lens of the eye begins to darken and grow opaque as a natural part of the ageing process, causing blurry vision and making the eyes more sensitive to glare. An eye doctor will perform a comprehensive eye examination to properly diagnose cataracts.

The antioxidants lutein, vitamin C and selenium, in particular, reduce the risk of cataracts. These nutrients can be found in supplements or in foods such as green leafy vegetables, citrus fruits, grains and seafood.

Alcohol increases the risk of cataracts, so drink only in moderation – no more than two drinks daily for men and one for women. (One drink equals 24 cl/8 fl.oz beer, 15 cl/5 fl.oz wine, or 4.5 cl/1.5 fl.oz distilled spirits.)

DIAGNOSIS

An eye doctor diagnoses cataracts based on age, symptoms and medical history, along with a comprehensive eye examination.

TREATMENTS

Surgery is the only cure for cataracts, but it is not always necessary, especially if the cataracts are mild. Visual aids can help improve eyesight. The good news is that it is never too late for surgery. If vision has been impaired by cataracts for a prolonged period, it will not decrease the effectiveness of the surgery.

• EYEGLASSES AND VISUAL AIDS
A stronger eyeglass prescription can improve visual acuity. Eyeglass lenses specially treated to reduce glare can help ease the discomfort caused by glare and bright sunlight. In addition, a hand-held magnifying lens or other low-vision aids can make it easier to read and do other close work.

• CATARACT SURGERY Doctors recommend surgery if cataracts are so severe that eyeglasses alone do not appreciably improve the ability to engage in everyday activi-ties such as working, reading and driving. Even if cataracts do not cause significant vision problems, doctors may recommend surgery if the disorder interferes with an eye examination or the treatment of another eye disorder.

During cataract surgery, an eye surgeon will remove the clouded lens and implant a clear plastic lens. The surgery can be done on one eye or both eyes, depending on how impaired vision is in each eye. Recovery from the surgery can take several days to several weeks.

• PHYSICAL ENVIRONMENT Using more light fixtures and brighter light bulbs at home and at work can improve vision by making images appear more distinct.

See also: Concussion, p.174 • Vision Problems, pp.36–9 • Diabetes, pp.338–41

VISION PROBLEMS

The eyes can have many problems, other than diseases, that result in blurring and distortions of vision. Some of the most common vision problems are difficulties with focusing, including myopia (nearsightedness), hyperopia (farsightedness), presbyopia (middle-age vision) and astigmatism. Others are strabismus (crossed eyes), amblyopia (lazy eye) and colour vision deficiency.

These problems may be present alone or in combination, in one or both eyes, and to a greater or lesser degree they may occur in each eye. Some of these conditions are preventable and most can be improved with eyeglasses, contact lenses or surgery.

CAUSES

Most vision problems that involve difficulties focusing stem from either an abnormal shape of one or several parts of the eye, or changes that take place with age – or both. Others may be hereditary.

Myopia (Nearsightedness)

When the distance between the front and back of the eyeball is abnormally long or the cornea (the clear membrane that covers the eyeball) has too much of a curve, myopia is the result. Distant objects appear out of focus because light entering the eye from afar is not refracted, or angled, to the proper spot on the inner eye for accurate interpretation. Instead of reaching the retina (the part of the eye responsible for focusing), the light lands in front of the retina. Close-up objects, such as the words in a book, appear sharp,

however, because light from them is refracted normally.

Myopia usually develops before the age of 20. It tends to run in families, suggesting that it may have a genetic component. Spending a lot of time reading and at other activities that require extensive, ongoing close vision are thought to increase the odds of developing myopia.

Hyperopia (Farsightedness)

This condition is the opposite of myopia. It occurs when either the distance between the front and back of the eye is too short, or the cornea does not have enough of a curve. The result is that light rays from close objects focus behind the retina, making it difficult to focus.

Symptoms of farsightedness include trouble sustaining a clear focus on printed words and other near objects, but not always. Close objects do not necessarily look blurred, because the muscles of the eye can often overcome the focusing problem by contracting and increasing the curvature of the cornea. But this additional work by the muscles contributes to other symptoms, including eye strain, headaches and fatigue when doing close work.

Presbyopia (Middle-Age Vision)

This condition is caused by a change in the crystalline lens of the eye that occurs as part of the normal ageing process. The muscles of the eye normally change the curvature of the crystalline lens to adjust its focus on objects at different distances. This adjustment, or accommodation, enables people to see clearly as the eyes shift between near and far sight – for example, from reading to looking across a room. By about the age of 45, the

healing hope My son was having trouble at school. It started with not paying attention. Then came the reading problems. He wasn't able to answer the teacher's questions, either. She suspected a learning disability. He also had headaches sometimes, so I took him to our doctor. She suggested a vision examination, and it turned out that my son's problems in school were caused by the fact that he couldn't see clearly! When he got his glasses, he finally realized that he hadn't been able to see the blackboard before, which is why he often couldn't respond properly to the teacher. It was also why his mind wandered sometimes and he ended up daydreaming. But not anymore.

Brian K.

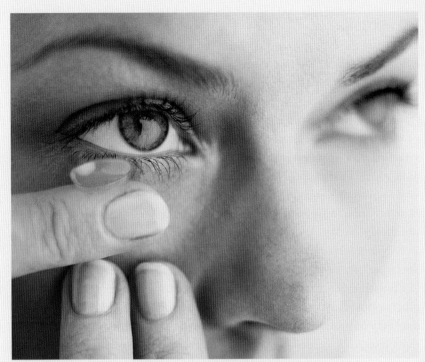

Contact lenses, compared to eyeglasses, offer better vision correction and less distortion. However, contact lenses require a longer initial examination and more follow-up visits to the optician to maintain good eye health.

crystalline lens gradually becomes less flexible, a change that makes close objects look blurred. The main symptom is difficulty reading at a normal distance.

Astigmatism

In a normal eye, the cornea is a regular sphere. Astigmatism is caused by bumps and waves in the curvature of the cornea. It is so common that most people have it to some degree. When astigmatism is mild, the symptoms include blurred vision only at certain distances, as well as headaches and eyestrain – a sense of fatigue in the eyes that can manifest itself as aching or burning, or even general fatigue. Symptoms of severe astigmatism are more consistently blurred or distorted vision, particularly seeing blurred lines.

Strabismus (Crossed Eyes)

With this condition, one or both of the eyes turns inwards toward the nose, outwards, or down. The underlying cause of this misalignment is usually inadequate control of the eye muscles. The problem develops in childhood, most often before the age of two. Left untreated, strabismus can lead to amblyopia, a cause of permanent vision impairment.

Amblyopia (Lazy Eye)

Amblyopia occurs when vision in the eye does not develop normally during the first few years of life. Specifically, the nerve connections between the brain and one eye do not develop properly, either because that eye is misaligned or because it does not focus as clearly as the other eye. The result is that the brain ignores the image from the weak eye and relies only on the image

from the strong eye. The conditon is not caused by an eye disease and cannot be corrected with glasses or contact lenses. The most common cause is strabismus, but other causes include trauma and a drooping eyelid. Toxic amblyopia is a rare form of the condition that appears to be caused by damage to the optic nerve from deficiencies of vitamin A and the B-complex vitamins.

Colour Vision Deficiency

This condition can take several forms, but basically it is the inability to distinguish between certain colours or to see colours in the same way as people with normal vision see them. Although some people are completely colour blind – able to see only in black, white, and shades of grey – this is extremely rare. Most people with colour vision deficiency have problems with particular colours. By far the most common is the inability to distinguish between certain reds and greens. Other people with colour vision deficiency have trouble distinguishing blue from yellow. The condition is

On Call

Have your eyes checked every two years if you are age 65 or older. Regular eye examinations can detect changes in your vision and signs of eye diseases such as glaucoma, which become more common with age. Yearly eye examinations are recommended for people of all ages with diabetes, because of the increased risk of vision problems.

caused by a defect in the cone cells in the eye, which are responsible for transmitting colour signals to the brain. Red-green colour deficiency affects many more males than females, because it is caused by a recessive gene located on the X chromosome. Males inherit just one copy of the X chromosome and females two copies of it. Therefore, females need two copies of the gene and males only one for it to be expressed as red-green colour blindness.

Other forms of colour vision deficiency are not linked to the X chromosome and therefore can affect males and females equally. In rare cases, some types of eye injuries may also cause colour vision deficiency.

Clinical Query

I work at a computer all day. How is this likely to affect my eyes and what can I do to protect them?

Working at a computer for many hours a day can cause eyestrain. To minimize the problem, reduce the light in the room so it does not create glare on the computer monitor. An anti-glare screen for your monitor can also help. In addition, adjust the brightness of the monitor and, if necessary, increase the size of the letters to make them stand out clearly. Finally, make a conscious effort to blink. People blink less frequently when working at a computer, which can cause the eyes to become dry and irritated.

PREVENTION

Protecting the eyes from injury can help guard against the rare forms of colour vision deficiency and amblyopia that can result from trauma. Getting adequate amounts of vitamin A and B-complex vitamins may help prevent toxic amblyopia. There appears to be no way to prevent nearsightedness, farsightedness, astigmatism or middle-age vision.

Supplements of nutrients that are important for healthy eyes, such as zinc, selenium, vitamin A and other antioxidants, and riboflavin, may help improve visual acuity, but more research is needed.

DIAGNOSIS

An ophthalmologist (a medical doctor trained in eye diseases) or an optometrist (a non-medical practitioner trained to diagnose and treat vision problems) can diagnose vision problems with a professional eye examination that measures visual acuity and looks at the structure of the eye. The symptoms of some vision problems, especially middle-age vision, are so obvious that they are usually recognized by the affected individuals. But other vision problems are subtle or do not cause symptoms at first. Therefore, it is important to have regular eye examinations to detect vision problems and get proper treatment.

TREATMENTS

For many vision problems, corrective lenses are used to improve visual acuity. But for some problems, surgery and other treatments are necessary.

• **EYEGLASSES** Prescription lenses made of plastic or glass can be ground into specific shapes and thickness to correct nearsightedness, farsightedness, middle-age vision and astigmatism. Lenses with prisms are sometimes used for double vision and crossed eyes. Non-prescription reading glasses that simply magnify images are an option for people with middle-age vision who do not have other vision problems.

There are many types of prescription lenses. They can be ground in such a way that they address just one focusing problem or several problems at once. Bifocals (two corrective surfaces set into the same lens) can correct for both nearsightedness and farsightedness or middle-age vision. The top half of the lens focuses distant objects

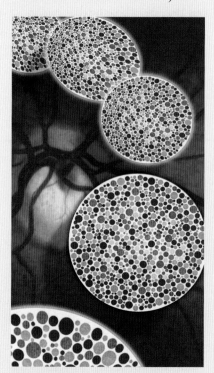

The way a person perceives patterns on Ishihara plates, which are made of dots composed of primary colours, can help detect problems with colour vision.

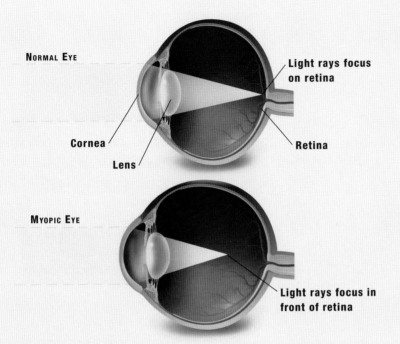

NORMAL EYE

Cornea

Lens

Light rays focus on retina

Retina

MYOPIC EYE

Light rays focus in front of retina

In a myopic eye (bottom image) the distance between the front and back of the eyeball is abnormally long and the cornea has too much curvature, forcing light rays to focus in front of the retina, instead of directly onto it as in the normal eye (top image).

and an area in the bottom half is designed for reading. Trifocals are divided into three fields: the top for distance, the middle for moderately close objects (about 1–2 m/ 3–6 ft away), and the bottom for reading. Progressive lenses are trifocals without pronounced lines that divide the different areas.

• CONTACT LENSES These are clear, thin plastic lenses that cover the cornea and can correct nearsightedness, farsightedness, and astigmatism. A tinted lens worn in one eye can sometimes help correct colour vision deficiency. Not everyone can wear contact lenses; some people never get used to the sensation of something being in the eye.

There are two basic types of contact lenses: gas-permeable hard lenses and soft contact lenses. The hard lenses offer the greatest improvements in vision because they can be crafted

to conform more precisely to the contours of the cornea. They may be the only option for people with severe astigmatism. Soft lenses may be more comfortable. Some soft contact lenses must be removed daily and others can be worn overnight. Still others are designed to be discarded each day.

• PATCHING To treat lazy eye, a patch is worn over the stronger eye for several weeks or months to prevent it from compensating for the weak eye. Forcing the weak eye to do all the work gradually improves its vision. To maintain this improvement, a patch may have to be worn off and on for several years.

• MEDICATION In addition to wearing a patch, children with lazy eye may be given eye drops in the strong eye to blur its vision and force the weak eye to work harder.

• SURGERY Surgery is often necessary to properly align crossed eyes.

Surgery can also treat nearsightedness and astigmatism, reducing and in some cases eliminating the need for corrective lenses.

Laser in situ keratomileusis (LASIK) reshapes the cornea to improve the eye's ability to focus. The procedure is effective for low to moderate nearsightedness, but the results are more variable in patients with severe nearsightedness. People with certain conditions, such as diabetes, autoimmune diseases, and inflammations of the eyelids, are not good candidates for this type of surgery.

The newest type of surgery for nearsightedness is the implantation of lenses. Implanted lenses are more effective than LASIK for people with moderate to severe nearsightedness. The surgery is done using a mild sedative and the patient can go home the same day.

• VISION THERAPY This is a sequence of individualized activities that aim to improve visual skills and processing in people with focusing difficulties, crossed eyes, lazy eye and other vision problems. The activities use therapeutic lenses, prisms, filters, patches, electronic targets, computer software, balance boards and other techniques, and are done under the direction of an optometrist or other eye-care professional.

There is controversy about the effectiveness of vision therapy, and it is considered an adjunct to, not a replacement for, standard therapies such as corrective lenses, patching, and surgery.

See also: Glaucoma, pp.42–3 • Headaches, pp.166–7 • Supplements, pp.532–41

Macular Degeneration

When the light-sensitive cells in the macula (the middle area of the retina that enables you to see minute details in the center field of vision) deteriorate, the result is blurry or distorted central vision, difficulty reading, and, eventually, a blind spot. Both eyes are usually affected by macular degeneration, which is a progressive disease that becomes increasingly common with age, and is the leading cause of blindness in people over 60 in North America and Europe.

CAUSES

Macular degeneration begins with deterioration of the retinal pigment epithelium, which is a membrane between the retina and the choroid, a layer of blood vessels behind the retina. This membrane acts as a filter for the retina, letting in beneficial nutrients from the blood and blocking harmful substances. When the filter breaks down, the retina suffers.

There are two forms of macular degeneration. The most common is the dry form, which is characterized by a thinning of the macula tissues and gradual vision loss. This is the first stage of the disorder. A small percentage of patients go on to develop the more severe wet form of macular degeneration, in which abnormal blood vessels grow beneath the retina and leak fluid or blood, destroying the retina's nerve tissue. Vision loss from wet macular degeneration often occurs quickly and is severe.

The precise cause of macular degeneration is unknown, but age-related changes in the eye play a key role. It affects mainly people over the age of 50 and its prevalence rises each subsequent decade.

PREVENTION

Although we have no control over age, there are risk factors that can be avoided. These include smoking and prolonged exposure to the sun.

• PHYSICAL ENVIRONMENT Stay indoors as much as possible during midday. When outdoors, wear a hat and sunglasses that block the full spectrum of ultraviolet light. Do not smoke and avoid second-hand smoke.

• NUTRITION A diet high in saturated fat and cholesterol may increase the risk of macular degeneration, while eating fish and nuts may reduce the risk slightly. Eating spinach and kale, vegetables with large amounts of antioxidants, may also lower the risk of macular degeneration.

• ANTIOXIDANTS Two antioxidants – lutein and zeaxanthin – may reduce the risk of developing macular degeneration. Research has found no preventative benefit from the antioxidants vitamin C, vitamin E, and zinc, although they may help reduce the progression of advanced disease.

DIAGNOSIS

Macular degeneration is diagnosed during an eye examination that includes a vision test and inspection of the macula. The vision test uses an Amsler grid, a chart that looks like graph paper with a black dot in the middle. The patient looks at the dot with one eye at a time. If the lines in any area of the grid look wavy, blurred, or dark, macular degeneration could be the cause.

Doctors often recommend that people with macular degeneration use an Amsler grid at home daily to detect changes in their vision that can give early warning signs of the disease progressing.

TREATMENTS

Though there is no cure for macular degeneration, several therapies can slow the progression of the disorder.

• **MEDICATION** Pegaptanib sodium is injected into the eye to treat wet macular degeneration. It inhibits the activity of a chemical that promotes blood vessel growth, reducing the formation of abnormal blood vessels that degrade the retina.

• **SURGERY** Laser photocoagulation, a procedure for wet macular degeneration, uses a thermal laser to burn the abnormal blood vessels behind the retina, stopping them from leaking and growing. A drawback of this surgery is that it often destroys healthy blood vessels as well.

• **PHOTODYNAMIC THERAPY** This is a relatively new treatment for wet macular degeneration that aims to staunch an area of blood or fluid leakage in the eye. It is less likely to damage healthy blood vessels in the eye. Photodynamic therapy is performed in a doctor's surgery. A light-sensitive medication is injected into the arm, which circulates throughout the body, including the blood vessels in the eyes. Then a non-thermal laser is directed at selected areas of the eyes. The laser beam interacts with the medication to destroy abnormal blood vessels.

• **SUPPLEMENTS** Antioxidant and zinc supplements are often prescribed to reduce the rate of deterioration and preserve eyesight. A large clinical trial in the United States, published in

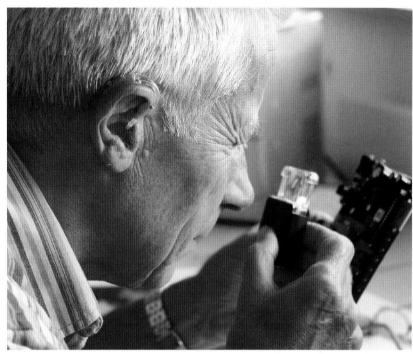
Low-vision aids like hand-held magnifying lenses and attachments for eyeglasses can help make reading and other everyday tasks easier for people with macular degeneration.

2001, found that people with moderate macular degeneration who took daily supplements of vitamin C, vitamin E, beta carotene and zinc reduced their risk of developing advanced macular degeneration by about 25 percent. In this study, taking the supplements did not reduce progression in people with early-stage disease.

• **PHYSICAL ENVIRONMENT** Various low-vision aids can help make reading easier for people with macular degeneration. They include strong reading glasses, magnifying-glasses, hand-held telescopes, telescopic lenses fitted into eyeglass frames and coloured lenses that reduce glare.

• **COUNSELLING** A randomized clinical trial conducted in the United States and published in 2005 found that a counselling programme could help improve daily

functions and prevent depression in people with advanced macular degeneration. In the 12-hour programme, patients learned behavioural strategies for coping with symptoms and practical problem-solving skills. These patients felt more self-confident and stronger emotionally than comparable patients who did not participate in the programme.

On Call

Eating foods rich in lutein and zeaxanthin may reduce the risk of developing macular degeneration. These foods include egg yolk, yellow corn, kiwi fruit, grapes, spinach, orange juice, courgettes and various kinds of squash.

See also: *Vision Problems, pp.36–9* • *Nutritional Supplements, pp.523–41* • *Obesity, pp.348–9*

Glaucoma

Glaucoma is characterized by damage to the optic nerve – the bundle of nerve fibres that connects the eye to the brain. This damage usually occurs as the result of an increase in pressure in the fluid within the eye. At first there may be no noticeable symptoms, but as the condition progresses, it causes a loss of peripheral vision, blurriness, the appearance of halos around lights and other vision problems.

Other symptoms include pain in the eye and face, headaches, sensitivity to light, watering and redness of the eyes. Glaucoma is increasingly common with age and is a leading cause of blindness among people aged 60 and older. It can be effectively managed to prevent blindness.

CAUSES

There are five main types of glaucoma, each with different causes. In open angle types, the drainage channel, or angle, between the iris and the cornea is open (as it should be to allow fluid to drain), but for some reason is blocked. With closed angle glaucoma, the angle between the iris and cornea closes, preventing normal fluid drainage.

Primary Open Angle Glaucoma

This most common form is a chronic condition that occurs when the vessels that drain fluid from the eye become partially clogged. The fluid, called the aqueous humour, cannot drain properly and builds up in these vessels, increasing pressure within the eye. This pressure squeezes the optic nerve and the retina, restricting blood flow. Deprived of adequate blood, cells in the optic nerve gradually die. Ageing appears to cause most cases of primary open angle glaucoma in adults.

Normal Tension Glaucoma

In this kind of open angle glaucoma, pressure in the eye is within normal limits. It is unclear why the optic nerve becomes damaged, but one theory is that the blood supply is reduced because of another medical condition, such as coronary artery disease. Though rare, normal tension glaucoma is most likely to affect people with a family history of the condition, a history of heart disease, or people of Japanese ancestry.

Closed Angle Glaucoma

This rare condition is also called acute glaucoma or narrow angle glaucoma. Eye pressure rises suddenly, in a matter of hours, when the drainage structure between the iris (the coloured part of the eye) and the cornea (the clear membrane surrounding the front of the eyeball) becomes clogged.

The problem often affects people born with an unusually narrow drainage structure (called the anterior chamber angle). Symptoms include pain, nausea and rapid vision loss. This is a medical emergency that must be treated promptly to avoid blindness.

Secondary Glaucoma

This is a complication of an eye injury or disease that increases eye pressure such as cataracts, diabetes or a tumour. Secondary glaucoma can also be a side-effect of steroids, which may interfere with the eye's drainage system.

Congenital Glaucoma

This birth defect is an abnormality in the drainage channels of the eye. It is usually diagnosed in the first year of life. Most cases are caused by genetic mutation.

WHO IS AT RISK?

The risk factors include:

- Over age 40
- Family history
- Mutation of the myocilin gene
- Eye injury
- Cataracts
- Eye tumours
- Diabetes
- Hypertension
- Heart disease
- Use of anti-cholinergic (neurotransmitter blockers) or steroid medication

PREVENTION

There is no way to prevent glaucoma. The risk of secondary glaucoma can be reduced by protecting the eyes from injury and avoiding high blood pressure (pp.236–9) and diabetes (pp.338–41). Regular eye examinations can ensure that glaucoma is diagnosed early and treated before it causes extensive damage. They can also determine if there is a risk of closed angle glaucoma.

DIAGNOSIS

Glaucoma can be diagnosed during an eye examination. An ophthalmoscope is used to examine the optic nerve. The front of the eyes are examined using a slitlamp, an instrument that uses a powerful microscope and a narrow light beam to view the cornea, lens, fluids, and anterior chamber of the eye.

A key test is tonometry which measures intraocular pressure. Normal pressure within the eye is 10–22 mm (¼–¾ in) of mercury. Higher pressure is often a sign of glaucoma. Other possible tests include checking for signs of vision loss, and gonioscopy, which examines the anterior chamber angle to see if it is abnormally narrow.

TREATMENTS

Glaucoma treatments aim to reduce the build-up of fluid in the eyes and lower intraocular pressure.

• **LASER TRABECULOPLASTY** This type of laser surgery is used to treat open angle glaucoma when medication is not sufficient.

The laser widens the fluid channels to improve drainage. Although the surgery usually succeeds in reducing eye pressure, many people still need to take medication.

• **LASER PERIPHERAL IRIDOTOMY** This is emergency surgery to treat closed angle glaucoma. A laser creates a tiny hole in the iris to make it easier for fluid to drain from the eye. This surgery is sometimes also used as a preventative measure for people at high risk of closed angle glaucoma.

• **ND:YAG LASER CYCLOPHOTO-COAGULATION (YAG CP)** Reserved for people with severe glaucoma, YAG CP surgery destroys a portion of the ciliary body, the structure of the eye that produces fluid. With less fluid, there is less pressure within the eye.

• **FILTERING MICROSURGERY** This conventional surgery involves cutting a small drainage hole in the white part of the eye. It is used

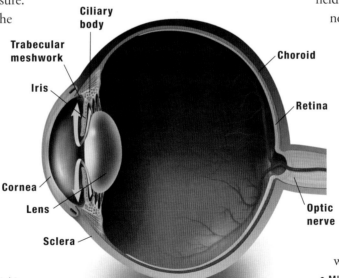

The fluid within the eye, or aqueous humour, normally circulates through openings around the iris. Glaucoma occurs when these openings become blocked. The fluid pressure in the eye increases, squeezing the optic nerve, often causing blindness.

when laser surgery does not lower eye pressure adequately or the benefits of laser surgery do not last.

• **ACUPUNCTURE** Acupuncture may reduce intraocular pressure, although results are not conclusive.

• **MEDICATION** Several kinds of medicine improve fluid drainage from the eyes, decrease fluid production, or both. Available eye drops, ointments and pills include adrenergics, alpha agonists, beta-blockers, carbonic anhydrase inhibitors, cholinergics, cholinesterase inhibitors and prostaglandin analogs. They can be used alone or in combination.

• **VITAMIN E** Vitamin E supplements enhance the effectiveness of glaucoma medications.

• **HERBAL REMEDIES** Marijuana temporarily lowers intraocular pressure markedly in some people. *Ginkgo biloba* may help treat normal tension glaucoma by improving the field of vision in people with normal tension glaucoma or by improving blood circulation to the eye. Ginkgo does not decrease intraocular pressure.

• **MOVEMENT AND EXERCISE** Exercising for about 40 minutes at least four times a week, by bicycling or walking briskly, can reduce intraocular pressure in people with glaucoma.

• **MIND-BODY CONNECTION** Relaxation techniques (pp.472–3) and biofeedback (pp.502–4) can help control eye pressure.

See also: *High Blood Pressure, pp.236–9 • Diabetes, pp. 338–41 • Meditation, pp.514–19*

Uveitis

The eye is a hollow ball made up of three layers. The outer layer is the sclera, a tough covering; the inner layer is the retina, which gathers light; and the middle layer is the uvea. Uveitis is an inflammation of the uvea layer of the eye between the sclera and the inner retina. The uvea is made up of three parts: the iris, the coloured part that regulates how much light enters the eye; the choroid, a layer of blood vessels that supply the retina; and the ciliary body, which connects the other two. Any of these parts may become inflamed.

The part of the uvea that is most often affected is the iris. This type of uveitis is called iritis. The inflammation can also affect other parts of the eye, including the retina, optic nerve and vitreous fluid. The condition can affect one or both eyes, and cause permanent vision loss.

CAUSES

In many cases, the cause of uveitis is unknown. But the risk of

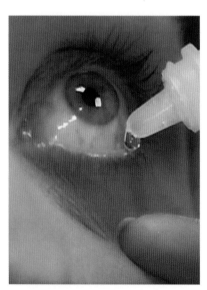

Special eye drops that dilate the pupil can relieve pain associated with uveitis.

developing it has been associated with a gene called HLA-B27, which also causes ankylosing spondylitis, an auto-immune disease of the spine and pelvis. There are many medical conditions that occur in association with uveitis. These include rheumatoid arthritis, sarcodiosis, Bechet's disease, infections such as toxoplasmosis, tuberculosis, HIV, and herpes zoster. Trauma to the eye, or even past eye injuries can lead to uveitis, as can exposure to snake venom. Uveitis can also be a complication of eye surgery.

PREVENTION

There is no way to prevent uveitis.

DIAGNOSIS

Symptoms often develop quickly and include redness in the eye, sensitivity to light, blurred vision, floaters and pain. The particular symptoms depend on the location of the inflammation. Anterior uveitis most often causes pain, redness and decreased vision, while intermediate and posterior uveitis most often present with floaters and decreased vision.

An eye doctor can diagnose uveitis by examining the eye with a slit lamp microscope for signs of inflammation.

TREATMENTS

Eye drops that dilate the pupil can relieve pain. Eye drops or ointment that contains a steroid can reduce inflammation. Other medication, such as antibiotics for an underlying infection and immune-suppressing drugs for uveitis associated with autoimmune diseases, may be needed. Even with treatment, uveitis often recurs.

See also: *Tuberculosis, p.212 • HIV, pp.316–17 • Blurred Vision, pp.36–9*

Retinitis Pigmentosa

This rare inherited degenerative disorder of the retina is characterized by damage to the rods (the cells that enable people to see in low light) and sometimes also the cones (the cells that detect colours and detail). Symptoms usually begin in adolescence or early adulthood, but they can occur in childhood. The first sign is night blindness – difficulty seeing in dim light. Next, there is a gradual deterioration of peripheral vision. By middle age, central vision is also impaired. Although retinitis pigmentosa usually does not cause complete blindness, the vision loss is permanent.

CAUSES

This disorder is caused by mutations of several genes. Damage from free radicals may augment the harm caused by the genetic mutations. Retinitis pigmentosa may occur alone or in conjunction with other inherited diseases.

It is more common in males because one pattern of inheritance is caused by a recessive gene on the X chromosome. Males inherit an X chromosome from their mothers and a Y chromosome from their fathers, while females inherit two X chromosomes. Therefore, males need to inherit only one recessive gene for it to be expressed as retinitis pigmentosa, whereas females need two.

PREVENTION

There is no way to prevent retinitis pigmentosa. However, antioxidant supplements may slow the course of the disease by reducing free radical damage to the retina.

DIAGNOSIS

An ophthalmologist can diagnose retinitis pigmentosa by looking for dark spots in the retina. In addition to a comprehensive eye examination, several specialized tests may be needed, including an ultrasound of the eye.

Clinical Query

My mother has retinitis pigmentosa. I know the disease is genetic, so what can I do to reduce my risk of getting it?

Unfortunately, there is no known way to prevent the disease. But vitamin A supplements can slow its development. And taking the omega-3 fatty acid docosahexaenoic acid, along with vitamin A, may be even better than vitamin A alone. This type of omega-3 is found in fatty fish, such as canned light tuna (not solid white), salmon, trout and pollock, as well as in fish oil supplements.

On Call

Free radicals are atoms that have an odd number of electrons, which makes them unstable and highly reactive. As they react with other free radicals, new radicals are created, and a chain reaction begins. This reaction is believed to cause tissue damage at the cellular level, harming our DNA, mitochondria (the site of cellular energy production), and cell membranes. Antioxidants are molecules that defend the body from cellular damage by ending the free radical chain reaction.

TREATMENTS

There is no cure, but there are strategies that may slow the progress of the disease. Regular visits to an ophthalmologist are recommended to monitor any development of cataracts or retinal swelling.

• SUPPLEMENTS Vitamin A supplements help delay the decline of vision in people with retinitis pigmentosa. Other antioxidant supplements, such as high doses of vitamin E, have not been found to be helpful and may, in fact, be harmful.

• PHYSICAL ENVIRONMENT Wearing sunglasses that protect against the full spectrum of ultraviolet light may help delay the disease.

See also: *Vision Problems, pp.36–9* • *Omega-3 Fatty Acids, pp.252–3* • *Nutritional Supplements, pp.523–41*

Ocular Cancers

Cancers of the eye are rare. The type of ocular cancer most likely to affect adults is malignant melanoma of the uveal tract, which encompasses the iris, blood vessels and muscles. Symptoms include vision loss, flashing lights and the appearance of specks (also known as floaters) crossing the field of vision. Retinoblastoma, or cancer of the retina, is the most common form of ocular cancer in children under the age of five. It can occur alone or in conjunction with other diseases.

Symptoms include crossed eyes and whiteness in the pupil. While removing the eye was once the almost universal treatment for ocular cancers, new treatments can often preserve sight.

CAUSES

Different types of ocular cancers have different causes and risk factors. However, the odds of developing a malignant melanoma of the eye are increased by regular, prolonged exposure to sunlight and certain chemicals, as well as a genetic predisposition for developing the disease. Light-coloured skin, eyes and hair are also risk factors.

Retinoblastoma is caused by mutations in the gene retinoblastoma-1. These mutations can be hereditary, or they can occur spontaneously, due to unknown causes. Hereditary retinoblastoma can affect one or both eyes, but retinoblastoma as the result of a spontaneous mutation will affect only one eye. Some ocular cancers are secondary tumours, meaning they arose elsewhere in the body and spread to the eye.

PREVENTION

Minimizing sun exposure, especially for people who live in hot climates, can help prevent malignant melanoma. When outdoors in midday, wear a hat and sunglasses that protect against the full spectrum of ultraviolet light.

While there is no known way to prevent retinoblastoma, early diagnosis and treatment can limit the damage it causes. If there is a

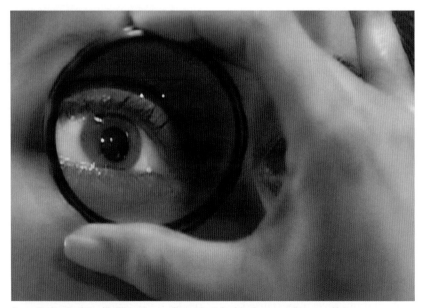

An opthalmologist will dilate the pupil and look inside the eye with magnifying equipment to detect tumors or other abnormalities. Occasionally, a secondary test such as an ultrasound will be used to confirm the diagnosis.

WHO IS AT RISK?

The risk factors include:

Retinoblastoma
- Mutation of the retinoblastoma-1 gene (retinoblastoma)
- Family history of the disease

Melanoma
- Family history
- Caucasian
- Light hair
- Blue or green eyes
- Regular, prolonged exposure to sunlight
- Exposure to certain industrial chemicals, such as polychlorinated biphenyls (PCBs)

family history of retinoblastoma, all babies should be examined by an ophthalmologist shortly after birth.

DIAGNOSIS

Ophthalmologists can diagnose ocular cancers using a variety of techniques. Sometimes there are readily visible signs, such as a growth on the surface of the eye or a bulge to the eyeball. But to see cancers within the eye, a doctor must dilate the pupil and look inside with magnifying equipment. If a tumour is seen, specialized imaging tests may be needed, including ultrasound, computed tomography (CT scan) and magnetic resonance imaging (MRI), to determine the tumour's precise location and characteristics.

TREATMENTS

For many years, the standard treatment for ocular cancer was to surgically remove the eye. But newer treatments aim to control the cancer and preserve the eye. The specific treatment chosen depends on the type of tumour, its size and its location.

More than 90 percent of children with retinoblastoma can be cured because the cancer is usually confined to the eye. The challenge is to target the treatment precisely so that blindness and other serious complications do not result.

• RADIATION THERAPY Many ocular melanomas and retinoblastomas can be treated with radiation therapy to kill cancer cells. Radiation therapy is as effective as surgical removal of the eyes, and the resulting quality of life is better because it preserves vision.

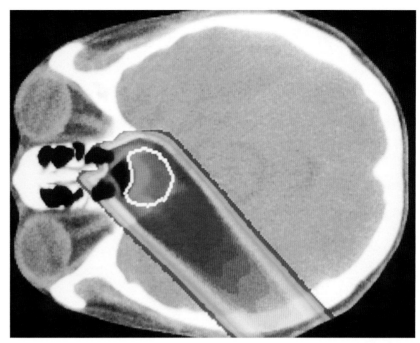

Radiation therapy, which uses focused beams of X-rays to target a tumour, can be used to treat many retinoblastomas. This computerized image of a CT scan shows the eyes and optic nerves (blue and green), the tumour (purple) and the radiation beam (yellow).

• GAMMA KNIFE RADIOSURGERY This type of radiation therapy, which delivers precise beams of radiation directly to the tumour, may be effective for treating small melanomas. The treatment has a relatively low risk of side-effects.

• LASER TREATMENTS Laser treatments may be used to combat ocular melanomas and retinoblastomas. Conventional laser treatment uses a hot laser beam to destroy ocular cancer cells. Although it is quick and painless, it often leads to permanent vision impairment. Photodynamic laser therapy is more finely targeted and less destructive to vision. A light-sensitive drug is injected intravenously, then a low-intensity laser is precisely targeted within the eye to kill the cancer cells without damaging the healthy cells. Transpupillary thermotherapy uses a warm laser beam delivered through the pupil.

• CRYOTHERAPY This procedure kills cancer cells by freezing them by using a cold probe. When the probe is touched to the outer wall of the eye, the freezing temperature passes through the eye wall and reaches the targeted inner region. Cryotherapy is used for some ocular melanomas and retinoblastomas.

• ENUCLEATION This surgery is performed in order to remove the entire eyeball. It is used for ocular melanomas and retino blastomas that are too large to be treated with more conservative procedures.

• CHEMOTHERAPY Cancer-fighting drugs are sometimes prescribed to be used along with surgery to prevent ocular cancers from metastasizing, or spreading to other tissues throughout the body.

See also: *Crossed Eyes, p.37*

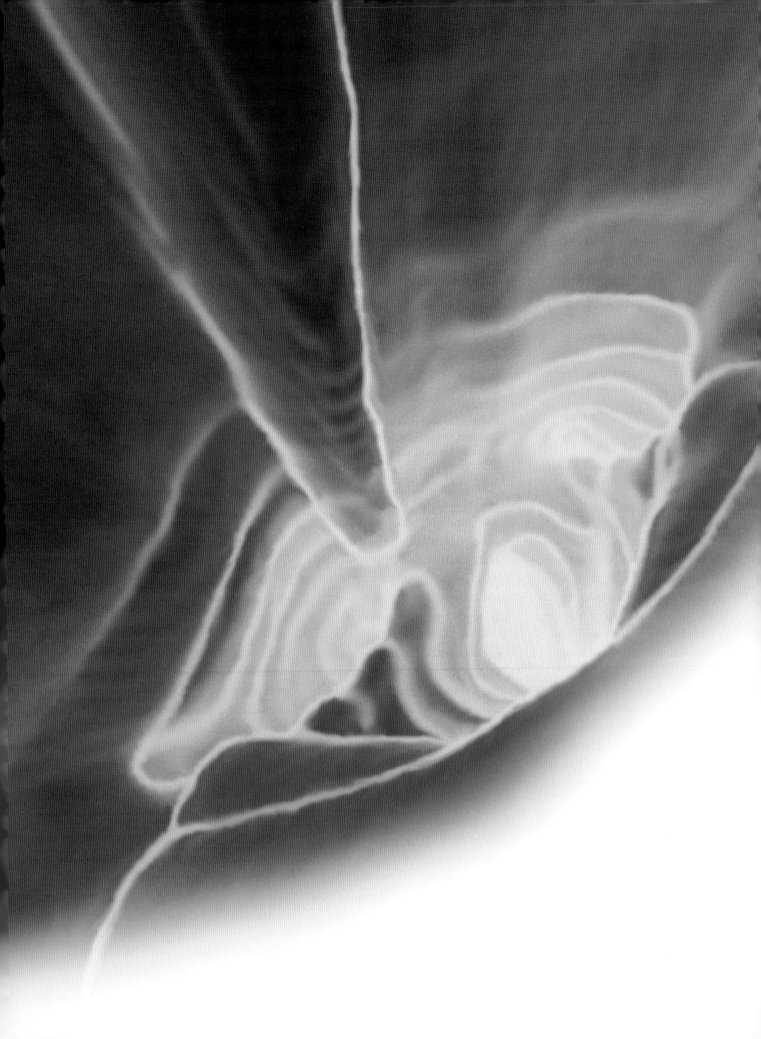

2 EARS, NOSE &THROAT

Except for conditions of the brain and eyes, diseases and illnesses above the shoulders are treated by an ear, nose and throat specialist, also called an ENT. The ears, nose and throat are delicate systems that are interconnected within the skull by passageways lined with mucous membranes. This interconnection means that illness in one system can affect the others, and sometimes the whole body.

Disorders of the ears, nose and throat can be more complicated than earache, sore throat and sinus infection. Seasonal conditions such as hay fever and pharyngitis can be managed with over-the-counter medications. But more serious conditions, such as epiglottitis and throat cancer, are medical emergencies.

These systems also involve balance, taste, smell, speech and language. Problems arising with any of these functions may be a sign of deeper problems and should be evaluated by a doctor.

Hay Fever

Also known as seasonal allergic rhinitis, hay fever is a nasal allergy to pollen. It happens at the times of year when trees and other plants flower and release pollen: spring for trees, summer for grasses, and summer and autumn for ragweed and other flowering plants. In mild climates, some plants flower and release pollen during the winter, as well. Symptoms of hay fever include runny nose, congestion, itchy and watery eyes, sneezing, and irritation of the throat and skin.

CAUSES

Like all allergies, hay fever occurs when a typically harmless substance – a type of pollen in this case – provokes a response from the immune system. The response starts after repeated exposure to the substance, when the immune system has become sensitized to it. The first response is to release antibodies to attack the foreign substance in the body. The type of antibody that is released during an allergy attack is immunoglobulin E (IgE). When IgE encounters an allergen, it floods the body with chemical weapons known as chemical mediators. These chemical mediators, which include histamine and leukotrienes, cause the allergy symptoms.

Hay fever runs in families, which suggests that it is at least partly genetic. Experts think people inherit a predisposition to the allergic response but not necessarily to a particular type of allergy. Environmental factors also play a role. Exposure to certain pollens when the immune system is weakened, such as during an illness or pregnancy, is believed to increase the chance of developing hay fever.

Having hay fever means a person has a tendency to develop allergies to plants. If they move to a different region where the plant they are allergic to does not grow, hay fever symptoms may go away for a few years, but not forever. It is likely they will eventually become allergic, instead, to pollen from one of the local trees, plants or weeds.

PREVENTION

Reduce the incidence and severity of hay fever by modifying the environment at home and, if necessary, taking allergy shots (see Treatments, right).

DIAGNOSIS

A doctor can diagnose hay fever based on the symptoms and the results of allergy tests. The doctor may ask a patient to record their symptoms over a period of time, including the season or seasons when they occur and the time of day when they are worst, to see if the symptoms suggest hay fever.

Two tests can identify the types of pollen to which a patient is allergic. One is a skin test in which a very small amount of different pollens is scratched or injected into the skin. Substances to which the patient is allergic will cause a mild localized inflammation. A blood test can also be used to identify which pollen is causing the hay fever.

TREATMENTS

The best way to control allergic rhinitis is to avoid the allergens that cause a reaction, but it is not possible to completely avoid inhaling pollen. There is no cure for hay fever, but treatments can reduce the incidence and severity of the symptoms.

• IMMUNOTHERAPY The purpose of immunotherapy is to desensitize a person's immune system to the allergens until it stops reacting to them. Injections of the allergens, commonly known as allergy shots, are given periodically over

WHO IS AT RISK?

The risk factors include:
- Having a parent with hay fever
- Having other allergies
- Being younger than 50

a period of three to five years. These injections contain progressively larger amounts of the pollens to which a patient is allergic.

• ACUPUNCTURE Acupuncture has been shown to reduce the severity of allergic rhinitis.

• HERBAL THERAPIES Butterbur (*Petasites hybridus*), stinging nettles (*Urtica dioica*) and nasal sprays containing southernwood (*Artemisia abrotanum*) can help relieve hay fever symptoms.

• PHARMACEUTICALS AND SUPPLEMENTS Several medications are used alone or in combination to control hay fever and other types of nasal allergies. Oral and inhaled antihistamines, which block the action of histamine, relieve runny nose and itching. Leukotriene modifiers accomplish the same thing by blocking the action of leukotrienes. Oral decongestants make it easier to breathe. If these medications do not provide enough relief, a doctor may prescribe a corticosteroid nasal spray to reduce inflammation in the nose. These nasal steroids do not enter the bloodstream, and so do not carry the same risk of side-effects as oral steroids. However, they do take several weeks to become effective.

• PHYSICAL ENVIRONMENT Limit or reduce exposure to pollens during allergy season(s). Keep the windows closed at home and in the car while driving, and use the air-conditioner on hot days. Clean air-conditioner filters regularly. Stay indoors as much as possible in the morning, when the pollen level is at its highest. Do not hang clothing, towels or bedding outdoors to dry. Avoid mowing the lawn and other outdoor activities that will result in exposure to pollen.

See also: *Acupuncture, pp.464–5* • *Supplements, pp.532–41* • *Homeopathy, pp.455–7*

On Call

Substances other than pollen can cause allergic rhinitis year-round, including dust mites, mould, and hairs, saliva and urine from pets. Control the symptoms with allergy medicines and by taking precautions to avoid the allergens:

• Use pillows with synthetic filling; they are less likely to harbour dust mites.
• Do not have wall-to-wall carpeting. Dust mites tend to collect there.
• Get a vacuum cleaner with a very fine filter, such as a HEPA (high-efficiency particulate air) filter, which keeps dust mites and other minute allergens out of the air. Have someone else vacuum your home, if possible.
• Consider using an air purifier.
• Use a dehumdifyer or an air-conditioner to dry out the air in your home; dust mites and mould thrive in moist environments.
• Avoid raking leaves to reduce your exposure to outdoor moulds. If you are outdoors when the mould count is high, cover your nose and mouth with a handkerchief or a face mask.
• If you are allergic to animals, avoid contact with them. If you touch a cat or dog, wash your hands immediately afterwards.

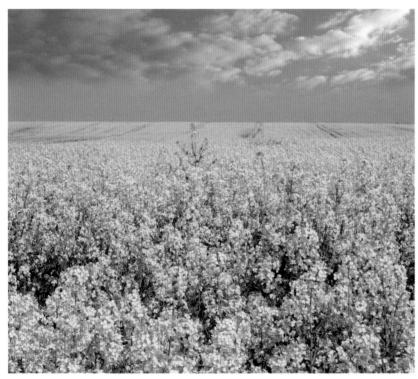
Hay fever occurs when pollen from trees and other flowering plants triggers an immune response in the body. Many people experience a runny nose, congestion, itchy and watery eyes, sneezing and irritation of the throat and skin.

EAR INFECTIONS

Infections can occur in the middle ear or the ear canal. Middle ear infection, called acute otitis media, causes inflammation behind the eardrum, especially the Eustachian tube, the vessel that connects the middle ear to the throat and back of the nose. Middle ear infections are most common in children, although adults get them, too. Symptoms include intensely painful earache and sometimes fever and difficulty hearing: they come on suddenly, usually following an upper respiratory infection or nasal allergy.

CAUSES

Bacteria and fungi may invade the ears in several ways, causing an infection.

Otitis media

Caused by a bacterial infection in the Eustachian tube, otitis media can be either acute or chronic, and usually follows soon after a viral infection.

Acute otitis media often occurs when an upper respiratory infection or nasal allergy causes the Eustachian tube to become inflamed. This inflammation blocks the Eustachian tube, preventing it from carrying out its normal function – which is to equalize pressure between the throat and the middle ear. Pressure decreases in the middle ear, causing earache and trapping mucus and pus, which often contains bacteria. Swelling from the infection causes pain.

Hearing may be impaired. This is because fluid in the Eustachian tube muffles sound, and swelling prevents the eardrum and the three tiny bones inside the middle ear from vibrating in response to incoming sounds and transmitting sound signals to the brain. Young children, especially boys, are most prone to middle ear infections because their Eustachian tubes are small and they tend to get upper respiratory infections frequently.

When fluid persists in the middle ear either after an infection has cleared up or in the absence of a middle ear infection, it is called serous otitis media (p.55).

Chronic otitis media is an ongoing abnormality in the middle ear. It can be an infection that persists or keeps recurring for many weeks or months, a perforation in the eardrum that does not heal, or a benign growth in the middle ear called a cholesteoma.

Acute otitis media can cause a perforation in the eardrum, and if the hole does not close by itself it can increase the risk of recurrent infections. Untreated, cholesteomas and eardrum perforations that cause recurrent ear infections can damage structures within the middle ear.

Otitis Externa

This condition, caused by a bacterial or fungal infection of the ear canal, causes itching, redness, pain and discharge. It is also known as swimmer's ear because it is frequently caused by swimming in water that contains bacteria. The bacteria or fungi in the water get into the skin of the ear canal.

Frequent use of earplugs or hairspray can also irritate the inside of the ear canal. Other risk

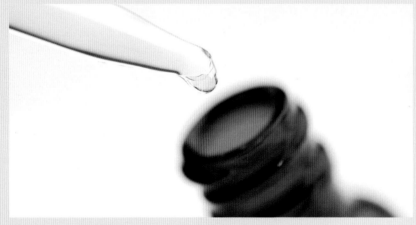

Homemade eardrops made from equal parts white vinegar and rubbing alcohol can help prevent otisis externa. The drops help by keeping the skin inside the ear canal dry and killing off any bacteria and fungi that are present.

factors are trauma to the ear canal, skin conditions such as eczema that allow bacteria or fungi to enter, and chronic otitis media with a perforated eardrum in which pus drains into the ear canal.

Malignant otitis externa is a rare complication in which the infection spreads from the floor of the ear canal to the adjacent tissues and into the bones of the base of the skull. The bones may be damaged or destroyed from the resulting infection, which may further spread and affect the cranial nerves, the brain or other parts of the body. Diabetics and people with compromised immune systems are particularly susceptible.

PREVENTION

Changes in physical environment, as well as several self-help measures, can reduce the risk of otitis media and otitis externa.

Otitis Media

Do not smoke, and avoid second-hand smoke. This can set the stage for middle ear infections by increasing the risk of colds as well as possibly altering the functioning of the Eustachian tubes.

Breast-feeding is believed to reduce the risk of otitis media in babies. Limit the use of a dummy, which may increase the risk of middle ear infections.

Vaccinations against *Pneumococcal* and *Haemophilus influenza* can help prevent otitis media.

Otitis Externa

Keeping the ear canals dry helps to reduce the risk of infection. To get water out of the ear canal after

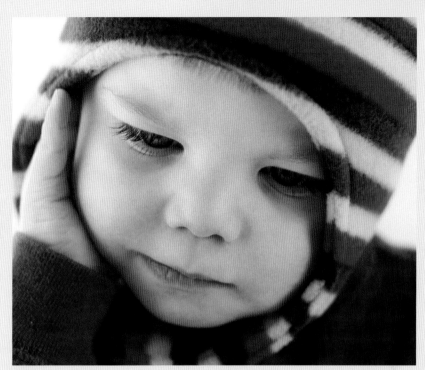

Middle ear infections occur most commonly in children, and three out of four children will experience an infection before the age of three. Symptoms can include painful earache, fever, difficulty hearing, or difficulty maintaining balance.

showering or swimming, tilt your head to one side and let the water run out while gently drying the opening with a towel. Then tilt your head to the other side to dry the other ear. As an added precaution while showering, apply petroleum jelly to two cotton balls and put a cotton ball in each ear.

Avoid injuring the ears. Scratches and other injuries increase the risk of otitis externa. One way to avoid this is not to use cotton swabs to clean the ear canals, because they can scratch the delicate skin.

A homemade solution of equal parts white vinegar and rubbing alcohol, used as eardrops, can help prevent otitis externa. Put a few drops in each ear after swimming. The drops make the skin of the outer ear resistant to infection by drying it out and killing off bacteria and fungi.

DIAGNOSIS

A doctor or nurse can diagnose ear infections by looking into the ear for telltale symptoms. Redness and fluid in the middle ear are signs of otitis media. Symptoms of otitis externa are swelling or redness of the skin of the ear canal, fluid draining into the ear canal and tenderness of the lymph nodes near the ear.

TREATMENTS

Treatment of both otitis media and otitis externa includes eliminating the infection, reducing inflammation, and making the patient more comfortable.

Otitis Media

With treatment, symptoms of acute otitis media are usually relieved within a day or two. However, it can take a month

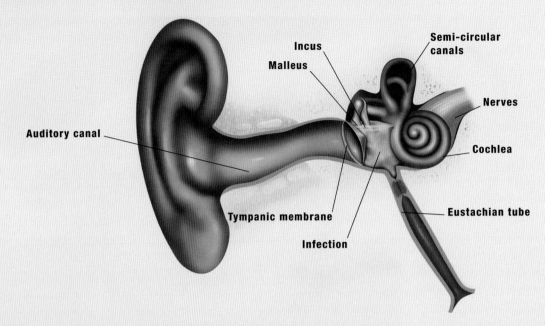

Incus

Malleus

Semi-circular
canals

Nerves

Auditory canal

Cochlea

Eustachian tube

Tympanic membrane

Infection

The ear is made up of the outer canal, the middle ear and Eustachian tube, which equalizes pressure between the ear and throat.
A middle ear infection occurs when the Eustachian tube becomes inflamed or blocked, preventing fluid from draining.

or longer for the fluid that is in the middle ear to drain or become absorbed by the body.

• MEDICATION Decongestants can help open the Eustachian tube and allow fluid to drain. Pain relievers such as acetaminophen or ibuprofen can help reduce the pain. Warm compresses on the ear can also relieve pain temporarily.

Although many middle ear infections go away on their own, antibiotics, applied orally or in eardrops, are often recommended because they lead to earlier resolution of symptoms and prevent infectious complications such as mastoiditis (inflammation of the bone and air space behind the ear canal). However, a 2004 study done at Temple University in Philadelphia, Pennsylvania, found that when patients use a broad-spectrum antibiotic eardrops, such as fluoroquinolone, it can lead to an increase in resistant bacteria

and fungi in the ear. To prevent bacteria from becoming antibiotic-resistant, the researchers recommend that patients receive antibiotics that are targeted specifically to the individual types of bacteria that are causing the infection.

• SURGERY Otitis media that recurs frequently or causes reduced hearing is often treated with myringotomy – surgery that helps fluid drain from the middle ear. A small opening is made in the eardrum and a drainage tube is inserted. For chronic otitis media, surgery may be needed to close a persistent hole in the eardrum or to remove a cholesteatoma.

• OSTEOPATHIC MANIPULATION THERAPY When it is used alongside conventional medicine, osteopathic manipulation therapy has proved to be effective. It has helped children who are prone to recurrent middle ear infections

to have fewer infections and fewer surgical procedures to drain fluid from the ear.

• HOMEOPATHY This has also been found to be effective and can substantially reduce the use of antibiotics in children with middle ear infections. Herbal eardrops that contain calendula, or marigold, can act as a mild anaesthetic and relieve pain from ear infections. But there are some questions about their safety, especially in children.

Otitis Externa

The main course of treatment for otitis externa is the use of eardrops that contain antibiotics to eliminate the infection and hydrocortisone to reduce inflammation. Symptoms of otitis externa usually begin to improve within three days with treatment.

See also: *Serous Otitis Media, p.55* • *Hay Fever, pp.50–1* • *Homeopathy, pp.455–7*

Serous Otitis Media

This condition, commonly known as fluid in the middle ear, is an accumulation of pus and/or mucus behind the eardrum. The fluid cannot drain because of persistent swelling or compression of the Eustachian tube, the channel for draining the ear. This problem is especially common in children under the age of three. Although the condition is usually painless, it is the most common cause of hearing loss in children and, if untreated, can cause recurrent middle ear infections and lead to delays in speech and language development.

WHO IS AT RISK?

The risk factors include:
- Otitis media
- Under 3 years old
- Nasal allergies
- Regular exposure to tobacco smoke or other air pollutants
- Cleft palate
- Infected tonsils or adenoids
- Gastrointestinal reflux disease

CAUSES

The most common cause is a middle ear infection (pp.52–4), which sets the stage for fluid in the middle ear by causing inflammation of the Eustachian tube. When the fluid accumulates as the result of recurrent ear infection, infections of the adenoids or tonsils (p.61) may be to blame. Other conditions that increase mucus production in the upper respiratory tract or impair the function of the Eustachian tube can also cause fluid build-up. These include nasal allergies (pp.50–1), colds, gastrointestinal reflux disease (pp.264–5) and cleft palate, a birth defect in which there is an opening in the roof of the mouth. Exposure to air pollution, including secondhand tobacco smoke, can also stimulate mucus production.

PREVENTION

Avoid exposure to secondhand smoke and to known allergens, such as dust mites and pollen.

DIAGNOSIS

Doctors will look into the ear and check for the presence of bubbles or fluid behind the eardrum. However, infections are sometimes difficult to diagnose; although the doctor can usually detect the fluid, there is no way to be sure it is infected. A tympanometer may be used to estimate the quantity and thickness of the fluid. This tool works by changing the air pressure in the ear canal and then measuring the eardrum's reaction. If the fluid has been present for six or more weeks, the doctor may also do a hearing test.

TREATMENTS

Fluid in the middle ear is treated with environmental changes and, if necessary, medicine and surgery. If an underlying illness, such as gastrointestinal reflux disease (GORD), is causing the fluid, treatment will also involve controlling that illness.

- **PHYSICAL ENVIRONMENT** The first line of treatment is to change environmental factors that may be promoting fluid in the middle ear, as described in the section on Prevention. This alone may help the fluid drain on its own.
- **MEDICATION** If the fluid persists for several weeks, a course of antibiotics may be given to stop a middle ear infection setting in.
- **SURGERY** When medication is not helpful and fluid remains after several months, a surgical procedure may be recommended in order to drain the fluid. A small incision is made in the eardrum and, in many cases, a ventilation tube is placed into the incision to help fluid drain. This will also prevent fluid from accumulating again.

If an infection of the adenoids or tonsils is the cause, surgery to remove them may be recommended.

See also: Ear Infections, pp.52–4 • Tonsillitis, p.61 • Hay Fever, pp.50–1

Pharyngitis

Pharyngitis, an inflammation of the tissue lining the pharynx (throat), is the medical name for a sore throat. It causes a feeling of scratchiness, burning or other pain, and tends to be at its worst first thing in the morning and when swallowing. In contrast to throat irritation due to factors such as smoking, nasal allergies and shouting, pharyngitis is caused by an infection. This condition usually goes away on its own within a week.

A sore throat that is unusually painful or persistent should be evaluated by a doctor, because it can be a symptom of a condition that needs medical treatment, such as strep throat (caused by *Streptococcus* bacteria), mononucleosis (p.319) or tonsillitis (p.61).

CAUSES

The most common cause of pharyngitis is an infection with a cold virus. A sore throat is usually the first symptom of a cold.

Cold viruses cause pharyngitis directly by infecting the throat and causing inflammation, or indirectly by increasing the production of mucus in the nasal passages, which then drips into the throat and causes irritation. Other viral infections in which pharyngitis is a symptom are influenza and mononucleosis.

Bacterial infections can cause sore throats, too. Strep throat must be treated with a course of antibiotics. The complications that occur if a bacterial infection is left untreated can be serious:

they include acute rheumatic fever (an inflammatory disease that can involve the heart, joints, skin and brain); nephritis, which is a kidney disorder (p.301); and other severe diseases such as bacteraemia and *streptococcal* toxic shock syndrome (in which bacteria enter and infect the bloodstream).

Sore throats are also a symptom of tonsillitis.

WHO IS AT RISK?

The risk factors include

- Colds
- Tonsillitis
- Strep throat

PREVENTION

Most cases of pharyngitis occur in the colder months, the season for respiratory disease. It often spreads among family members. Risk of contracting pharyngitis can be reduced by taking precautions against colds and other respiratory infections. Extra precautions include washing hands frequently, especially after having been in a public place, and not rubbing eyes or putting fingers in the mouth.

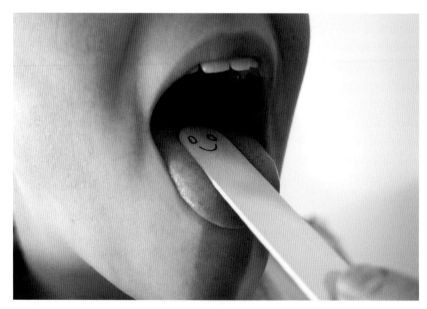

Pharyngitis has many causes including irratation from mucus drainage to bacterial or viral infections. A doctor will perform an examination of the pharynx to look for drainage or coating. A throat culture can determine if the irritation is caused by infection.

healing hope

I've had mild sore throats before, but never used to think much of them. They always went away a few hours after I woke up, unless I was really sick. But last winter I started getting them all the time. I was sure I had an infection. Ibuprofen helped, but I couldn't figure out how to keep them from coming back.

My doctor did some tests which ruled out strep throat. So she suggested I try gargling with salt water and sleeping with a vaporizer to raise the moisture level in the bedroom. Turns out these two simple things pretty much cured the problem. The doctor said that dehydration was probably causing drainage, which was keeping my throat sore. Now whenever I feel even a little stuffy, I gargle with salt-water and I use the vaporizer to keep my nasal passages moist while I sleep.

Sarah M.

DIAGNOSIS

Pharyngitis can be diagnosed based on the symptoms, the appearance of the throat and a throat culture. A doctor will examine the pharynx to look for drainage or a coating of mucus. The skin, eyes and lymph nodes in the neck may also be examined for any signs of inflammation and swelling.

Strep throat is often more severe than a sore throat caused by a viral infection, and is characterized by white spots on the throat, a temperature, tender lymph nodes in the sides of the neck, headaches and the absence of cold-like symptoms. However, strep throat can only be definitively diagnosed by taking a throat culture, in which a lab test is used to identify the organisms infecting the throat. Additional throat cultures or blood tests may be performed, depending on which organism is suspected of causing the infection.

Redness and mucus in the throat are typical symptoms of a viral infection. Viral pharyngitis may also be associated with runny nose and postnasal drip, or drainage from the sinuses into the back of the throat. Severe cases may be accompanied by difficulty swallowing and, rarely, difficulty breathing.

TREATMENTS

The treatment of pharyngitis depends on the underlying cause of the inflammation. Viral infections are managed with warm salt water gargles, pain relievers and fluids. Antibiotics are needed if strep throat is diagnosed. Most cases of pharyngitis go away on their own, without complications.

CAUTION

See a doctor if you have had a sore throat for two weeks or if it is accompanied by a rash, high temperature, swollen lymph nodes in the neck or difficulty breathing. These can be signs of a condition that needs prompt medical treatment. If you have a sore throat and experience difficulty breathing, seek medical care immediately.

• **MEDICATION** Regardless of the cause of a sore throat, you can temporarily ease the pain with over-the-counter pain relievers such as ibuprofen and acetaminophen, and topical preparations that contain a local anaesthetic. Antibiotics are necessary to treat bacterial infections such as strep throat and to prevent complications.

• **THROAT LOZENGES** A variety of throat lozenges can offer relief from symptoms of inflammation by lubricating the throat and numbing inflamed tissues. Lozenges that contain zinc may help relieve symptoms as well.

• **HERBAL MEDICINE** Lozenges and liquid solutions made of slippery elm (*Ulmus fulva*) bark, which comes from a tree that is native to North America, help to reduce sore throat pain.

See also: *Mononucleosis, p.319* • *Tonsillitis, p.61* • *Nephritis, p.301*

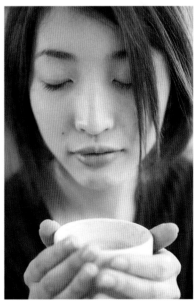

Drinking tea and other hot liquids, and gargling with a solution of salt water can help relieve the pain of a sore throat.

Sinusitis

This very common condition is an infection in the sinuses (the spaces in the bones around the nose), which causes inflammation of the membranes that line the sinuses. Symptoms include tenderness in the face, aching behind the eyes, nasal congestion and difficulty breathing through the nose, headaches and in severe cases, fever. Reduced sense of smell, aching in the upper jaw and teeth, bad breath and ear pain are other symptoms.

Agents that cause these sinus infections include bacteria, viruses and fungi. The infections can either be acute – lasting several days to a week – or chronic – requiring treatment for extended periods of time. Serious complications can result, including the spread of the infection to the skull bone, eye or brain covering (meningitis), and the formation of an abscess or blood clot.

CAUSES

The sinuses normally drain into the nose through small openings called ostia. When the ostia become blocked and the sinuses cannot drain, mucus builds up in the sinuses making them into a breeding ground for bacteria, viruses and fungi.

The most common causes of this kind of blockage are head colds and allergies. But sinusitis can also result from nasal polyps (p.76), a dental abscess, infected water inhaled while swimming or diving, an injury to the face, overuse of over-the-counter nasal decongestant sprays, altitude changes and foreign objects lodged inside the nose. A deviated septum (p.71) can increase the odds of developing sinusitis.

PREVENTON

Some people are especially prone to sinusitis—once they have had it, they tend to get it again, especially after a cold. But some simple precautions can help prevent it.

First of all, take steps to avoid catching a cold, especially by washing hands frequently. In addition, do not smoke (and avoid secondhand smoke). Inhaling smoke increases the risk of upper-respiratory infections and allergies. When blowing the nose, do so gently, one nostril at a time; blowing forcefully can set the

CAUTION

Never use decongestant sprays for more than three days in a row, unless directed by your healthcare provider. Overuse of decongestants can actually increase mucus production.

WHO IS AT RISK?

The risk factors include:

- Colds
- Respiratory or food allergies
- Dental abscess (an infection in the tissue surrounding the root of an upper tooth near a sinus cavity)
- Swimming in infected water
- Inhaling water infected with bacteria or other microbes
- Severe facial injury that results in difficulty breathing through one or both nostrils

stage for a sinus infection by causing nasal inflammation.

If suffering from respiratory allergies, reduce the risk of sinusitis by finding out what the allergy is to and avoiding exposure to it. Chronic sinusitis is sometimes

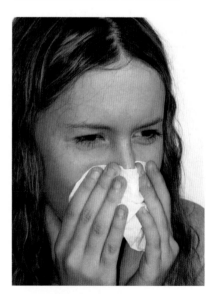

Blow your nose gently, one nostril at a time. Blowing forcefully can inflame nasal passages and lead to infection.

thought to be a complication of food allergies. An elimination diet, in which certain foods are avoided for several days to see if symptoms improve, can help identify foods that may be causing sinusitis. Such a diet yields the best results if it is done under the guidance of a doctor. A prescription steroid-based nasal spray to prevent inflammation of the nasal passages and to enable mucus to drain normally can also be helpful.

• PHYSICAL ENVIRONMENT Having a humidifier in the bedroom during the winter can help prevent respiratory infections by keeping the nasal passages moist and therefore resistant to germs. It is best to avoid flying or scuba diving when congested from a respiratory infection or allergy, because changes in air pressure can push mucus up into the sinuses. If flying is unavoidable, use a decongestant ahead of time and follow up with a nasal spray half an hour or so before landing.

• NUTRITION A healthy diet can reduce the risk of sinusitis by

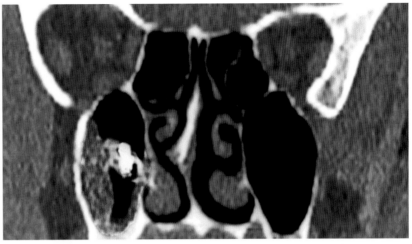

This is a CT scan of the face of a patient with sinusitis, a very common condition that causes inflammation of the membranes that line the sinuses. The right maxillary sinus contains mucus (shown as orange) resulting from the infection.

reducing the risk of colds. In particular, foods that are rich in antioxidants, such as many kinds of fruits and vegetables, help stave off infections. Drink at least 1.4 litres (48 fl.oz) of water a day, as well. Plenty of fluids help keep the mucus thin enough to flow freely. Alcohol also can cause the sinus membranes to swell.

• MIND–BODY CONNECTION Reducing stress is an important factor in preventing sinusitis.

DIAGNOSIS

A doctor or other health professional can often diagnose sinusitis based on symptoms and a medical history. Chronic sinusitis can be difficult to diagnose, however, because the symptoms may be similar to colds or allergies. Symptoms may include nasal congestion, headache, tooth pain beneath the cheeks, green discharge from the nose and a temperature. X-rays are sometimes taken to see the location and extent of the sinus infection. The practitioner may also take a fluid sample from the sinuses to determine the cause of the infection. Nasal endoscopy, in which a thin, flexible tube with a fibre-optic light is inserted into the nose, may also be used to enable the doctor to visually inspect the inside of the sinuses.

If someone has recurrent sinusitis, the practitioner may examine the nasal passages to see if there is a structural blockage, such as a deviated septum (p.71), that is contributing to the problem.

healing hope I used to get sinus infections that lasted for weeks. The pain was terrible – it felt like I had marbles rolling around in my head. I'd take antibiotics, as well as decongestants and painkillers, just to be able to function normally. But no sooner did I get rid of one sinus infection then I'd get another one. I didn't like the idea of taking medication so often, but my doctor said the only alternative was surgery. Then I sought a second opinion from a doctor who recommended acupuncture.

I was sceptical at first – and scared. But I went to an acupuncturist my doctor knew. She put needles around my nose and forehead, as well as my ears and other places. She also applied essential oils to these areas and had me inhale some herbs. I went back about three times. That was a year ago. I still get sinus infections, but not nearly as often as I used to. And they go away a lot faster.   *Brad S.*

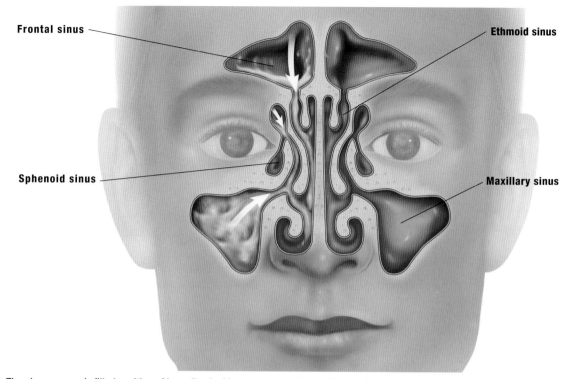

Frontal sinus

Ethmoid sinus

Sphenoid sinus

Maxillary sinus

The sinuses are air-filled cavities of bone lined with mucous membranes that drain into the nose through tiny holes called ostia. Infection occurs when bacteria, viruses, fungi or foreign matter enter the sinuses.

TREATMENTS

It is important to relieve pain and congestion, and fight off the infection. Chronic sinusitis can often require a long course of treatment.

• HYDROTHERAPY Contrast hydrotherapy (pp.482–3), in which alternating hot and cold compresses are placed over the sinuses, helps reduce congestion and pain. Start with three minutes of hot, followed by 30 seconds of cold, repeated three times and ending with the cold compress. Inhaling warm steam also helps open the sinuses.

• SURGERY This may be recommended when a structural abnormality in the nose, such as a deviated septum, contributes to sinusitis by interfering with breathing.

• ACUPUNCTURE The World Health Organization lists sinusitis as one of the many common conditions that acupuncture (pp.464–5) can help.

• NATUROPATHY This type of therapy (pp.443–5) works to relieve the symptoms of sinusitis, as well as possibly increase the immune system's ability to fight an infection and prevent future infections. Herbs that may be ingested include a mixture of goldenseal (*Hydrastis canadensis*), yarrow (*Achillea millefolium*), echinacea (*Echinacea purpurea*) and wild indigo (*Baptisia tinctoria*). Goldenseal may be mixed with a nasal wash of salt water to help clear the nasal passages.

• AYURVEDA This therapy (pp.451–4) can bring about improvement in chronic sinusitis.

• VITAMINS The antioxidants A, C and E may relieve sinus inflammation. These compounds may also help prevent infections by boosting the immune system.

• ZINC This mineral has been shown to reduce the severity and duration of colds and therefore may reduce the chance of developing sinusitis.

• ANTIBIOTICS If bacteria is the cause of sinusitis, antibiotics can eliminate the infection.

• STEROID NASAL SPRAYS These sprays are sometimes used for chronic or severe sinusitis to reduce inflammation. In this kind of nasal spray, the steroids do not enter the bloodstream, and so do not carry the risk of side-effects that oral steroids do. However, steroid nasal sprays do have to be used for several weeks to reach maximum effectiveness.

See also: *Nasal Polyps, p.76 • Deviated Septum, p.71 • Hydrotherapy, pp.482–3*

Tonsillitis

Tonsillitis is an inflammation of the tonsils, two oval lymphatic tissue structures on either side of the back of the mouth and the throat. The inflammation is the result of an infection. Symptoms include sore throats, difficulty swallowing, temperatures, chills, aches, swollen glands in the neck, bad breath and laryngitis (p.69). Tonsillitis is especially common in children. Recurrent tonsillitis causes problems such as difficulty breathing, and an increased risk of other infections, including middle ear infections. In such cases, surgery to remove the tonsils may be recommended.

WHO IS AT RISK?

The risk factors include:

- Children ages 5 to 10
- Exposure to *Streptococcus* bacteria
- Upper respiratory infection

CAUSES

Tonsillitis occurs when the tonsils, which normally filter germs from the throat before they cause infection, become infected. The most common causes are viruses and the *Streptococcus* bacteria.

PREVENTION

Reduce the risk of tonsillitis by avoiding contact with people with upper respiratory infections, and wash hands frequently.

DIAGNOSIS

A doctor or other healthcare professional can diagnose tonsillitis based on symptoms and the appearance of the tonsils. The tonsils will be red and swollen and may be covered with white specks, or a white or yellow coating. The lymph nodes in the neck may be swollen and painful when touched. A culture of cells from the tonsils can determine if the cause is *Streptococcus* or another bacteria.

TREATMENTS

The treatment of tonsillitis depends on the cause. If it is viral, the goal of treatment is to relieve the symptoms until the infection goes away on its own. A bacterial infection requires the use of antibiotics.

- **MEDICATION** Antibiotics are necessary to cure a bacterial infection and prevent complications. Pain relievers, such as nonsteroidal anti-inflammatory agents, can help ease the pain and reduce fever.
- **LOZENGES** Throat lozenges may provide additional pain relief.
- **FLUIDS** Gargling with salt water and drinking either hot or cold fluids can soothe pain from tonsillitis. Eating soft foods can help avoid irritating the throat and aggravating the symptoms.
- **HOMEOPATHY** Homeopathic tablets or liquids made from a combination of American pokeweed (*Phytolacca americana*), lignum vitae (*Guajacum officinale*) and paprika (*Capsicum annuum*) can reduce symptoms of tonsillitis.

- **SURGERY** A tonsillectomy, or the surgical removal of the tonsils, is considered when tonsillitis recurs several times in a year, is severe or causes complications such as abscesses on the tonsils, obstructed breathing, difficulty swallowing or recurrent middle ear infections. Although the operation reduces the number of throat infections, it does not eliminate them.

See also: *Laryngitis, p.69* • *Ear Infections, pp.52–4* • *Homeopathy, pp.455–7*

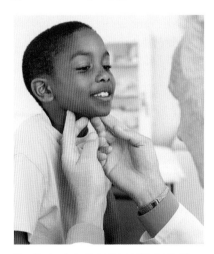

Tonsils are lymph nodes at the back of the throat that normally filter bacteria and viruses. When inflamed, they become swollen and tender.

Snoring

The loud, grating sounds of snoring occur when there is an obstruction to the free flow of air through the passages at the back of the mouth and nose. This is where the tongue and upper throat meet the soft palate and uvula. Snoring occurs when these structures strike each other and vibrate during breathing. About a quarter of adults snore regularly and nearly half snore occasionally. Because of the noise, snoring can sometimes affect the sleeping partner more seriously than it affects the snorer.

CAUSES

Colds, sinus infections, nasal allergies and asthma can all lead to snoring by causing congestion and swelling of the nasal passages. Congestion forces a person to breathe through the mouth instead of the nose, and snoring is more common with mouth breathing.

Antihistamines used to relieve allergy and cold symptoms can also contribute to snoring because of their sedative effect, which can relax the muscles in the tongue and throat so that they sag and partially block the airway. Other sedatives, as well as heavy alcohol use, can have the same effect.

Snoring can also result from structural abnormalities in the nose and throat that partially obstruct airflow. These include a deviated septum (p.71), an unusually large uvula (the dangling tissue in the back of the throat) or tongue, and large tonsils or adenoids. Being overweight (pp.348–9) can increase the risk of snoring by adding girth to the neck – the thicker the neck, the more likely it is to press against the airways. Snoring becomes more common in women during the last month of pregnancy because the airways tend to thicken.

Snoring can also be a symptom of obstructive sleep apnoea (pp.214–15), a serious condition in which a sleeper stops breathing for several seconds at a time.

PREVENTION

Reduce the risk of snoring by maintaining a normal weight and not consuming excessive amounts of alcohol. Even if you drink moderately, avoiding alcohol before bedtime may help prevent snoring. In addition, do not use sedative medications, such as sleeping pills, unless they are absolutely necessary.

DIAGNOSIS

Snoring is usually diagnosed by a partner or housemate who hears it during the night. The underlying cause can be determined by a doctor, who will do a physical examination and take a medical history.

TREATMENTS

Snoring can usually be alleviated with some changes in behaviour, diet and activity. If the snoring is severe and leads to other medical problems, surgical procedures can help alleviate the condition. Treatments for sleep apnoea include a mask that keeps the airways open during sleep and, in severe cases, surgery.

On Call

If you snore and are also are experiencing any of the following symptoms, consider a medical evaluation because you may have sleep apnoea.

- Falling asleep during normal waking hours
- Increased irritability
- Loss of concentration

WHO IS AT RISK?

The risk factors include:
- Overweight
- Upper respiratory infections
- Respiratory allergies
- Asthma
- Sedative medications
- Deviated septum
- Large tongue
- Large tonsils or adenoids
- Ninth month of pregnancy
- Sleep apnoea

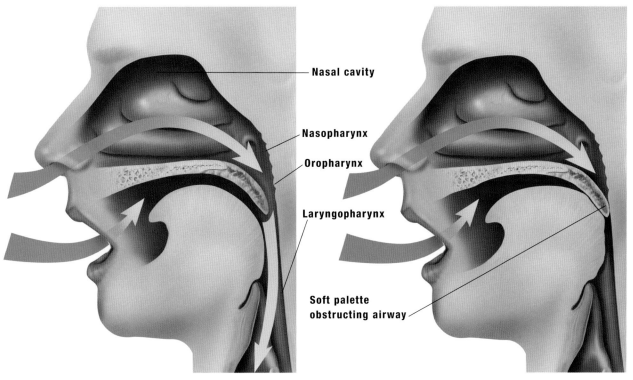

Nasal cavity

Nasopharynx

Oropharynx

Laryngopharynx

Soft palette
obstructing airway

Structural abnormalities in the nose and throat can partially obstruct airflow and cause snoring. As sleep progresses and becomes deeper, these tissues relax and the airway narrows, causing the tissues to vibrate against one other. Sometimes the airway becomes so relaxed and narrow that breathing stops completely, a serious condition called apnoea.

• **PHYSICAL ENVIRONMENT** Sleep on the side rather than the back, because in that position the throat is less likely to obstruct breathing. Raise the head – sleeping on two pillows may reduce snoring because it takes some of the weight off airways.

• **NASAL DILATOR STRIPS** These sticky little strips fit across the bridge of the nose and help hold open the nostrils. By making it easier to breathe through the nose, the strips may prevent breathing through the mouth while sleeping.

• **DIET** Drink in moderation – not more than one or two alcoholic drinks a day. (One drink is equal to 0.2 litres/8 fl.oz of beer, 0.1 litre/5 fl.oz of wine, or 4.4. cl/ 1.5 fl oz of distilled spirits.) Lose weight by reducing calories, increasing physical activity, or both.

• **SPRAYS AND GARGLES** Snoring can be significantly reduced by using either a gargle or a throat spray made of a variety of essential oils, including mint, lemon, cloves, pine, fennel, thyme, citronella, eucalyptus and lavender.

• **SINGING EXERCISES** A pilot research project conducted on 20 patients by voice teacher Alise Ojay in conjunction with the University of Exeter, England, found that doing 20 minutes of singing exercises every day for three months reduces the levels of snoring by about 20 percent. Ojay suggests that singing exercises can reduce snoring by toning lax muscles in the upper throat.

• **OTHER MEASURES** If these self-help measures are not sufficient, professional treatment may be needed. A dentist can create an

appliance, to be worn while asleep, that keeps the tongue from blocking the throat. If there is a deviated septum, surgery may be necessary.

• **LAUP PROCEDURE** If snoring is habitual and disruptive to others, laser assisted uvula palatoplasty (LAUP) may be an option. In this procedure, a laser is used to vaporize the uvula and a portion of the palate in a series of one to five small procedures spaced four to eight weeks apart. The uvula is thereby shortened, eliminating the obstruction that has contributed to the snoring. Each procedure is performed on an outpatient basis under local anaesthetic. Discomfort similar to a severe sore throat may last up to ten days.

See also: *Deviated Septum, p.71 • Sleep Apnoea, pp.214–15 • Obesity, pp.348–9*

Croup

Croup is an inflammation of the airways, trachea and larynx that narrows the airways. The word comes from the Anglo-Saxon *kropan*, which means 'to cry aloud'. The main symptom is a deep cough that sounds like a dog's bark. Croup is most common in children aged five and younger, and boys contract it more often than girls. It often follows a cold in autumn and winter, but can also develop alongside respiratory allergies or bacterial infections.

CAUSES

The leading cause of croup is a viral infection, usually from the viruses that cause colds or flu. The virus spreads to the larynx and trachea, causing the barking cough. The infection makes the airways swell and secrete excess fluid, sometimes leading to stridor, a condition characterized by noisy breathing during inhalation. Other causes of croup are bacterial infections, allergies, inhaled substances that irritate the airways and gastrointestinal reflux disease (pp.264–5).

PREVENTION

Immunization (pp.314–15) against diphtheria and measles prevent some of the most serious causes of croup. To guard against other causes, take measures to prevent colds and flu, including washing hands frequently (especially after being in public places) and avoiding contact with infected people.

DIAGNOSIS

Even though the disease is usually mild and can be treated at home, it is best to call the doctor if your child has the signs of croup because there is a chance the condition can cause breathing difficulties and other severe respiratory symptoms. Croup can also be confused with more serious conditions, such as epiglottitis (p.65).

The signs of croup may include the characteristic cough, mild to moderate difficulty breathing that is especially noisy when inhaling, a temperature and a hoarse voice. Symptoms may diminish during the day and get worse at night. Croup is usually preceded by symptoms similar to those of a cold.

A doctor may want to listen to a child cough over the phone. In an office visit, the doctor may listen to a child's chest through a stethoscope to hear the telltale wheezing. When croup symptoms are severe, diagnostic tests such as X-rays may be needed.

In rare cases, croup is serious enough to be considered a medical emergency. Such symptoms include extreme difficulty breathing, a whistling sound when breathing, a blue tint to the mouth and fingertips and drooling. If a child has these symptoms, go to the nearest hospital.

TREATMENTS

Croup usually goes away on its own in three to seven days.

• **STEAM TREATMENT** In the meantime, symptoms can generally be relieved with exposure to humid air. Turn on the hot water in the shower to steam up the bathroom, then have a child stay in the steamy room for 15 to 20 minutes. Use a humidifier or cool water vaporizer in the bedroom to help maintain improvements in breathing.

• **MEDICATION** If exposure to humid air is not sufficient, glucocorticoid, given orally or intravenously, can decrease the inflammation in the airways. Steroids such as dexamethasone can lessen symptoms and decrease the number of hospitalizations for this condition.

See also: GORD, pp.264–5 • Epiglottitis, p.65 • Hay Fever, pp.50–1

Epiglottitis

This is an infection and inflammation of the epiglottis, the cartilage that covers the windpipe when swallowing to keep food from entering. Epiglottitis is a medical emergency, because the inflammation can cause suffocation unless it is treated immediately. Symptoms are an extremely sore throat that starts suddenly and is soon followed by a temperature, noisy and laboured breathing and difficulty swallowing.

People with these symptoms should go to a hospital emergency room immediately. Epiglottitis is a rare condition that affects mainly children, but also occurs in adults.

CAUSES

The most common cause of epiglottitis is infection with the *Haemophilus influenza* type *b* bacteria, but other bacteria, including *Streptococcus* and *Staphylococcus*, and some viruses can also cause the condition. The *Haemophilus* vaccine has reduced the number of cases caused by this organism. Having an immune system weakened by disease or immuno-suppressive medication such as prednisone increases the risk of epiglottitis.

PREVENTION

Being immunized with the *Haemophilus influenza* type *b* (HIB) vaccine can prevent the most common cause of epiglottitis. Also, avoid contact with anyone who has epiglottitis or any other upper respiratory infection. If exposed to someone with epiglottitis, a visit to a doctor is advisable.

DIAGNOSIS

Doctors diagnose by examining the larynx to see whether the epiglottis is red and swollen. Neck X-rays may be used to see the epiglottis. A throat culture and blood tests may be done to determine the specific cause of the infection. Do not examine a child's (or anyone else's) throat if epiglottitis is suspected. Pressing on the tongue to view the throat can cause a throat spasm and block the windpipe.

TREATMENTS

Immediate treatment is essential to prevent the infection from suffocating the patient or spreading to the brain, lungs and other areas. Epiglottitis must be treated in the hospital. The first priority is to improve breathing. A mist of oxygen delivered through a facemask can often help with breathing, but if this is not sufficient, it may be necessary to insert a breathing tube through the nose or mouth.
 • TRACHEOSTOMY If the throat is too swollen to accommodate a breathing tube, doctors will do a tracheostomy, a surgical procedure that places a breathing tube through an incision in the neck. Antibiotics are given to fight the infection and corticosteroids may be used to decrease the swelling in the windpipe. If treated promptly, epiglottitis can usually be cured.

See also: *Immunization, pp.314–15* • *HIV/AIDS, pp.316–17*

See also: Immunization, pp.314–15 • HIV/AIDS, pp.316–17

WHO IS AT RISK?
The risk factors include:
- Children ages 2 to 6
- Exposure to someone with epiglottitis or another upper respiratory infection
- Suppressed immune system from illnesses such as cancer and HIV, or because of immune-suppressive medication

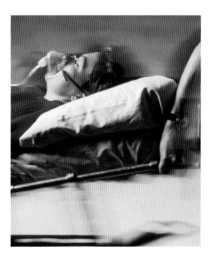

Inflammation of the epiglottis is a medical emergency requiring immediate attention. Supplemental oxygen may be used to prevent suffocation.

Hearing Loss

Hearing loss is a decreased ability to detect and identify sounds. The loss can affect one or both ears, and it can be partial or total. There are two basic types of hearing loss: conductive, in which sound waves are blocked from travelling through the ear; and sensorineural, in which the nerves or sensory cells in the ear are destroyed. Sensorineural hearing loss is by far the most common type, and it is permanent, whereas conductive hearing loss is often reversible. Both types of hearing loss are preventable in some cases and often can be improved with hearing aids and other treatments.

CAUSES

• **AGEING** By far the leading cause of hearing loss is the normal ageing process. Age-related hearing loss, called presbycusis, is a form of sensorineural hearing loss. It occurs because hair cells, the tiny hair-like sensory cells in the inner ear, die off over time and are not replaced.

• **LOUD NOISE** Regular exposure to loud noise over a period of many years causes sensorineural hearing loss by damaging hair cells. Sounds louder than 80 decibels have the potential to cause hearing loss. They include rock concert music, sirens, jackhammers, electric drills and lawnmowers.

• **EAR WAX** This is a normal secretion in the outer part of the ear, but if too much of it accumulates or if it gets pushed too deeply into the ear canal, it can cause conductive hearing loss.

• **INJURIES** Accidents and traumas that damage structures of the ear can cause conductive and sensorineural hearing loss. These include serious injuries such as skull fractures and concussions, and less serious events such as eardrums torn by cotton swabs and ruptures of the inner ear caused by changes in air pressure while flying in an airplane. Hearing loss caused by injuries may be temporary if the injuries heal on their own or can be surgically repaired.

• **INFECTIONS** Infections of the ear (pp.52–4) can lead to conductive hearing loss by causing either fluid or swelling within the ear that obstructs sound waves. They include middle ear and external ear infections, and labrynthitis (pp.72–3). Meningitis (p.180), a brain infection, can cause sensorineural hearing loss.

• **MENIÈRE'S DISEASE** With this condition (pp.72–3), there is a build-up of fluid in the inner ear that causes intermittent hearing loss, as well as dizziness and ringing in the ears.

• **MEDICATION** Hearing loss can be a side-effect of several common medications, including high doses of aspirin, certain antibiotics and cisplatin for cancer.

• **GENES** Several genes can predispose a person to hearing loss by affecting the development of the ears and the function of the sensory hair cells.

• **BIRTH DEFECTS** Babies can be born with impaired hearing for a variety of reasons, including pregnancy complications, intrauterine infections and premature birth.

• **OTOSCLEROSIS** This is excess bone growth in the inner ear. It is among the most common causes of conductive hearing loss.

• **TUMOURS** Benign or malignant tumours of the ear or brain can affect hearing.

• AUTOIMMUNE DISEASES Auto-immune diseases, in which the immune system attacks the body, can cause hearing loss if the attack affects the ears. Autoimmune diseases that can affect hearing include lupus (pp.324–5) and multiple sclerosis (pp.182–3).

PREVENTION

The most important way to prevent hearing loss is to protect the ears from loud noises. When using noisy equipment, use earplugs or guards to muffle the sound. When listening to music, turn the volume down. MP3 players pose a special risk because they can play hundreds of hours of music without pause. Duration determines the damage to hearing caused by high volume, and

On Call

Cumulative exposure to noises louder than 80 decibels is a major cause of permanent hearing loss. Here are the decibel levels of some common sounds.

150 Decibels: Rock music at its loudest

140 Decibels: Firearms, air raid sirens

130 Decibels: Jackhammer

120 Decibels: Jet plane taking off, amplified rock music 1.2–1.8 m (4–6 ft) away

106 Decibels: Drum roll

100 Decibels: Snowmobile, pneumatic drill, chain saw

90 Decibels: Lawnmower, shop tools, truck traffic, underground train

80 Decibels: Alarm clock, busy street.

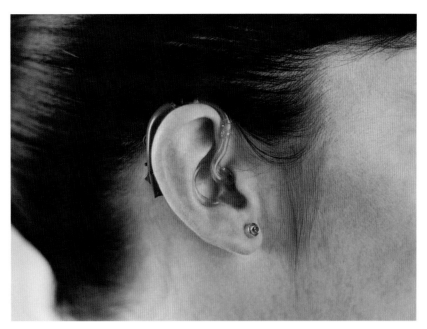

Hearing aids are battery-operated devices that amplify sound and are the main treatment for sensorineural hearing loss. Many new hearing aids are programmable, allowing the wearer to choose different settings for a variety of sound environments.

continuous listening, even at a seemingly reasonable level, can damage the delicate hair cells in the inner ear that transmit sound impulses to the brain. A five-minute rest period for every hour of listening is recommended.

DIAGNOSIS

The first step is to have a medical examination by a doctor who specializes in hearing disorders. By asking questions about symptoms, taking a health history, and examining the ears and ear canals, the doctor can diagnose problems of the ear. The next step is hearing tests to determine how severe the hearing loss is and which sound frequencies are most affected. In these tests, the patient listens to a range of sounds and indicates which ones they hear. Some hearing tests are conducted by doctors, others by audiologists (medical professionals who are trained to administer hearing tests).

The medical examination and hearing tests will determine whether the hearing loss is conductive, sensorineural, or both. It will also identify which kinds of sounds the patient has the most trouble hearing. It is not unusual to have moderate or severe hearing loss in the high frequency range and nearly normal hearing in the low frequency range.

TREATMENTS

Treatment depends on the type and extent of the hearing loss. Depending on the underlying cause, the goal of treatment may be to restore hearing or to use devices that make it easier to hear.

• HEARING AIDS These devices are the main treatment for sensorineural hearing loss. They amplify incoming sounds. Hearing aids come in many styles. Some rest on the outer ear with a section that fits partially in the ear canal, and others

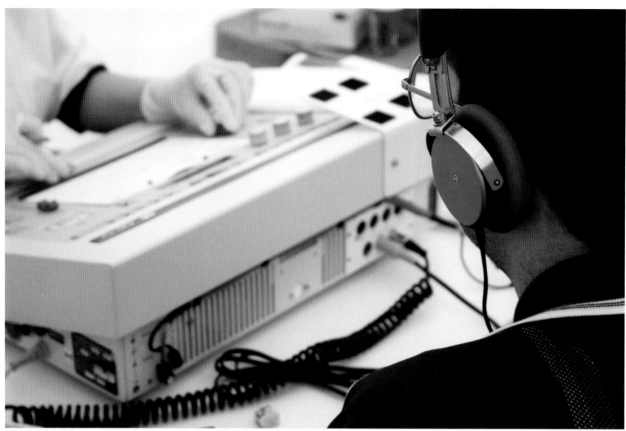

A hearing test can be used to measure the severity of hearing loss and help determine which treatments to use. Doctors will often use this type of test to determine if a more detailed test, such as an MRI, should be used to more precisely diagnose the nature of hearing loss.

fit completely inside the ear. Older hearing aids are large devices that are visible either inside or behind the ear, but more smaller, modern models are often difficult to see.

There are different options for circuitry that amplify different types or ranges of sounds, as well. Analogue hearing aids use the oldest type of circuitry, and amplify all sounds in a particular frequency range. Programmable hearing aids also have analog circuitry but can be programmed to boost some sounds more than others. For example, there could be one setting for a noisy restaurant, where the patient wants to hear conversation at the table but not background noise, and another setting for home, where they want to amplify a greater vari-

ety of sounds. Digital hearing aids are the newest technology. Their programming can be fine-tuned to a greater degree than analogue programmable hearing aids.

• SURGERY Several surgical procedures are used to treat for hearing loss. The simplest of them is surgery to drain fluid from the middle ear, if that is the cause. There are also various procedures to repair structural abnormalities within the ear.

• COCHLEAR IMPLANTS For people with sensorineural hearing loss that is too severe to be helped by hearing aids, devices can be implanted in the inner ear to increase residual hearing. The most widely used is the cochlear implant. It improves hearing by

sending electrical signals directly to the auditory nerve, which connects the ear to the brain.

• MEDICATION Antibiotics may be needed to cure middle ear or outer ear infections, as well as to help drain fluid in the middle ear.

• REDUCING EAR WAX If there is excess wax build-up in one or both ears, clear some of it away by putting baby oil, mineral oil, hydrogen peroxide or a commercial ear wax softener into the ear with a medicine dropper. These substances loosen ear wax to help it drain out. If it is not possible to get rid of the ear wax in this way, a doctor can help.

See also: *Ear Infections, pp.52–4* • *Meningitis, p.180* • *Menière's Disease, pp.72–3*

Laryngitis

This inflammation of the larynx, or voice box, causes hoarseness or temporary loss of the voice, throat pain, and sometimes fever. Vibration of the vocal cords, (two folds of tissue within the larynx) creates the sound of the voice. But the inflammation of laryngitis constricts the vocal cords, preventing them from vibrating properly when speaking.

Laryngitis is especially common during or after a cold, or if the voice has been over-used. It is usually a minor illness that goes away on its own in a few days with self-care.

CAUSES

Largynitis can be caused by an infection or an irritation. The most common cause is the same kind of viral infection that causes colds. Other causes of laryngitis are bacterial infections, respiratory allergies, smoking, inhaling irritating chemicals, overuse of the voice (such as shouting, giving speeches or singing for an extended period of time) and, for some people, drinking alcohol. Using inhalers to treat asthma may also cause laryngitis.

PREVENTION

There are several ways to reduce the risk of laryngitis. First of all, take precautions against upper respiratory infections by washing hands after being in public places, and avoid close contact with people who have colds. In addition, do not smoke and limit exposure to secondhand smoke.

Cut back on alcohol consumption if it is found that it leads to laryngitis. Finally, try not to strain the voice. If speaking or singing for long periods is unavoidable, rest the voice by not speaking. A vocal coach can also teach techniques that will enable people to use their voices in this way without straining them.

DIAGNOSIS

Laryngitis can usually be diagnosed based on the characteristic hoarseness or loss of voice, and a physical examination of the throat. If it lasts longer than a few days or is accompanied by other symptoms, see a doctor, because several other more serious conditions can cause hoarseness. These include tonsillitis (p.61), croup (mainly in children, p.64), vocal cord nodules and polyps (p.76) and throat cancer (p.74).

TREATMENTS

Laryngitis treatments focus mainly on reducing the inflammation of the larynx. Drink six or more glasses of water or tea a day, apply a warm compress to the throat and use a humidifier when you

sleep. In addition, rest the vocal cords by speaking softly and only when necessary. Avoid exposure to smoke and other substances that can irritate the larynx. Antibiotics are appropriate only if the cause is a bacterial infection.

See also: *Tonsillitis, p.61 • Throat Cancer, p.74 • Vocal Cord Nodules & Polyps, p.77*

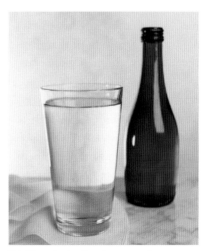

Drinking plenty of water can reduce inflammation of the larynx and help keep throat mucus thin and easy to clear.

Nosebleeds

Occasional bleeding from inside a nostril is common. Blood may appear in a small trickle or in a heavy flow that lasts 15 minutes or longer. A nosebleed may be an isolated event or it may recur. Some people are especially prone to nosebleeds, such as people with a deviated septum (p.71), a deformity of the cartilage between the nostrils. Nosebleeds are usually harmless and are easily stopped, but frequent, heavy nosebleeds warrant a trip to the doctor.

CAUSES

Nosebleeds are especially common during the winter because two of the main causes are dry air and colds. Indoor air, made extremely dry by heating systems, can cause the nasal membranes to dry out, increasing the risk that their fragile blood vessels will break. Colds cause inflammation of the nasal passages, which can also damage the blood vessels. Blowing the nose frequently and hard also causes nosebleeds.

Other causes of nosebleeds are respiratory allergies, trauma to the nose, inhaling irritating chemicals and taking medications that thin the blood. In children, nose picking and foreign objects in the nose often lead to nosebleeds. In rare cases, frequent nosebleeds are a sign of an underlying illness, such as high blood pressure, a problem with blood-clotting or an abnormal growth in the nose.

PREVENTION

Increasing the humidity of the indoor air in the winter with either a central air humidifier or a room humidifier. To moisten the nasal passages, place a small dab of petroleum jelly inside each nostril once a day or use saline nose drops. Take precautions against getting colds, such as washing hands frequently, and blowing noses gently.

DIAGNOSIS

In most cases, a formal diagnosis is unnecessary because the symptoms are obvious and the condition is minor and short-lived. In the case of frequent or severe nosebleeds, visit a doctor to find out the underlying cause.

TREATMENTS

Most nosebleeds can be stopped at home with simple treatments.
• HOME REMEDIES Cover the nose with a tissue while pinching the end of the nose with the fingers and tilting the head forward. Do this for at least five minutes before checking to see if the bleeding has stopped. Applying a cold compress to the bridge of the nose may help stop the bleeding even faster.

WHO IS AT RISK?

The risk factors include:
- Deviated septum
- Colds
- Respiratory allergy
- Dry air
- Trauma to the nose
- Blowing the nose too hard
- Foreign body in the nose
- Nose picking
- Irritating chemicals in the air
- Medication that thins the blood, such as coumadin and nonsteroidal anti-inflammatory agents
- High blood pressure
- Clotting disorders
- Abnormal growths in the nose
- Hereditary haemorrhagic telangiectagia (HHT; also called Osler–Weber–Rendu syndrome)

• MEDICAL TREATMENTS Recurrent or severe nosebleeds may require medical treatment. The doctor may cauterize a weakened blood vessel with heat or silver nitrate to seal it. Other treatments include packing the nostril or nostrils with gauze to stop the bleeding, reducing or eliminating the use of blood-thinning medications, and controlling conditions such as high blood pressure that may be causing recurrent nosebleeds.

See also: *Deviated Septum, p.71* • *High Blood Pressure, pp.236–9* • *Hay Fever, pp.50–1*

Deviated Septum

This is a pronounced curve of the septum, which is the bone and cartilage that separates the nostrils. The septum should run straight down the centre of the nose; the nostrils are then equal in size and able to accommodate the same amount of airflow. In most people, the septum is a little bit off-centre, but the asymmetry is so slight that it is not visible and does not cause any problems.

In a person with a deviated septum, the septum is so crooked that one nostril is noticeably larger than the other. As a result, airflow through one nostril may be partially blocked, causing chronic congestion.

CAUSES

A deviated septum can be caused by a broken nose or other injury to the nose. Some people are born with a deviated septum because of trauma to the nose during birth or for unknown reasons.

PREVENTION

Prevent deviated septum by protecting yourself from facial injuries. This includes wearing seatbelts when travelling in a car and appropriate headgear when playing contact sports.

DIAGNOSIS

A deviated septum is diagnosed by a physical examination of the nose. Symptoms can include facial pain, headaches and post-nasal drip. The airflow blockage may interfere with sinus drainage,

setting the stage for recurrent sinus infections (pp.58–60). A deviated septum also increases the risk of recurrent nosebleeds, because the abnormal airflow in the nose can cause the septum to become dry and cracked. The symptoms are usually worse on one side, and sometimes actually occur on the side opposite the bend.

TREATMENTS

Correction of the deviation is not needed if a deviated septum does not cause symptoms.

WHO IS AT RISK?

The risk factors include:
- Severe injury to the nose
- Trauma during birth

• SURGERY A deviated septum can be corrected with surgery called septoplasty, in which the septum is straightened by removing any excess cartilage on the curved side. This surgery can be done in an outpatient facility. It is performed entirely through the nostrils, so there is no bruising or external evidence of the procedure. A child with a deviated septum must wait to have the surgery until they become a teenager and their nose has finished growing.

See also: *Sinusitis, pp.58–60 • Headaches, pp.166–7*

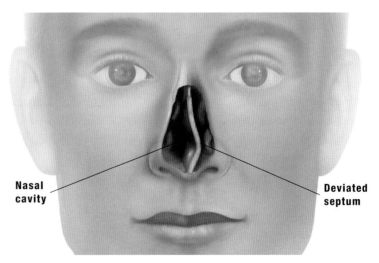

Nasal cavity · Deviated septum

Severe cases of deviated septum can disrupt airflow through the nose, causing difficulty breathing and chronic sinusitis.

TINNITUS

This is a persistent noise in the ears that has no external cause. Although this noise is more commonly known as ringing in the ears, the term is somewhat misleading because the sound is not always a ring; it can also be a buzz, a whistle or some other type of noise. Nearly everyone has had tinnitus for a few seconds or minutes after hearing an extremely loud noise, such as a siren or a jackhammer, or after attending a loud rock concert.

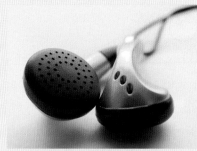

Protect your ears from loud noises and keep the volume at a moderate level when listening to headphones.

Tinnitus is also a symptom of ear disorders such as Menière's disease, which is caused by fluid imbalance in the inner ear, and labyrinthitis, an inflammation of the inner ear. Tinnitus often goes away on its own, but it can be recurrent.

CAUSES

The main cause of tinnitus is nerve damage in the inner ear, usually from exposure to loud noise. Tinnitus can also be a symptom of a wide range of medical conditions, including excess ear wax, perforated eardrum, respiratory allergies (pp.50–1), sinus infections (pp.58–60), high or low blood pressure (pp.236–9), diabetes (pp.338–41), cardiovascular disease (pp.234–5) head or neck injuries, and brain tumours (p.196). It can be a side-effect of several medications, including aminoglycoside antibiotics, quinidine for irregular heartbeat, cicplatin for cancer, and aspirin. It is more common in people over 55.

Menière's Disease

This disorder is characterized by episodes of tinnitus, vertigo, hearing loss and nausea. The symptoms occur when the labyrinth (the network of fluid-filled channels in the inner ear that regulate balance) fills up with so much fluid that the surrounding membranes rupture and damage nearby sensory cells. The cause of this fluid build-up is unknown, but it may be influenced by several factors, including respiratory or middle ear infections, head injuries and heavy alcohol use. Menière's disease is most common in women. The pattern and severity of the symptoms varies considerably, with some people having attacks every few hours and other people having them every few years. Menière's disease usually affects just one ear.

Labyrinthitis

This condition is caused by an inflammation of the labyrinth in the inner ear caused by an infection, usually viral. The infection may originate in the middle ear and then spread to the labyrinth. Other sources of infection include bacterial meningitis, influenza, measles, herpes and hepatitis. Symptoms include tinnitus, hearing loss, vertigo, nausea and vomiting.

PREVENTION

The most effective way to avoid ringing in the ears is to protect the ears from loud noises. Wear protective earplugs or guards when operating loud machinery. Keep music at a moderate volume, especially when wearing head-phones. In addition, guard against head injuries by wearing seatbelts when in cars and using protective headgear for sports such as cycling, skiing and hockey. Getting prompt treatment for ear infections and upper respiratory infections can reduce the risk of labyrinthitis. Other measures that may reduce the occurrence of tinnitus include controlling respiratory allergies, avoiding smoking, taking precautions against cardiovascular disease by exercising regularly and eating a healthy diet, and reducing intake of salt, alcohol and caffeine.

DIAGNOSIS

A doctor will ask about symptoms and medical history and examine the ears to diagnose causes such as ear wax build-up or an ear infection. Further examination by an otolaryngolotist (a doctor who specializes in ear disorders) and hearing tests by an audiologist may be needed to diagnose other disorders. Other tests, such as a head MRI or CT and angiography, may be done to detect structural abnormalities or blockages in blood vessels.

TREATMENTS

The treatment depends on the cause. Medical treatment is often needed when the cause is an ear disorder. There is no cure for Menière's disease, but some treatments can relieve the symptoms.

• **REMOVING EAR WAX** This can be done at home with mineral oil, hydrogen peroxide, or store-bought ear wax removal preparations.

• **TINNITUS MASKERS AND HEARING AIDS** Tinnitus maskers fit into the ear like hearing aids and generate a low, pleasing sound that masks the bothersome noise inside the head. When tinnitus is related to

hearing loss, a hearing aid may help by amplifying incoming sounds so that they drown out the inner sounds.

• **PRESSURE TREATMENT** Portable devices that increase pressure in the ear can ease symptoms of Menière's disease.

• **SURGERY** When Menière's disease is the cause of tinnitus and the symptoms cannot be controlled by other treatments, surgery may be recommended. One surgical procedure entails creating a drainage hole in the inner ear to eliminate excess fluid. Another involves cutting the vestibular nerve, which helps control balance. Because Menière's disease affects just one ear, this forces the balance apparatus in the other ear (which is usually unimpaired), to take over. Although surgery is effective, it can cause deafness.

• **MEDICATION** Antibiotics can cure labyrinthitis and other bacterial infections. Topical antibiotics in the

ear have also been found to relieve Menière's disease. Antihistamines can control respiratory allergies. Antihistamines and diuretics can relieve Menière's disease by reducing the amount of fluid in the inner ear. Ringing in the ears can also cause depression (pp.364–5) and insomnia (pp.170–1). There are many treatment options for these conditions, including cognitive-behavioural therapy, antidepressants, dietary modification and meditation.

• **PHYSICAL THERAPY** Because the symptoms of Menière's disease can intensify when the body is in certain positions, physical therapy can help by teaching you ways to make these positions less uncomfortable.

• **TINNITUS RETRAINING THERAPY** This therapy aims to help people get so accustomed to the sounds of their tinnitus that they stop noticing them. This is accomplished with counselling and the use of a device that generates background sound, such as a tinnitus masker, for at least eight hours a day. Tinnitus retraining therapy can take 12 to 24 months before the in-the-ear device is no longer needed.

• **RELAXATION TECHNIQUES** Stress can intensify tinnitus, and biofeedback (pp.504–7) and other relaxation techniques may ease the symptoms. Hypnosis (pp.508–13) is also sometimes used for tinnitus.

• **COUNSELLING** This can help control depression associated with recurrent tinnitus. Support groups for people with tinnitus give techniques to help them cope with the symptoms and reduce stress.

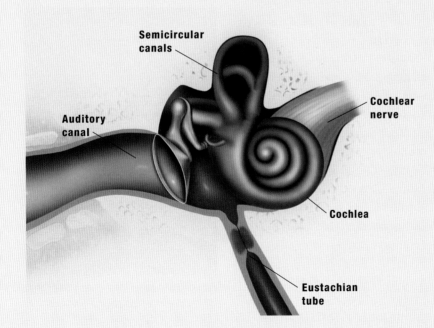

Semicircular canals

Auditory canal

Cochlear nerve

Cochlea

Eustachian tube

The semicircular canals are a fluid-filled labyrinth of channels in the inner ear that regulate balance. Tinnitus can be caused by conditions that damage or inflame these structures.

See also: *Hay Fever, pp.50–1 • Sinusitis, pp.58–60 • Hypnotherapy, pp.508–511*

Throat Cancer

Any malignant tumour of the larynx, vocal cords or other areas of the throat is throat cancer. Symptoms include a sore throat that lasts longer than two weeks despite antibiotic treatment, a persistent cough, hoarseness, pain in the neck or ears, and difficulty swallowing. It is most common in men age 50 and older, especially if they smoke or used to smoke. Throat cancer is curable if it is detected early.

CAUSES

Most people with throat cancer are current or former smokers. Heavy alcohol intake is another major risk factor, especially for people who smoke, because alcohol increases the cancer-causing effects of tobacco. Other risk factors are occupational exposure to asbestos or smoke, human papilloma virus infection and gastroesophogeal reflux disease (pp.264–5).

PREVENTION

Dramatically reduce the risk of throat cancer by not smoking and not drinking alcoholic beverages in excess. There is some evidence that taking adequate amounts of vitamin A and beta-carotene may also help prevent the disease.

DIAGNOSIS

A doctor can diagnose throat cancer by examining the throat using imaging tests such as a CT scan and an MRI to detect abnormal growths. A biopsy is taken of unusual tissue for laboratory analysis. If cancer is found, further tests are done to determine its particular stage and grade. (The stage is

how widespread the cancer is and whether it has invaded any lymph nodes. The grade identifies the characteristics of the cancer, such as how quickly it is growing.)

TREATMENTS

Treatment depends on the stage and grade of the cancer. The prospects for recovery also depend on these factors, as well as overall health and whether the cancer has recurred. Continuing to smoke and drink alcohol reduces the odds of recovery.

• **RADIATION** Radiation therapy to kill cancer cells can be delivered using an external beam aimed at the throat or by implanting radio-active substances into the tumour.

• **SURGERY** Laser surgery may be used to excise small tumours. When cancer has spread to the larynx or beyond, surgery may be done to remove the vocal cords, part or all of the larynx, and part or all of the thyroid. Artificial vocal cords may be implanted to make speech possible. If the cancer has invaded any lymph nodes, they may be surgically removed as well. If the vocal cords have been removed, speech

therapy can help teach alternative methods of speaking.

• **CHEMOTHERAPY** Medication to kill cancer cells is often given in addition to surgery to reduce the risk of recurrence.

WHO IS AT RISK?

The risk factors include:

• Current or former smoker (this dramatically increases the odds)
• Heavy drinking
• Ages 50 and older
• Occupational exposure to asbestos or smoke
• Human papilloma virus infection
• Gastroesophogeal reflux disease

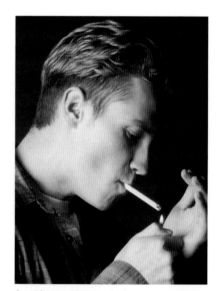

Smoking and heavy alcohol consumption greatly increase the risk of throat cancer.

See also: *Gastroesophageal Reflux Disease, pp.264–5 • Smoking Cessation, pp.216–17*

Sinus Cancer

This malignancy, also called paranasal sinus cancer, affects either the sinuses (the cavities inside and around the nose) or the nasal cavity (the airway behind the nose leading to the throat). Symptoms include congestion, frequent nosebleeds, a lump inside the nose, frequent headaches or sinus pain, pain in the teeth and a bulging eye. It is important to see a doctor if there are any of these symptoms, because the earlier the cancer is diagnosed and treated, the greater the chance of recovery.

WHO IS AT RISK?

The risk factors include:

- Smoking
- Occupational exposure to smoke, metals and chemicals
- Chronic sinusitis

CAUSES

The cause of sinus cancer is not known, but smoking and exposure to certain pollutants increase the risk of developing the disease. Sinus cancer is most common among people with jobs that expose them to dust from wood, textiles and leather, as well as mustard gas, isopropyl oils, volatile hydrocarbons, and metals such as nickel and chromium. Exposure occurs most commonly in the textile production, leather tanning, nickel mining and carpentry industries. Having chronic sinusitis may also increase the odds of developing sinus cancer. Smoking is a risk factor for the most common form of sinus cancer (squamous cell carcinoma), although the role of tobacco in other types of sinus cancer is less clear.

PREVENTION

Quit smoking. In addition, minimizing exposure to secondhand smoke and other pollutants that have been associated with sinus cancer may help prevent the disease.

DIAGNOSIS

A doctor diagnoses sinus cancer based on the symptoms and several medical tests. A CT scan or an MRI of the head can reveal abnormal growths inside the nose. An imaging instrument called a rhinoscope or nasoscope may be placed inside the nose to detect growths. The doctor will take a biopsy of any abnormal growth and have it analysed in a laboratory for the presence of cancer cells. If cancer is found, further testing will be done to determine the stage of the cancer (that is, whether it has spread within or beyond the sinuses or the nasal cavity).

TREATMENTS

Sinus cancer treatment depends on its stage and location.
- **SURGERY** For most stages of sinus cancer, surgery is done to remove the cancerous tissue, along with a margin of healthy tissue. Because the sinuses are so close to the eyes, mouth and throat, these areas may be affected as well. Depending on where and how extensive the cancer is, surgery may involve the removal of portions of nasal tissue and bone, as well as the eye. If the cancer has spread to the lymph nodes in the neck, they must also be surgically removed. Plastic surgery afterwards can help to restore the appearance of the face.
- **RADIATION** Radiation therapy to kill cancer cells can be delivered using an external beam aimed at the site of the cancer or by injecting radioactive substances into the tumor. Radiation therapy is sometimes used before surgery to shrink the tumour and reduce the likelihood of having to remove healthy bone and tissue. It may also be given after surgery to destroy any cancer cells that may still remain.
- **CHEMOTHERAPY** Medication designed to kill cancer cells is often given orally or by injection in addition to surgery, radiation, or both, for maximum effectiveness.

See also: *Smoking Cessation, pp.216–17*

Nasal Polyps

Nasal polyps are small single or clustered growths that start in the sinus cavities and descend into the nostrils. They can cause congestion and runny nose, interfere with the sense of smell and lead to recurrent sinus infections. Sometimes, they appear during a cold, and go away or shrink once the infection ends. Polyps are most common in people with chronic respiratory conditions such as nasal allergies, asthma and cystic fibrosis. A significant number of people with nasal polyps are allergic to aspirin.

WHO IS AT RISK?

The risk factors include:

- Respiratory allergies
- Asthma
- Cystic fibrosis
- Colds and other upper respiratory infections
- Family history
- Low levels of antioxidants

CAUSES

Nasal polyps form as a result of chronic inflammation of the mucus membrane lining the nose. The polyps themselves are composed of inflamed tissue. Cystic fibrosis is a major cause of nasal polyps, but any chronic condition that causes nasal inflammation also increases the risk of polyps. The tendency to develop polyps runs in families, suggesting that genes may play a role.

A preliminary study of 58 patients published in the July 2004 issue of *Laryngoscope* found that people with nasal polyps had lower levels of certain antioxidant nutrients (vitamins A, E and C, and beta-carotene) than a control group. This finding suggests that free-radical damage may be a cause of nasal polyps.

PREVENTION

Using decongestants and anti-his-tamines for either a cold or a respiratory allergy can help prevent nasal polyps by reducing nasal in-

flammation. Increasing the intake of antioxidants, either in foods such as fruit and vegetables, or in supplements (pp.532–41), may help prevent nasal polyps by combating destructive free radicals.

DIAGNOSIS

A doctor can diagnose nasal polyps by looking inside the nostrils. A biopsy may be taken and sent to a laboratory to check for signs of cancer. Nasal polyps can be either benign or cancerous, but cancerous nasal polyps are very rare. Having benign nasal polyps does not increase the risk of developing nasal cancer.

TREATMENTS

• **MEDICATION** The first line of treatment is corticosteroid medication to shrink the polyps. Corticosteroids can be given in a nasal spray, oral preparations or injections.

• **SURGERY** If corticosteroids do not reduce polyps enough to relieve the symptoms, or if the polyps disappear and then recur,

they can be surgically removed. This is usually done with an endoscope, an instrument that is inserted through the nostrils. Surgery usually relieves the symptoms, but polyps may grow back unless the underlying condition that causes chronic inflammation of the nasal cavity is controlled.

A 2003 study of 170 patients at the University of Siena Medical School in Italy found furosemide (a drug that decreases the reabsorption of sodium and chloride in the respiratory epithelial cells) nasal spray to be effective at preventing relapses of nasal polyps after surgery. After one month of taking the medication, only 17.5 percent of the patients treated with furosemide experienced a recurrence, as compared to 24 percent who were treated with mometasone (a corticosteroid), and 30 percent who received no follow-up treatment.

See also: *Hay Fever, pp.50–1* • *Asthma, pp.206–9* • *Cystic Fibrosis, p.218*

Vocal Cord Nodules and Polyps

These benign growths cause changes in the voice, such as hoarseness, cracking, lower pitch, difficulty or inability to reach high notes, and the frequent need to clear the throat. Nodules are callous-like lesions that form on both sides of the vocal cords. Polyps are fluid-filled lesions that usually appear on just one side of the vocal cords.

Nodules and polyps are most common among singers and other people who often need to project their voices for extended periods.

CAUSES
Irritation of the vocal cords causes nodules and polyps to develop. The irritation can come from voice strain, respiratory allergies, smoking, inhaling polluted air or fumes, and drinking alcohol or caffeinated beverages (which can dry out the vocal cords). The backflow of stomach acid into the throat, as occurs with gastroesophogeal reflux disease (pp.264–5), can also cause nodules or polyps.

PREVENTION
Reducing voice strain and eliminating sources of airborne chemical irritation (such as tobacco smoke) are the best ways to avoid nodules and polyps. Speak softly when possible and, when using the voice a lot, rest it afterwards. Drink water regularly, because when the throat is dry, it is more susceptible to strain than when it is moist. Avoid excess consumption of alcohol and caffeine.

DIAGNOSIS
An ear, nose and throat specialist can see vocal cord nodules and polyps by looking down the throat.

TREATMENTS
Nodules are treated differently from polyps, and the treatments used depend on the severity of the symptoms and on the requirements of the individual. A singer, for example, may need more intensive therapy than someone who does not rely so heavily on their voice.
- RESTING THE VOICE The most basic treatment for nodules is to use the voice as little as possible. This alone can often make nodules shrink. Resting the voice does not reduce existing polyps, but it may help prevent new ones from forming.
- SPEECH THERAPY A speech and language pathologist can teach a variety of techniques to minimize straining the vocal cords such as modulating the pitch of the voice. The goal is to improve voice quality, help shrink nodules, and prevent new nodules and polyps from growing.

Speech therapy techniques include modulating the pitch of the voice, doing exercises to improve voice production, and practising 'vocal hygiene' to keep the vocal cords healthy. Vocal hygiene strategies include avoiding smoking and other irritating substances in the air, drinking water throughout the day, and reducing the habit of clearing the throat, which strains the vocal cords.
- OTHER TREATMENTS If nodules and polyps are the result of acid reflux or respiratory allergies, controlling these underlying medical problems may improve voice quality.
- SURGERY If the previous measures do not lead to enough of an improvement in the voice, surgery may be needed to remove nodules. Surgery is the only way to eliminate polyps.

See also: *Gastroesophageal Reflux Disease, pp.264–5 • Smoking Cessation, pp.216–17 • Hay Fever, pp.50–51*

WHO IS AT RISK?
The risk factors include:
- Voice strain
- Smoking
- Regular exposure to airborne chemical irritants
- Respiratory allergies
- Gastroesophogeal reflux disease
- Excess consumption of alcohol and caffeine

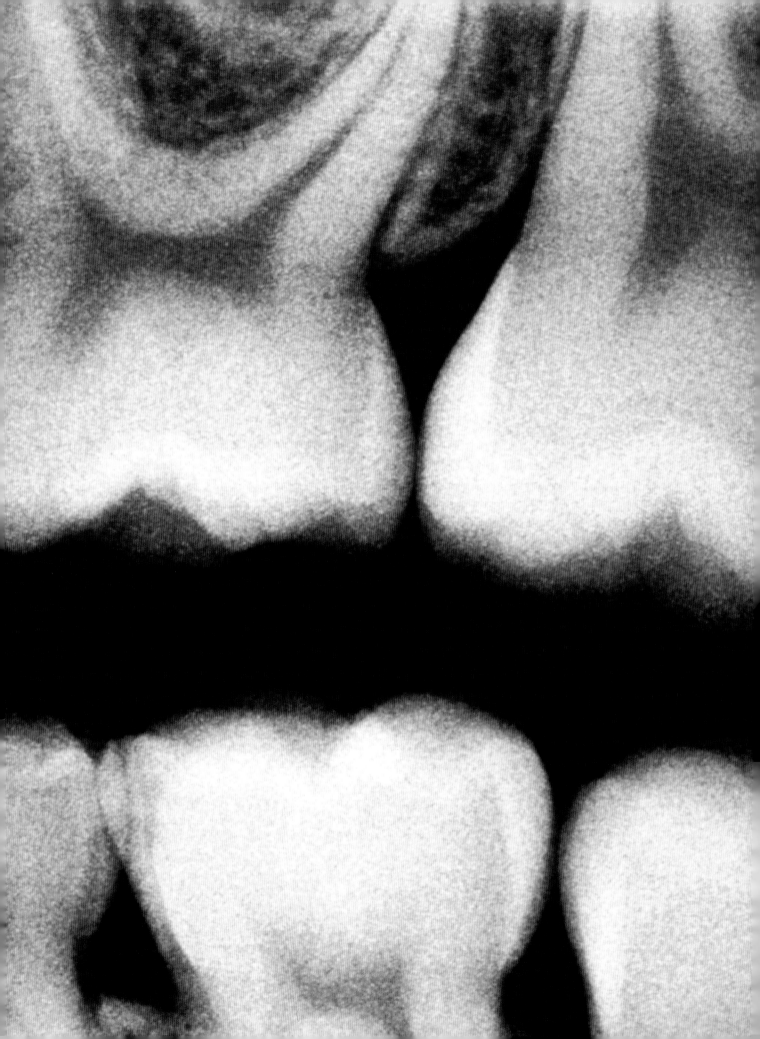

3 | MOUTH & TEETH

An unhealthy mouth and teeth can take a serious toll on our overall health. But for many of the conditions that affect the mouth, prevention is the key. Good hygiene and regular dental check-ups can go a long way to maintaining a healthy mouth and avoiding the need for medical attention.

Certain oral disorders, however, do require the attention of a specialist. Mouth cancer, for example – although it is highly preventable – spreads rapidly and is often fatal, so early detection and treatment are crucial. Other conditions, such as cold sores that are caused by viruses, are more difficult to prevent, but easier to treat.

A dentist can advise on care and prevention of most oral health issues. Brushing and flossing daily and avoiding smoking can help prevent common disorders such as gingivitis, cavities and halitosis. But more serious conditions such as temporomandibular joint disorders may require medical attention.

Gingivitis & Periodontitis

Gum disease, an inflammation and infection of the tissue that supports the teeth, occurs in two stages: gingivitis and periodontitis. Gingivitis, the earliest stage, affects only gum tissue – the gingiva. The gums become red and swollen, and bleed easily when the teeth are brushed. Gingivitis is reversible with treatment and good oral hygiene.

Periodontitis occurs if gingivitis is untreated or inadequately treated. It is an infection and inflammation of the ligaments that hold the teeth to the jawbone, as well as the jawbone itself. The infections cause the gums to pull away from the teeth, eventually causing the teeth to loosen. Periodontitis is the leading cause of tooth loss.

CAUSES

The main cause of both gingivitis and periodontitis is the accumulation of plaque (a sticky substance made of bacteria, saliva and bits of food) on the teeth. Plaque that is not removed by brushing and flossing turns into a hard material called tartar, which becomes trapped between the gums and the teeth, forming pockets. Bacteria in the tartar and plaque, as well as toxins the bacteria produce, irritate and infect the gums, causing gingivitis. If the tartar and plaque are not removed, they create deeper and deeper pockets beneath the gums, causing the gums to pull away from the teeth, and infecting the ligaments and bone around the teeth – this is periodontitis.

Poor dental hygiene greatly increases the risk of developing gingivitis. However, brushing or flossing too hard can promote gingivitis by injuring the gums, which increases their vulnerability to plaque damage. Other causes of gum irritation that can lead to gingivitis are misaligned teeth and ill-fitting dental bridges, crowns and orthodontic appliances.

Hormonal changes during puberty and pregnancy increase the risk of gingivitis by increasing the sensitivity of the gums. Other risk factors include uncontrolled

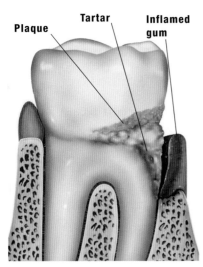

Plaque **Tartar** **Inflamed gum**

Bacteria in plaque and tartar irritates and infects the gums, causing gingivitis, which can cause the gums to recede from the tooth and expose the roots.

WHO IS AT RISK?

The risk factors include:

- Poor oral hygiene
- Smoking or chewing tobacco
- Brushing or flossing so hard that the teeth are damaged
- Poor diet
- Misaligned teeth
- Ill-fitting crowns, bridges, or orthodontic appliances
- Diabetes
- Puberty
- Pregnancy
- Medications such as oral contraceptives and steroids

diabetes, a diet high in sugary and starchy foods, certain medications (such as oral contraceptives and steroids), and smoking or chewing tobacco.

PREVENTION

Good oral hygiene is the most effective way to prevent gingivitis and periodontitis. Brush the teeth twice a day with a soft-bristled toothbrush. Floss at least once a day to remove plaque from between the teeth. In addition, eat a balanced diet and do not smoke or chew tobacco.

Regular dental checkups to professionally clean the teeth help prevent gum disease or treat it before it becomes irreversible. Regular medical checkups can detect health problems such as diabetes (pp.338–41), which can increase the risk of gum disease.

A sufferer from diabetes should make sure it is controlled with diet and, if necessary, medication.

Untreated, periodontal disease may lead to heart disease. A 2003 study by researchers at the University of Aarhus in Denmark found a correlation between the severity of periodontal problems and the incidence of heart disease in patients hospitalized for heart problems in Chile. And another study is currently under way at the University of Indiana in the United States to study the possible link between gingivitis and heart disease.

DIAGNOSIS

A dentist can diagnose gingivitis and periodontitis based on the appearance of the gums. Dental X-rays may be needed to reveal the extent of damage to the jawbone from periodontitis. A dentist may also use a periodontal probe to measure the depth of the pockets of plaque and tarter beneath the gum line. This measurement indicates the extent of the disease and determines whether gum surgery is needed.

TREATMENTS

There are different treatments for gingivitis and periodontitis.

Gingivitis

The condition can often be reversed within a few weeks with regular brushing and flossing to remove plaque. A dental procedure called scaling, in which tartar is scraped away from the teeth and gums, can also help control gingivitis. Dental groups recommend checkups twice a year for scaling, professional cleaning, and examination of the gums and teeth.

• RINSES AND GELS Antibiotic mouthwashes and gels, when used with regular brushing and flossing, control gingivitis better than brushing and flossing alone. Preparations containing various essential oils have also been found to be effective. For example, a gel containing tea tree oil, applied to affected gums, can reduced bleeding and other symptoms of gingivitis.

• DENTAL WORK Orthodontic treatment to straighten teeth may be recommended if misaligned teeth are promoting gingivitis. Replacing poorly fitting crowns or other dental appliances can also help prevent the recurrence of the problem.

Periodontitis

This condition can be stopped with a combination of good oral hygiene and dental treatment. Scaling and professional cleanings may be needed more than twice a year to keep periodontitis from getting worse.

• MEDICATION Dentists prescribe oral or topical antibiotics to treat abscesses (pus-filled infections around teeth that often occur with periodontitis).

• SURGERY Minor surgery is done to clean bacteria-laden plaque and tartar from beneath the gums. Gingevectomy involves removing the soft tissue of the gum that surrounds a pocket of plaque or tartar. If the bone is infected, a surgical procedure cleans and

On Call

It is crucial to get proper treatment at the first sign of gingivitis not only to keep it from developing into periodontitis, but also to prevent other health problems. The bacteria involved in periodontal disease may play a role in heart disease and stroke.

reshapes the bone. Another surgical procedure is done to reconstruct the root of a tooth that has been degraded by gum disease. The damaged root is replaced with a synthetic material bonded to the tooth. Other types of surgery are performed to stabilize loose teeth.

• TOOTH EXTRACTION Teeth that are drastically loosened by periodontitis may have to be pulled.

• TRADITIONAL CHINESE MEDICINE Chinese herbs have been used for hundreds of years to treat periodontal disease, and they effectively inhibit bacterial growth.

• PROPOLIS EXTRACT Irrigating the gums with propolis extract, a sticky brown, resinous substance collected by honeybees from various plants, is a beneficial addition to periodontal treatment.

• HYPERBARIC OXYGEN TREATMENT For severe periodontitis, hyperbaric oxygen treatment (p.579), which uses a high-pressure chamber to increase the oxygen supply to the tissues surrounding the teeth, can increase the effectiveness of conventional therapy such as scaling and root surgery.

See also: *Diabetes, pp.338–41* • *Oxygen Therapy, pp.579* • *Traditional Chinese Medicine, pp.446–50*

MOUTH ULCERS & COLD SORES

Small, painful lesions in and around the mouth can be either mouth ulcers or cold sores. Mouth ulcers, sometimes referred to as aphthous ulcers, are breaks in the mucous membranes. The most common type of mouth ulcer is a canker sore, which can be very uncomfortable but is not serious. Cold sores, also called fever blisters, are small blisters inside the mouth, mainly on the lips, that are caused by infections, including the herpes simplex virus.

A burning or tingling is the first sign that a cold sore is forming. Two days later, a painful blister or cluster of blisters emerges. After several days, the blister breaks and forms a scab. The pain caused by mouth ulcers and cold sores can be relieved with home remedies, as well as topical and oral medications. The lesions usually go away on their own within about two weeks, but if they persist, a doctor or dentist should be consulted.

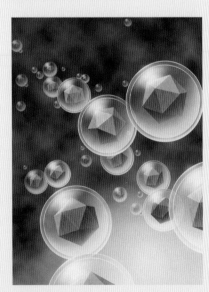

The herpes simplex 1 virus, which causes cold sores, lies dormant in nerve tissue between outbreaks.

CAUSES

Mouth ulcers, also called aphthous ulcers, and cold sores have different causes. Injury to the gums or to the inside of the mouth appears to be the most common cause of mouth ulcers. The injury can come from dental work, a jagged tooth or a dental appliance that rubs against the tongue, lip or the inside of the cheek. It is unknown what else causes mouth ulcers, but several factors are known to be important, including fatigue, stress, allergies, tobacco, depressed immune function and infections. Despite the possible role of infections, however, mouth ulcers are not contagious.

Mouth ulcers are also a common side-effect of chemotherapy and radiation treatments administered to cancer patients.

Though most mouth ulcers are benign lesions, leukoplakia, one type of mouth ulcer, can potentially lead to cancer.

Cold sores are infections caused by the herpes simplex type 1 virus, and they are highly contagious. Cold sores usually

appear around the edge of the lips, but they can also develop on the chin under the nose, and on the fingers. Once a person has had a cold sore, the virus lies dormant in the nerve cells in the skin where it may reemerge as an active infection at times when the immune system is weakened from causes such as stress, injury, sunburn, fever or other infections.

PREVENTION

Good oral hygiene can help reduce the risk of developing mouth ulcers: brush teeth twice a day, floss once a day and have regular dental check-ups. In addition, avoid injury to the mouth by having the dentist file down jagged teeth and replace broken or ill-fitting dental appliances. Not smoking or chewing tobacco and getting a good night's sleep may also reduce the risk of developing mouth ulcers.

To prevent cold sores, avoid kissing people who have cold sores or other direct contact with the sores caused by herpes virus infections, such as during oral sex.

Because stress can promote mouth ulcers and recurrences of cold sores, an important means of prevention is to reduce stress with techniques such as guided imagery (pp.520–2), meditation (pp.514–15) and yoga (pp.476–9).

DIAGNOSIS

A dentist or primary care physician can diagnose mouth ulcers and cold sores based on their appearance and location. If leukoplakia – a special type of mouth ulcer that appears as raised white patches – is suspected, then the dentist may take a biopsy because some of these mouth ulcers are premalignant and can lead to cancer.

TREATMENTS

The main goal of treating mouth ulcers is to relieve the pain. For leukoplakia, close monitoring for signs of cancer is crucial. Treatment of cold sores focuses on relieving the symptoms, preventing the infection from spreading, and shortening the duration of the infection.

Mouth Ulcers

Rinsing the mouth with a solution of salt and soda is effective to relieve pain. Avoiding spicy foods can help reduce mouth irritation.

• PAIN RELIEVERS Various mouth rinses and topical pain relievers applied to mouth ulcers can temporarily reduce the symptoms. Amlexanox paste reduces pain and decreases healing time.

• SUPPLEMENTS A small clinical trial found that oral supplements of lycopene (an antioxidant and also the pigment that gives vegetables and fruits, such as tomatoes and watermelons, their red colour) were more effective than a placebo in treating leukoplakia.

• PROBIOTICS *Lactobacillus*, a beneficial bacterium found in yogurt, may hasten the healing of mouth sores. Make sure to eat yogurt that contains live active cultures. Alternatively, *Lactobacillus* is available in capsule form.

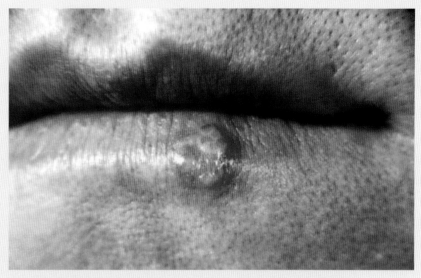

Cold sores, also called fever blisters, are caused by the herpes simplex 1 virus and are highly contagious. They usually appear around the edge of the lips, but they can also develop on the chin, under the nose or on the fingers.

Cold Sores

• MEDICATION Cold sores usually go away on their own within two weeks. Topical or oral antiviral medications can help hasten recovery from the infection, ease the symptoms, and reduce the risk of a recurrence. Topical pain relievers can also decrease the symptoms. To prevent the cold sore from spreading to other areas around the mouth, wash them daily with soap and water.

• TOPICAL CREAMS A small clinical trial showed that a herbal cream made of rhubarb and sage applied to cold sores shortened the duration of the symptoms. Another trial compared a cream made from zinc oxide with a placebo cream in treating cold sores. Cold sores went away faster with the zinc oxide cream than with the placebo. A cream made of mint balm has also been shown to be effective in relieving cold sore symptoms and speeding healing of the lesions.

• LIGHT THERAPY A five-minute treatment of light therapy (p.564), in which a low-powered laser is focused on the infection, will eliminate cold sores in four days, twice as fast as a topical antiviral medication.

• SUPPLEMENTS Taking 1,000 mg a day of lysine, an amino acid, helps reduce the recurrences of cold sores. Lysine supplements should be used only when an active cold sore is present, not as a regular supplement.

See also: *Guided Imagery, pp.520–2 • Meditation, pp.514–19 • Light Therapy, p.564*

CAUTION

See your dentist or doctor if you have had a mouth ulcer or a cold sore for more than two weeks. Such a lesion could be a sign of a serious infection, such as a bacterial infection of the mouth, or a symptom of mouth cancer (p.91).

Temporomandibular Joint Disorders (TMJ)

There are several conditions that cause discomfort and difficulty moving the jaw: myofascial pain, which is pain in the muscles that control jaw movement; dislocation or some other structural abnormality of the joint; and degenerative joint disease. Collectively, these conditions are known as temporomandibular joint disorders (TMJ).

The two temporomandibular joints are located in front of each ear where the jawbone meets the skull. The joints enable the jaw to move up and down, back and forth, rotate and glide as a person speaks, chews and swallows. Soft discs in each joint keep its movement smooth and cushion it from the force of chewing. TMJ occurs when there is a problem with one of the joints or discs, or with the ligaments and muscles that support the joints and guide their movement. Symptoms include aching in the jaw or neck, pain near the ears, clicking or popping noises when the mouth is opened, and headaches. TMJ is most common among women who are of childbearing age, although it is not known why this is.

CAUSES
There has been a lot of controversy about the causes of TMJ. It is known that an injury that fractures or dislocates the jaw, or damages the discs, can cause pain and impair jaw movement.

Most people with TMJ whose jaws make clicking or popping sounds have a displaced disc in one of their temporomandibular joints. In addition, arthritis of a temporomandibular joint can cause the degenerative form of TMJ. Teeth grinding and clenching (p.90) can make the problem worse by putting undue mechanical stress on the jaw muscles.

Stress also plays a role by leading to teeth grinding and clenching. At one time, dentists believed malocclusion (improper alignment)

WHO IS AT RISK?
The risk factors include:

- Female
- Injury to the jaw
- Arthritis of the temporomandibular joint
- Stress

of the upper and lower teeth caused TMJ, but recent research has not supported a connection.

PREVENTION
Protecting the jaw from injury and controlling stress may reduce the risk of developing TMJ. Wear a mouth guard when playing contact sports such as basketball, football or hockey. Explore the many effective strategies for reducing daily stress, including

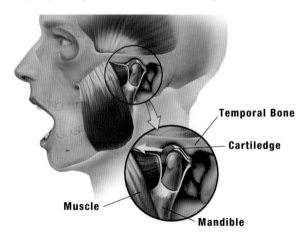

Temporal Bone

Cartiledge

Muscle

Mandible

The temporomandibular joint is the hinge where the lower jaw meets the skull. TMJ pain is usually caused by a disorder of the ligaments, muscles or the soft discs inside each joint.

Clinical Query

Does chewing gum cause TMJ?

There is no scientific evidence that chewing gum causes TMJ. However, if you have TMJ, gum chewing can aggravate the symptoms by putting stress on the temporomandibular joint. A simple and effective way to relieve facial pain is to stop chewing gum until the symptoms disappear completely.

yoga (pp.464–9), exercise, massage (pp.468–73), and meditation (pp.514–19).

DIAGNOSIS

TMJ can be diagnosed by a dentist or a doctor who specializes in facial pain. Although there is no consensus on how to make a diagnosis, it is usually done based on symptoms, a medical and dental history, and a physical examination. The examination involves feeling the jaw and face for painful areas, listening for sounds as the jaw moves, and evaluating the range of motion of the jaw. Dental X-rays are not useful in diagnosing TMJ. However, if arthritis appears to be the cause other imaging tests, such as joint X-rays and MRI, can help with the diagnosis.

TREATMENTS

This is usually a temporary condition that can be relieved with self-care. Treatment focuses on alleviating the pain and other symptoms, and reducing stress on the jaw. Relaxation techniques discussed under Prevention may also

help relieve symptoms. It is best to use conservative treatments, such as those listed here, which have a success rate of 75 to 90 percent, according to a study done at Columbia University in New York and published in the August 2002 issue of *Dentistry Today*. More complicated and invasive treatments are unproved and may make the problem worse. These include orthodontia, placing dental crowns and bridges in the mouth to change the bite, filing down teeth, and surgery to replace a temporomandibular joint.

• **HYDROTHERAPY** Applying an ice pack to the jaw right after an injury can reduce swelling. Afterwards, warm compresses applied periodically throughout the day can temporarily improve range of motion and reduce pain by increasing circulation. Warm compresses can also be helpful for TJM that was not caused by a jaw injury.

• **ORAL SPLINT** This dental appliance, which fits over the upper or lower teeth, is intended to reduce or eliminate teeth clenching. Wearing an oral splint can sometimes increase jaw discomfort. If this happens, stop using it and tell a health practitioner.

• **MEDICATION** Nonsteroidal anti-inflammatory agents can reduce pain. Muscle relaxants can improve the range of jaw movement.

• **OTHER THERAPIES** Dozens of treatments are used for TMJ and several have been studied. These therapies use a broad range of approaches to relieve symptoms or reduce underlying structural causes of TMJ. They include

methods to improve posture such as the Alexander technique (pp.488–9), chiropractic manipulation (pp.446–7), transcutaneous electrical nerve stimulation (TENS, p.443) to improve nerve function, acupuncture (pp.464–5), and injections of glucosamine-chondroitin (a nutritional supplement used to treat osteoarthritis) or hyaluronate (a muscle relaxant used to treat osteoarthritis). But there is either insufficient or conflicting evidence on the effectiveness of these measures.

• **NUTRITION** Eating soft foods can minimize the stress that is placed on the temporomandibular joint while chewing.

• **MOVEMENT AND EXERCISE** Taking care not to overuse or overextend the jaw can ease the discomfort of TMJ. Avoid chewing gum or opening the mouth wide when yawning. Exercises in which the jaw muscles are gently stretched and consciously relaxed may also help.

See also: *Teeth Grinding & Clenching, p.90 • Massage, pp.468–73 • Acupuncture, pp.464–5*

On Call

A clicking sound and a popping sensation when you chew can be worrying, but they do not mean there is something seriously wrong with your jaw. In fact, if these are the only symptoms of TMJ that you experience, you do not need any treatment at all. Treatment is only necessary if you are in pain or have difficulty moving your jaw.

Cavities

Tooth decay is among the most common health conditions. Cavities are holes in the teeth made by acids that are created through the interaction of bacteria in the mouth and sugars from food. Cavities are most likely to form on the chewing surfaces of molars. They first damage the outer layers of the teeth, but if they are not treated they can penetrate the pulp (the inner structure that contains nerves), causing pain, especially when something hot, cold or sweet is consumed.

Although it is widely assumed that cavities mainly affect children, they are also common among adults. Unless they are treated, cavities can cause complications such as dental abscesses, which are bacterial infections that produce pus and can spread and destroy the teeth.

CAUSES
Cavities are formed by the buildup of plaque on the surface of the teeth. Plaque is a sticky substance composed of food debris, saliva and bacteria that coat the teeth after eating. Bacteria that normally live in the mouth help break down food particles into sugars, a process that forms acids. If the acids remain in contact with the teeth longer than about 20 minutes, they begin to eat away at the tooth enamel (the outer surface). Eating starchy and sugary foods increase the risk of developing cavities.

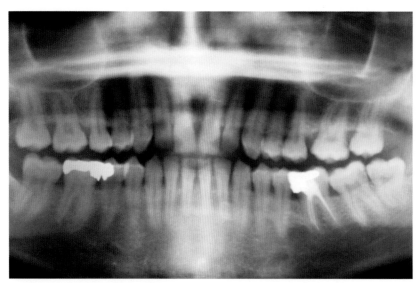

X-rays help dentists identify cavities that are hidden or difficult to see, as well as showing the overall condition of the teeth, roots and jawbone.

WHO IS AT RISK?
The risk factors include:
Cavities
- Poor oral hygiene
- Diet high in sweet and starchy foods
- Frequent snacking

Dental abscesses
- Untreated cavities
- Injury to a tooth

PREVENTION
Routine dental check-ups are essential for diagnosing and treating cavities, and to prevent them from becoming abscesses.

Self-Care
Brush teeth twice a day with a toothpaste that contains fluoride, a mineral that makes teeth resistant to cavities by strengthening tooth enamel. Floss once a day to remove debris from between the teeth. Daily use of fluoride rinses and gels provides added protection. Limit consumption of sugary and starchy foods (especially those that are sticky) and drink water with meals and snacks to rinse food off the teeth. Do not chew gum that contains sugar. Drinking green tea may also help prevent cavities because it has antibacterial properties.

Dental Care
Fluoride treatments by a dentist offer more protection against

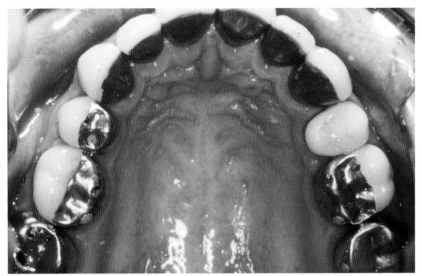

Amalgam fillings (above) are made from a mixture of mercury and an alloy of silver, tin, and copper. They are typically less expensive than composite fillings (not shown), which are a tooth-coloured plastic made of resin and glass.

cavities than fluoride toothpaste and rinses or gels alone. For children, dental sealants are also a proven way of protecting the chewing surfaces of the back teeth – the areas that are most prone to tooth decay. Sealants, which are made of plastic resin, are painted onto the teeth.

DIAGNOSIS

A dentist can diagnose cavities based on the appearance of the teeth and symptoms described. X-rays can identify those that are hidden or difficult to see, and show how deeply they have penetrated the teeth.

TREATMENTS

The aim of treatment is to prevent further tooth damage by removing the decayed portion of a tooth. Dental abscesses must be treated with antibiotics to eliminate the infection.

• FILLINGS The standard treatment is for a dentist to clean out the decayed area of the tooth with a dental drill and then fill it in with a material such as amalgam (a mixture of mercury, and an alloy of silver, tin, and copper), or a tooth-coloured composite resin or porcelain.

• CROWNS If a cavity has destroyed so much of a tooth that there is not enough of it left to fill, a crown is used. This is an artificial replacement of the visible part of a tooth. First, the dentist cleans the decayed area of tooth, and then files down the remaining area into a stub. A crown is created to fit over the stub and fill the space between the adjoining teeth.

• ROOT CANAL This procedure may be necessary when tooth decay reaches the pulp, which contains nerves, blood vessels and lymph vessels, and causes an infection there. First, the tooth decay and infected pulp are eliminated and the area (which is called the root canal) may be filled with antibiotic paste to prevent further infection. Next, a filling material is put into the root canal and a crown is fitted. A root canal requires two or more visits to a dentist or an endodontist (a dentist who specializes in root canal procedures).

• ANTIBIOTICS Oral antibiotics are prescribed to treat a dental abscess, as well as to prevent infection following a root canal procedure.

• SURGERY If a dental abscess is severe and painful, surgery may be performed to drain it.

• OZONE THERAPY Regular exposure of cavities to ozone air may help reverse cavities. Ozone therapy (p.579) is believed to have antimicrobial properties.

See also: *Teeth Grinding & Clenching, p.90* • *Ozone Therapy, p.579*

Clinical Query

What is baby bottle tooth decay?

Infants are more likely to get cavities if they often fall asleep while sucking on a bottle, or if they routinely drink fruit juice from a bottle. Tooth decay is especially likely when a baby falls asleep with a bottle in their mouth, allowing the sugary liquids to pool in the mouth. Bacteria in the mouth interact with sugars in the liquids to produce acid, which can cause the developing teeth to decay. In the most severe cases, the teeth may have to be removed. The spaces left by the lost baby teeth can cause the permanent teeth to grow in crooked. To prevent baby bottle tooth decay, do not let your infant sleep with a bottle, and avoid putting juice in a bottle at any time. Try to wean your child from a bottle to a cup when they are about 18 months old.

Dry Mouth

An inadequate flow of saliva that leaves the mouth feeling uncomfortably parched is called dry mouth. It is a symptom of several illnesses as well as a side-effect of many medications and medical treatments. The condition may be temporary or permanent, depending on the cause. Apart from being uncomfortable, dry mouth can cause several different health problems.

Cavities and mouth infections become more common because of the lack of saliva to clear away food particles. When it is severe, dry mouth can interfere with swallowing, leading to nutritional deficiencies. Although it affects people of all ages, dry mouth becomes increasingly common as people get older.

CAUSES

Drinking too little water can make the mouth feel dry. Several illnesses can reduce saliva production, including Sjogren syndrome, an autoimmune disease, as well as Parkinson's disease (p.181), stroke (pp.168–9), Alzheimer's disease (pp.178–9), depression (pp.364–5), and anxiety.

Hundreds of medications can temporarily reduce saliva production, including antihistamines, antidepressants, tranquillizers, painkillers and blood pressure medicines. Chemotherapy for cancer can affect the chemistry of saliva, making the mouth feel dry. Radiation treatments for cancers of the head and neck can permanently damage the salivary glands.

Surgery of the head or neck can cause dry mouth by severing the nerves that prompt the salivary glands to secrete saliva.

Salivary stones that block a salivary gland duct can cause dry mouth by blocking the flow of saliva. Salivary stones form when salts and other chemicals in the saliva clump together.

PREVENTION

Reducing the risk of the many conditions that can cause dry mouth can help prevent the problem. In addition, drink at least eight glasses of water a day and limit consumption of dehydrating foods and beverages such as coffee, tea, alcohol, and spicy or salty foods.

If you are taking medication that can cause dry mouth, or if dry mouth is a chronic problem for another reason, it is important to take action to prevent dental problems by practising good dental hygiene.

DIAGNOSIS

A doctor or a dentist can diagnose the underlying cause based on symptoms and a physical examination. They may squeeze the salivary glands (which are located in pairs on either side of the jaw, beneath the jaw and beneath the tongue) to stimulate saliva flow and see if it appears normal or inadequate, as well as to feel for any swellings or blockages that may be interfering with the functioning of the gland.

TREATMENTS

In most cases, treatment involves temporarily relieving the symptoms with the prevention measures listed earlier, as well as several self-help strategies:

• ACUPUNCTURE This Traditional Chinese Medicine (pp.446–50) technique, using needles placed in the face, may alleviate dry mouth.

• MOISTURE Use a humidifyer in the bedroom, because moist air helps the body conserve moisture. Drink water when talking for an extended period. Taking sips of water can replenish the moisture that is lost while speaking.

• DIET Chew sugarless gum. Chewing gum helps stimulate saliva production and sugarless gum does not harm the teeth. Sucking on hard sweets in moderation can also stimulate the salivary glands.

• SURGERY If a salivary stone is the cause, it can be removed either manually or surgically.

See also: *Stroke, pp.168–9 • Anxiety, pp.354–5 • Chinese Medicine, pp.446–50*

Halitosis

A foul odour that comes from the mouth is halitosis. The odour can be caused by eating pungent foods, such as garlic, or it can be a symptom of a number of health problems, including infections in the mouth and elsewhere, and anatomical problems with the gastrointestinal tract. It can also be a side-effect of smoking and certain medications.

CAUSES

Bad breath has a wide variety of causes. The most common one is food that has a strong taste or odour. Not only do chemicals from these foods remain in the mouth, but they also get into the bloodstream during digestion and eventually reach the lungs. When a person exhales, the odours from these foods are expelled from the lungs out through the mouth. The odours persist until the food is fully digested. Smoking and heavy alcohol consumption contribute to the problem by adding their own odours.

Another cause of bad breath is poor dental hygiene. When a person does not brush or floss regularly, food particles linger on the teeth, tongue and gums, and as they decompose they give off a foul odour. Poor hygiene also leads to cavities (pp.86–7), tooth abscesses, and gum disease, conditions that can cause bad breath. Dry mouth (p.88), in which there is a lack of saliva, can also cause bad breath.

Bad breath can be a side-effect of some medications, such as insulin injections for diabetes, inhaled anaesthetics and paraldehyde (an anticonvulsant).

PREVENTION

Good oral hygiene is the most effective way to prevent bad breath. Brush the teeth twice a day and floss once a day. Brush the tongue, as well, to clean off food and bacteria that may have formed a coating. Antimicrobial mouth rinses can help by reducing the risk of cavities and gum disease. See a dentist regularly for checkups to clean the teeth and identify cavities and other oral health problems that can contribute to bad breath.

Drinking water regularly throughout the day can also prevent bad breath by washing away food debris and bacteria. Avoid smoking, drinking alcohol and foods that give people bad breath, such as onions and garlic.

WHO IS AT RISK?

Risk factors include:

- Allergies
- Sinus infections and abnormal sinus anatomy
- Post-nasal drip
- Tonsillitis
- Lung diseases
- Kidney diseases
- Liver diseases
- Blood disorders
- Diabetes
- Gallbladder dysfunction
- Menstruation
- Carcinomas
- Extensive tooth decay
- Periodontal disease
- Oral infections or abscesses
- Oral cancers
- Dry mouth

DIAGNOSIS

Bad breath itself is easy to recognize, but the underlying cause is not always obvious. If prevention does not control the problem, consult a doctor or dentist.

TREATMENTS

While using breath mints and mouthwashes can temporarily get rid of bad breath, the only way to eliminate it is to identify and treat the underlying cause.

See also: *Cavities, pp.86–7 • Gum Disease, pp.80–1*

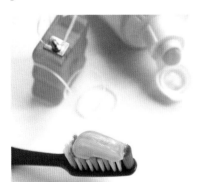

Good oral hygiene and regular dental check-ups are essential for preventing bad breath.

Teeth Grinding & Clenching

Involuntarily grinding of the teeth side to side or clenching of the teeth is called bruxism. It is most likely to happen during sleep, but can also be a habit during the day that is brought on by stress. The grinding can be so loud that it awakens a bed partner. Other symptoms are an aching in the jaw or a headache upon waking, tooth pain, facial pain and the wearing down of the biting surfaces of some teeth. Teeth grinding can lead to temporomandibular joint disorders (TMJ, pp.84–5).

CAUSES

Bruxism is often the result of stress, anxiety, tension, suppressed anger or frustration, or a competitive or hyperactive personality. Other causes are the abnormal alignment of the upper and lower teeth, which forces some of the upper and lower teeth to press against each other.

In children, bruxism may occur when the top and bottom teeth do not fit together comfortably. Children may also grind their teeth as a result of tension, anger, allergy problems, or as a response to pain caused by an earache or teething.

PREVENTION

Reducing stress with relaxation techniques such as yoga (pp.476–9), meditation (pp.514–19), and massage (pp.468–73), can help prevent grinding and clenching of the teeth. If a person has crooked or missing teeth, correcting these problems can prevent grinding and clenching.

DIAGNOSIS

A dentist or family physician can identify bruxisms based on the symptoms and an examination of the teeth.

TREATMENTS

Treatment focuses on reducing the incidence of grinding and clenching, and relieving the discomfort they cause.

• **MOUTH GUARD** This is a flexible plastic device that fits over the upper or lower teeth and is used while sleeping. The mouth guard absorbs the force of jaw clenching and prevents the top and bottom teeth from grinding against each other. Mouth guards can be custom-made by a dentist.

• **ORAL SPLINT** This device is usually worn on the top teeth. Some oral splints are designed to relax the jaw, and others to prevent the rear top and bottom teeth from touching, which can reduce grinding.

• **ACUPUNCTURE** This therapy can reduce the muscle tension associated with bruxism.

• **DENTAL PROCEDURES** Orthodontic adjustment may be used to correct a misalignment of the jaw or teeth contributing to bruxism. Oral surgery is an option if other treatments do not relieve bruxism.

• **RELAXATION** In addition to using strategies to cope with and reduce daily stress, take time to relax the muscles in the face several times each day. After a while, facial relaxation will become a habit, and may reduce the tendency to clench or grind the teeth.

• **BIOFEEDBACK** This therapy (pp.504–7), which helps you learn to control involuntary body functions, is sometimes recommended to reduce grinding and clenching during the day by helping to control muscle activity in the jaw. A biofeedback device for use during sleep reduces grinding and clenching at night by alerting the patient when the jaw muscles are clenched.

• **COUNSELLING** Counselling with a psychologist or other mental health professional may be needed to deal with ongoing tension and anxiety.

See also: *Yoga, pp.476–9 • Meditation, pp.514–19 • Massage, pp.468–73*

WHO IS AT RISK?

Risk factors include:
• Stress
• Misaligned or missing teeth

Oral Cancers

A lump on the gums or lips that does not heal, or bleeding or persistent pain in the mouth are signs of oral cancer. These malignancies occur most often on the lips and tongue. Cancer on the tongue may cause pain while eating and drinking, and affect speech. Some oral cancers begin as mouth ulcers (pp.82–3). They are among the deadliest of all cancers, but they are also among the most preventable because of their strong link with tobacco use.

CAUSES

Most oral cancers are caused by tobacco. The smoke and heat from cigarettes, cigars and pipes irritate mouth tissue. Chemicals from chewing tobacco or taking snuff also cause irritation.

PREVENTION

The risk of developing oral cancer can be dramatically lowered by avoiding tobacco in all forms and moderating alcohol consumption. Other important preventive measures are brushing teeth twice a day and flossing every day, receiving regular dental check-ups, protecting skin from the sun and, if any dental appliances are being used, telling the dentist if they hurt because irritations from ill-fitting appliances can lead to oral cancers. Drinking green tea may also reduce the risk of oral cancers.

DIAGNOSIS

Oral cancers are often diagnosed during routine dental check-ups. A dentist or doctor can diagnose oral cancers based on their appearance and other symptoms. Imaging tests such as X-rays, CT scanning or MRI may also be done. Biopsies are taken of abnormal-looking tissue to examine it for cancer cells.

TREATMENTS

Treatment depends on the stage of the cancer and whether it is recurrent. The stage is determined by the cancer's size, whether it has infiltrated lymph nodes in the neck and how extensive this infiltration is, and whether it has spread beyond the mouth.

• SURGERY The cancer and a margin of healthy tissue are cut out. Any cancerous lymph nodes are removed as well. Reconstructive surgery can be performed if a portion of the mouth or lip has to be removed.

• RADIATION Radiation therapy to kill cancer cells can be delivered using an external beam aimed at the site of the cancer or by injecting or infusing radioactive substances into the cancerous areas of the mouth.

• HYPERTHERMIA This experimental treatment uses a heat-generating machine to kill cancer cells and shrink tumours. (Cancer cells are

more vulnerable to damage by heat than normal cells.)

• SPEECH AND OCCUPATIONAL THERAPIES Speech therapy may be needed if speaking is impaired by oral cancer or surgery. Occupational therapy is useful if the ability to swallow is affected. Both therapies help a patient either regain the ability to speak and swallow, or learn new ways to do these things.

See also: *Mouth Ulcers, pp.82–3* • *Smoking Cessation, pp.216–17* • *Substance Abuse, pp.358–60*

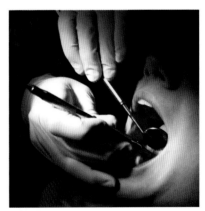

Oral cancer is a fast-spreading disease that can occur in the mouth or pharynx. It affects twice as many men as women.

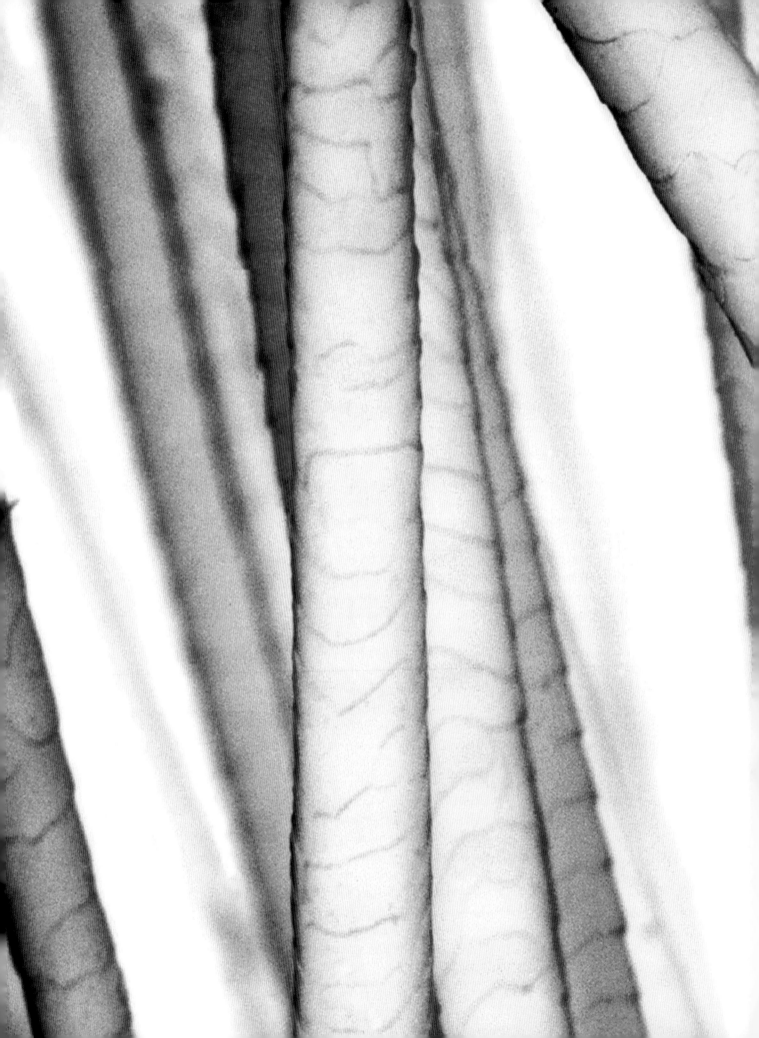

4 SKIN, HAIR & NAILS

The skin is the body's largest organ, accounting for about seven percent of body weight. It is the boundary that separates us from the outside world, screening out harmful substances and protecting us from heat and dehydration. The organ we call the skin includes the hair, nails, and sweat glands.

A variety of conditions affect the skin – bacterial and viral invaders can lead to chronic conditions such as acne, impetigo and boils, and exposure to the sun can cause skin cancer. But other conditions, such as psoriasis and dermatitis, may result from a variety of causes. A dermatologist can treat these conditions with oral medication, creams or injections, and may also advise lifestyle changes that may help avoid recurrence.

Without the skin's complex network of sensory nerves, we would be unable to detect changes in temperature and pressure, or feel pain. Simple injuries could be fatal. The skin's real role may be in protecting us from ourselves.

Bacterial Skin Infections

The three main types of bacterial skin infections are impetigo, boils and cellulitis. Impetigo, which affects mainly children, is very contagious. It begins as a red patch, most often around the nose or mouth and, a day or two later, develops into a cluster of tiny blisters which then form a yellow–brown scab. Other symptoms may include fever and swollen lymph glands in the face or neck.

Boils, known as furuncles, are painful inflammations of the hair follicles and the tissue beneath them. They are red bumps filled with pus that appear most often on the face, neck, armpits, buttocks and thighs.

Cellulitis is the most serious of the bacterial skin infections because it can lead to blood poisoning. It affects deeper levels of the skin, extending to connective tissue, causing the skin to become red, swollen, tender and warm to the touch, often with red streaks extending to nearby swollen lymph nodes. The infection can cause fever and chills.

CAUSES

Many of the same types of bacteria cause impetigo, boils and cellulitis, but the infections affect different skin structures.

Impetigo

The cause of impetigo is usually an infection of *Staphylococcus*, *Streptococcus*, or both bacteria in the top layers of skin. The infection may follow a respiratory infection or occur when bacteria infect a minor skin lesion, such as a cut or an insect bite. Because impetigo is highly contagious, it can also be spread by contact with the skin of an infected person or towels and other personal items the person has used.

Boils

These are usually caused by *Staphylococcus* migrating from the surface of the skin into the hair follicles and the surrounding tissue in the dermis layer. To fight off the infection, the immune system sends white blood cells to the follicles, causing inflammation and forming pus. Boils can occur alone or in groups. A cluster of boils is called a carbuncle. Atopic dermatitis (pp.102–3), a skin inflammation that is caused by an allergy or a sensitivity to a particular substance, increases the risk of developing boils. Recurrent boils are especially common in people with diabetes and conditions that weaken the immune system. As with impetigo, boils can be spread by touching an infected person or the personal items they have used.

WHO IS AT RISK?

The risk factors include:

Impetigo
- Children
- Recent upper respiratory infections
- Skin lesions such as cuts and insect bites

Boils
- Diabetes
- Atopic dermatitis
- Weakened immune system

Cellulitis
- Skin injury
- Recent surgery
- Peripheral vascular disease
- Diabetes
- Suppressed immune system

Cellulitis

Several types of bacteria can cause cellulitis, but the most common are *Staphylococcus* and *Streptococcus*. The infection usually follows a skin injury such as a burn, bite, sore or surgical incision, but it can also begin with exposure to bacteria in water (such as fish tanks or pond water) or on animals. The risk of developing cellulitis is increased by medication or illnesses that suppress the immune system, and by illnesses that reduce blood circulation, including diabetes (pp.338–41) and peripheral vascular disease (pp.254–5). Cellulitis can occur anywhere on the body, but is especially common on the legs, feet, trunk, arms and

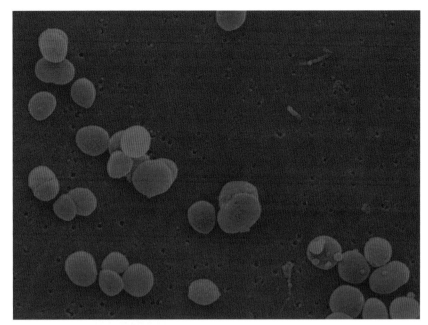

Some of the same types of bacteria, including *Staphylococcus* and *Streptococcus*, cause impetigo, boils, and cellulitis. But these infections each affect the skin differently. However, impetigo can be highly contagious, while boils and cellulitis usually are not.

face. Cellulitis of the skin around the eye sockets is seen most often in children. Unless it is treated quickly, this type of cellulitis can spread to the brain. Cellulitis in other areas of the body can spread through the lymphatic system into the bloodstream, causing blood poisoning and gangrene.

PREVENTION

Good hygiene can help prevent bacterial skin infections from forming and spreading. Prevent skin injuries by wearing gloves when gardening and working outdoors and by not walking barefoot outdoors. All cuts, bites and other wounds should be cleaned with soap and water. Try not to scratch itchy rashes or insect bites – doing so can make them worse and increase the odds of infection.

Avoid contact with people who have bacterial infections. If a bacterial infection develops, prevent it from spreading to others within the household by washing sheets and pillowcases daily and keeping personal items such as towels, washcloths and soap away from other people. Never try to drain a bacterial skin infection on your own, because this can spread the infection.

DIAGNOSIS

A doctor can diagnose bacterial skin infections based on appearance and a health history. If an infection is draining fluid or pus, the doctor may take a sample to identify the type of bacteria.

TREATMENTS

The goal of treatment is to cure the infection and prevent complications, as well as to prevent the infection from spreading to others. Although boils often heal on their own, the other bacterial skin infections need to be treated with antibiotics.

Impetigo

• ANTIBIOTICS Topical creams usually eliminate impetigo, but oral antibiotics are sometimes used. The affected areas of skin should be washed several times a day to clear away the crust and draining fluid.

Boils

• COMPRESSES Warm, moist compresses applied several times a day can help small boils drain and heal, usually within two weeks. As they drain, the boils should be washed often and covered with sterile dressings. Wash hands afterwards to avoid spreading the infection. Never drain a boil: doing so can spread the infection.

• SURGERY Medical attention is needed for boils on the face or spine, large boils or carbuncles, and boils that do not heal after two weeks or are accompanied by a temperature or other symptoms. A doctor may drain these surgically and prescribe oral antibiotics.

Cellulitis

• ANTIBIOTICS These are needed to prevent blood poisoning and other serious complications. Mild cases of cellulitis can often be cured with oral antibiotics taken at home. Severe cases require intravenous antibiotics given in hospital.

• COMPRESSES Warm compresses can speed recovery by improving blood flow to the affected area.

See also: *Diabetes, pp.338–41* • *Peripheral Vascular Disease, pp.254–5* • *Atopic Dermatitis, pp.102–3*

Bites & Stings

Bites from insects or arachnids (a group that includes spiders and mites) and stings from bees are among the most common wounds. A bite is a scratch, tear or puncture inflicted by the teeth or other mouthparts of an insect or arachnid. A sting is a skin puncture from a stinger. Although many bites and stings are minor and can be treated at home, some are life-threatening emergencies.

CAUSES

Certain insects and arachnids, such as mosquitoes, ticks and spiders, frequently bite humans. Stings can come from insects, such as bees, wasps, hornets and scorpions, or from marine animals, such as jellyfish, stingrays, sea urchins and Portuguese men-o-war.

PREVENTION

To prevent insect bites and stings, use insect repellents when in backyards and other natural areas during mild weather. Permethrin, when applied to clothing and used in addition to an insect repellent on the skin, is also effective in reducing insect bites. However, it is not effective when applied to the skin.

Some herbal repellents also appear to be effective at repelling pests, although the research is preliminary. Essential oil of *Zanthoxylum limonella* fruit (from the ma-kwaen tree, native to Thailand), key lime (*Citrus aurantifolia*) leaves, and petroleum ether extract of *Zanthoxylum limonella* fruits each afford several hours of protection against mosquito bites—with the oil of *Zanthoxylum limonella* preventing them for the longest period. An extract of curcuma aromatica, the source of the spice turmeric, can protect against mosquito bites for three and a half hours. Lemon eucalyptus (*Eucalyptus citriodora*) extract protects against tick bites.

When in wooded or grassy areas, wear trousers and socks for extra protection against ticks. At the beach, avoid jellyfish and other stinging animals; even dead animals can inject their venom if they are touched.

DIAGNOSIS

Most bites and stings leave a laceration, rash, bump or some other mark on the skin. Other symptoms may indicate an allergic reaction or an infection, such as muscle cramps, nausea, vomiting, chills, dizziness and difficulty breathing.

Bites and stings can be diagnosed by their appearance and a history of recent exposure to particular arachnids and insects. For bites or stings that cause serious allergic reactions, immediate medical attention is necessary. Urine tests, blood tests and other laboratory tests may be done to look for signs of infection or allergic reaction.

TREATMENTS

The way bites and stings are treated depends on their cause.

Insect and Arachnid Bites

Mosquito bites are usually mild. The itchiness can be relieved with calamine lotion or

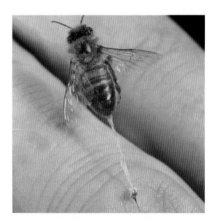

Venom from stinging insects like bees can cause a painful immune reaction but is usually not dangerous.

hydrocortisone cream. Applying an ice cube or witch hazel (a liquid distilled from the plant *Hamamelis virginiana*) can give temporary relief, as well.

Bites from spiders or ticks have the potential to be serious. Bites from black widow spiders and brown recluse spiders are poisonous and require emergency medical attention. Both types of spiders live in dark, dry places such as garages or piles of wood, rock or brush. Symptoms of a black widow spider bite include intense pain and stiffness and possibly nausea, fever, chills and abdominal pain. Symptoms of a brown recluse spider bite include blistering and intense pain, along with fever, chills and nausea. If someone thinks they have a spider bite, they should go to the nearest hospital, keeping the area of the bite below the level of the heart to slow the spread of the venom and covering the bite with an ice pack to relieve the symptoms.

Most tick bites are not dangerous, but in some areas ticks can carry organisms that cause serious infections, such as Lyme disease and Rocky Mountain spotted fever (pp.94–5). If bitten by a tick, remove it with tweezers. (In an area where tick-borne illnesses occur, save the tick in a sealed plastic bag or a glass jar for analysis by a laboratory to see if it carries an infectious organism). Wash the area of the tick bite and apply an antiseptic ointment to prevent infection. The signs of a tick-borne illness, which include a rash or flu-like symptoms, can take several days

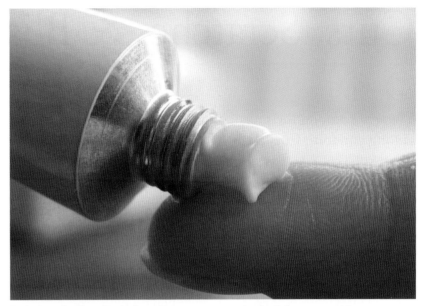

Topical medications like hydrocortisone cream or calamine lotion can provide relief from the irriation of mosquito bites and insect stings. Ointments should be applied gently to prevent further irritation and to avoid infection.

or weeks to develop. See a doctor if these symptoms develop.

Insect Stings

Some home remedies can soothe bee and wasp stings. A poultice of meat tenderizer reduces swelling and pain by neutralizing the venom from the sting. Make a thick paste by mixing warm water or rubbing alcohol with powdered meat tenderizer, then put the paste on the bee sting. Baking soda can also help relieve pain from a bee sting and vinegar or lemon juice can reduce the pain from wasp stings.

Some people are allergic to insect stings, and for these people, one sting can cause life-threatening anaphylactic shock, in which widespread histamine release causes respiratory distress, heart failure, circulatory collapse and, sometimes, death. People with known allergies to stings often carry an injectable form of

epinephrine, a hormone that increases breathing and heart rate.

Marine Animal Stings

Stings from marine animals are poisonous, and those from a Portuguese man-o-war are potentially life-threatening. If someone has been stung by a Portuguese man-o-war, call an ambulance or go immediately to a nearby hospital. Do not pull out attached stingers – doing so can spread the venom to the hands.

Any marine animal sting that is bleeding or causes breathing difficulties or other generalized symptoms also requires emergency medical care. Stings from jellyfish that cause pain but no other symptoms can be relieved with calamine lotion and a cold compress. If other symptoms develop, call a doctor.

See also: *Fever, p.318 • Lyme Disease, pp.326–7 • Homeopathy, pp.455–7*

Cuts, Scratches & Blisters

These are among the most common skin injuries, especially among children. Cuts are breaks in the skin and underlying tissue that cause bleeding. Scrapes and scratches are abrasions of the top layer of skin, the difference being that scratches are thin and scrapes are wide. Blisters are bubbles under the top layers of skin that are filled with fluid.

CAUSES

Cuts are caused by sharp objects such as knives, scissors or even the edges of paper. Scrapes are usually caused by falling or sliding against a rough surface, as happens when children fall on pavement and scrape their knees. Scratches are often caused by animal claws or even human nails, but accidents with other sharp objects can also leave scratches. Blisters most often develop because of friction on an area of skin. Poor-fitting shoes can cause blisters on the feet. Sports and other activities that involve firmly grasping a bat or other hard object can cause blisters on the hands. Other causes of blisters are burns, contact with strong industrial chemicals such as kerosene, and allergic reactions to plants such as poison ivy.

PREVENTION

Taking precautions against accidents can reduce the risk of most cuts, scrapes and scratches. Wear kneepads when skating or Rollerblading. To prevent blisters, wear shoes that fit well and appropriate gloves for activities that can irritate the hands. Cuts and scratches carry the risk of tetanus, a bacterial infection that causes nerve damage. To prevent tetanus, have a tetanus shot every 10 years.

DIAGNOSIS

These skin lesions can be diagnosed based on their appearance. A doctor should examine a cut or scratch that is more than about 0.64 cm (¼ in) deep, does not stop bleeding after about 20 minutes, or is on the face. If the wound remains red and swollen for more than two days, visit a doctor to check for infection.

TREATMENTS

Most of these skin injuries can be treated at home. The main goal of treatment is to prevent infection.

• **CLEANING AND BANDAGING** Clean all wounds with running water and soap. If the bleeding doesn't stop on its own within a few minutes, firmly press a clean cloth or bandage over it for five to ten minutes. Apply antibacterial ointment and cover a bandage. Cover blisters with a bandage to help prevent infection.

WHO IS AT RISK?

The risk factors include:
• Children
• Having a pet
• Wearing tight-fitting shoes
• An active lifestyle
• Exposure to irritating plants, such as poison ivy

• **STITCHES** These may be needed for deep cuts and scratches, as well as for cuts on the face, to help avoid scarring.

• **MEDICATION** Any skin wound that becomes infected should be treated with antibiotics. Topical antibiotic ointments may be applied to minor cuts and scratches as a preventative measure.

• **COMPLEMENTARY TREATMENTS** Many complementary treatments speed skin healing. Aloe vera contains compounds that have been found to be especially beneficial for healing wounds in people with diabetes (pp.338–41). Ethanol extract from the bark of the cinnamon tree (*Cinnamonum zeylanicum*), electrical stimulation of the skin, acupuncture (pp.464–5), hypnosis (pp.508–13), guided imagery (pp.520–2), energy healing (pp.560–73), and relaxation (pp.474–5) have also been found effective in helping skin heal rapidly.

See also: *Energy Healing, pp.560–73* • *Acupuncture, pp.464–5* • *Hypnosis, pp.508–11*

Acne & Rosacea

Both of these conditions mark the face with red blotches that can be persistent and difficult to clear up. It was once assumed that rosacea was a type of acne – it was even known as adult acne because it is most common in adults. However, acne and rosacea are different skin disorders.

Acne is a disease of the pilosebaceous units (PSUs). Found over most of the body, PSUs consist of a sebaceous (oil-secreting) gland connected to a canal, called a follicle, that contains a fine hair. When the PSUs are plugged, sebum produced by the sebaceous glands cannot escape and pimples erupt. There may be just a few small pimples on the face or, in severe cases, large or clustered pimples on the face, neck, upper chest, and back. Acne is most common among teenagers, although it can also affect children and adults.

Rosacea is a widening of the small blood vessels of the face that causes chronic redness, especially of the cheeks, nose, forehead and chin. At first the redness has a 'spider web' appearance, formed by dilated blood vessels beneath the skin's surface. But if the condition persists, small pimples may develop. In severe cases, the nose becomes red and bulbous.

CAUSES

Acne and rosacea have different causes. Acne is caused mainly by an increase in sex hormones, especially androgens, which stimulate the sebaceous glands beneath the hair follicles to secrete oil. A surge in sex hormones is common during puberty and, in females, just before menstruation each month. When the sebaceous glands secrete

too much oil, it can clog the pores. Plugs of dried oil, skin cells and bacteria form pimples.

There are different types of pimples. Blackheads are the tiny dark specks of dried oil and skin cells that develop mainly on the nose, cheeks and chin. Whiteheads, which have a white top, are clogged pores that are infected and filled with pus. Other causes of acne are stress and corticosteroid medication.

Rosacea is most common in women in their 30s and 40s. It is caused by certain foods, emotions and environmental factors that increase blood flow and make the blood vessels in the face expand. Foods include alcohol, hot

WHO IS AT RISK?

The risk factors include:

Acne
- Teenagers
- The surge in sex hormones each month before menstruation
- Stress
- Corticosteroids

Rosacea
- Fair skin
- Women in their 30s and 40s
- Stress
- Anger
- Exposure to sun
- Exposure to extreme hot or cold temperatures
- Cosmetics or creams that irritate the skin

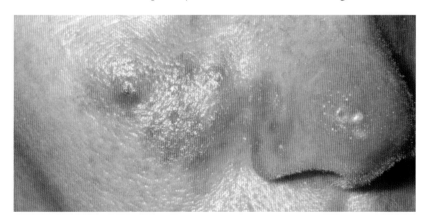

Rosacea appears as persistent redness of the cheeks and nose and in severe cases can affect the eyes. Although there is no cure for rosacea, a dermatologist can help patients control the condition and improve the appearance of the skin.

beverages and spicy foods; emotions include stress and anger; and environmental factors include sun exposure, very hot or very cold temperatures, and vigorous exercise. Some topical products can also lead to rosacea, including hydrocortisone cream, alpha-hydroxy acid lotions, facial scrubs, and cosmetics that irritate the skin.

PREVENTION

There are several ways to reduce the occurrence and severity of both acne and rosacea. Controlling emotional stress can help prevent both conditions. In addition, to minimize acne use oil-free cosmetics and lotions, wash faces and other affected areas once or twice a day with mild cleanser, and wash hair regularly to keep it from spreading oil to the face. Acne pimples can be prevented from spreading and scarring by not squeezing or touching them.

To prevent rosacea flare-ups, avoid environmental exposures and foods that dilate or damage the blood vessels. Protect face and head from the sun by using sunscreen and wearing a hat on sunny days. Stay away from foods and drinks that often spark rosacea, including spicy foods, sharp cheeses, hot drinks and alcohol. Faces should be washed only with a mild cleanser; harsh agents such as astringents and alcohol can irritate the skin and may promote flare-ups of rosacea.

DIAGNOSIS

A doctor can diagnose acne and rosacea based on the appearance of the skin and a medical history.

TREATMENTS

Although they are different conditions, acne and rosacea respond to some of the same treatments. Combinations of treatments often yield the best results.

• TOPICAL PREPARATIONS Several lotions and creams are used to treat acne and rosacea. Acne preparations contain one or more of the following active ingredients: benzoyl peroxide, resorcinol, salicylic acid, azelaid acid or sulphur. Some of these agents kill bacteria and others reduce inflammation. They are less effective than topical retinol (see below), but they may be all that is needed for mild acne. Azelaic acid cream, an acne preparation, also relieves symptoms of moderate rosacea. Herbal preparations include tea tree oil, a distillation from *Melaleuca alternifolia*, the tea tree, which grows in Australia. It can reduce the number of acne pimples.

• SURGERY There are several surgical procedures for acne and rosacea. A dermatologist can drain and remove individual pimples. For superficial acne scars, a chemical peel using mild acid can be applied to burn off the top layer of skin.

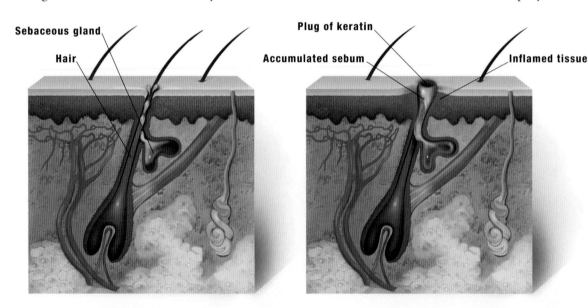

Sebaceous gland

Hair

Plug of keratin

Accumulated sebum

Inflamed tissue

The sebaceous glands beneath the surface of the skin produce a lubricating oil called sebum that is secreted out of the hair follicle. This oil can clump together with hair and dead skin cells, plugging the opening of the follicle. When bacteria on the skin infects and grows within the plugged follicle, the follicle becomes inflamed and swollen, and an acne pimple forms.

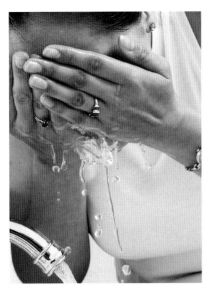

Washing your face is essential for keeping pores from clogging, but eccessive scrubbing can make acne worse.

Options for deep acne scars are dermabrasion, which uses a wire brush to remove damaged skin, and laser skin resurfacing, which uses pulses of laser light to remove layers of damaged skin. For severe rosacea that causes a red, bulbous appearance of the nose, laser surgery can remove excess tissue.

• TRADITIONAL CHINESE MEDICINE Acupuncture (pp.464–5) may help clear up acne. A herbal remedy called compound oldenlandis mixture has also been found to be effective. In a study done at the China Academy of Traditional Chinese Medicine in Beijing, 86 cases of acne were treated with compound oldenlandis mixture and 34 cases assigned to a control group. The study found 73 percent of the people who used the compound showed marked improvement, compared with just 47 percent of the people in the control group.

• AYURVEDA. Several Ayurvedic (pp.451–4) herbal preparations may be effective in controlling acne. A mixture of seven Ayurvedic herbs, taken orally or applied in a cream, have been found to be effective: aloe (*Aloe barbadensis*), neem (*Azardirachta indica*), turmeric (*Curcuma longa*), hemidesmus (*Hemidesmus indicus*), chebulic myrobalan (*Terminalia chebula*), arjuna (*Terminalia arjuna*) and winter cherry (*Withania somnifera*). Tablets of sunder vati, taken three times a day, can also be effective in controlling acne. Sunder vati contains Indian gooseberry (*Emblica officinalis*), false black pepper (*Embelia ribes*), tellicherry bark (*Holarrhena antidysenterica*) and ginger (*Zingiberis officinale*). A small clinical trial (published in 1994 in the *Journal of Dermatololgy*) randomly assigned 20 people with acne to receive the antibiotic tetracycline or gugulipid, an Ayurvedic herbal preparation, for three months. Both therapies achieved comparable results: a 65 percent reduction in acne lesions in the group given tetracycline and a 68 percent reduction in the group given gugulipid. The patients with oily faces responded much better to gugulipid.

• ANTIBIOTICS Taken orally or applied to the skin, antibiotics can help control acne by killing bacteria that cause inflammation. Even though bacterial infection does not contribute to rosacea, as it does to acne, oral antibiotics have been found effective for rosacea because they reduce inflammation. Topical preparations of an antibiotic and benzoyl peroxide, an acne medicine, also appear to be helpful for rosacea.

On Call

It is widely assumed that greasy foods and chocolate cause acne, but there is no evidence that this is true. Food does not cause acne. However, spicy foods, hot beverages, and alcohol are common triggers of rosacea.

• RETINOIDS These medications, derived from vitamin A, are effective in controlling both acne and rosacea. Topical retinoids help loosen hardened oil plugs and open pores. One side-effect is increased sensitivity to the sun, so it is important to protect the skin with sunscreen and wear a hat when outdoors. When topical retinoids are not effective, an oral retinoid called isotretinoin may be prescribed. It is highly effective in reducing pimples, but the drug causes severe birth defects. To avoid this complication, women who are sexually active must use birth control while using this drug and must stop taking it at least one month before planning to become pregnant.

• ORAL CONTRACEPTIVES These can help reduce the occurrence of acne in women because they reduce the amount of androgen that is available. (Just how this works depends on the specific hormone combination in a particular oral contraceptive.)

• HYPNOSIS This therapy (pp.508–13) may improve or even resolve acne and other dermatological conditions.

See also: *Acupuncture, pp.464–5* • *Ayurveda, pp.451–4* • *Hypnosis, pp.508–11*

Dermatitis

A rash that is not caused by an infection is called dermatitis, or eczema. There are several types of dermatitis. Some are chronic conditions and others are acute allergic reactions or irritations. Typical symptoms include redness, itchiness and a thickening of the affected skin. However, the symptoms can vary considerably, depending on the type of dermatitis and the individual who is affected.

CAUSES

Each type of dermatitis has its own set of causes.

Atopic Dermatitis

Hay fever or asthma increases the tendency to develop atopic dermatitis, a chronic, itchy rash; another risk factor is dry, sensitive skin. It often flares up in response to exposure to common allergens, such as pollen, ragweed, dust mites, moulds and animal hairs. Stress can be another trigger. Scratching can also promote atopic dermatitis.

Contact Dermatitis

Contact dermatitis is redness and irritation that develops on an area of skin when a person touches an allergen or irritating substance, such as nickel in jewellery, certain antibiotics, cosmetics, harsh soaps, detergents, chemicals and irritating plants such as poison ivy. Having allergies or asthma increases the risk of contact dermatitis.

Dermatitis Herpetiformis

This is a chronic disease in which clusters of itchy, painful bumps

form in a symmetrical arrangement on the scalp, shoulders, elbows, buttocks and knees. People who are allergic to gluten (Coeliac disease), a protein in wheat, rye and other grains, are prone to this form of dermatitis.

Seborrhoeic Dermatitis

The sebaceous (oil-producing) glands of the skin are the targets of seborrhoeic dermatitis. It is a chronic condition that makes the skin red and oily with a covering of light, dry flakes. It often occurs on the scalp, where it is called dandruff (p.113), although it can also affect the eyebrows and the sides of the nose.

PREVENTION

There are several ways to prevent or reduce the severity of dermatitis. Breast-feeding babies lowers their risk of developing it throughout life. Delaying the introduction of solid foods until a baby is at least four month old can also help prevent dermatitis.

Dermatitis is an inflammation of the skin marked by redness, itching and a thickening of the skin in the affected area. Scratching will worsen the condition, and is especially a problem during sleep when conscious control of scratching is lost.

Both measures are thought to help prevent a child from developing food allergies.

If you know what causes your dermatitis, minimize exposure as best you can. In addition, follow these general preventative measures to keep the skin from becoming irritated:

• Stay away from irritating plants, such as poison ivy, poison oak, poison sumac and nettles.

• Protect the hands when using harsh chemicals such as ammonia and when gardening.

• Do not let the skin become too dry, as this can promote atopic dermatitis. Use a moisturizer several times a day and avoid taking long, hot showers or baths.

• Keep the humidity level moderate in your home. Air that is too dry or too humid can lead to dermatitis.

• Wear loose-fitting clothes to avoid irritating the skin.

• When your skin itches, only scratch it lightly so as not to cause dermatitis. If necessary, relieve the itch by other means, such as applying a cool compress.

• Control stress with regular exercise, meditation (pp.514–19), yoga (pp.476–9), guided imagery (pp.520–2) or whatever methods work for you.

DIAGNOSIS

Dermatitis can be diagnosed by its appearance and by carefully documenting any pattern of exposure to allergens and irritants. If dermatitis is chronic and appears to be due to an allergy, a doctor may perform a skin patch test. For this test, potential allergens are briefly placed on the skin to see if a rash develops.

TREATMENTS

The various forms of dermatitis can often be controlled by following the preventative measures discussed earlier. In addition, soothing skin lotions and topical and oral medication can help relieve the symptoms and reduce flare-ups.

• HYDROTHERAPY Cold compresses (pp.482–3) can help temporarily reduce inflammation and relieve itching. Oatmeal baths have been found to be effective for rashes that cover a large area of the body.

• TRADITIONAL CHINESE MEDICINE Acupuncture (pp.464–5) treatments can alleviate atopic dermatitis. Chinese herbal mixtures may also be effective for treating atopic dermatitis.

• PHOTOTHERAPY Exposure to low levels of ultraviolet light (p.564) is used to treat dermatitis that will not not respond to other treatments. Patients come to a doctor's office for treatments several times a week for about a month. A medication that increases the body's sensitivity to ultraviolet light may be given to enhance the therapy's effectiveness. Like exposure to the sun, phototherapy can cause skin cancer; therefore, it is considered only for short-term use.

• TOPICAL TREATMENTS Topical steroid creams have long been the mainstay of treatment to reduce itching and inflammation. New topical medications, called immunomodulators, reduce inflammation without steroids. These medications include pimerolimus and tacrolimus.

• MEDICATION If topical medicines are not effective, oral antihistamines can be prescribed. Oral steroids may also be prescribed for short-term use to reduce severe inflammation. Long-term use of steroids, however, carries a high risk of side effects. Antibiotics may be used to treat bacterial infections that develop as a complication from dermatitis.

• HERBAL SUPPLEMENTS Supplements of evening primrose oil are a standard treatment for dermatitis in several Asian countries.

• PROBIOTICS Probiotics (pp.550–1), which are foods or supplements that contain beneficial bacteria, may help reduce the occurrence of dermatitis. But more research is needed to establish the effectiveness of probiotic foods and supplements (pp.532–41), as well as the doses.

See also: *Dandruff, p.113 • Meditation, pp.514–19 • Hydrotherapy, pp.482–3*

On Call

These substances often cause allergies and sensitivities that lead to dermatitis:

• Soaps and detergents
• Fabric softeners
• Chlorine
• Perfumes
• Glues in artificial nails
• Solvents
• Wool clothing
• Rubber
• Nickel and other metals
• Topical antibiotics and anaesthetics
• Irritating plants

Fungal Skin Infections

Fungi that live in the environment and the human body can infect the skin, causing itchy, painful rashes. Tinea and candida are the fungi that are most often responsible. Tinea infections are caused by dermatophytes, a type of fungus similar to mould. It is also known as ringworm because of the raised, ring-shaped rash it causes, but it is not a worm. The infected area of skin usually itches and looks red and scaly, sometimes with blisters, but the particular symptoms vary with the different types of tinea.

Tinea can occur on the groin, face, nails, scalp, arms and legs. Athlete's foot is a tinea infection on the toes and bottoms of the feet.

Candida is a type of yeast that normally lives harmlessly in the mouth, digestive tract and vagina. But when it proliferates, it can infect mucous membranes and moist areas of skin. Candida infects mucous membranes and moist skin, including the vagina, penis, underarms and mouth.

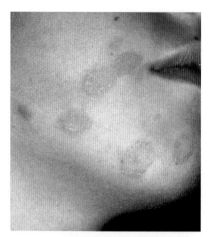

Ringworm is a fungal infection that creates a ring-shaped rash as it spreads. It is not generally a serious condition and can be treated with anti-fungal medication.

Candida is extremely common among infants, and is the cause of nappy rash.

CAUSE

Because tinea thrive in warm, moist areas, they are most likely to develop in the summer. They are highly contagious and can be transmitted by infected people and pets, as well as contaminated surfaces such as swimming-pools, public showers, towels and combs. Poor hygiene and having cuts or other lesions on the skin increase the risk of contracting tinea infections. Walking barefoot, particularly in locker rooms and common shower areas, increases the risk of developing athlete's foot.

Candida proliferation has a variety of causes, including humid conditions, tight-fitting clothing, poor hygiene and inflammatory skin diseases such as psoriasis (pp.120–1). Antibiotics can cause the number of candida to rise because antibiotics kill off

WHO IS AT RISK?
The risk factors include
Tinea:
- Children
- Poor hygiene
- Summer
- Walking barefoot in public places
- Close contact with someone who has a tinea infection
- Sharing personal care items

Candida
- Tight-fitting clothing
- Pregnancy
- Birth control pills
- Antibiotics
- Diabetes
- Obesity

the bacteria that normally keep candida in check. Pregnancy, oral contraceptives, obesity and diabetes also increase the risk of developing candida infections.

PREVENTION

Good hygiene can help prevent fungal skin infections. Wear sandals or shoes outdoors, around swimming-pools, and in locker rooms. Wash feet daily and keep them dry. Wash hair regularly. Do not share personal items, such as combs, brushes, towels and nail clippers. Do not touch pets who have patches of fur missing, since this could be a sign of a fungal infection, and take them to be treated at the vet. Maintaining a normal weight through diet, exercise or both can also reduce the risk of candida infections.

DIAGNOSIS

A doctor can diagnose fungal skin infections based on their appearance and the result of a skin test. One test involves shining a blue light on the affected area; if fungi are present, the skin tends to appear fluorescent. The definitive test is a skin scraping, in which a small skin sample is scraped off with a blade and analysed under a microscope for the presence of fungi.

TREATMENTS

Most fungal skin infections are mild and can be cured within a month with antifungal medications and careful hygiene. Scalp infections take the longer to treat than other fungal skin infections.

• TOPICAL TREATMENTS Topical antifungal lotions, creams and powders are first-line treatments for most fungal skin infections, except those of the scalp. Candida infections that do not respond to topical antifungal treatments can often be cured with gentian violet, a purple dye that is applied to the affected skin.

• MEDICATION Oral antifungal medications are used for scalp ringworm and for body ringworm that does not respond to topical treatment, as well as some candida infections. Antibiotics are necessary if a bacterial infection develops as a complication of a fungal skin infection. Corticosteroids are sometimes given to control itching.

• OZONE THERAPY Topical application of ozonized sunflower oil, which is sunflower oil that has been exposed to ozone gas, can be effective for athlete's foot. Ozone therapy (p.579) is thought to have antimicrobial effects.

• HERBAL MEDICINE A topical application of tea tree oil, which is derived from *Mecaleuca alternifolia*, a tree that grows in Australia, can be effective against tinea. Herbal preparations made from plants in the Solanum species – the nightshade family – and oil of bitter orange (*Citrus aurantium*), is also effective.

• PROBIOTICS *Lactobacillus* (pp.548–9), a beneficial bacterium found in yogurt, speeds the recovery from vaginal yeast infections when used with conventional antifungal medication. The bacterium helps restore the body's natural flora, which hold the yeast in check.

• HYGIENE For tinea infections, bed sheets should be changed daily to help keep the infection from spreading to other parts of the body and to other people in the household. For ringworm infecting the scalp, a medicated shampoo may also reduce the spread of infection. For candida, keeping the skin dry can help eliminate the infection and prevent a recurrence.

See also: *Psoriasis, pp.120–1 • Ozone Therapy, p.579 • Obesity, pp.348–9*

Common Fungal Infections

Infection	Signs and Symptoms
Athlete's foot	Red, scaly rash, caused by tinea pedis, that itches and burns; most often appears between the toes
Scalp ringworm	Red or grey scaly patches on the scalp, caused by tinea capitis, that may itch; sometimes bald spots appear instead of a rash; most common in black children
Jock itch	Scaly, itchy rash with a pink border, caused by tinea cruris, that appears on the groin and thigh; most common in men
Body ringworm	Doughnut-shaped rash with a scaly pink edge, caused by tinea corporis; appears on exposed parts of the body, including arms, legs, face and uncovered areas of the trunk
Vaginal candidiasis	Yeast infection of the vagina, characterized by itching and burning of the external areas and a white or yellow discharge
Penile candidiasis	Painful red yeast rash on the head of the penis or the scrotum
Thrush	Candida infection inside the mouth characterized by painful white patches on the tongue and sides of the mouth
Nappy rash	Candida infection that causes a red rash on the skin underneath an infant's nappy

Urticaria

Oval welts on the skin are the characteristic symptom of urticaria, a common rash more often known as hives. The welts are usually red, but they can also be white or flesh-coloured and are often itchy. Hives occur when immune system cells in the skin called mast cells release histamine, a chemical that causes inflammation. Hives are especially common on the arms and legs. They are usually mild and go away within a few hours or days, but they can also remain or recur for months or years. Treatment depends on the pattern and severity of the symptoms.

CAUSES

An estimated 20 percent of people are affected by hives at some point in their lives. Hives are often caused by an allergic reaction to pollen, animal hair, mould, insect stings or bites or foods. Foods such as eggs, shell-fish, and tree nuts are common causes. Hives can also be a side-effect of several kinds of medication, including nonsteroidal anti-inflammatory agents, penicillin and other antibiotics. When a medication is the culprit, hives emerge within minutes or hours of taking the drug. A variety of other conditions can trigger hives, including: infections; irritations to the skin from latex, cosmetics or other chemicals; environmental factors such as heat, cold and sunlight; exercise; physical trauma; and stress. In many cases of hives, the cause is never identified.

PREVENTION

Prevent hives by identifying and avoiding substances or conditions that have caused you to break out in hives in the past. This may require closely reading food labels to be sure to eliminate allergy triggers. To reduce the risk of recurrent hives, wear loose-fitting clothes and take warm, but not hot, showers – measures that minimize irritation to the skin. If someone is allergic to insect venom, the doctor may advise carrying an injectable pen of

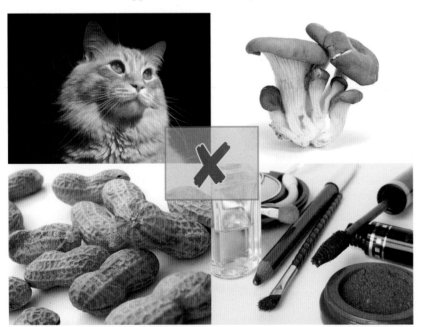

Hives can be triggered by a variety of allergens including pollen, animal hairs, mould, cosmetic products, insect stings and certain foods. The easiest way to control hives that are caused by allergic reactions is to identify and eliminate the cause.

epinephrine. Epinephrine is a medication used to prevent anaphylactic shock, a life-threatening allergic reaction that is characterized by difficulty breathing that can sometimes develop along with hives.

DIAGNOSIS

Hives can be diagnosed by anyone based on their appearance. See a doctor if the hives are persistent or recurrent, or if there are any other symptoms, such as difficulty breathing or tightness in the chest. Doctors can diagnose hives based on their appearance and a medical history, with special attention paid to whether there are any allergies, recent medications or new foods that may have caused them. If an allergy is suspected to be a factor, keeping a food diary can be a helpful way to track which foods may be the cause. With recurrent hives, the doctor may take blood tests or perform skin tests to diagnose allergies.

TREATMENTS

The preventative measures described above are the first line of treatment. Mild cases of hives usually go away on their own

CAUTION

If hives are accompanied by difficulty breathing or a swelling of the throat or tightness in the chest, go to the nearest hospital. This life-threatening emergency is an allergic reaction called anaphylaxis, and requires immediate medical treatment.

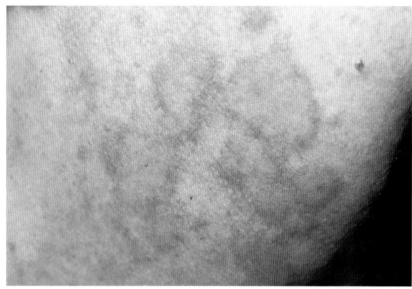

Hives are itchy red, white, or flesh-coloured oval welts on the skin that occur when immune system cells in the skin, called mast cells, release histamine, a chemical that causes inflammation. Hives usually go away on their own within a few hours or days.

within a few hours. The main goal of treatment is to reduce itching. This is important not only to relieve discomfort but also because scratching can cause the hives to spread. If hives are severe, persistent or recurrent, and especially if there are any other symptoms, medical treatment to stop the immune system's over-reaction may be needed.

• HYDROTHERAPY Applying cool compresses to the hives may reduce inflammation and discomfort. If hives cover a large area of the body, take cool baths.

• TOPICAL MEDICATIONS The itchiness of hives can usually be relieved with calamine lotion or hydrocortisone cream.

• ORAL MEDICATIONS Oral antihistamines can ease symptoms by temporarily interrupting the release of histamine, the chemical that causes hives, although these medications may cause drowsiness. If antihistamines do not

offer sufficient relief, an H2 receptor blocker (normally used to treat ulcers) may be prescribed. For severe or recurrent cases of hives, corticosteroids may be needed to suppress the immune system.

• STRESS REDUCTION In cases where hives are made worse by external events or environments, find ways to calm responses to stressful situations. Many complementary therapies have been shown to be effective, including yoga (pp.476–9), meditation (pp.514–19), guided imagery (pp.520–2), and biofeedback (pp.504–7).

• HYPNOSIS This therapy (pp.508–13) may be helpful because it has been shown to improve or resolve numerous skin conditions, including dermatitis and rosacea, as well as reduce the anxiety and pain associated with stressful dermatologic procedures.

See also: *Yoga, pp.476–9 • Guided Imagery, pp.520–1 • Biofeedback, pp.504–7*

HEAT INJURIES & SUNBURN

The body has natural defences against heat and sun. Even when a person feels hot on a summer day, their body is normally able to maintain a constant internal temperature using mechanisms such as sweating. The body's defence against the sun's burning rays is melanin, the skin's pigment and natural sunscreen. However, when someone spends too much time in very hot or sunny conditions, the body's natural defences may break down, leading to sunburn, heat exhaustion or heat stroke.

Skin becomes sunburned when it has been exposed for a long period to the damaging ultraviolet rays of the sun. Sunburned skin is red, painful and in severe cases, blistered. Heat exhaustion is characterized by fever of up to 40°C (104°F), headaches, nausea, fatigue and muscle cramps. Heatstroke can be life-threatening. Symptoms include a temperature, absence of sweating, and neurological symptoms such as mental confusion and loss of consciousness due to the failure of the body's temperature-regulating mechanisms.

CAUSES

Heat injuries are the result of dehydration caused by spending too much time in heat without replacing fluids and electrolytes lost through perspiration. Dehydration impairs the functioning of the body's cooling mechanism, resulting in heat exhaustion. If this is not treated, it can progress to heatstroke. Some medications increase the risk of heat injuries by promoting dehydration, including diuretics for high blood pressure (pp.236–9), some antipsychotic drugs, and some sedatives.

Sunburn is caused by ultraviolet light from the sun. The amount of time it takes to cause sunburn depends on the shade of the skin and the time of day. Light-colored skin burns faster than dark skin because it has less melanin. Regardless of skin type, sunburn occurs faster during midday, when the sun's rays are strongest. Several medications can increase the skin's sensitivity to the sun and the risk of sunburn, including topical retinoic acid for acne, oral contraceptives, tricyclic antidepressants, and some antibiotics (tetracycline and quinolones).

PREVENTION

To prevent heat injuries, take precautions against becoming

Clinical Query

Is it a good idea to give salt tablets to someone with heat exhaustion?

No. Even though heat exhaustion is caused by a loss of fluids and salts (electrolytes), the large amount of salt in salt tablets can make the problem worse by causing further dehydration. It is beneficial, however, for the person to drink a fluid with some salt in it, such as electrolyte solution or lightly salted water.

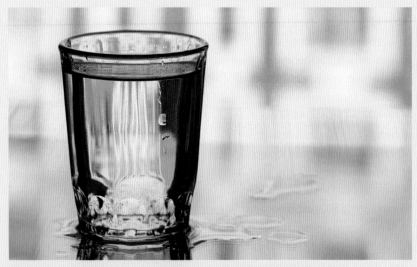

To prevent heat injuries, take precautions against becoming overheated and dehydrated. It is very important to drink plenty of water, but also replace any missing minerals and electrolytes. Do this by taking a sports drink.

dehydrated and overheated. Be especially vigilant about preventative measures if taking a medication that increases the risk of dehydration. Drink plenty of water throughout the day, but be careful to also replace needed minerals and electrolytes if you are exercising by drinking a sports drink or taking a specially formulated supplement. Reduce consumption of caffeine and alcohol on hot days, because they promote dehydration. On hot days, wear lightweight clothing and limit strenuous activities at midday. If active, take periodic breaks.

If someone develops any of the symptoms of heat exhaustion, such as headaches or nausea, they should cool themselves by drinking an electrolyte solution or sports drink to replace lost fluids and salts, and by taking a swim or going into the shade or an air-conditioned building.

To prevent sunburn, limit the amount of time spent outdoors from 10 a.m. to 2 p.m., when the risk of sunburn is greatest. When outdoors during the day, use a sunscreen that protects against the full spectrum of ultraviolet light that causes sunburn: ultraviolet A and ultraviolet B light. Sunscreen does not completely prevent sunburn; it merely delays the time that it would otherwise take for the skin to burn. So it is still important to limit sun exposure and to wear a hat on sunny days for added protection.

Green tea, as well as beta-carotene and lycopene, two antioxidant nutrients, may reduce the risk of sunburn. However, because re-

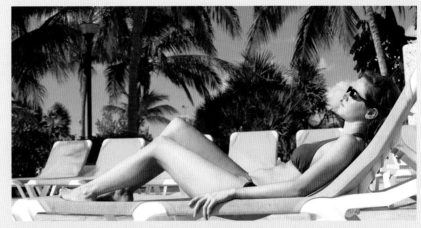

Tanning occurs when the skin produces the pigment melanin in response to damage caused by exposure to ultraviolet radiation. Sun exposure can also lead to more serious heatlh conditions such as cataracts, a reduced immune system, and skin cancer.

search on these alternative remedies is not definitive, they should not be considered a replacement for proven measures to prevent sunburn.

DIAGNOSIS

Heat injuries and sunburn can be diagnosed from the symptoms. See a doctor immediately or go to the nearest hospital with symptoms of heatstroke. Further testing may be needed to detect complications such as muscle damage.

TREATMENTS

First aid is usually sufficient to treat heat exhaustion and sunburn. Heatstroke often requires medical treatment.

Heat Exhaustion

The preventative measures discussed earlier are often sufficient. In addition, loosen or remove unnecessary clothing and apply cool compresses to the skin. If symptoms do not improve, call a doctor.

Heatstroke

This is an emergency. Before reaching the hospital, first aid

to cool the body can be helpful, such as wrapping in wet sheets. Do not use fever-reducing medicines, such as paracetomol or ibuprofen – they cannot lower the fever. Other medications may be needed for complications, such as seizures (pp.176–7).

Sunburn

Cool compresses can relieve discomfort. If blisters form, cover them with bandages to prevent infection. Ibuprofen or paracetomol can be helpful to lower temperature if there is a fever.

See also: *Acne, pp.99–101 • High Blood Pressure, pp.236–9 • Epilepsy & Seizure, pp.176–7*

CAUTION

Get emergency medical assistance for the following symptoms of heatstroke:
• Loss of consciousness
• Seizures
• Mental impairment such as confusion
• Rapid pulse or breathing

Burns

Contact with hot liquids or vapours, fire, electricity, hot objects, or corrosive chemicals can cause burns. Symptoms depend on the severity of the wound and include pain and swelling of the skin. Because burns impair the skin's ability to shield the body from germs, they increase the potential for infections. While superficial burns affect only the surface of the skin, severe burns can penetrate to muscle and bone.

CAUSES

Burns are usually caused by accidents. The specific cause varies with the type of burn.

Thermal Burns

The most common burns occur when the skin comes in contact with something hot: fire, hot liquids, steam or hot objects. Common causes are handling hot dishes and pots while cooking, house fires, road accidents, and electrical malfunctions. A scald is a burn caused by hot liquid. Inhaling smoke or very hot steam can cause a thermal burn in the airways.

Chemical Burns

Most chemical burns are caused by corrosive agents such as acids and alkalis. These kinds of chemicals cause a reaction with the skin in which chemical energy is converted to heat. Household cleaning fluids such as ammonia, paint strippers and garden chemicals, as well as industrial chemicals, can cause chemical burns. Inhaling toxic chemicals can also burn the airways.

Electrical Burns

Contact with a source of electricity, such as electrical outlets, defective electrical appliances, power lines and lightning, causes these burns.

PREVENTION

Install smoke detectors in the home and keep a fire extinguisher in the kitchen. Keep children away from matches and other sources of fire. When cooking, turn pot handles away from the edge of the stove to prevent scalding liquid from spilling and to avoid accidentally touching them. To prevent chemical burns, keep household chemicals stored safely and wear protective gloves when using corrosive chemicals.

DIAGNOSIS

Burns can be diagnosed and categorized based on their appearance. A doctor should be called immediately to diagnose burns that are larger than the palm of a hand, look deep, are caused by chemicals, electricity or smoke inhalation, are oozing pus, or are accompanied by other symptoms, such as fever or shock.

TREATMENTS

First-degree burns and most second-degree burns that are smaller than 7.6 cm (3 in) in diameter can be treated at home with first aid. Larger or more severe burns require immediate medical attention.

- **FIRST AID** Hold the affected skin under cold water for about five minutes to reduce the pain. An ice cube or even a bag of frozen vegetables can also be used as a cold compress. Then dry the skin and cover the area with a bandage to protect it from irritation and infection. Over-the-counter pain relief such as ibuprofen or paracetomol can be taken to relieve discomfort.
- **SUPPLEMENTS** Selenium, phosphorus and vitamin B_5 may reduce the time it takes for burns to heal. There is also some scientific evidence supporting the use of supplements of arginine, which dilates blood vessels, but more research is needed.
- **HERBAL REMEDIES** Topical preparations made from the pulp of leaves from the aloe vera plant are often used to ease the pain of minor burns, and may speed up healing time. Dashen, a herb used in Traditional Chinese Medicine (pp.446–7) that is swallowed or injected, may also speed recovery from burns.

See also: *Traditional Chinese Medicine, pp.446–7 • Supplements, pp.532–43*

Dry Skin

Skin that lacks enough water beneath its surface to make it supple and soft becomes rough, scaly, and more wrinkled than usual. Nearly everyone occasionally has areas of dry skin, but it becomes more common with age because oil glands beneath the skin become less active. With less oil, moisture in the skin evaporates faster. Areas that are most often affected are the arms, legs and sides of the abdomen.

CAUSES

Apart from ageing, seasonal and environmental factors are the most common causes of dry skin. Dry skin tends to be worse during the winter because cold, dry outdoor air and hot, dry indoor air can deplete the skin of its natural moisture. During the summer, sunburn can make the skin dry and flaky. Dry skin is also a symptom of a wide range of ailments: thyroid and parathyroid disorders (p.350), Coeliac disease, lymphoma (p.328), rheumatoid arthritis (pp.136–7), and dermatitis (pp.102–3). It can also be a side-effect of medication such as topical retinoic acid and creams and lotions used to treat acne (pp.99–101).

PREVENTION

Prevent dry skin by using a moisturizer or bath oil regularly. Moisturizers, which are oil-based lubricants, help conserve water beneath the skin by preventing it from evaporating. The best time to apply moisturizer is after a bath or shower, when the skin is damp.

When bathing or showering, use warm instead of hot water. Avoid alkaline soaps, which can dry the skin. Instead, use soaps with a high fat content, such as glycerin soaps.

Other measures include using a humidifier at home if the indoor air is very dry. Protect skin from sunburn by using sunscreen and wearing a hat when outdoors. Drinking several glasses of water each day is beneficial, too, because it replenishes moisture in the body.

DIAGNOSIS

Dry skin is diagnosed by its appearance. See a doctor if the skin is so dry and itchy that it prevents sleep, there are open wounds from scratching, or itchiness without a rash. The doctor may do a physical examination and ask questions about health history and symptoms, including those that are not skin-related, to discover if the dry skin is due to an underlying illness.

TREATMENTS

The goal of treatment is to prevent the skin from losing water. Follow the preventative measures outlined above. Creams and lotions that contain hydrocortisone can help reduce inflammation if the skin becomes irritated. Topical preparations that contain lactic acid, salicylic acid or urea are highly effective for very dry, scaly skin.

If an underlying illness is the cause of dry skin, treating the illness also reduces the dryness.

See also: *Acne, pp.99–101 • Dermatitis, pp.102–3 • Thyroid Disorders, pp.344–7*

WHO IS AT RISK?

The risk factors include:

- Regular exposure to dry air, indoors or outdoors
- Sunburn
- Hot baths and showers
- Alkaline soap
- Thyroid disorders, rheumatoid arthritis, and Coeliac disease
- Medications such as retinoic acid and other acne treatments

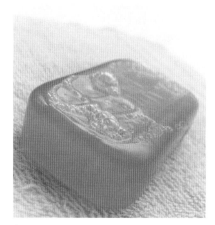

Soap may aggravate dry skin, but using a product with a high fat content, such as glycerin, can help alleviate the condition.

Calluses & Corns

Areas of hard, thick skin can be either calluses or corns. Corns develop on the toes, while calluses form most often on the bottoms of the feet, the heels, and the hands. Both are made from keratin, a strong, fibrous protein that grows on the skin in response to repeated friction, forming a kind of armour to protect the skin. Calluses and corns are not dangerous, but the skin beneath them is sometimes painful.

CAUSES

Corns are most commonly caused by ill-fitting shoes that rub against the toes. Calluses are caused by any activity that causes repeated pressure against an area of skin, including sports, gardening and other manual labour, walking barefoot or playing a musical instrument. Having a bunion, an abnormal bony protrusion from the big toe, increases the risk of developing calluses because the bunion is likely to rub against the shoe.

PREVENTION

Anything that protects the skin from repeated friction will reduce the risk of calluses and corns. Wear gloves when playing sports or digging in the garden or doing other manual work. Wear shoes that fit properly. Do not walk barefoot on rough surfaces.

DIAGNOSIS

Calluses and corns can be diagnosed by their appearance and location. People should see a doctor if the skin beneath a callus or corn is particularly painful, if it seems inflamed or infected, or if they have diabetes (pp.338–41); diabetes sufferers are prone to infections and skin ulcers from circulatory problems in the hands and feet.

TREATMENTS

Simple self-care measures can often reduce or eliminate calluses and corns. If corns are painful, cover them with corn pads – doughnut-shaped cushions designed to relieve pressure on corns when walking. Switching to comfortable shoes can, by itself, often get rid of corns within a few weeks. Moisturizers can help soften calluses. For bunions, flat, extra wide shoes can minimize friction. If these measures are insufficient, consider seeing a podiatrist. They may recommend orthodics – custom shoe inserts designed to reduce pressure and friction.

• **ABRASION** Make corns and calluses flatter by rubbing them gently with a pumice stone when the skin is soft after bathing or by applying a topical preparation to soften them, such as salicylic acid plaster. However, these preparations risk damaging the skin.

• **MEDICATION** Calluses and corns that become infected may need to be treated with a full course of antibiotics in order to heal them completely.

• **SURGERY** Calluses and corns that are very large, hard and painful can be cut away by a dermatologist or podiatrist. Large bunions may need to be reduced with foot surgery. Treating bunions usually prevents more calluses.

See also: *Diabetes, pp.338–41*

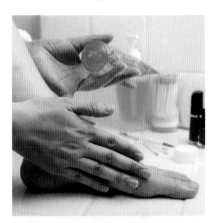

Corns can be treated by soaking feet and using a pumice stone when skin is soft. A topical preparation such as salicylic acid can also be used to treat corns.

Dandruff

Scalp skin replaces itself, on average, about once every 28 days. If disease causes the turnover to speed up to every 11 days, dandruff – dry, flaky skin that sheds from the scalp – results. It is the most common type of seborrhoeic dermatitis, or seborrhoea (pp.102–3), which is characterized by patches of itchy red skin with large flakes scattered about the scalp, hairline, eyebrows and even in the ears.

Among adults, dandruff affects men more often than women. It is also common among infants, in which case it is called cradle cap. Dandruff is a harmless condition and can be controlled with special shampoos, but it tends to recur.

CAUSES

Dandruff runs in families, which suggests that there it has a hereditary component. People with oily hair or skin, acne (pp.99–101), or psoriasis (pp.120–1) are especially prone to developing dandruff. For reasons that are not clear, people with various other medical conditions also tend to develop dandruff, including obesity, Parkinson's disease (p.181), stroke (pp.168–9), head injury and HIV (pp.316–17). In addition, flare-ups of dandruff are often brought on by extremely hot or cold weather, emotional stress, and fatigue.

Inadequate washing of the hair and other aspects of personal hygiene do not cause dandruff. However, shampooing the hair too infrequently can cause a flare-up of dandruff if a person is already prone to the condition.

PREVENTION

It is possible to reduce the incidence and severity of dandruff by reducing the controllable risk factors. Shampoo hair only often enough to keep it from getting oily. Maintain a normal weight by eating a healthy diet and getting regular exercise. If suffering from acne or psoriasis, see a doctor for treatment. Control stress with proven strategies, such as progressive muscle relaxation (pp.474–5), yoga (pp.476–7), meditation (pp.514–19) and exercise.

DIAGNOSIS

Dandruff is diagnosed by appearance. Call a doctor if there are signs of infection, such as painful red patches on the scalp, with fluid or pus.

TREATMENTS

The treatment is different for adults and infants.

Adults

Dandruff can usually be controlled with a medicated shampoo that contains salicylic acid, coal tar, zinc, resorcin or selenium. Use the shampoo daily and scrub the scalp for about five minutes. Shampoo containing 5 percent tea tree oil is also effective. If this does not work, a doctor may prescribe a shampoo that contains a ketoconazole, an antifungal medicine and corticosteroids. An oral homeopathic remedy consisting of potassium bromide, sodium bromide, nickel sulphate, and sodium chloride has also proven helpful.

Infants

Shampooing an infant's hair daily with a mild shampoo or soap can often get rid of cradle cap. If this is insufficient, massage the baby's scalp with mineral oil and cover it with a warm, moist towel for an hour before shampooing.

See also: *Acne, pp.99–101 • Psoriasis, pp.120–1 • Progressive Muscle Relaxation, pp.474–5*

WHO IS AT RISK?

The risk factors include:

- Family history
- Infrequent shampooing
- Oily skin
- Acne
- Psoriasis
- Obesity
- Stress
- Fatigue
- Very hot or cold weather
- Neurological conditions (head trauma, stroke, Parkinson's disease)
- HIV

Frostbite

When the skin and, sometimes, the underlying tissue freeze, the injury is called frostbite. It can be temporary or it can cause lasting damage, depending on the severity. There are four degrees of frostbite. First-degree affects only the surface of the skin, causing it to turn white, swell and become temporarily numb. Second-degree also affects the skin's surface, but with more severe damage characterized by a firm or waxy texture and blisters filled with clear fluid.

Third-degree frostbite affects all layers of the skin. The skin turns blue and forms blisters with dark, bloody fluid. Fourth-degree affects the muscle and bone and carries the risk of gangrene (tissue death). Frostbite is most likely to occur on the exposed extremities – the hands, feet, nose and ears. Do not begin to thaw frostbitten skin until indoors or sufficiently protected from freezing temperatures. If the thawed skin gets frostbitten again, it can suffer additional damage.

CAUSES

Frostbite occurs when skin is inadequately protected against extreme cold or when a person spends too much time outdoors when the temperature is below freezing. Wind increases the risk because it accelerates heat loss. Especially vulnerable are people with illnesses that impair circulation, including diabetes (pp.338–41), peripheral vascular disease (pp.254–5), and Raynaud's disease (p.243). Beta-blockers, medication taken for

high blood pressure (pp.236–9), also reduce circulation to the extremities, increasing susceptibility.

PREVENTION

Dress warmly, paying special attention to the extremities, and do not stay outdoors if gloves, socks and other clothing become wet, because wet clothing accelerates heat loss. Do not wear tight-fitting clothing because it can restrict blood circulation. Limit time spent outdoors if you have a condition that impairs blood circulation or if taking beta-blockers. Smoking and drinking alcohol before going outdoors in freezing weather can hasten frostbite, because those activities dilate the blood vessels, so avoid them.

DIAGNOSIS

Frostbite is diagnosed by the symptoms and the appearance of the skin. Tingling, throbbing or aching in an area of skin are early signs of frostbite; go indoors and warm up immediately if experiencing these warning signs.

WHO IS AT RISK?

The risk factors include:
- Prolonged exposure to freezing temperatures
- Illnesses that impair blood circulation, including diabetes, peripheral vascular disease, and Raynaud's disease
- Beta-blockers
- Drinking alcohol shortly before going outdoors in freezing weather
- Smoking

TREATMENTS

First aid to warm the body and thaw the affected area is often all that is needed. Go indoors and either wrap the frostbitten skin in a warm cloth or immerse it in warm water. Do not use hot water or rub the skin, as these can cause further damage. Continue warming until the skin regains sensation and softness. Warm drinks can help warm the body and prevent dehydration.

• MEDICATION Treat any blisters with an antibiotic ointment and cover them with a sterile bandage to prevent infection. If needed, relieve discomfort and reduce inflammation with topical aloe vera or by taking a nonsteroidal anti-inflammatory agent such as ibuprofen. Emergency medical care is needed if the skin does not regain sensation and normal colour following first-aid.

See also: *Diabetes, pp.338–41* • *Raynaud's disease, p.243* • *Smoking Cessation, pp.216–17*

Fungal Nail Infections

Ringworm, the same mould-like fungus that causes skin infections, can also infect the fingernails and toenails. Fungal nail infections are called onychomycosis. They are most common in toenails and they frequently follow a bout of athlete's foot, a fungal skin infection (p.105). Fungal infections cause nails to become thick and deformed and can make them pull away from the skin, crumble and even fall off. These infections occur mainly in adults and can be difficult to treat, but good hygiene can prevent them.

CAUSES

Fungal nail infections are caused by dermatophytes, a type of fungus. Walking barefoot in locker rooms, around public swimming-pools, and in other warm, moist public places increases the risk of developing fungal toenail infections. Diabetes and other conditions that reduce blood circulation to the hands and feet also increase the risk.

PREVENTION

Wearing sandals or shoes can prevent fungal infections of the toenails. Prompt treatment may prevent athlete's foot from spreading to the nails. Once a nail infection is cured, a nail lacquer that contains an antifungal agent can be used prophylactically to help prevent a recurrence.

DIAGNOSIS

A doctor may scrape part of the nail for laboratory analysis to confirm an initial diagnosis based on the appearance of the nail.

TREATMENTS

Antifungal medication is used to treat these infections. It can take three months or longer to cure a fungal infection, and even then they often recur. An antifungal nail lacquer is sometimes sufficient for mild to moderate nail infections, but oral antifungal medicine is needed to treat severe or recurrent nail infections. Oral antifungal medications should be used with caution, however, because they can be toxic to the liver.

See also: *Fungal Skin Infection, pp.104–5* • *Diabetes, pp.338–41*

On Call

Changes in one or more nails are signs of fungal infection.

- Discoloration
- Texture changes (brittleness or thickening)
- Distorted shape
- Crumbling
- Debris beneath the nail
- Pulling away from the skin or falling off

WHO IS AT RISK?

The risk factors include:

- Walking barefoot in public areas
- Athlete's foot
- Diabetes
- Poor circulation

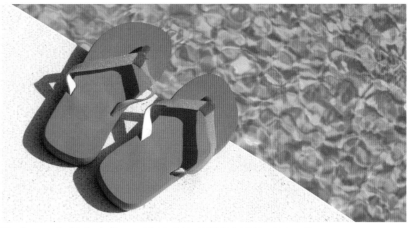

The fungus that infects fingernails and toenails thrives in warm, wet environments. Wearing shoes or sandals around public swimming-pools and locker rooms can reduce the risk of getting these fungal infections.

Alopecia

A partial or complete loss of hair from the head or other areas where it normally grows is called alopecia. It occurs when old hair strands fall out faster than new ones can grow to replace them. The most common type of hair loss is a gradually receding hairline in the middle of the scalp, leaving a fringe of hair on either side. This is called male-pattern baldness because it mostly affects men. In women, the hair usually thins hair throughout the scalp. Hair loss can be temporary or permanent, and can be scarring or non-scarring, depending on the cause.

WHO IS AT RISK?
The risk factors include:
- Advancing age
- Male
- Family history of baldness
- Ringworm of the scalp
- Chemotherapy and radiation treatments for cancer
- Stress
- Childbirth
- End of pregnancy
- Oral contraceptives

CAUSES
Baldness becomes more common as people age. The tendency to become bald runs in families, as well, which suggests a genetic cause. Testosterone and its conversion to 5 alpha testosterone, the sex hormone that is most abundant in men, causes male-pattern baldness. Other sex hormones may play a role in baldness in women, because they tend to experience hair loss after childbirth and menopause when levels of oestrogen and other hormones are changing. Temporary hair loss can also be caused by the rapid hormonal changes associated with childbirth, terminating a pregnancy, and starting or stopping oral contraceptives.

Certain illnesses and medical treatments can also cause hair loss. A dysfunction of the immune system is believed to cause alopecia areata, which is the temporary loss of hair in patches on the scalp, beard, and sometimes the eyebrows and eyelashes; this condition can be very difficult to treat. Tinea capitis, or ringworm of the scalp (p.105), also causes bald patches on the head. Systemic diseases such as lupus (pp.324–5) can cause hair loss. Chemotherapy and radiation treatments for cancer can cause temporary hair loss.

Physical and emotional stress can cause hair to fall out at an increased rate, a temporary condition that is called telogen effluvium. Some people lose hair because they have a nervous habit of pulling it out.

PREVENTION
Good hygiene can reduce the risk of developing ringworm of the scalp. Avoid sharing hairbrushes and other personal care items. Strategies to control emotional stress can help prevent hair loss. These include relaxation techniques, meditation (pp.514–19), yoga (pp.476-9), guided imagery (pp.520–2) and exercise.

DIAGNOSIS
A doctor can diagnose the cause of hair loss by examining the pattern of baldness and by asking about other symptoms and taking a health history. A skin biopsy may be needed if a rash or other skin changes accompany hair loss.

TREATMENTS
The treatment for all forms of alopecia depends on what is causing the hair loss. Some causes require no treatment because the

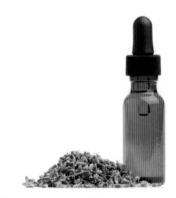

Alopecia areata, which causes patchy baldness on the head and body, may respond to some herbal treatments.

hair loss is temporary, such as thinning hair following childbirth and menopause.

• **SURGERY** Hair transplant surgery is a permanent treatment for male-pattern baldness or other hair loss that does not affect the entire scalp. A doctor removes small plugs of hair, skin and underlying tissue from donor areas – areas with ample hair growth – and transplants them to the bald, or recipient areas.

• **ESSENTIAL OILS** Rubbing essential oils containing cedarwood, lavender, rosemary and thyme into the scalp may promote hair growth for people with alopecia areata. Onion juice also appears to be beneficial.

• **MEDICATION** Two medications can promote new hair growth for people with male-pattern baldness. Minoxidil is a topical medication that stimulates hair growth within about six months. Finasteride is an oral medication for men only that changes the action of testosterone by inhibiting the enzyme that converts testosterone to its more active form at the hair follicle.

Scalp ringworm is treated with a course of oral antifungal drugs.

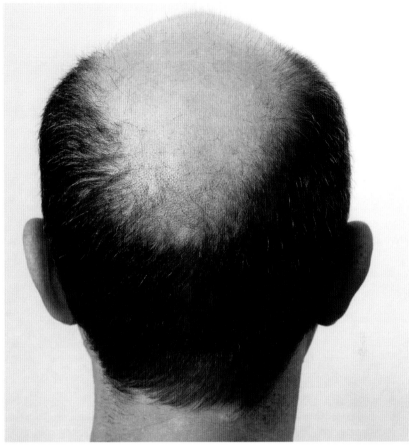

Androgenetic alopecia, or male-pattern baldness, is the most common type of hair loss, affecting 30 to 40 percent of both men and women. The condition creates a gradually receding hairline and is often the result of hormonal changes within the hair follicle.

For alopecia areata, injected steroids can be used to reduce the underlying inflammation, but this treatment is not uniformly effective at halting hair loss or promoting regrowth.

• **LIGHT THERAPY** This treatment (p.564), which uses a low-powered laser to stimulate cells, is also used for alopecia areata, but its effectiveness is also limited.

• **MELATONIN** In a pilot study conducted in 2004 at Friedrich-Schiller University in Jena, Germany, 40 women with male-pattern baldness had significantly more hair after applying a topical solution of melatonin applied daily for six months. In contrast, there was no increase in hair growth in a control group. Melatonin is a hormone that controls the body's inner clock.

See also: *Lupus, pp.324–5 • Meditation, pp.514–19 • Yoga, pp.476–9*

healing hope

Two years ago I decided to get my hair cut short, but after I did I noticed my hair seemed thinner all over than I remembered. Then last year I went through a stressful episode with my job, and my hair started coming out in clumps. Every morning my pillow was covered with hair that had fallen out while I slept. I'm only 26 – too young to be going bald, I thought.

I went to a dermatologist who suggested I try a special shampoo for hair loss, which did nothing. Then she gave me a prescription, and after about seven months I realized my hair loss had stopped. But so far it has only barely started growing back. My dermatologist said it might take some time. Even though I'm still anxious to see if my hair will come back, it's such a relief at least to know that it has stopped falling out.   *Bill C.*

Scabies & Lice

Scabies are small mites that tunnel beneath the skin to lay their eggs, often leaving a visible mark in their wake. The first symptom is itching that is most intense at night, followed by a red rash that may form a crust. Scabies is most likely to affect the hands, wrists, genitals and abdomen, although in very young children an infestation may occur anywhere on the body.

Lice are insects that feed on blood and lay their eggs (called nits) on the skin's surface or clothing. They can affect the scalp (head lice), pubic hair (pubic lice) or the entire body (body lice). Lice also cause itching and sometimes a rash. Both scabies and lice are highly contagious.

CAUSES
Both of these pests can be picked up via contact with an infested person. Head lice can also be caused by contact with hats, combs and brushes used by someone who is infested. Pubic lice are transmitted during sexual relations with an infested person,

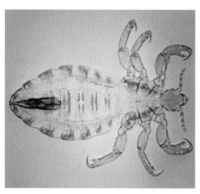
Body lice live on the body and in clothing or bedding. Adult lice are greyish–white and are about the size of a sesame seed.

as well as contact with infested bedding. Poor hygiene, living in close quarters, and contact with infested bedding also increase the risk of body lice.

PREVENTION
Reduce the risk of being infested with lice or scabies by avoiding contact with infested people, as well as their clothing and bed sheets. Do not share personal items, such as hats, combs, brushes and towels.

DIAGNOSIS
Scabies and lice can be diagnosed by a physical examination.

TREATMENTS
Medication and vigilant hygiene can eliminate both kinds of infestation.
• **INSECTICIDES** Scabies can often be eliminated with one treatment of a cream that contains permethrin, an insecticide. If this does not work, ivermectin, an oral drug that kills parasites, may be prescribed. Head lice and pubic lice are treated with a shampoo that contains permethrin or pyrethrin and piperonyl butox-

WHO IS AT RISK?
The risk factors include:
• Contact with an infected person
• Contact with infested bedding or clothing
• Sharing personal care items such as combs and brushes
• Poor hygiene

ide, and body lice with a cream or wash containing the same anti-parasite ingredients.
• **HERBAL TREATMENT** A topical preparation of turmeric and the herb neem (*Azadirachta indica*) is effective for eliminating scabies.
• **ESSENTIAL OILS** A combination of coconut oil, anise oil and ylang ylang oil applied to the scalp can be used to control head lice. A topical preparation made from citronella can also prevent a re-infestation of head lice. An essential oil made from the leaves of *Lippia multiflora* 'Moldenke' (also known as bush tea) is effective against scabies.
• **PHYSICAL ENVIRONMENT** For head lice and pubic lice, a fine-tooth comb is needed to remove nits, the lice eggs, because they are not affected by insecticides. Wash all affected clothing and bedding in hot water or dry clean them to prevent lice and scabies from spreading.

See also: *Homeopathy, pp.455–7 • Traditional Chinese Medicine, pp.446–7*

Bedsores

Painful ulcers that form on areas of skin subject to constant pressure are called bedsores. They are most common among elderly or disabled people who are bedridden or who sit for many hours in wheelchairs. Bedsores form on bony areas such as the base of the neck, the shoulders and shoulder blades, base of the spine, elbows, hips, sides of the knees and sides of the feet. They can be minor or life-threatening, and are easier to prevent than to treat.

WHO IS AT RISK?
The risk factors include:
- Advanced age
- Being bedridden
- Regular use of a wheelchair
- Diabetes
- Peripheral vascular disease
- Poor nutrition

CAUSES
Bedsores are often caused by lying or sitting in the same position. Unremitting pressure restricts the flow of blood to an area of skin, starving it of oxygen and nutrients. After about two to three hours, the skin may develop open sores. Moisture compounds the damage.

Other conditions, such as diabetes (pp.338–41) and peripheral vascular disease (pp.254–5), reduce blood flow to the extremeties. Poor nutrition can lower the immune system's ability to fight infections and also reduces the amount of cushioning body fat and can deprive the skin of vital nutrients.

PREVENTION
Change position frequently when sitting or lying down. Sprinkle powder on the sheets, regularly wash and dry the skin, and apply a cream or ointment that protects the skin from moisture. Also, for people who are bedridden or in wheelchairs, check the condition of the skin regularly for redness and other early signs of bedsores.

Use pillows or cushions to relieve pressure areas. Good nutrition can help fortify the skin.

DIAGNOSIS
Bedsores can be diagnosed at home by their appearance. Sores that are red, inflamed or foul-smelling should be examined by a doctor for infection.

TREATMENTS
Treatment depends on the severity of the bedsore. Rinse very superficial bedsores with salt water and cover them. Relieve pressure on the affected area.
- **DEBRIDMENT** For bedsores that are oozing, a doctor will remove dead cells. A promising complementary therapy is the use of sterilized bottle fly maggots (*Phaenicia sericata*). When applied to wounds, maggots remove the dead cells, which accelerates healing.
- **WOUND CLOSURE** Newer treatments include vacuum-assisted devices that close a wound with suction; injection of growth-factors, which are proteins that

stimulate new cell growth; hyperbaric oxygen treatment to increase the oxygen supply to the tissues; and, for advanced sores that do not heal, skin grafting.
- **MEDICATION** Oral antibiotics may be needed to control infections.
- **NUTRITION** Deficiencies of protein, vitamin C and zinc can impair the skin's ability to heal. A high-protein diet and a daily multivitamin and mineral supplement may improve wound healing.

See also: *Diabetes, pp.338–41* • *Peripheral Vascular Disease, pp.254–5*

Bedsores are categorized by stages of severity.

Stage 1 A red area that does not turn white when pressed; this is a superficial sore.

Stage 2 A sore with a blister.

Stage 3 A sore that is indented, indicating damage to tissue beneath the skin.

Stage 4 A white or black sore with a foul odour; it has damaged the muscle or bone and can cause a fatal blood infection.

Psoriasis

When scaly, inflamed patches of skin come and go, the cause could be psoriasis, a common chronic skin condition. The patches often burn and itch. While psoriasis can occur anywhere on the body, it is most common on the scalp, elbows, knees, hands and lower back. It is not contagious. Although there is no cure, there are several treatments that can control the condition.

CAUSES

Experts think psoriasis occurs when the immune system malfunctions and signals skin cells to grow and replace themselves abnormally quickly. When this happens, an overabundance of dead cells accumulates on the surface of the skin and form thick scales. A genetic predisposition is thought to be the underlying cause of the immune system abnormality, because many people with psoriasis have relatives with the condition. But for people who are genetically predisposed, several physical and emotional triggers appear to trigger the condition. Medications such as beta-blockers, antimalarial drugs and lithium can cause flare-ups. Infections such as strep throat, skin injuries such as scratches and allergies can bring on psoriasis. Although moderate amounts of sunlight can actually help, too much exposure, and especially sunburn, can bring on the condition. So can exposure to toxic chemicals. Cold weather is another trigger. And because stress affects the immune system, it can also cause flare-ups.

One possible complication of psoriasis is psoriatic arthritis, in which the abnormal immune response causes inflammation in the joints as well as overproduction of skin cells.

PREVENTION

There is no known way to prevent psoriasis, but it may be possible to reduce the incidence of flare-ups. Prevent sunburn by limiting exposure to the sun and wearing sunscreen and a hat when outdoors in midday. In addition, control daily stress with proven strategies such as meditation (pp.514–19), yoga (pp.476–9), exercise, and relaxation techniques.

DIAGNOSIS

There are several types of psoriasis, each with different symptoms:
• Plaque psoriasis, the most common form, causes round or oval plaques on the skin. About 10 percent of affected people also have arthritis symptoms.
• Psoriasis vulgaris causes silvery scales.
• Guttate is characterized by small, dot-like lesions.

• Pustular has weeping lesions and intense scaling.
• Inverse causes intense inflammation.
• Erythrodermic is marked by intense shedding and redness of the skin.

A doctor can diagnose psoriasis by its appearance. The doctor may take a biopsy of the affected skin to confirm that the cause is psoriasis and not dermatitis (pp.102–3), which can look similar.

TREATMENTS

The treatment used depends on the type of psoriasis and how severe it is. Treatment can be complex, because psoriasis flares up and then symptoms recede, but the flare-ups cannot always be attributed to a specific cause. Similarly, not all treatments work for all cases, and people can become resistant to a specific treatment over time. Several treatments are often combined or used in rotation, with the goal of achieving the lowest possible cell turnover with the fewest side effects.
• MOISTURIZERS AND TOPICAL TREATMENTS These are first-line

WHO IS AT RISK?

The risk factors include:
• Family history
• Sunburn or other skin injury
• Exposure to cold air
• Systemic infection
• Stress

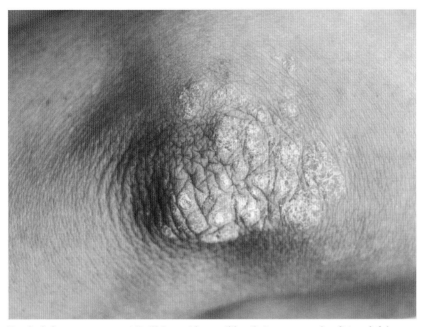

Psoriasis is a common, usually lifelong skin condition that causes scaly, often painful patches of skin that appear most often on the scalp, elbows, knees, hands and lower back. A majority of sufferers also experience joint pain associated with psoriasis.

treatments for psoriasis. Moisturizers such as petroleum jelly are used to relieve redness and itching. Preparations made from coal tar have been used for hundreds of years to reduce inflammation and relieve itching and redness. Corticosteroids reduce inflammation. Other topical medicines that are used to reduce or remove scales include calciprtriol, a synthetic form of vitamin D, salicylic acid and retinoids.

• PHOTOTHERAPY Ultraviolet light treatment, also called phototherapy (p.564), slows down the rate of skin cell growth. It is used when psoriasis does not respond adequately to topical preparations. There are three kinds of phototherapy.

Ultraviolet B uses lamps that emit the ultraviolet B spectrum of light. The patient is exposed several times a week. This is the mildest type of light therapy, and

it can be given in a doctor's surgery or at home. It does not cause skin cancer or other adverse effects.

Psoralen plus ultraviolet A light (PUVA) is used when ultraviolet B light does not work. The patient is exposed to light in the ultraviolet A spectrum and takes psoralen, a light-sensitive drug. The drawback of PUVA therapy is that it can only be used for a few months because exposure to UVA light increases the risk of developing skin cancer.

Lasers are the newest delivery system for phototherapy, and are used on relatively small patches of psoriasis. Because lasers can be focused to specific areas, they can deliver high amounts of ultraviolet B light without risking harm to surrounding healthy skin.

• MEDICATION Oral retinoids help clear away skin scales. Cyclosporine suppresses the immune system, thereby reducing the

inflammation that causes psoriasis. Methotrexate slows down the rate of skin cell growth. Biologics, the newest medications for psoriasis, are made from proteins that affect cells or chemicals that are involved in the psoriasis process. These oral medications have severe side effects and, therefore, are prescribed only when other treatments are not effective. Oral retinoids should not be used by women who are or may become pregnant because of the potential for birth defects.

• HERBAL REMEDIES Many herbal preparations are used for psoriasis, in studies: aloe vera cream; oatmeal baths; and oral preparations made from extracts of polypodiaceae, a fern species that grows in South America and Europe.

• CLIMATOTHERAPY Treating an illness by spending time in a particular region is called climatotherapy. Exposure to seawater, a type of climatotherapy, can help clear up psoriasis. The beneficial effect of exposure to water from the Dead Sea, which is high in mineral salts, has been established clinically. A study published in Acta Dermatoverol Croatia in 2004 found that treatment in Veli Losinj in Croatia, a beach resort that also has water fed by a mountain spring, led to long-lasting remission without the use of corticosteroids.

• STRESS REDUCTION Meditation (pp.514–19) and hypnosis (pp.508–13) may help clear up psoriasis, when used with conventional therapies.

See also: *Meditation, pp.514–19 • Yoga, pp.476–9 • Dermatitis, pp.102–3*

Melanoma

Worldwide, the incidence of melanoma is growing faster than it is for any other form of cancer. Melanoma is cancer of the melanocytes, the cells that give the skin its colour. It is most common on the skin, but also occurs in the pigment-producing cells of the eyes (pp.46–7). Early detection is crucial because melanoma is the most aggressive form of skin cancer. It looks like a freckle or mole, but it is more than one shade of brown or black, is asymmetrical, and changes colour and shape.

In addition, a melanoma often itches, bleeds or oozes fluid, and similar spots may appear around it. Unlike most other types of cancer, melanoma is common among young adults. In men, melanoma is most likely to develop on the back, chest, neck or face, and on women it is most common on the arms and legs.

CAUSES

There are several environmental and biological causes of melanoma. An important cause is an overexposure to ultraviolet light, either from the sun or tanning beds. One or more blistering sunburns during childhood is believed to initiate melanoma formation. Another cause is the presence of large number of moles (more than 50) or moles of an unusual shape. Other risk factors are blond or red hair, fair skin and light-coloured eyes, and living in a warm, sunny region.

PREVENTION

As with other forms of skin cancer (pp.127–9), reduce the risk of melanoma by avoiding sunburn.

DIAGNOSIS

If a doctor suspects melanoma, a biopsy will be analysed for the presence of cancer cells. If melanoma is found, other tests determine whether it has spread to surrounding skin cells, invaded any lymph nodes or spread to distant areas of the body. The doctor will remove a margin of skin around the melanoma to check for cancer cells. In addition, the doctor may do blood and urine tests, imaging studies of the lymph nodes, chest X-rays, and CT or other scans to look for evidence of cancer that has spread.

The results of these tests indicate the stage of melanoma: how large the tumour is, whether it is

Overexposure to ultraviolet light, from the sun or tanning beds, increases the risk of developing melanoma, which is a skin cancer that affects the cells that gives skin its colour. Unlike other cancers, melanoma is common among young adults.

WHO IS AT RISK?

The risk factors include:

- Sunburn
- Unusual or numerous moles
- Light skin, hair, and eyes
- Living in a warm, sunny region

Clinical Query

(See *On Call*, right.)

What should I look for in a mole or lesion that might make it suspect?

Melanoma is often recognized by using the ABCDE guideline:
Asymmetry A melanoma skin lesion is usually an irregular shape.
Border The outline of a melanoma is ragged rather than smoothly defined.
Colour There is a variation of colour within the lesion.
Diameter The lesion is bigger than 6 mm (2½ in) across, has increased in size recently, or both (6 mm/2½ in is about the size of a rubber on the end of a pencil).
Elevation The lesion is raised above the surface of the skin.

ulcerated (cracked or broken on the surface), and the extent of its spread. The higher the stage, the more advanced the cancer. (See *On Call*, right.)

TREATMENTS

All melanomas are treated with surgery. Other approaches include chemotherapy, radiation, and biological therapy (p.583) to stimulate the immune system, increase the odds of survival and ease discomfort. The combination of therapies used depends on the stage of the cancer. Other therapies, such as melanoma vaccines, are currently being investigated.
• **SURGERY** Different types of surgical procedures are used for melanoma. Local excision – removing the melanoma and a margin of normal tissue around it

– is used for small tumours. Wide excision is used for tumours that are too large for local excision. It may involve removing cancerous lymph nodes. In a lymphadenectomy, lymph nodes are removed and analysed for signs of cancer. A sentinel node biopsy is the removal of only the lymph node closest to the tumour to see if it contains cancer cells. Skin grafting. is a type of reconstructive surgery in which skin from another part of the body is used to cover an area of skin that was disfigured by cancer surgery.
• **CHEMOTHERAPY** Medications are given to destroy cancer cells throughout the body or to prevent them from multiplying. The drugs may be taken orally or injected into a vein or muscle. For melanoma in an arm or leg, an option is to deliver a high dose of chemotherapy directly to the site injecting the drugs in a warmed solution into the limb. Chemotherapy may be given for stages I through IV melanomas, as well as for recurrent melanoma.
• **RADIATION THERAPY** X-rays or radioactive substances are used to destroy cancer cells in a local area. Radiation therapy may be given externally or internally. External radiation uses a machine to generate X-rays and direct them to an area of the body. Internal radiation uses various techniques to implant radioactive substances in or near the cancer. Radiation therapy may be used for stages I, III, IV, and recurrent melanomas.
• **BIOLOGICAL THERAPY** Biological therapy, also called immunotherapy, uses chemicals derived from

On Call

Melanoma is diagnosed according to the following stages, which are degrees of severity.

Stage 0 (Melanoma *in situ*): Melanoma is confined to the epidermis, or outer layer of skin.

Stage IA The tumour is no more than 1 mm thick and has no ulceration. It is confined to the epidermis and the upper layer of the dermis, just below the epidermis.

Stage IIB The tumour is either no more than 1 mm thick, has ulceration, and may have spread to the dermis or tissue beneath the skin, or the tumour is 1–2 mm thick without ulceration.

Stage IIA The tumour is either 1 to 2 mm thick with ulceration or 2 to 4 mm thick without ulceration.

Stage IIB The tumour is either 2 to 4 mm thick with ulceration or more than 4 mm thick without ulceration.

Stage IIC The tumour is more than 4 mm thick with ulceration.

Stage III The tumour may be any thickness with or without ulceration and has spread to one or more lymph nodes, has spread into the nearby lymph system but not into any lymph nodes, or is surrounded by satellite tumours 2 cm or less away.

Stage IV The tumour is of any thickness, with or without ulceration, has spread to at least one lymph node, and has spread to a distant area of the body.

the human body to stimulate the immune system to fight cancer. Interleukin 2 and interferon are agents used in biological therapy. Biological therapy may be administered for stages II, III, IV and recurrent melanomas.

See also: *Skin Cancer, pp.127–9* • *Ocular Cancers, pp.46–7*

VIRAL SKIN INFECTIONS

Small, hard bumps on the surface of the skin can be signs of a viral skin infection. Unlike other viral infections that cause rashes, such as chickenpox, viral skin infections affect only the skin and may not cause fever or other symptoms. Common viral skin infections include molluscum contagiosum and verruca, or warts.

An infection with molluscum contagiosum causes painless flesh-coloured bumps with either a depression or a raised head in the centre. They can appear anywhere on the body except for the soles of the feet and palms of the hands. Warts are round or oval growths that are either darker or lighter than the surrounding skin. Plantar warts, among the most common types, usually grow on the soles of the feet and can be painful. Genital warts are sexually transmitted diseases. (Herpes, another common viral skin infection, is discussed in the entry on sexually transmitted diseases/STDs, pp.422–3). Other kinds of warts can appear on the hands, face, or near the fingernails and toenails. Although molluscum contagiosum and warts are harmless, they can take many months to go away and may recur.

CAUSES
Molluscum contagiosum is caused by a virus called molluscipox virus. Warts are caused by human papillomavirus, which stimulates the rapid growth of cells of the outer layer of the skin. Because warts shed viral particles of HPV, new warts can

appear as quickly as old ones go away. There is also a potential to infect others, although this generally requires repeated contact. Wart viruses can also be spread between areas of the body, usually from broken skin such as a scratch or an open sore.

Molluscum contagiosum infection is more contagious than warts and can be transmitted during contact sports such as wrestling, as well as coming into contact with contaminated towels and other personal items, swimming in infected pools, and receiving a massage under conditions of poor hygiene. People with AIDS and other conditions

that suppress the immune system are at increased risk of molluscum contagiosum infection. Both types of viral skin infections can be transmitted sexually.

PREVENTION
Prevent contracting viral skin infections by not touching the affected skin or personal items of infected people. Do not brush, shave, clip or comb affected areas in order to avoid spreading the virus. Condoms do not completely protect against the sexual transmission of viral skin infections.

DIAGNOSIS
A doctor can diagnose molluscum contagiosum and warts by their appearance. The doctor may take a biopsy of the affected skin to confirm the diagnosis. In some cases of suspected genital wart infection, a doctor may apply a special acetic acid (vinegar) solution to whiten any warts that are difficult to see.

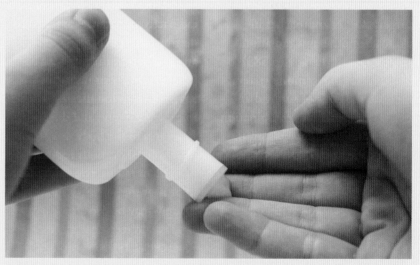

Treatment with creams and other topical preparations that contain salicylic acid, retinoic acid or 5-fluorouracil may help accelerate healing of viral infections by peeling away infected skin.

TREATMENTS

Medicine and minor surgery can hasten recovery from viral skin infections and prevent them from spreading. Without treatment, the infections can take months or even years to resolve.

• **TOPICAL TREATMENTS** Several creams and other topical preparations can help cure a molluscum contagiosum infection by peeling away affected skin. These preparations may contain chemicals such as salicylic acid, retinoic acid, or 5-fluorouracil. Warts on the hands and feet are usually treated with salicylic acid, and flat warts on the hands or face are treated with retinoic acid. Imiquimod cream is a standard treatment for genital skin infections and is increasingly being prescribed for use on other areas. Topical medications must be applied repeatedly for several weeks. Some can be used at home, but others can harm healthy tissue and must be applied by doctors or other health professionals.

• **MEDICATION** For molluscum contagiosum, some doctors prescribe high doses of cimetidine, an oral drug usually used to treat stomach ulcers, because it seems to be effective against the skin infections as well.

On Call

Immunotherapies, which prompt the immune system to fight off viral skin infections, are currently under development and may soon be used to treat these infections.

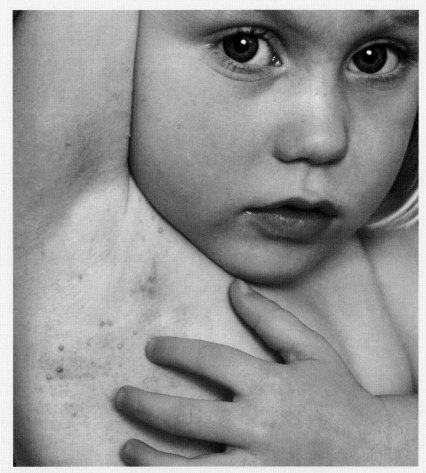

Molluscum contagiosum is a common viral infection that causes painless flesh-coloured bumps that can persist from two weeks to as long as four years. Typically the condition affects children more commonly than adults.

• **SURGERY** Viral skin infections that do not respond to medication or are too large can be surgically removed. The doctor can remove warts by cutting, using a special tool and a local anaesthesia. Freezing, or cryotherapy, involves the application of a small amount of a freezing liquid, such as liquid nitrogen, which causes a blister to form around the wart. The blister then sloughs off as new skin forms. A doctor may also scrape away and cauterize the wart, using a procedure called electrodesiccation and curettage. Surgery to remove warts usually requires several surgery visits.

• **ESSENTIAL OILS** A topical application of Australian lemon myrtle oil is effective for treating molluscum contagiosum.

• **SELF-CARE** Placing duct tape over warts on the fingers may help them disappear. Cover the warts with duct tape for six days, then removed the tape, wet the wart and scrape the outer layers with a nail file. The next morning, cover the wart agains. This procedure can be continued for up to two months, and is as effective as surgery done by freezing the wart.

See also: *STD, pp.392–3* • *AIDS, pp.316–17*

Folliculitis

A combination of irritation to the skin and an infection of the hair follicle causes folliculitis. Symptoms include a red rash, pimples or pustules around a follicle, and itching. The condition occurs most often on the scalp, beard area, thighs, underarms and groin. Folliculitis is usually a mild condition of the top layer of skin, but sometimes it can penetrate to the lower layers. Antibiotics and other medications are often needed to treat the condition.

CAUSES

The process often starts with friction to an area of skin – from shaving, tight-fitting clothing or skin folds rubbing against each other. Friction creates scrapes and nicks, which can open up a follicle to infection.

There are different types of folliculitis. Whirlpool folliculitis is typically caused by pseudomonas aeruginosa, bacteria that colonize in inadequately chlorinated whirlpools, hot tubs and warm swimming-pools. It causes an itchy rash on areas of the body covered by a bathing suit. Three types of folliculitis are triggered by shaving: barber's itch (caused by *Staphylococcus* bacteria); tinea barbae (caused by fungus); and pseudofolliculitis, which develops when shaving causes an ingrown hair by pushing the end of a beard hair into a follicle. Pseudofolliculitis is most common in black men.

PREVENTION

Reducing friction against the skin and minimizing exposure to bacteria and fungus can help prevent folliculitis. Wear clothes that are comfortable and do not irritate any areas of skin. If using a hot tub, whirlpool or swimming-pool, make sure that it is chlorinated well enough to eliminate bacteria. Do not share razors, towels, or other personal care items.

If suffering from folliculitis, avoid shaving the affected area or discard the razor after each use so as not to spread the infection.

Shaving can cause several types of folliculitis. Avoid shaving against the grain to prevent cutting hairs too short, which can lodge inside pores and become infected.

WHO IS AT RISK?

The risk factors include:
- Shaving
- Wearing tight-fitting clothing
- Using hot tubs, whirlpools, and swimming pools
- Obesity
- Male
- Black skin
- Diabetes
- Suppressed immune system

Obese people are at elevated risk of folliculitis because skin folds create friction.

DIAGNOSIS

A doctor can diagnose folliculitis by its appearance. The doctor may take a culture of the affected skin to identify the bacteria responsible for the infection.

TREATMENTS

• COMPRESSES Warm, moist compresses help pustules drain. Washing the affected area with antibacterial soap can eliminate mild cases.

• ANTIBIOTICS Topical antibiotics often eliminate folliculitis in a small area, but oral antibiotics may be needed if folliculitis covers a large area or is unresponsive to topical medications. Oral antifungal medicine may be needed for tinea barbae (pp.104–5).

See also: *Obesity, pp.348–9.* • *Diabetes, pp.338–41*

Skin Cancer & Premalignant Lesions

The most common form of cancer is skin cancer. There are three main types: basal cell carcinoma, squamous cell carcinoma, and melanoma. In contrast with melanoma (pp.122–3), which is an aggressive form of cancer, the other two skin cancers tend to be slow growing. Squamous cell carcinoma frequently begins as a premalignant skin lesion called actinic keratosis. Squamous cell cancer can be life-threatening, but only if left untreated for long periods. Basal cell cancers rarely spread and tend not to be life-threatening.

WHO IS AT RISK?

The risk factors include:

- Extensive exposure to sunlight or ultraviolet light in tanning beds
- Fair hair and skin
- Light-coloured eyes
- Repeated exposure to X-rays
- Exposure to chemical pollutants such as arsenic

Skin cancer develops most often on areas of skin exposed to the sun, such as the face, arms, legs and back. Basal cell carcinoma, the most common form, occurs in the basal cells, which are in the lowest layer of the epidermis. It can appear as a small open sore, a red patch, a shiny bump or a waxy patch that resembles a scar. Squamous cell carcinoma, the second most common skin cancer, affects the squamous cells, which appear in the uppermost layers of the epidermis. It looks rough and scaly, and is more likely to spread than basal cell carcinoma. Actinic keratosis, the most common type of premalignant skin lesion, is scaly or crusty; it may disappear and then re-emerge. Early treatment can prevent actinic keratosis from becoming cancerous.

tanning beds, is the main cause of skin cancer and premalignant skin lesions. Another cause is extensive exposure to X-rays and other sources of radiation. Fair skin and light-coloured hair and eyes increase the risk of developing skin cancer, because people with these features are most prone to sunburn and other sun damage.

Two additional factors apply specifically to the risk of developing squamous cell carcinoma. One of them is exposure to certain chemical pollutants, such as arsenic, which is found in some herbicides. The other is an untreated actinic keratosis. Nutritional deficiencies of the

CAUSES

Excessive exposure to ultraviolet light, either from the sun or from

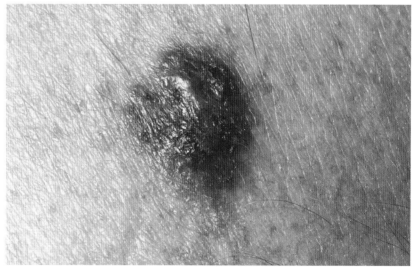

Basal cell carcinoma is the most common form of skin cancer, accounting for 80 percent of all diagnosed cases. But with proper diagnosis and treatment, this type of cancer has a cure rate of 95 percent.

antioxidants lutein, zeaxanthin and beta-cryptoxanthin may also increase the risk of developing squamous cell carcinoma.

PREVENTION

Most skin cancers and precancerous skin lesions can be prevented by limiting exposure to the sun and tanning beds. Avoid being in direct sun between the hours of 10 a.m. and 2 p.m., when the sun is strongest. When spending time outdoors, use a sunscreen that protects against ultraviolet A and ultraviolet B light – the complete spectrum of ultraviolet light that damages skin. For extra protection, wear a hat. Re-apply sunscreen after swimming or perspiring heavily, enough to wet the skin. A class of agents known as oligosaccharins – complex carbohydrates found in plants – can also protect the skin from sun

damage. *Tamarind xylogucan*, one such agent, may become an important ingredient in sunscreens.

In addition, certain nutrients can help protect the skin from sun damage either by absorbing ultraviolet light or modulating its effect on the skin. Dietary protection is provided by carotenoids, tocopherols (vitamin E), ascorbate (vitamin C and magnesium), flavonoids, and omega-3 fatty acids (pp.252–5).

Medical treatment can prevent an actinic keratosis from progressing to a squamous cell carcinoma. High doses of vitamin A supplements may also reduce the risk of squamous cell carcinoma in people with actinic keratosis.

DIAGNOSIS

If an area of skin looks cancerous or premalignant, a doctor can make a diagnosis by taking a biopsy for laboratory analysis to check for the presence of cancer cells. Because there is a risk that melanoma and, to a lesser degree, squamous cell carcinoma, can spread to the lymph nodes, a lymph node biopsy may also be done to rule it out. Other tests may be necessary for melanoma. Based on the examination and laboratory tests, the doctor will determine the stage of the cancer (see *On Call*, left).

TREATMENTS

Surgery is required to remove all skin cancers and some premalignant skin lesions. There are several surgical procedures for skin cancer and premalignant skin lesions. Most skin cancers are also

Clinical Query

What does 'carcinoma *in situ*' mean? Is it less serious?

In situ is Latin for 'in position'. The phrase is used to describe non-invasive cancers that have not spread to the surrounding tissues or other parts of the body. They can, however, develop into or raise your risk for a more serious, invasive cancer.

treated with medication and other therapies. The combination of treatments used depends on the stage of the cancer.

• MOHS MICROGRAPHIC SURGERY This is the least invasive type of skin cancer surgery, often used for basal cell and squamous cell carcinomas on the face to minimize disfigurement. Thin layers of the tumour are removed and analysed in a laboratory, one at a time, until no more cancer cells are found.

• EXCISION In this procedure, the tumour is removed along with a margin of healthy tissue. This procedure may be used for melanoma and non-melanoma skin cancers, and actinic keratosis.

• ELECTRODESICCATION AND CURETTAGE A curette, which is a cup-shaped cutting tool, first removes the cancer and then another instrument is used to deliver an electric current to the surrounding area to kill remaining cancer cells and help the surgical wound heal. This surgery may be used for basal cell and squamous cell carcinomas, and actinic keratosis.

On Call

These stages (degrees of severity) are used to categorize basal cell carcinoma and squamous cell carcinoma.

Stage 0 (Carcinoma *in situ*): Cancer is found only in the epidermis, the top layer of skin.

Stage I The tumour is 2 cm (1 in) or smaller.

Stage II The tumour is larger than 2 cm (1 in).

Stage III Cancer has spread beneath the skin to the cartilage, muscle or bone, or to nearby lymph nodes, but not to other parts of the body.

Stage IV Cancer has spread to other parts of the body.

• **CRYOSURGERY** This surgery is often used for Stage 0 basal cell or squamous cell carcinoma, and actinic keratosis. A tool freezes the tumour and removes it along with surrounding abnormal tissue.

• **LASER SURGERY** A laser beam is used to cut away cancerous tissue from the surface of the skin. This procedure may be used for basal cell or squamous cell carcinomas, and actinic keratosis.

• **DERMABRASION** The top layer of skin is scraped away using the friction from a device with a rotating wheel. This procedure may be used to remove lesions of actinic keratosis.

• **CHEMOTHERAPY** Topical medication that destroys cancer cells applied to the skin to treat basal and squamous cell carcinomas, and actinic keratosis.

• **RADIATION THERAPY** X-rays or other radioactive sources are used to kill cancer cells. External radiation uses a machine called a linear particle accelerator to direct beams of X-rays or other radiation energy into the body. Internal radiation involves injecting or implanting radioactive wafers or pellets in and around a tumour. Radiation therapy may be used for all types of melanoma and non-melanoma skin cancers.

• **PHOTODYNAMIC THERAPY** This procedure uses anticancer drugs that become activated in the presence of a special laser light. First the medication, which is designed to concentrate more in cancer cells than in normal cells, is injected into a vein. Then laser light is focused onto the cancer cells to active the medication.

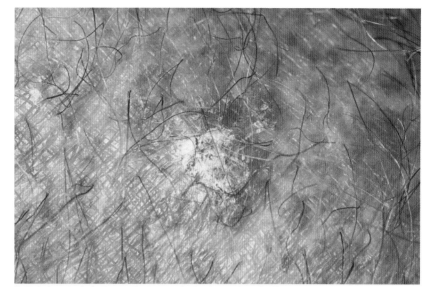

Actinic keratosis is the earliest stage in the formation of skin cancer and can progress to squamous cell carcinoma if left untreated. Lesions appear as rough, brownish scaly patches on skin most often exposed to the sun, including the back of the hands and the face.

Photodynamic therapy may be used on basal cell carcinoma and actinic keratosis. Research suggests that it is beneficial for basal cell carcinoma.

• **BIOLOGICAL THERAPY** This type of therapy involves substances that stimulate the immune system to fight cancer. It is a standard treatment for melanoma and has been used experimentally for non-melanoma skin cancers.

• **RETINOIDS** Topical or oral retinoids – medication chemically derived from vitamin A – are sometimes administered to prevent the formation of non-melanoma skin cancer. These compounds are also being used experimentally to treat squamous cell carcinoma.

See also: *Melanoma, pp.122–3 • Omega-3 Fatty Acids, pp.252–3*

healing hope I used to be a sun worshipper, back when looking tan meant looking healthy. I think back on those days in college when I'd be out on the dorm roof trying so hard to lay in my 'base tan' in May, and I wonder what I was thinking.

Anyway, last year I noticed this flat round little spot of scaly skin on my leg that would not wash away and didn't get softer, even with moisturizer. Eventually, I went to my doctor about it. Tests revealed squamous cell carcinoma – skin cancer!

It was still stage 0 – just in the top layer of my skin – and it was easily removed, but that was a wake-up call for me. Now I am a shade worshipper. And I know light clothes don't always protect you from the sun, so I am oiled up with sunscreen before I ever leave the house. So are my kids, because I don't ever want them to have the scare that I had.   *Kelley S.*

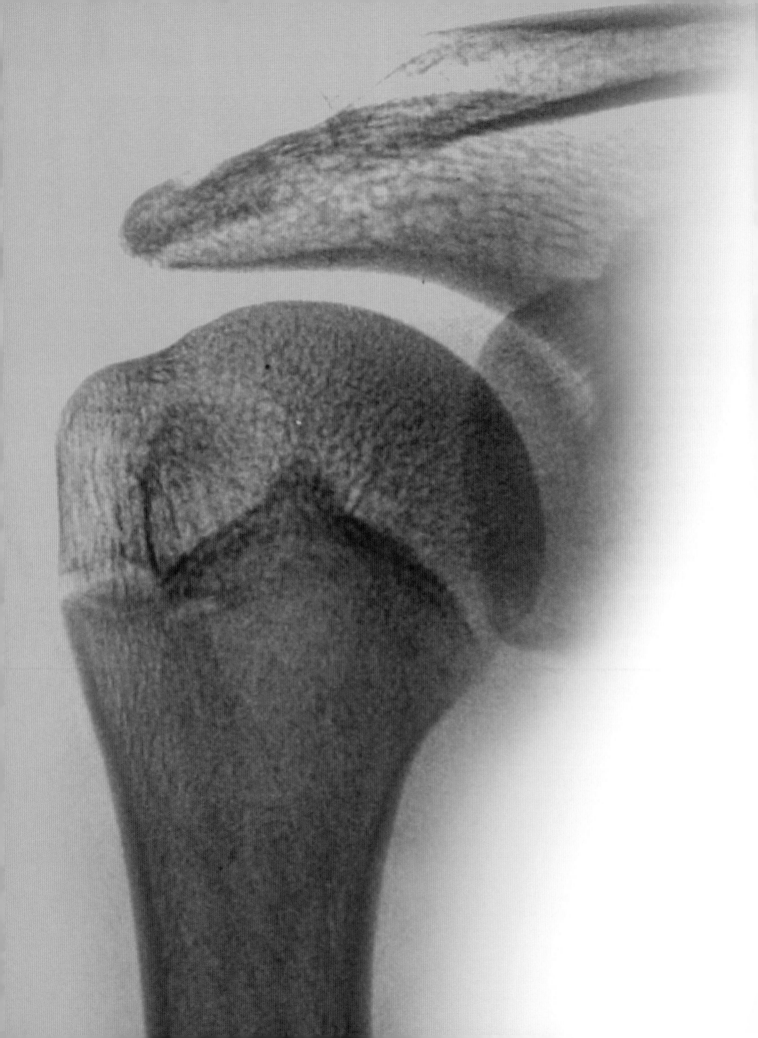

BONES, JOINTS & MUSCLES

5

Our skeletons, muscles and joints give humans the framework that allows them to walk and move and interact with the physical world. Problems with any of these systems can take a heavy toll on quality of life. But many problems are preventable or treatable.

Muscle injuries such as strains and cramps can cause discomfort that may require pain relief and rest. Issues with bones and joints, however, can have a more serious impact on mobility. Chronic conditions such as tendonitis and arthritis can cause lingering pain, and bone fractures are a medical emergency.

Preventing injuries to bones and muscles is often a simple matter. By stretching and warming up properly before exertion strains and sprains may be prevented. A healthy diet and regular exercise can minimize the risk of gout and bone fractures resulting from osteoporosis. However, conditions such as broken bones and osteomyelitis must be treated by a doctor.

Back Pain

A dull ache just above the waist, a sharp pain between the shoulder blades, stiffness when waking up in the morning – these are some of the many symptoms of back pain. It can be mild or severe, constant or intermittent. It can be felt anywhere along the spine, although it is most common in the lower back.

Back pain can be acute or chronic. Acute back pain can last from one day to several weeks and is often caused by an injury to the back. Chronic back pain persists or recurs for three months or longer and is often progressive. In its many forms, back pain is one of the most common health problems and a leading reason for absence from work.

CAUSES

One of the most common causes of back pain is injury, which can result from sports, manual labour, or movements such as reaching for an object on a shelf or lifting something heavy. Injuries or accidents can strain muscles, causing painful muscle spasms, which may press on nerves in and around the spine.

Another cause is a slipped or herniated disk. The disk that provides cushioning between each vertebra slides towards the spinal canal (that is, it becomes herniated) and presses on nerves. Causes of a slipped disk include injury, bending, lifting a heavy object and age-related changes in disks.

Arthritis (pp.136–9) is a common joint disease that can also cause back pain. Osteoarthritis can occur in the spine as well as along the joints that link the vertebrae. Ankylosing spondylitis, a form of rheumatoid arthritis, causes inflammation and stiffness starting in the lower back and progressing along the spine.

There are other factors that may increase the risk of back pain. Obesity (pp.348–9) puts undue pressure on the spine, which can cause pain and arthritis. Lack of exercise weakens abdominal muscles, which also adds to the pressure on the spine. Poor posture may lead to misalignment of the vertebrae, which may then cause muscle strain or press against nerves. Emotional stress can increase the risk of back pain and delay recovery.

Back pain can accompany many conditions, including fibromyalgia (pp.144–5), osteoporosis (pp.146–7), hernia in the groin, testicular torsion (p.427), ovarian cysts (p.389), pregnancy (pp.398–400), infections, primary spinal tumours, and some cancers.

PREVENTION

Avoid unusual stress on the spine and reduce your risk of injury. Regular exercise can reduce stress on the spine by strengthening the muscles in the back and the abdomen. Beneficial exercises that strengthen the back include walking, cycling, swimming, weightlifting and stretching. Maintaining good posture, or improving posture if necessary, can minimize back strain. Losing weight can also help prevent back pain by reducing any stress on the spine. Other preventative measures include:

• Avoid standing or sitting for prolonged periods.
• When driving for extended periods, stop every hour or so to walk around.
• Do not wear high-heeled shoes – they can strain the back and increase the risk of falling.
• Do not lift objects that are too heavy for you. When you must lift something heavy, stand close to the object, spread your feet apart, bend your knees,

WHO IS AT RISK?

The risk factors include:
• Age
• Manual labour
• Obesity
• Lack of exercise
• Arthritis
• Osteoporosis
• Fibromyalgia
• Pregnancy
• Disorders of the pelvic region (such as testicular torsion, ovarian cysts and ovarian cancer)

and tighten your abdominal muscles as you lift the object and put it down.

- Reduce emotional stress with proven techniques such as yoga (pp.476–9), meditation (page 514–19), exercise and relaxation.

DIAGNOSIS

A doctor can diagnose back pain and, often, its underlying cause by doing a physical examination and taking a medical history. X-rays or other imaging tests may be needed to diagnose a herniated disk.

TREATMENTS

Most back pain goes away within six weeks. In the meantime, several self-care and other therapies may relieve pain and improve mobility. Surgery is not helpful for most back pain. There are various types of back surgery, but they are reserved for people who are not helped by other therapies.

- MEDICATION Nonsteroidal anti-inflammatory medication can temporarily relieve pain and reduce inflammation of the nerves in the back. For severe lower back pain, doctors may prescribe muscle relaxants or, if the nerves in the spine are

CAUTION

It is extremely important to recognize when back pain may be caused by a more serious condition. Signs include pain that does not resolve within two to four weeks, pain that does not improve with rest, loss of function or sensation in an extremity, fever, a history of cancer, or a history of using intravenous drugs.

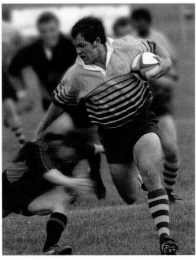
Acute back pain is often caused by injury, which can occur while playing sports, but can also result from ordinary movements such as turning or lifting.

inflamed, they may inject analgesics or steroids directly into the spinal canal to reduce the inflammation.

- EXERCISE Regular exercise helps relieve chronic low-back pain. Start exercising gradually two to three weeks after an injury.
- SELF-CARE Reduce physical activity for the first few days after an injury to reduce pain and inflammation of the joints along the spine. Do not lift anything and avoid movements that involve twisting the back. Apply ice to the affected area for the first three days to reduce inflammation, and thereafter apply heat to the area to improve mobility. Bed rest, particularly longer than two days, is not helpful.
- BEHAVIOURAL THERAPIES Cognitive behavioural therapy and progressive muscle relaxation (page pp.474–5) can help relieve back pain by reducing stress and tension.
- EDUCATION Back schools are patient education courses that are designed to prevent and reduce back pain. They include information on the anatomy of the spine

and practical advice on how to stand, sit and function in daily life without straining the back.

- SPINAL MANIPULATION AND PHYSICAL THERAPY Hands-on techniques to manipulate the spine can help relieve acute back pain, including chiropractic (pp.446–7) and osteopathy (pp.438–40).
- MASSAGE Chronic low-back pain can be relieved with massage (pp.468–73). It is unclear whether one type of massage is superior to another.
- TRANSCUTANEOUS ELECTRICAL NERVE STIMULATION TENS (pp.443) blocks pain signals by placing electrodes that deliver electrical impulses to a painful area. It is a standard treatment for back pain and other muscle pain.
- ACUPUNCTURE This therapy (pp.464–5) can provide short-term relief from back pain.
- HERBAL REMEDIES A herbal remedy made from an extract from the dried roots of the Devil's claw plant (*Harpagophytum procumbens*), is an analgesic and anti-inflammatory agent that is widely used for back and joint pain.
- NEURO-REFLEXOTHERAPY This novel therapy involves stimulating nerve cells in the skin as a means of reducing pain, inflammation and muscle spasms in the back. The nerve stimulation comes from surgical staples implanted just beneath the skin's surface and left in place for three months. Neuro-reflexotherapy is effective for chronic lower back pain and has no adverse effects.

See also: *Yoga, pp.476–9 • Massage, pp.468–73 • Acupuncture, pp.464–5*

Muscle Sprains, Strains & Pain

Everyone has aches, pains, soreness and stiffness in their muscles from time to time, and the culprit is often a strain or sprain. Strains are overstretched muscles, also called pulled muscles. Sprains are a more serious condition in which the ligaments (tissue that holds a joint together) are severely stretched or torn. Sprains often cause swelling and may also cause bruising of the surrounding blood vessels. Ankles are the most common locations for sprains.

Diffuse muscle pain can be a symptom of a wide range of conditions, including infections, hormonal problems such as an underactive or overactive thyroid (pp.344–7), drug side effects, and emotional stress.

CAUSES

Strains and sprains occur with sports and other physical activity, as well as accidents such as falls or twisting an ankle while walking. They are especially common among those who play contact sports such as football and sports that involve a lot of quick, sudden moves, such as basketball, volleyball, and tennis. Muscle strains in the back and abdomen often result from lifting heavy objects.

Muscle pain has many, varied causes, including:
- Overuse injuries (using the muscle too much, too often or too soon after another injury)
- Infections, such as flu, Lyme disease (pp.326–7) and malaria
- Lupus (pp.324–5)
- Fibromyalgia (pp.144–5)
- Arthritis (pp.136–9)
- Thyroid disorders (pp.344–7)
- Neuromuscular disorders (such as polymytositis, dermato-mytositis, and polymyaligia rheumatica)
- Electrolyte imbalances, such as a deficiency of calcium or potassium
- Several medications, including statins for high cholesterol and ACE inhibitors for high blood pressure
- Some recreational drugs
- Emotional stress

PREVENTION

It is easier to prevent strains and sprains than other causes of muscle pain. To reduce the risk of injury, warm up before engaging in sports and other physical activities. Only stretch after you have had at least a 10-minute warm-up. Do not increase the intensity or duration of exercise quickly, which can lead to strains or sprains. Maintain good posture to prevent resting too much weight on one area of the body. Keep your body weight within normal limits; obesity can strain muscles in the lower body. To reduce the risk of twisting an ankle or falling, wear comfortable shoes and avoid high heels.

In addition, take precautions against infections and other causes of muscular aches. During flu season, stay away from people who are infected and wash your hands frequently. If you live in an area with Lyme disease, use tick repellent when outdoors. Do not use cocaine – it can irritate the kidneys and aggravate back pain. Practise proven strategies for managing stress, such as meditation (pp.514–19), yoga (pp.476–9) and guided imagery (pp.520–2).

DIAGNOSIS

If the pain is related to an injury, the doctor can often determine whether the cause is a strain or

WHO IS AT RISK?

The risk factors include:
- Physical activity and sports
- Heavy lifting
- Poor-fitting shoes
- High heels
- Obesity
- Emotional stress
- Illnesses such as flu, Lyme disease, and muscular disorders
- Medications such as statins for cholesterol and ACE inhibitors for high blood pressure
- Some recreational drugs

BONES, JOINTS & MUSCLES

sprain based on a physical examination, the mobility of a joint, the strength of a muscle, and the presence of swelling or bruising. X-rays may be taken if the doctor suspects a fracture or broken bone.

The doctor can narrow down the cause of other muscle pain by determining when the pain began, whether there is a pattern to it, what other symptoms are present, and if you recently began taking medication. When muscle pain is caused by an infection or other illness, there may also be symptoms such as fever or headache. A blood test is needed to diagnose Lyme disease, and specialized muscular tests may be carried out if muscle disorders are suspected.

TREATMENTS

The treatment of muscle pain depends on the cause. Pain relievers can reduce pain due to flu, arthritis, and some muscular disorders such as polymyalgia rheumatica. Stronger medications

such as steroids, as well as physical therapy, may be needed for dermatosyositis and polymyositis.

For muscle sprains and strains, there are a variety of options.

• **FIRST AID** This is often sufficient to treat strains and sprains. Rest the injured muscle by avoiding sports and other physical activities for at least a few days. For the first 24 hours after an injury, apply ice or a cold compress to the affected area to reduce swelling. Apply the compresses for 30 minutes at a time, and then take a break for 30 minutes. In addition, immediately after the injury, compress the affected joint with an elastic bandage to stabilize it and reduce swelling. Elevate the area to further reduce swelling and to encourage blood to circulate throughout the body, not just to the injury.

For a sprained wrist, elbow or shoulder, placing the arm in a sling can help keep it elevated. Be careful not to immobilize the

limb for more than a few hours without doing passive range of motion exercises, such as letting the limb hang loose and gently swinging it, to prevent stiffness. After 24 hours, periodically use warm compresses or soak the affected area in warm water to relieve pain and improve mobility.

• **MEDICATION** Pain relievers such as acetaminophen or nonsteroidal anti-inflammatory drugs, such as ibuprofen, can ease discomfort and swelling. A topical gel that contains lecithin, a fatty substance that occurs naturally in plants and animals, has been found to relieve pain from knee, ankle and muscle injuries. For severe pain, a doctor may prescribe muscle relaxants.

• **MASSAGE** Friction massage can improve range of motion and reduce pain from frozen shoulder, a condition in which the range of motion of the shoulder joint is restricted. Massage may also provide temporary relief of other types of muscle pain.

• **HOMEOPATHY** Two double-blind placebo-controlled studies published in *The Journal Homeopathy* in 2003 tested the effectiveness of Arnica D30, homeopathic pills made from the flowers of the herb *Arnica montana*, on 82 marathon runners. Runners who took the pills before and after participating in marathons reported less muscle pain afterward than did runners who took a placebo. However, cell damage was similar in the two groups.

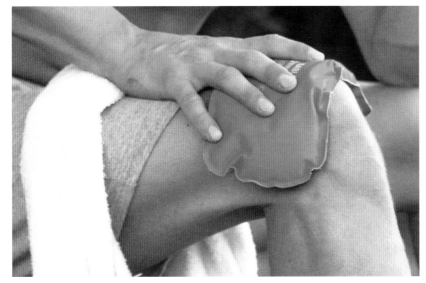

Minor muscle and joint injuries should first be treated with ice or a cold compress to reduce swelling. Rest and apply heat to the injury after the first 24 hours to improve circulation and speed healing. Avoid physical activity for at least a few days.

See also: Arthritis, pp.136–9 • Yoga, pp.476–9 • Guided Imagery, pp.520–2

ARTHRITIS

Arthritis is an inflammation of one or more joints, often accompanied by pain, swelling, stiffness and redness. Symptoms vary widely, ranging from mild aching to extreme deformity. It is one of the most prevalent health problems and causes of disability. It can occur as an isolated problem or secondary to other conditions, such as colitis or psoriasis, or infections such as gonorrhoea.

There is no cure for arthritis, but pain and disability can be significantly relieved with an holistic approach, including pharmaceuticals and supplements, exercise, mind–body techniques, nutrition therapy and acupuncture.

CAUSES

There are more than 100 types of arthritis, but the most prevalent ones are osteoarthritis and rheumatoid arthritis. Other types include ankylosing spondylitis (an inflammation of the spine), scleroderma (a connective tissue disease that causes the skin to thicken and harden) and lupus (pp.324–5).

Osteoarthritis is the most common form of arthritis. It occurs mainly in people over age 60 and is characterized by a progressive wearing away of the cartilage of the joints due to excess wear and tear. As the protective cartilage is worn away, bare bone is exposed within the joint, causing pain. Several factors can contribute to this wear and tear. One is obesity, which places undue stress on weight-bearing joints, such as those in the lower back, knees and hips. The heavier a person is, the more pressure is placed on the joints, causing the cartilage around them to break down more quickly.

Physical inactivity can also be as harmful to the joints as overuse. A lack of exercise or other physical activity can weaken the muscles that support the joints and decrease joint flexibility. These problems increase the risk of injury, which can lead to osteoarthritis.

Injuries, inflammatory diseases such as gout (pp.150–1), and congenital joint deformities can also increase the risk of developing osteoarthritis. (Gout is a metabolic disorder that causes episodes of arthritis.)

Rheumatoid arthritis is an auto-immune disorder – a condition in which the immune system attacks the body itself. The areas most often affected are the fingers, wrists, shoulders, knees, hips and neck. Rheumatoid arthritis, like other autoimmune disorders, strikes two to three times more women than men. It usually starts in early adulthood or middle age, but it can develop later in life.

Although emotional and psychological stress does not cause arthritis, they may cause flare-ups of the symptoms because the muscles become tense under stress, and this muscle tension can increase arthritis pain.

PREVENTION

There is no way to prevent rheumatoid arthritis, but people can reduce the odds of developing

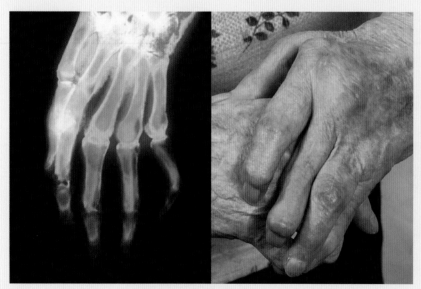

Rheumatoid arthritis is an inflammatory disease that can lead to joint deformities, most commonly affecting the hands, feet and knees. Early and aggressive treatment can minimize joint damage and help patients continue to lead productive lives.

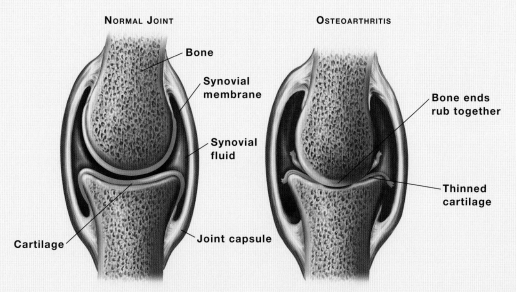

NORMAL JOINT   OSTEOARTHRITIS

Bone

Synovial
membrane

Synovial
fluid

Cartilage

Joint capsule

Bone ends
rub together

Thinned
cartilage

Osteoarthritis results from wear and tear on the joints and most commonly affects weight-bearing joints such as the lower back and knees. In a healthy joint (left), cartilage cushions the ends of the bones and reduces friction during movement. Osteoarthritis (right) occurs when the protective cartilage wears away and the ends of the bones rub together, causing pain.

osteoarthritis and possibly gout. To help guard against rheumatoid arthritis, try to avoid anything that puts abnormal stress on weight-bearing joints. This includes being overweight (pp.348–9).

It is also important to reduce the risk of injuries when engaging in physical activity by wearing protective gear, seeking good care for any overuse injury, and allowing plenty of time for any such injury to heal. This is because a variety of injuries, particularly during sports activity, may lead to osteo-arthritis later in life. Among them are ligament damage that causes instability to a joint and injury to the cartilage that leads to degen-erative damage. A fracture may also cause abnormalities in the alignment of the lower limbs that force a joint to bear weight asym-metrically, leading to uneven wear of the cartilage. Direct injury to the joint or joint structures – most commonly the meniscus or ante-rior cruciate ligament (ACL) in

the knee, or a hip injury – can also contribute to osteoarthritis. While upper-extremity arthritis as a result of injury does occur, because the upper extremities are not weight-bearing, it is less likely to alter the functioning of the patient.

Eating a healthy diet may help prevent gout. Gout (pp.150–1) occurs when uric acid, a protein waste product normally eliminated in urine, builds up in the body, either because it is being over-produced by the body or insuffi-ciently eliminated by the kidneys. The high levels of uric acid in the body form crystals in the joints, most often the big toes, causing pain and inflammation.

Uric acid results from the breakdown of purines, which are compounds that are part of all human tissue and are found in many foods. Consuming a lot of alcohol and foods rich in purines, such as organ meats, herring, anchovies and sardines, increases the risk of gout.

DIAGNOSIS

The earlier arthritis is diagnosed, the better, because the disease is progressive and treatment can

Clinical Query

How will I be able to tell if I have arthritis?

If you have any of the following symptoms, you may have arthritis and should see your doctor:
• Stiff joints in the morning that may ease once you start moving.
• Joint pain that continues throughout the day and some-times interferes with sleep.
• Joint pain and stiffness that starts or intensifies after exercise.
• Pain along with a grating sen-sation or a cracking noise when the affected joints move.
• Warmth around a joint.
• Swelling around joints.
• Unexplained weight loss, fever, or weakness that accompanies joint pain.

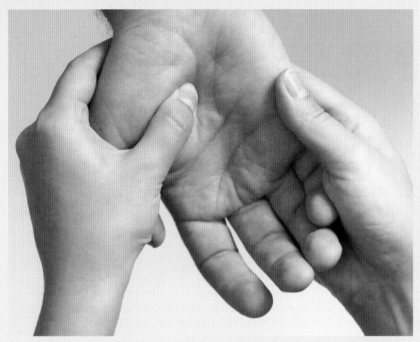

Treatments such as hydrotherapy, yoga, massage, chiropractic and kinesiology are often used to relieve arthritis symptoms. These methods, called bodywork therapies, can improve joint function and diminish pain and inflammation by helping patients relax.

help slow or prevent further damage to the joints. Doctors can usually diagnose arthritis based on symptoms and physical signs of the disease, such as fluid around the affected joint, as well as swelling, tenderness or warmth in the area. Sometimes tests are used to identify the type and extent of the arthritis, including blood and urine tests, as well as X-rays of the joints.

TREATMENTS

Although there is no cure for arthritis, many integrative treatments can help reduce discomfort and help prevent further damage over the long term.

• SURGERY When arthritis is severe and other therapies do not help, surgery may be needed to fuse, smooth or reposition bones or to replace a joint with an artificial one.

• TRADITIONAL CHINESE MEDICINE AND ACUPUNCTURE Acupuncture (pp.464–5) can relieve pain from osteoarthritis of the knee.

• HOMEOPATHY Homeopathic treatment (pp.455–7) of rheumatoid arthritis reduces pain and stiffness and improves grip strength.

• AYURVEDA Some herbs used in this natural medicine system from India (pp.451–4) are used to relieve arthritis pain. They include winter cherry (*Withania somnifera*), boswellia (*Boswellia serrata*), turmeric (*Cucurma longa*), and ginger (*Zingiberis officinale*). Some of the herbs are applied to the skin and others are ingested.

• BODYWORK This encompasses therapies that use hands-on methods and movement awareness to help a patient relax and improve the structure and functioning of the body. Hydrotherapy (pp.482–3), yoga (pp.476–9), massage

(pp.468–73), chiropractic (pp.466–7) and kinesiology (pp.484–5) are bodywork treatments used to relieve arthritis symptoms.

• ANALGESICS Drugs such as aceta-minophen are used to relieve arthritis pain. Nonsteroidal anti-inflammatory drugs (NSAIDs), such as ibuprofen, can reduce inflammation and pain.

• BIOLOGICAL RESPONSE MODIFIERS These drugs reduce inflammation and damage to the joints by blocking the action of tumour necrosis factor, a protein that is involved in the immune response that characterizes rheumatoid arthritis. Such drugs include etanercept, infliximab and ankinra.

• CORTICOSTEROIDS These drugs decrease inflammation and suppress the immune system. They include prednisone and cortisone, and are usually

CAUTION

Vitamin C is an antioxidant that has been heralded for its ability to slow the progression of osteoarthritis, but an eight-month study done at Duke University and published in the June 2004 issue of *Arthritis & Rheumatism* revealed that prolonged ingestion of high doses of vitamin C (about 2 g per day) may actually worsen the condition. The study was conducted on guinea pigs, which are considered good models for studying osteoarthritis treatments for humans. The authors concluded that vitamin C intake should not exceed 90 mg per day for men and 75 mg per day for women with arthritis.

prescribed for short-term use during a bout of intense discomfort. They are only prescribed for short-term use because they can cause serious side-effects, including swelling, weight gain and mood swings. These effects usually go away once the drug is no longer being taken.

- **DISEASE-MODIFYING ANTIRHEUMATIC DRUGS** DMARDs may have the effect of slowing or stopping the progression of rheumatoid arthritis. This class of drugs includes methotrexate and leflu-nomide. Omega-3 fatty acids are poly-unsaturated fatty acids that may slow the progress of rheumatoid arthritis, as well as decrease symptoms (pp.252–3).

- **GLUCOSAMINE SULPHATE** This nutrient has anti-inflammatory properties but with significantly less toxicity than nonsteroidal anti-inflammatory agents such as ibuprofen and naproxen. It may also help prevent further loss of cartilage, particularly in osteoarthritis, and, over the long term, may delay or even prevent the need for joint replacement.

- **VITAMINS** Supplements of vitamins A, B$_1$, B$_3$, B$_6$ and E may lead to increased flexibility and help prevent arthritis.

- **BORON** This mineral is needed for healthy bones and aids in the absorption of calcium. A supplement of 6 mg of boron a day may help to relieve the discomfort of osteoarthritis.

- **NUTRITION** There are several dietary strategies that can help to prevent arthritis or minimize symptoms. Maintaining a normal weight, or losing weight

healing hope I was an avid runner for many years, but when I was about 50, I developed osteoarthritis in my knees. My doctor said it was probably caused in part by the pounding that my knees took from running. The doctor told me I had to give up running, but he advised me to keep active because the right exercises can actually decrease arthritis symptoms. He recommended activities that are easy on the joints, like swimming, walking and low-impact aerobics, or even elliptical trainers (they're workout machines that simulate the motion of cross-country skiing).

At first I couldn't exercise at all because my knees hurt so much. So I used glucosamine sulfate every day to reduce inflammation and ease the pain enough to get started. I decided to swim twice a week and walk with a friend twice a week. That was three months ago. Now my knees feel much better – there's less stiffness and pain. And I don't even need medicine on most days.

John C.

if necessary, prevents excess strain on the joints. In addition, certain foods and supplements have been shown to be helpful. Eating fatty fish (high in omega-3 fatty acids) such as salmon, mackerel and sardines, can decrease inflammation. Alcohol can interfere with some of the medications prescribed for rheumatoid arthritis, so reduced alcohol consumption is recommended.

- **EXERCISE** For many years, people with arthritis were advised to avoid exercise to reduce the risk that it would further damage their joints. Now, doctors know that the right kind of exercise is one of the best treatments for arthritis. Exercise can reduce joint pain and stiffness, increase muscle strength, and improve flexibility. It can also help prevent further damage by strengthening the joints themselves.

A doctor or physical therapist can recommend an exercise programme – the type and amount of exercise will depend on which joints are affected, how stable or swollen they are, and whether you have had joint replacement surgery. In general, three types of exercises are usually included. Range-of-motion exercises help to reduce stiffness and improve flexibility of the joints and the tendons and ligaments that support them. Strengthening exercises help maintain or increase muscle strength. Low-impact aerobic exercises, such as walking, swimming or cycling increase endurance. However, sufferers are advised to scale back their exercise regimen and get more rest during a bout of inflammation.

- **KEEPING A DIARY** Writing a diary of thoughts and feelings has been shown to decrease the symptoms of arthritis and the need for pain medication among people with rheumatoid arthritis. This is possibly because it helps to reduce stress.

See also: *Lupus, pp.324–5* • *Acupuncture, pp.464–5* • *Ayurveda, pp.451–4*

Tendonitis and Bursitis

Pain in a shoulder, elbow, knee or other joint can be a sign of tendonitis or bursitis. Tendonitis is an inflammation of or small tear in a tendon – the fibrous tissue that connects muscles to bones. Common sites of tendonitis include the Achilles tendon in the ankle and the rotator cuff in the shoulder, as well as in the elbow, knee and wrist.

Bursitis is an inflammation of the bursa – sacs of fluid around a joint that cushion the muscle, bone and ligaments from friction when the joint moves. Bursitis is most likely to affect the shoulder, elbow, hip or knee.

CAUSES

Both conditions often occur with repetitive physical activity, as is common with sports such as tennis, swimming, golf and baseball, as well as manual labour such as carpentry. Tendonitis can also be caused by infections, such

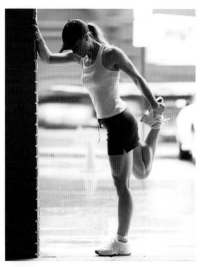

Tendonitis is usually caused by overuse or strain of the elastic tissues – the tendons – that connect muscles to the bones.

as gonorrhoea (pp.424–5), and rheumatoid arthritis (pp.136–9). Bursitis is sometimes caused by trauma, rheumatoid arthritis, gout (pp.150–1), and infections of organisms such as *Staphylococcus*. Being overweight increases the risk of developing bursitis in the joints of the legs, because it puts increased pressure on them.

PREVENTION

Avoid tendonitis by warming up before exercising. Avoid abruptly increasing the intensity of an exercise routine because doing so can irritate or tear the tendons. For sports with repetitive motions, such as tennis, that have a high risk of tendonitis, coaching in proper technique can also reduce the risk of injury. Comfortable athletic shoes can help prevent tendonitis of the Achilles tendon and knees. To protect yourself from gonorrhoea, avoid sexual relations with someone who is infected and use condoms during intercourse.

To prevent bursitis, avoid moving the same joint over and over again for prolonged periods. Use protective gear when engaging in manual work and other activities

WHO IS AT RISK?

The risk factors include:

Tendonitis
- Sports (especially tennis, swimming, golf and baseball)
- Manual labour, such as carpentry, painting or welding
- Rheumatoid arthritis

Bursitis
- Sports
- Manual labour
- Overweight
- Trauma
- Rheumatoid arthritis
- Gout

that put ongoing pressure on a joint. For example, wear kneepads while working in the garden for an afternoon. Try to maintain a normal weight.

DIAGNOSIS

A doctor can diagnose tendonitis and bursitis by reviewing a patient's medical history, evaluating their symptoms and examining the affected area. Questions about sports and other physical activity, as well as sexual relations, can help narrow down the cause.

To diagnose tendonitis, the doctor will examine the area for swelling and tenderness and ask the patient to move the limb or joint to test its range of motion and strength against resistance. Specific resistance tests are used for particular tendons. X-rays may be

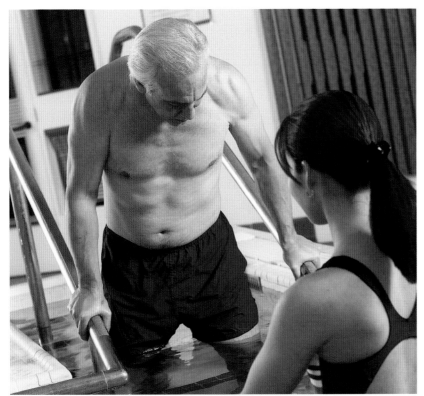

Treatment for tendonitis may include wearing a splint or brace to stabilize an injured knee to help reduce swelling. Massage and water therapy can help restore mobility to injured joints and improve strength of the muscles that surround and stabilize them.

taken to rule out a broken bone. For Achilles tendonitis, ultrasound or magnetic resonance imaging (MRI) may be needed to evaluate the extent of the injury.

To diagnose bursitis, the doctor will press on the painful area to determine if the pain is coming from a bursa. Blood tests may be done to look for signs of infection or rheumatoid arthritis. The doctor may also drain fluid from the bursa and have it analysed for signs of infection.

TREATMENTS

The goal of treatment is to relieve pain and reduce inflammation.

• SELF-CARE For the first day, apply ice to the affected joint or limb for about 20 minutes several times a day to ease swelling. Thereafter, apply heat to improve range of motion. Rest the joint or limb for several days or weeks to allow it to heal, avoiding activity that causes pain. A sling may help rest an arm or wrist with tendonitis and a splint or brace can help stabilize an ankle or knee and reduce swelling. Gradually resume normal activity and exercise when the pain stops.

• MEDICATION Ibuprofen, aspirin, and other anti-inflammatory agents can reduce inflammation and pain. Antibiotics are needed for gonorrhoea. For severe tendonitis and bursitis, a doctor may recommend injections of corticosteroid medication into the affected area for a short period of time.

• PHYSICAL THERAPY Severe non-infectious tendonitis and bursitis can be treated with techniques such as massage (pp.468–73) and hydrotherapy (pp.482–3) to restore mobility to the joints. A carefully planned exercise programme may also help. For tendonitis, physical therapy also involves stretching and strengthening the muscles and tendons.

• SURGERY This may be needed to remove fluid from a bursa to relieve the inflammation. Other types of surgery may be recommended to repair an injured bursa or to remove inflamed tissue around a tendon affected by tendonitis. But surgery is used only in the rare cases when tendonitis and bursitis do not respond to other treatments.

• ACUPUNCTURE This Traditional Chinese Medicine (pp.446–50) technique is effective in treating tendonitis, especially tendonitis of the elbow (tennis elbow) and the shoulder (rotator cuff tendonitis).

See also: *Arthritis, pp.136–9 • Massage, pp.468–73 • Water Therapy, pp.482–3*

Clinical Query

How do I know if I have tendonitis or bursitis?

The symptoms of tendonitis are:
• Pain in a heel, near a knee, in an arm or in a wrist
• Pain that gets worse with movement and at night
• Red skin above the painful area

The symptoms of bursitis are:
• Pain around a joint, especially when it moves or is pressed
• Swelling of the affected joint
• Warmth or redness of the joint

Muscle Cramps

When a muscle or muscle group contracts suddenly and feels hard and painful, that is a cramp. Muscle cramps generally come in waves, lasting for several seconds at a time and then recurring. They are especially common during and after exercise, as well as with menstruation and pregnancy. Cramps are usually harmless, but they can be a sign of nutritional deficiencies and other health conditions.

CAUSES

Muscle cramps can occur for no apparent reason. Leg cramps, for example, can strike when you lie down or sleep. But a common cause is exercise. Lactic acid, a byproduct of glucose metabolism, rises during exercise, and a build-up in a muscle can cause cramps. Dehydration and low levels of potassium, sodium and other electrolytes can increase the risk of cramps from exercise. Overuse of muscles can cause cramps, and can occur not only with exercise, but also with simple activities such as writing. Stress can also cause some muscles to tense up and cramp.

Abdominal cramps are common just before and during menstruation and at the end of pregnancy. Leg cramps can be a symptom of poor blood circulation due to atherosclerosis (pp.230–3) or peripheral vascular disease (pp.254–5). Muscle twitches can trigger cramps; causes include hypothyroidism (p.350), alcoholism (pp.358–60), caffeine, anxiety (pp.354–5), side effects of medications such as diuretics, and kidney failure (pp.306–7).

PREVENTION

Stretch before exercising to make the muscles more flexible. Do not stop exercising suddenly – this can trigger a spasm. Instead, cool down by walking or doing some other moderate movement. Drink enough fluids to avoid dehydration, but do not drink large amounts of water. Sports drinks containing electrolytes may help prevent both cramps and central nervous system complications, including seizures, caused by electrolyte disturbances.

Use proven techniques to control emotional stress, such as meditation (pp.514–19), yoga (pp.476–9) and guided imagery (pp.520–2). For anxiety, seek help from a mental health professional. If there are frequent muscle cramps that have no apparent cause, cut back on caffeine and alcohol and avoid taking any stimulating medications.

DIAGNOSIS

Cramps that persist should be evaluated by a doctor, who may ask about alcohol use, exercise and other habits that can lead to cramps. Blood tests may be done for electrolyte levels, as well as for kidney and thyroid function, and pregnancy. If a muscle or nerve disorder is suspected, spinal X-rays or CT scans and specialized nerve and muscle testing may be done.

TREATMENTS

Muscle cramps usually go away on their own, but the discomfort can be relieved with self-care measures. Warm or cold compresses can ease the pain. Stretching can help stop cramps and prevent them from occurring. Massage can ease cramps by relaxing the muscles. Pain relievers such as ibuprofen or acetaminophen can reduce pain from menstrual cramps.

See also: *Kidney Failure, pp.306–7 • Atherosclerosis, pp.230–3 • Anxiety, pp.354–5*

WHO IS AT RISK?

The risk factors include:

- Exercise, especially without warming up and cooling down
- Dehydration
- Deficiency in potassium, sodium and other electrolytes
- Menstruation
- Pregnancy
- Peripheral vascular disease
- Atherosclerosis
- Medications, such as diuretics and stimulants
- Emotional stress
- Anxiety

Bone Fractures

Any break or crack in a bone is a fracture. A broken bone that punctures the skin is an open, or compound, fracture. This is more serious than a simple, or closed, fracture in which the bone does not protrude. All fractures require immediate medical attention.

CAUSES

Fractures occur when bones receive more pressure than they can withstand. Common causes are falls, collisions in sports and car accidents. The continuous pounding on the feet from running can cause thin breaks, called hairline fractures, in the feet, ankles, shinbones and hips. Osteoporosis (pp.146–7), a weakening and thinning of the bones, increases the risk of fractures.

PREVENTION

Wear protective gear when playing sports. Use common sense to guard against accidents at home:

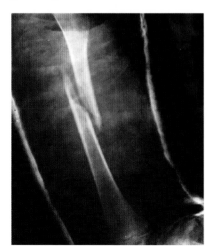

A severe fracture may require surgery to properly align and fuse the broken bone so that it heals correctly.

eliminate floor clutter, use handrails when taking stairs, and repair broken steps and walkways. To reduce your risk of osteoporosis, get enough calcium and vitamin D from diet or supplements and do weight-bearing exercises regularly, such as walking and weight-lifting.

DIAGNOSIS

A swollen or misshapen limb following an injury or a joint that cannot bear weight may be fractured. A doctor uses X-rays for a definitive diagnosis. CT scans or an MRI may also be needed to see minute details of joint fractures and damage to the surrounding tissue.

TREATMENTS

If a closed bone fracture is suspected, seek immediate medical attention. A closed fracture can often be treated in the doctor's surgery. Open fractures are medical emergencies. Aspirin or any other nonsteroidal anti-inflammatory agents should not be taken to relieve pain from fractures because they promote bleeding; instead, apply an ice pack.
• IMMOBILIZATION This is the main treatment for most closed fractures. A cast or splint is used to hold the broken bone in place until new

bone grows. A sling may be enough for a fractured shoulder or elbow.
• SURGERY Open fractures may require surgery to clean the broken bone and surrounding tissue. Open or closed fractures that involve multiple breaks require stabilization by surgically fusing the bones with metal rods, pins, screws and plates.
• TRACTION The fractured limb is held taut with ropes and pulleys to keep the bone properly aligned as it heals. In children, traction is may be used instead of surgery so as not to damage the growing tissue at the ends of long bones. In adults, traction may be used before surgery or casting to improve the odds of successful treatment.
• ANTIBIOTICS These prevent infection from open fractures.
• PHYSICAL THERAPY After the bone heals, physical therapy can help restore range of motion and function.
• MAGNET THERAPY Pulsed electromagnetic fields are widely used in North America and Europe to help heal leg fractures.

See also: *Osteoporosis, pp.146–47, Magnet Therapy, p.572*

WHO IS AT RISK?

The risk factors include:
• Sports or activities that involve contact, speed or repetitive stress
• Difficulty walking
• Climbing
• Osteoporosis

FIBROMYALGIA, CHRONIC FATIGUE SYNDROME & CHRONIC PAIN

Many illnesses cause pain and fatigue for a few days or weeks, but with fibromyalgia, chronic fatigue syndrome, and chronic pain, the symptoms last far longer and are less responsive to treatment. Fibromyalgia is pain and stiffness in 11 to 18 specific tender points of soft tissue throughout the body that last for at least three months.

Chronic fatigue syndrome causes extreme fatigue, and often, joint pain and other symptoms that last for at least six months. Chronic pain can strike anywhere, but is especially common in the back, head and extremities.

CAUSES

Although there is considerable overlap among the conditions, they each have different risk factors. For reasons that are unclear, these conditions are far more common in women.

Fibromyalgia

Experts are not sure what causes fibromyalgia. One theory is that it is an abnormal pain response. The condition runs in families, so genetics may be involved. Physical trauma, emotional stress and insomnia may also play a role. Fibromyalgia is sometimes a complication of a musculoskeletal disorder, such as rheumatoid arthritis (pp.136–9) or lupus (pp.324–5).

Chronic Fatigue Syndrome

The cause is also unknown, but there are several theories based on limited scientific evidence.

One theory is that it is caused by a virus such as the Epstein-Barr virus or human herpes virus 6, or is triggered by some prior illness. Another theory is that an allergy or some other immune system abnormality causes inflammation in pathways of neurons (nerve cells). More than half of people with chronic fatigue syndrome also have a history of allergies, which is another immune system disorder. Social support also appears important – people with chronic fatigue syndrome who lacked positive relationships had worse symptoms than patients with supportive relationships, according to a 2004 study at the University Medical Center in Nigmegan, Netherlands. Other possible causes are genetic predisposition, stress or inadequate blood flow to the brain.

Chronic Pain

The main causes of chronic pain are chronic conditions, including cancer, arthritis and back pain (pp.132–3). Fibromyalgia and chronic fatigue syndrome are also common causes. An acute injury, such as a sprained back or a severe infection, can cause residual pain even after the problem has resolved. Sometimes chronic pain has no physical cause and is thought to be due to emotional and psychological factors, such as stress or depression.

PREVENTION

Managing stress with techniques such as meditation (pp.514–19) and yoga (pp.476–9) may reduce the risk of developing all three conditions. Taking precautions against injuries can prevent chronic pain and, possibly, fibromyalgia.

Clinical Query

How can I distinguish fibromyalgia and chronic fatigue syndrome from other types of fatigue and pain?

What sets fibromyalgia apart from chronic fatigue is that the pain lasts at least three months and occurs in 11 to 18 tender points in the neck, shoulders, chest, rib cage, lower back, thighs, knees, elbows and buttocks.

It is the severity and the persistence of the fatigue that distinguishes chronic fatigue syndrome. Look for these signs:

- Profound fatigue or tiredness that lasts at least six months and is not relieved by resting or sleeping.
- Fatigue that starts with half the amount of exertion that typically made you feel tired before the illness started.

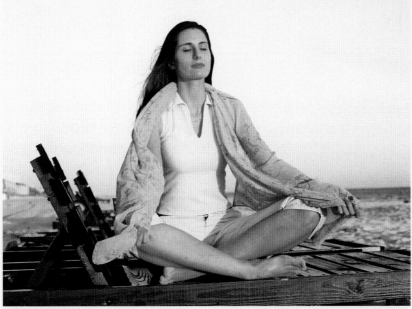

Fibromyalgia and chronic fatigue syndrome can cause long-lasting or recurring pain and extreme fatigue. Meditation and yoga may help relieve symptoms of these disorders.

DIAGNOSIS

A doctor can diagnose fibromyalgia and chronic fatigue syndrome based on the symptoms, their duration and a physical examination. Pain is considered chronic if it lasts longer than three months.

Diagnosing fibromyalgia and chronic fatigue syndrome involves ruling out other disorders that can cause the symptoms. The doctor may order blood tests and X-rays to check for rheumatoid arthritis, lupus, Lyme disease (pp.326–7), hepatitis (p.269) and thyroid disorders (pp.344–7). There may also be tests for depression (pp.364–5) and anxiety (pp.354–5). In addition, to diagnose fibromyalgia, the doctor will check for tender points in the neck, shoulders, lower back and other areas. For chronic fatigue, the doctor will look for a low-grade fever (101°F/39°C), tenderness in the lymph nodes, muscle weakness and pain, and joint pain that moves and is not accompanied by any inflammation.

TREATMENTS

An integrated approach can relieve the pain and other disabling symptoms of all three disorders.

• **MEDICATION** Pain-relieving medicines, such as nonsteroidal anti-inflammatory agents, can help all three conditions temporarily.

• **EXERCISE** Aerobic exercise can improve functioning, mood and pain from fibromyalgia for up to one year. A graded exercise programme yields short-term gains in energy for people with chronic fatigue syndrome.

• **SUPPLEMENTS** L-carnitine, an amino acid, reduced physical and mental fatigue in a study published in *Psychosomatic Medicine* in 2004. In an Italian study in 1992, half of the 50 fibromyalgia patients who took 5 HTP (5-hydroxy-L-tryptophan) reported good or fair improvement of symptoms, such as tender point pain, anxiety, and difficulty sleeping, and that improvements lasted for 90 days. Studies of SAMe (s-adenosylmethionine) supplements for fibromyalgia are mixed, with some studies showing improved symptoms and others showing no benefit. Doctors who have used it also disagree about its effectiveness.

• **COGNITIVE BEHAVIOURAL THERAPY** This form of psychotherapy, which focuses on a person's thought patterns and behaviour as a means of resolving emotional strife, improves functioning and activity levels in people with chronic fatigue syndrome and fibromyalgia.

• **CHIROPRACTIC** Chiropractic manipulation (pp.446–7) can alleviate chronic pain, although its effectiveness for fibromyalgia and chronic fatigue syndrome is unclear.

• **HYPNOTHERAPY** This can relieve chronic pain (pp.508–11).

• **KEEPING A DIARY** Writing about thoughts and feelings helped reduce pain and improve energy in women with fibromyalgia in a study published in *Psychosomatic Medicine* in 2005. However, the benefits lasted only four months.

• **THERAPEUTIC TOUCH** This therapy, which incorporates the laying on of hands with other energy techniques, can decrease muscle and joint pain and reduce the reliance on pain medication.

• **ACUPUNCTURE** This therapy (pp.464–5) relieves some kinds of chronic pain. Its effectiveness for fibromyalgia is unclear.

See also: *Arthritis, pp.136–9* • *Back Pain, pp.132–3* • *Hypnotherapy, pp.508–11*

Osteoporosis

Osteoporosis, a leading cause of bone fractures, is a metabolic disease in which the structure of bone tissue breaks down, leaving bones thin and brittle. As part of the natural life-cycle of bone, old bone tissue is continuously being reabsorbed and new bone is forming. Until about age 30, bone mass increases because new bone forms faster than old bone breaks down. After 30, the rate of new bone formation gradually declines, leading to overall loss of bone mass.

Osteoporosis is caused by an accelerated rate of bone loss. It is most common among post-menopausal women, although it also affects men and younger people of both sexes. The wrists, hips and spine are most often affected.

CAUSES

Ageing is the major cause of osteoporosis. It is more common in women than in men because oestrogen, a female sex hormone, helps supply bones with calcium, a mineral that is essential for new bone formation. The drop in oestrogen that occurs during and after menopause increases the risk of osteoporosis. The danger is especially high in women who experience early menopause, whether natural or induced.

Inadequate consumption of calcium appears to be a major preventable cause, because calcium is essential for new bone formation. Lack of vitamin D can also lead to osteoporosis because vitamin D assists in the absorption of calcium. Smoking accelerates bone loss by lowering oestrogen levels and

possibly interfering with calcium absorption. Alcohol (more than 59 ml/2 fl.oz distilled spirits a day) promotes bone loss and can lead to fractures even in young adults. Women who exercise too strenuously lower their oestrogen levels, which can cause osteoporosis.

PREVENTION

Eating a balanced diet with adequate calcium and vitamin D, and exercising daily can help prevent osteoporosis. Recommendations for daily calcium intake from the National Academy of Sciences in the United States are 1,300 mg a day for children ages 9 to 13, 1,000 mg for adults ages 19 to 50, and 1,200 mg for adults ages 51 and older. Recommendations for vitamin D are 400 to 800 IU (international units) each day. Good sources of dietary calcium are non-fat or low-fat milk and yogurt; tofu; leafy green vegetables such as greens and broccoli; sardines and salmon with bones; and citrus juices fortified with calcium. Vitamin D can be obtained from foods such as

fortified milk and cereals, as well as from exposure to sunlight. Fifteen minutes a day will ensure adequate levels of vitamin D.

Doing weight-bearing exercises encourages the formation of new bone, and include walking, tennis, cycling, cross-country skiing and dancing. Osteoporosis can also be prevented by not smoking and drinking fewer than two alcoholic beverages a day. (One drink equals 355 ml/12 fl.oz of beer, 148 ml/5 fl.oz of wine, or 44 ml/ 1.5 fl.oz of distilled spirits.)

To prevent fractures, take commonsense precautions against falls, such as wearing comfortable shoes, using handrails when walking up and down stairs, and removing clutter from the floors. If you are

WHO IS AT RISK?

The risk factors include:

- Women over 50 years old
- Family history of osteoporosis
- Caucasian or Asian
- Inadequate calcium and vitamin D intake
- Smoking
- Excess alcohol consumption
- Underweight
- Small frame
- Long-term use of medications such as steroids, anticonvulsants, and high doses of thyroid medication
- Hyperthyroidism and hypothyroidism
- Cushing's disease

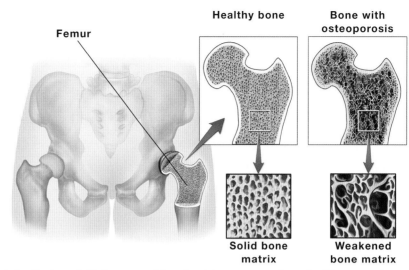

In healthy bone (left), the spongy internal matrix appears regular and solid, compared to bone with osteoporosis (right), in which the matrix is weakened. Loss of bone mass leaves bones thin and brittle and vulnerable to fractures.

taking a medication that causes bone loss, your doctor may prescribe one of the drugs that slows or reverses bone loss and increases bone density (see Treatments).

DIAGNOSIS

Osteoporosis is most often diagnosed with dual energy X-ray absorptiometry (DEXA), which measures the mineral content of bone, an indicator of its density and strength. DEXA can be used to give a baseline reading of bone density, to confirm a diagnosis of osteoporosis in someone who has had a fracture, and to show changes in bone density over time. Women should start having routine bone density tests by age 65, or earlier if they have a family history of osteoporosis.

TREATMENTS

The aim of treatment is to help maintain bone density by increasing the rate of new bone production, slowing the rate of bone loss, or both. Calcium and vitamin D alone, however, cannot increase

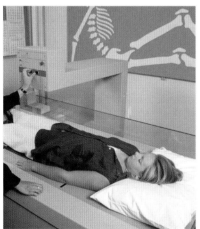

Osteoporosis is caused by accelerated bone loss. The condition can be diagnosed using a bone density test, which measures the mineral content of bones.

bone density in a person suffering from osteoporosis. Many doctors recommend one of the following medications to increase bone density.

• **HORMONES** Oestrogen replacement therapy consists of pills or skin patches that supplement oestrogen in post-menopausal women. It reduces bone loss and lowers the risk of fractures. However, hormone replacement therapy has significant side effects, including an increased risk of breast cancer, heart disease, and possibly Alzheimer's disease.

Calcitonin is a hormone that regulates calcium metabolism. Given by injection or nasal spray, it increases the density of the spine. It is prescribed for men and women when bisphosphonates, Selective oestrogen receptor modulators (SERMs), and oestrogen therapy are not effective or cannot be used.

Teriparatide is a supplement of parathyroid hormone, a naturally occurring hormone that helps maintain calcium levels in the blood. It increases new bone for-

mation in the hips and spine. The drug is given by injection to men and post-menopausal women who are at high risk of bone fractures.

• **MEDICATION** SERMs are drugs that do not contain oestrogen but function like oestrogen in the body. They appear to have fewer dangerous side effects than oestrogen replacement therapy. Raloxifene is a SERM that reduces the risk of fractures in the vertebrae and is believed to prevent bone loss in the spine, hips and other bones. It is prescribed for post-menopausal women. It may also decrease the risk of developing breast cancer.

Bisphosphonates, which do not contain or act like oestrogen in the body, inhibit bone loss. They are prescribed to increase bone density in the hips and spine and reduce the risk of fractures. Medications in this category include alendronate and risedronate.

See also: *Smoking Cessation, pp.216–17 • Menopause, pp.406–8 • Thyroid Disorders, pp.344–7*

Scoliosis

A normal spine is curved from front to back, but is straight from side to side. A sideways curvature of the spine, one in which the curve looks like an S or a C, is sign of scoliosis, a musculoskeletal disorder. Scoliosis can occur at any age, but is often diagnosed in children and adolescents. In infants and young children, equal numbers of boys and girls are affected, but adolescent girls are most likely to have a curvature that is pronounced enough to require treatment.

Severe scoliosis requires treatment for more than cosmetic reasons: it can help prevent serious complications, such as spinal cord or nerve damage, lower-back arthritis and respiratory problems.

CAUSES

For most people the cause of the scoliosis is idiopathic, or unknown. However, the condition runs in families, suggesting that it may be partly genetic. Other causes include differences in limb length; neuromuscular disorders including muscular dystrophy (p.158) and cerebral palsy; Marfan's syndrome, an inherited disorder affecting the body's connective tissue; and structural birth defects of the spine. People who have a family history of spinal deformity also have a greater risk for developing the condition.

PREVENTION

There is no known way to prevent scoliosis.

DIAGNOSIS

Screening for scoliosis is part of a standard paediatric checkup. A doctor examines the spine when the child is bending forwards. When the child is standing straight, the doctor notes any asymmetries, such as one shoulder being higher than the other, the head being off-centre or posture that leans to one side. X-rays of the spine are usually taken to measure the angle of the curve, which helps determine whether treatment is necessary.

TREATMENTS

Most people who have idiopathic scoliosis require no treatment

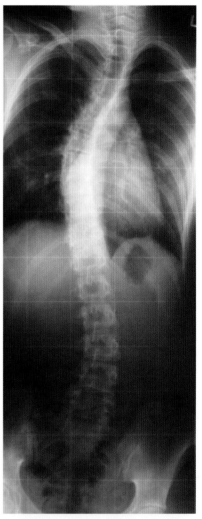

Scoliosis is a side-to-side curvature of the spine that requires medical attention. X-rays help measure the curve and determine the course of treatment.

because the curve is minor. If treatment is required, the degree and location of curvature, the person's age, and whether he or she is still growing will determine the treatment recommended.

• **OBSERVATION** Some cases of scoliosis – those in which the curve is slight, for instance – have

WHO IS AT RISK?

The risk factors include:

• Family history
• Female
• Neuromuscular disorders, such as muscular dystrophy and cerebral palsy
• Marfan's syndrome
• Birth defects of the spine

healing hope My youngest daughter is a very active teenager. Last year she wanted to go out for cheerleading and track at the same time, and we've always encouraged her to do the best she can.

But I noticed something peculiar when she was trying on new school clothes last summer. Every time she tried on a pair of jeans, one leg was shorter. We soon realized her shoulders were uneven too. We talked to a doctor, and after an X-ray and an examination, he told us she has scoliosis.

My grandmother had scoliosis, and I worried my daughter might have to forget about track and cheerleading. I didn't want her having the kind of back problems my grandmother had. But the doctor assured us she could continue with sports, and that it might actually keep the condition from getting worse. We've made sure to keep a close eye on her back as she grows, but so far the scoliosis hasn't caused her any more problems. *Kelen T.*

getting worse or has not responded to bracing, surgery may be the only option. Surgical procedures straighten the spine by fusing some of the vertebrae in the curve and securing them with metal rods, hooks and screws. Surgery can be performed on children who are still growing and also on adults. Recovery from surgery varies depending on the type of procedure performed. It may take several months; however, most patients can eventually resume normal activities.

a low risk of progressing, making observation the wisest choice. Medical checkups every four to six months may be recommended for a child who is still growing and has a curvature of less than 25 degrees. In cases of idiopathic scoliosis that affect the thoracic (upper) spine in an adolescent, doctors should check to see whether respiratory function is impaired, especially if the scoliosis is severe.

• **BACK BRACE** For children who are still growing and whose spinal curvature is greater than 25 degrees, doctors often recommend that a back brace be worn to prevent the curvature from worsening. A back brace is also considered an option when the curvature is 20 degrees or more and is getting worse, or if the child is a girl who is at least two years away from her first menstrual period. (Girls are more likely than boys to develop severe curvatures when they reach puberty.) Different types of braces are available to correct curvatures in different parts of the spine. A brace is worn for a specified number of hours each

day until the child stops growing.

• **SURGERY** When the curvature is more than 45 degrees and is

See also: *Muscular Dystrophy, p.158* • *Arthritis, pp.136–9*

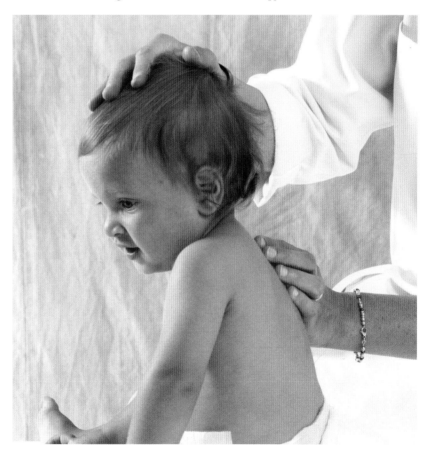

Although scoliosis can occur at any age, it is often diagnosed in childhood. Causes can include congenital spine deformities, genetic disorders, neuromuscular conditions and a difference in limb length. However, in the majority of cases, there is no known cause. Screening for scoliosis is now a standard part of paediatric checkups.

Gout

Swelling, redness and severe pain in a joint that comes on suddenly and lasts for about a week are signs of gout, a form of arthritis (pp.136–9). The big toe is the most common site, but gout can also affect the ankles, knees, wrists and hands. Attacks of gout sometimes include a temperature and general malaise. Gout is most common in men who are middle-aged and older, but it also affects women. About one-fifth of people with gout develop kidney damage.

CAUSES

Gout is the result of excess uric acid, a by-product of the break-down of protein and other compounds. Either the metabolism, for unknown reasons, produces an excess of uric acid or the kidneys do not eliminate enough uric acid in the urine. This excess uric acid then leads to the formation of crystals in a joint. Irritation from these crystals causes pain and inflammation.

There are several risk factors for gout. Certain foods increase the production of uric acid because they are high in purines – chemicals that the body converts to uric acid. These foods include organ meats, brains, anchovies, asparagus and mushrooms. Alcohol increases uric acid production and hampers kidney function. A diet that is heavy in these foods and in alcohol can trigger gout. Other illnesses can cause gout, including obesity (pp.348–9), hypothyroidism (p.350), diabetes (pp.338–41), leukaemia (p.335) and kidney failure (pp.304–7). Radiation treatments and medications that slow kidney function also increase the risk, including diuretics for high blood pressure and warfarin for stroke.

PREVENTION

Avoiding obesity and foods high in purines, and moderating alcohol consumption can help prevent gout from developing or recurring. Drinking six to eight glasses of water a day can dilute uric acid, possibly preventing attacks of gout.

WHO IS AT RISK?

The risk factors include:
- Men middle-aged and older
- Obesity
- High alcohol consumption
- High consumption of purine-rich foods (including organ meats, brains, anchovies and mushrooms)
- Kidney disease
- Hypothyroidism
- Diabetes
- Leukaemia
- Medications (diuretics, warfarin)
- Radiation treatments

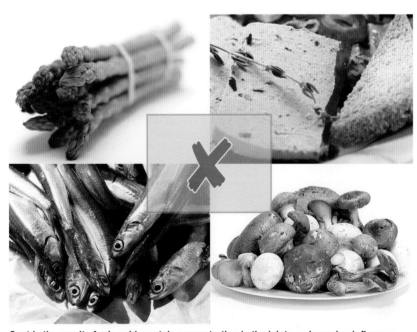

Gout is the result of uric acid crystals concentrating in the joints and causing inflammation. Foods such as asparagus, organ meat, sardines and mushrooms are high in purines, which can lead to uric acid build-up in the blood and cause gout.

On Call

The following homeopathic remedies may help alleviate pain from gout. The dose is usually three to five pellets of a 12x to 30c remedy every one to four hours until the symptoms improve.

- Aconite for sudden onset of burning pain, anxiety, restlessness and attacks that come after a shock or injury.
- Belladonna for intense pain that may be throbbing; pain is made worse by any motion and better by pressure; joint is very hot.
- Bryonia for pain made much worse by any kind of motion; pain is better with pressure and heat.
- Colchicum for pain made worse by motion and changes of weather, especially if there is any nausea associated with the attacks.
- Ledum when joints become mottled, purple and swollen; pain is much better with cold applications and is worse when overheated.

DIAGNOSIS

A doctor can diagnose gout based on the symptoms and on a physical examination of the joints to look for swelling and restricted range of motion. Blood tests can reveal high levels of uric acid, but high levels are found in only 50 percent of people suffering from gout. Blood tests can also reveal elevated white blood cell count, a sign of inflammation, which can be caused by crystals in the joints. The doctor may also collect fluid from a joint and have it analysed for signs of crystals. X-rays may be taken to look for the presence of joint damage.

TREATMENTS

There is no cure for gout, but the frequency of attacks and their symptoms can be decreased with diet and medication.

- **NUTRITION** Avoiding alcohol and restricting foods that contain purines can help reduce the incidence of attacks of gout. People who are obese should lose weight gradually. An extreme restriction of calories can increase uric acid production.
- **MEDICATION** Pain relievers such as nonsteroidal anti-inflammatory agents and acetaminophen can reduce pain from gout. Colchicine, which decreases joint inflammation, can relieve discomfort and help prevent attacks. Other medications can lower levels of uric acid in the blood: uricosuric drugs, such as probenecid and sulfinpyrazone, increase excretion of uric acid in the urine; and allopurinol reduces uric acid production. For severe attacks, corticosteroids may be given to reduce swelling.

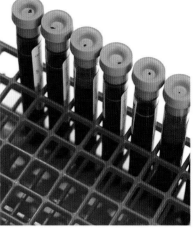

A blood test can reveal high levels of uric acid or an elevated white blood cell count, both of which are possible signs of gout.

- **ACUPUNCTURE** A small study in the *Journal of Traditional Chinese Medicine* in 2004 found that people who had one month of acupuncture (pp.446–50) treatment had greater reduction of uric acid and other markers for gout than did a control group. The researchers concluded that acupuncture may help prevent kidney damage from gout.
- **HOMEOPATHY** Homeopathic remedies (pp.455–7) may help relieve pain from gout.

See also: *Arthritis, pp.136–9* • *Obesity, pp.348–9* • *Acupuncture, pp.464–5*

healing hope

Several years ago my wrists and ankles started bothering me at night, and my doctor said it may be arthritis. I've been taking aspirin to keep the pain down. But then last month I woke up in the middle of the night and my big toe was killing me. It was so swollen and red, I couldn't really bear to walk for a few days. The doctor took some blood, and he said I have gout. He said my arthritis is caused by crystals in my blood that build up in my joints.

The pain went away after a few days, and now I take medicine to help keep the attacks from hitting me again. But the doctor also said certain foods can cause the crystals to build up faster, and now I have to cut out one of my favourite things to eat – liver. Although I know my grandkids will be happy to hear that.
Cory H.

Heel Spurs

Abnormal hook-shaped bones that grow from the bottom of the heel are heel spurs. The condition is common, especially in middle age. Although heel spurs are not usually painful, they often occur along with another condition, plantar fasciitis (an inflammation of the ligament that connects the heel to the toes, p.153), that does cause a sharp pain when weight or pressure is placed on the heel. Heel spurs sometimes also lead to bursitis (pp.140–1), a painful inflammation of the bursae (sacs of fluid that help reduce joint friction).

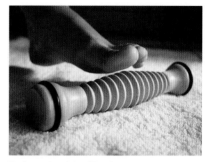

Reduce the risk of heel spurs by doing exercises to stretch and increase the flexibility of the plantar fascia ligament.

CAUSES

Heel spurs occur when the plantar fascia, the connective tissue that is between the heel and toes, pulls too tightly on the heel. A heel spur grows in response to the excess stress. Several factors can increase the risk of heel spurs, including poor-fitting shoes, obesity and osteomalacia, a bone deformity usually caused by vitamin D deficiency.

PREVENTION

There are several ways to reduce the risk of heel spurs. Wear comfortable shoes. Maintain a normal weight to avoid putting excess pressure on the feet. Do foot exercises to stretch and increase the flexibility of the plantar fascia. For example, stand with the foot on a cylinder and roll the foot around it. Another exercise is to grab the front of the foot (near the toes) and pull towards yourself.

DIAGNOSIS

A doctor can diagnose heel spurs by taking X-rays of the affected heel and examining them for signs of the telltale claw-shaped projection of bone.

TREATMENTS

Heel spurs only require treatment if they cause pain, which is often the case when they are associated with plantar fasciitis. Even then, simple self-help measures are usually sufficient.

• **SELF-HELP** Rest the foot for a few days by limiting the amount of time spent standing, walking or running to reduce the inflammation and pain of plantar fasciitis. Putting ice on the affected area can further reduce these symptoms. The foot-stretching exercises described in Prevention are also helpful.

• **MEDICATION** Nonsteroidal anti-inflammatory agents (NSAIDs) can temporarily ease pain and inflammation. For severe pain that does not respond to more conservative treatment, a steroid may be injected into the heel to reduce inflammation.

• **SHOE INSERTS** Gel heel cups can reduce heel pain and pressure on the plantar fascia when you stand, walk or exercise. It is unclear whether orthodics, which are custom-made shoe inserts, are superior to generic inserts.

• **SURGERY** This is rarely used to treat heel spurs because the results are unpredictable. But it may be considered as a last resort if pain is constant and does not respond to other treatments. Surgery involves removing either the bone spur or the plantar fascia.

See also: *Plantar Faciitis, p.153* • *Bursitis, pp.140–1*

WHO IS AT RISK?

The risk factors include:

• Poor-fitting shoes
• Excessive pressure on the feet
• Obesity
• Rheumatoid arthritis, gout or ankylosing spondylitis

Plantar Fasciitis

Heel pain first thing in the morning that diminishes when you begin walking around is a sign of plantar fasciitis, an inflammation in the soft tissue on the bottom of the foot. The inflammation is in the plantar fascia, a thick swath of tissue that functions as a shock absorber and an arch support. The heel may be red and slightly inflamed. Plantar fasciitis often occurs with heel spurs (p.152) and is most common among athletic adults age 40 and older. It usually goes away with rest.

CAUSES

Small tears in the plantar fascia cause plantar fasciitis. The tears often result from repetitive injury caused by running, dancing and occupations that require standing for many hours. Other risk factors include flat feet, unusually high arches, obesity (pp.348–9), rheumatoid arthritis (pp.136–9), fibromyalgia (pp.144–5) and psoriasis (pp.120–1).

PREVENTION

Exercises that stretch the calves and the plantar fascia can help prevent plantar fasciitis. They include rolling the arch of each foot over a tennis ball and, while sitting, using the hands to pull the front of each foot toward you. Wearing comfortable shoes can also reduce the risk.

DIAGNOSIS

A doctor can diagnose plantar fasciitis by examining the heel and arch for symptoms including tenderness, redness and swelling.

TREATMENTS

About 90 percent of people will get better within nine months if they:

- Cut back on running and other activities that put pressure on the feet.
- Apply ice to the feet after activity.
- Wear comfortable shoes; cushioning in the midsole is especially helpful.
- Do exercises that stretch the calf muscles and the plantar fascia.

• **SHOE INSERTS** Arch supports can help relieve plantar fasciitis in people who have flat feet. The supports, which fit inside the shoes, decrease the stress placed on the plantar fascia. Orthotics are also helpful because they can correct various biomechanical problems that put stress on the plantar fascia, such as the tendency to turn in the foot.

• **SPLINTS** When worn on the affected foot while sleeping, splints that keep the foot in a flexed position, stretching the calf and plantar fascia, can help to relieve the condition.

WHO IS AT RISK?

The risk factors include:
- Running or other physical activities that put stress on the feet
- Age 40 and over
- Ill-fitting shoes
- Flat feet
- Unusually high arches
- Obesity
- Rheumatoid arthritis
- Fibromyalgia
- Psoriasis

• **EXTRACORPOREAL SHOCKWAVE THERAPY** This experimental treatment uses pulses of energy to stimulate healing of inflamed tissue. A German study in the journal *Foot and Ankle International* in 2003 found that more than 90 percent of people with plantar fasciitis who had the therapy experienced less pain and improved walking time for up to two years after treatment. But other studies do not show positive results, leaving the therapy's effectiveness in question.

• **STEROIDS** Injections into the heel relieve pain in about half of the people for whom more conservative treatments are not helpful.

• **SURGERY** An operation to loosen the plantar fascia is performed when other treatments have failed, relieving pain in 70 to 90 percent of patients.

See also: *Heel Spurs, p.152 • Obesity, pp.348–9 • Fibromyalgia, pp.144–5*

Whiplash Injuries

A sudden force that thrusts the head back and forth in a whip-like motion can injure the bones and soft tissue in and around the neck. These are called whiplash injuries. Symptoms include neck pain and stiffness, as well as headache, pain in the back or shoulder, and dizziness. Some patients also report associated problems such as anxiety, depression, fatigue, sleep disturbance and difficulty with memory or concentration. The symptoms can begin immediately after the injury or several days later.

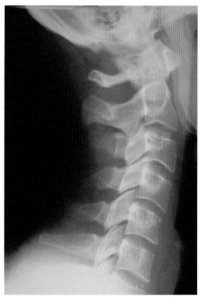

A sudden movement of the neck that strains muscles, joints and nerves, such as during a car accident, can cause whiplash. An X-ray may be used to check for fractures in the bones of the neck.

CAUSES

Car crashes are a major cause of whiplash injuries. A rear crash or a sudden stop forces the driver's and passengers' heads forwards and backwards beyond their normal range of motion. This motion can strain muscles, ligaments and connective tissue in the neck, and injure the vertebrae. Other causes of whiplash injuries include roller-coasters and other fast amusement park rides that start and stop abruptly; contact sports such as football; and physical fights that involve punching or shaking.

PREVENTION

Headrests in cars can reduce the risk of receiving whiplash from rear-end collisions. Adjust the headrest so that it is high enough to cushion your head.

DIAGNOSIS

Whiplash may be suspected based on the symptoms, especially if the patient was involved in an accident.

If there is any question about the seriousness of the symptoms, it is wise to see a doctor to confirm the diagnosis and receive advice and treatment.
See a doctor if:
- The force involved in the injury was great.
- You have severe or persistent neck pain.
- You lost consciousness following the injury.
- The pain went away and then returned.
- A shoulder or an arm hurts or feels numb.
- You feel pain when you move your head.

These symptoms can suggest that your injuries are more serious and extensive than whiplash. A doctor should also be consulted for whiplash injuries in babies (see Clinical Query).

TREATMENTS

Whiplash injuries can often be successfully treated with first aid and rest, but may require medical care.

- REST Do not lift anything, play sports, or engage in other activities that strain the neck for two to three weeks – the time it usually takes for whiplash injuries to heal. Avoid all activities that require you to tilt the head backwards.
- HOT COMPRESSES Applying a heating pad or hot water bottle to the painful area of the neck can

WHO IS AT RISK?

The risk factors include:
- Motor vehicle accident
- Roller-coasters and other fast amusement park rides
- Contact sports
- Physical fights

ease the pain, relax neck muscles and improve blood flow to the injured area.

• MEDICATION Pain relievers such as nonsteroidal anti-inflammatory agents (NSAIDs) and acetaminophen can temporarily relieve pain. If these medications are not effective or if you have muscle spasms when you move the head, muscle relaxants may be prescribed. Preliminary research suggests that a steroid (methylprednisolone) given intravenously may be beneficial when used in the early stages of acute whiplash, and that injecting lidocaine, a local anaesthetic, into the tender areas of muscle (called trigger points) may relieve chronic neck pain.

• CERVICAL COLLAR If the neck hurts when you move your head from side to side, a doctor may recommend that you wear a soft collar around the neck for two to three weeks. The collar may relieve the pain by taking the pressure off of the strained neck muscles and joints, giving them time to heal.

• PHYSICAL THERAPY Various techniques may be used to promote healing, reduce pain, and restore range of motion to the neck, including ultrasound, traction, massage (pp.468–73), active mobilization, exercises, and pulsed electromagnetic therapy, as well as localized heat and ice treatment and cervical collar immobilization. Scientific assessments have suggested that using a combination of these active treatments may be better than collars and rest alone, and that either is better than no treatment. When physical therapy techniques do help relieve symptoms, it may be a result of promoting muscle relaxation, although the precise benefits are not certain.

Clinical Query

What is shaken baby syndrome?

This is a severe and life-threatening whiplash injury to an infant that occurs when the baby is deliberately shaken. It is most common in infants six months old and younger. Their necks are not strong enough to support their heads, which are heavy in relation to their bodies. Shaking a baby can injure the upper spine, causing blindness, brain damage and possibly death. When holding an infant, be sure to support the head and avoid jumping, excessive jiggling and other abrupt movements.

• CHIROPRACTIC Many patients seek chiropractic care (pp.446–7). As with physical therapy techniques (many of which may be included in chiropractic treatment), conclusive scientific evidence proving chiropractic treaments provide a measurable therapeutic benefit is lacking, but it suggests potential for relieving pain and improving range of motion.

• NECK EXERCISES Once the whiplash injuries have begun to heal, a doctor may suggest exercises to stretch the neck muscles.

• ACUPUNCTURE Whiplash and other types of chronic neck pain are common reasons for patients to seek acupuncture (pp.464–5), but there is a lack of scientific proof of this treament is effective in relieving this type of pain.

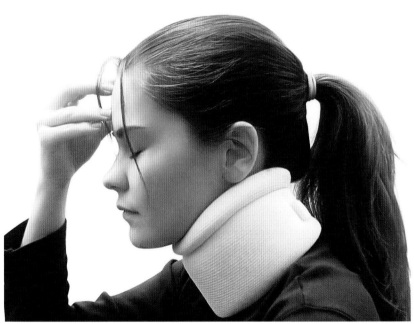

A soft cervical collar worn for several weeks can help relieve neck pain associated with whiplash. Studies suggest that when combined with other therapeutic techniques, such as massage and ultrasound, healing occurs more quickly than with a collar and rest alone.

See also: *Massage, pp.468–73* • *Magnet Therapy, p.572* • *Acupuncture, pp.464–5*

Shin Splints

Shin splints are small tears in the muscles at the front of the lower leg, sometimes referred to as medial tibial stress syndrome. Pain along several inches of the shinbones of both legs the day after jogging or running is the classic sign of shin splints. The calves may also look red and swollen. Shin splints are most common in people who spend many hours on their feet, including joggers, dancers, athletes and soldiers.

CAUSES

Repeated pounding of the feet on hard surfaces causes inflammation of the tendons connecting the muscles to the shins. Anterolateral shin splints are the most common type, affecting the anterior tibial muscle, which is in front of the shin. Posteromedial shin splints affect the muscles in the back of or along the inner sides of the shins.

Running uphill and a tendency to roll the feet outwards increases the risk of posteromedial shin splints. Other risk factors are knock knees and bow legs (anatomical abnormalities that put undue stress on the outside of the feet), and wearing poorly cushioned athletic shoes.

PREVENTION

Stretching before engaging in physical activities that involve being on your feet for a long time can reduce the risk. Running shoes that have a rigid heel and arch supports can help by keeping the foot from rolling outwards. In addition, avoid exercise that is beyond your fitness level; increase the rigour and duration of your exercise routine gradually.

DIAGNOSIS

Many people can diagnose shin splints on their own based on the symptoms and when they occur. If you are unsure or if the pain is severe and persistent, see a doctor. With a physical examination, medical history, and possibly X-rays, a bone scan or an MRI, the doctor can determine if the pain is due to shin splints or another cause, such as a stress fracture (p.143).

TREATMENTS

Though uncomfortable, shin splints are usually minor and go away within several days to several weeks. The main way to treat them is simply to rest the affected muscles. In fact, research among United States Navy midshipmen with shin splints suggests that rest alone works better than any combination of other treatments. Do not run until the pain is gone.

• HOME REMEDIES Meanwhile, relieve pain by periodically applying ice to the affected area and taking pain relievers such as nonsteroidal anti-inflammatory medicines. When resuming activity, start with a shorter, easier routine than you were accustomed to and then gradually increase the intensity.

• EXERCISE Simple exercises performed to stretch and strengthen the shin muscles may help heal and prevent shin splints. Stand on the toes and then gradually lower the heels to the floor. Do two sets of 10 repetitions of this exercise. Stand with the feet flat on the floor and roll them outward and back again. Do three sets of 10 repetitions.

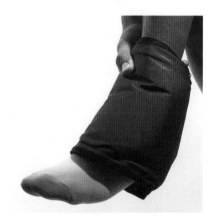

See also: *Bone Fractures, p.143*

WHO IS AT RISK?

The risk factors include:

- Running
- Aerobic dancing
- Military training
- Bow legs, knock knees or flat feet
- Wearing athletic shoes with inadequate padding and support

Ice can help relieve the pain associated with shin splints, but studies have shown the best treatment to heal the condition is rest.

Osteomyelitis

Because of their hard exterior bones are normally shielded from infections. But poor blood circulation, trauma and other problems can make them vulnerable to osteomyelitis, an infection of the bone or bone marrow. Symptoms include pain in the affected bone, swelling, fever, and sometimes pus draining through the skin over the bone. Osteomyelitis is most common in children with chronic diseases and in elderly people.

CAUSES

Bacteria and fungus cause osteomyelitis. They often gain entry to bones that have open fractures (p.143) or surgery. An artificial joint may harbour bacteria or fungus and spread it to the adjoining bone. Infections elsewhere in the body can spread through the bloodstream to the bone. Such blood-borne infections are most likely to affect people who are already weakened by other diseases and treatments, including cancer, radiation therapy, and poor blood circulation from diabetes (pp.338–41) and other conditions. Intravenous drug abuse is a source of infections that can spread to the bones.

PREVENTION

Taking precautions against accidents that cause broken bones can reduce the risk of osteomyelitis. These include wearing seat belts when travelling in a car, wearing wrist guards and shin guards when using inline skates, and using handrails when walking up and down stairs. If you have an artificial joint, metal rods or other synthetic material implanted in your body, you are at increased risk of osteomyelitis following future surgeries. Reduce this risk by taking antibiotics before any surgical procedure, including dental surgery.

DIAGNOSIS

A doctor can make a preliminary diagnosis based on symptoms such as bone pain and fever. Other tests are usually done to confirm the diagnosis, including blood tests for elevated white blood cell count and other signs of infection; imaging tests such as CT scans, bone scans, and MRI; and biopsies of the tissue surrounding the affected bone or of the bone itself.

TREATMENTS

The goal of treatment is to cure.
• MEDICATION For a bacterial infection, antibiotics are usually prescribed for a minimum of one to two months. Antifungal medications may be needed for several months to control an infection of fungal osteomyelitis.
• SURGERY Different surgical procedures may be required for osteomyelitis, depending on the cause and location. If there is pus (which means that there is an abscess in nearby tissue), the pus is surgically drained. When osteomyelitis is around an artificial joint, the joint is removed and replaced. When the affected bone has dead tissue – as often happens with diabetes – the dead tissue is removed and replaced with a graft.
• HYPERBARIC OXYGEN THERAPY This treatment (p.579) may help eliminate chronic osteomyelitis and prevent recurrences, when used with surgery.
• MAGGOT THERAPY A 16th-century treatment, in which fly larvae are were placed on an open wound, has made a comeback in conventional medicine for treating osteomyelitis that is unresponsive to medicine and surgery. Maggots sterilize the wounds and promote healing by eating bacteria and secreting therapeutic substances.

See also: *Bone fractures, p.143* • *Diabetes, pp.338–41* • *Oxygen Therapy, p.579*

WHO IS AT RISK?

The risk factors include:
- Bone fracture
- Bone surgery
- Joint replacement
- Diabetes
- Cancer
- Radiation therapy

Muscular Dystrophy

A gradual weakening and deterioration of some muscles is the main symptom of muscular dystrophy. There are nine forms of the disease, each attacking different muscles, starting in different age groups, and resulting in varying degrees of disability. Duchenne muscular dystrophy, the most common form, occurs almost exclusively in boys, but other forms affect both males and females.

CAUSES

All forms of muscular dystrophy are genetic, but each is caused by a different genetic defect and has a different pattern of inheritance.

Duchenne and Becker-type muscular dystrophy are caused by a defect in the gene responsible for regulating dystrophin, a protein that helps maintain muscle fibre. Inadequate levels of the protein cause muscle fibres to deteriorate. This gene is passed on the X chromosome from mother to son. Females inherit one X chromosome from each parent – a normal gene from the father cancels out a defective gene from the mother.

Other forms of muscular dystrophy are not linked to the X chromosome and are inherited equally among males and females.

PREVENTION

There is no known way to prevent muscular dystrophy.

DIAGNOSIS

A doctor can diagnose muscular dystrophy and identify the form of the disease based on a physical examamination, blood tests and tests of the muscles. The most common forms, their age of onset and their symptoms are:

• DUCHENNE Symptoms begin between ages two and four. Leg muscles become weak, leading to difficulty walking and running. The calf muscles become enlarged. Scoliosis, or curvature of the spine, often develops. Most of those affected cannot walk by age 12.

• MYOTONIC This form begins any-time from infancy to early adult-hood. Prolonged muscle spasms occur in the hands, wrists and facial muscles. The eyelids droop and the face appears elongated. Other symptoms include abnormal gait, heart problems, cataracts and hormonal disturbances.

• FACIOSCAPULOHUMERAL Usually starts in adolescence. The first sign is weakness of the facial muscles. This form of the disease progresses slowly. Symptoms can be mild or cause disability, with the leg and arm muscles growing weak.

TREATMENTS

Although muscular dystrophy is incurable, integrative treatments can help relieve the symptoms and relieve complications. There is currently no way to slow the progress of the disease.

• MEDICATION Corticosteroids, such as prednisone, are often prescribed to temporarily improve muscle strength. For myotonic muscular dystrophy, medications that reduce muscle contractions may be used, including phenytoin and carbamazepine.

• SUPPLEMENTS Several small studies suggest that supplements of creatine, a chemical found in human muscle, may increase muscle strength. Supplements of coenzyme Q10, an enzyme produced by the human body, increase exercise capacity in people with muscular dystrophy.

• PHYSICAL THERAPY AND EXERCISE Exercises that stretch the muscles in the arms and legs can help prevent the tendons and muscles from contracting around the joints, a painful and disabling symptom of the disease.

• SURGERY When muscle contraction around joints is disabling, surgery can be performed to loosen the muscles.

See also: *Supplements, pp.532–43* • *Yoga, pp.476–9* • *Scoliosis, pp.148–9*

WHO IS AT RISK?

The risk factors include:

• Family history of muscular dystrophy

Bone Cancer

Cancers often spread, or metastasize, to the bones from other parts of the body. Less common are cancers that originate in bone or cartilage. Among these primary bone cancers, the most common is osteosarcoma, which usually occurs in the knees, upper legs and upper arms. Ewing's sarcoma affects mainly the pelvis, upper legs, ribs and arms.

Chondrosarcoma is cancer of the cartilage, usually in the pelvis. Symptoms of bone cancer include pain, swelling and a lump in the affected area, and often fatigue, a temperature and weight loss. Osteosarcoma and Ewing's sarcoma are most likely to strike children and young adults; chondrosarcoma is most common in people ages 50 to 60.

CAUSES

It is not clear what causes primary bone cancer, but there are several risk factors. In children, having had radiation and chemotherapy for other types of cancer increases the odds of developing bone cancers. Retinoblastoma (pp.46–7), a cancer

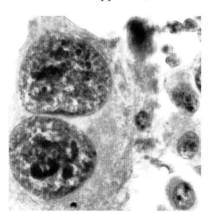

Malignant osteosarcoma (bone cancer) mostly affects children and young adults, when bones are growing rapidly.

of the eye, predisposes children to osteosarcoma. In adults, a risk factor for bone cancers is Paget's disease, a noncancerous condition in which bone cells grow too quickly.

PREVENTION

Experts know of no way to prevent bone cancer.

DIAGNOSIS

Doctors diagnose bone cancer with a physical examination and tests. X-rays can show whether a tumour is present; if so, imaging tests of higher resolution, such as CT scans or magnetic resonance imaging (MRI) may reveal more detail. If tests suggest bone cancer, a bone biopsy may be recommended, in which a small amount of bone is removed and examined under a microscope. Bone biopsies are usually done by orthopedic specialists.

TREATMENTS

Bone cancer is usually treated with a combination of surgery, chemotherapy and radiation.
 • SURGERY Most primary bone cancers are removed surgically. Relatively small cancers can be taken out along with a margin

WHO IS AT RISK?

The risk factors include:

- Osteosarcoma and Ewing's sarcoma are most common in people age 10 to 25; chondrosarcoma is most common in people 50 to 60 years old
- Previous chemotherapy or radiation therapy
- Retinoblastoma
- Paget's disease

of healthy tissue. However, an arm or leg with a large tumour may require amputation of all or part of the limb. Surgery may also be done to remove cancer that has spread to other areas of the body.
 • CHEMOTHERAPY This treatment uses drugs to kill cancer cells throughout the body. The drugs may be in the form of a pill, or injected into a vein or into the site of the cancer. Chemotherapy is given after surgery to destroy any remaining cancer cells. For osteosarcoma, it may also be used before surgery to shrink a cancer on an arm or leg bone and make it small enough to remove without amputation.
 • RADIATION THERAPY A machine generates X-rays or other sources of radiation to the site of the cancer to destroy cancer cells in that area. Like chemotherapy, radiation can be used to shrink large tumours before surgery, or to kill cancer cells that may remain after surgery.

See also: *Ocular Cancer, pp.46–7*

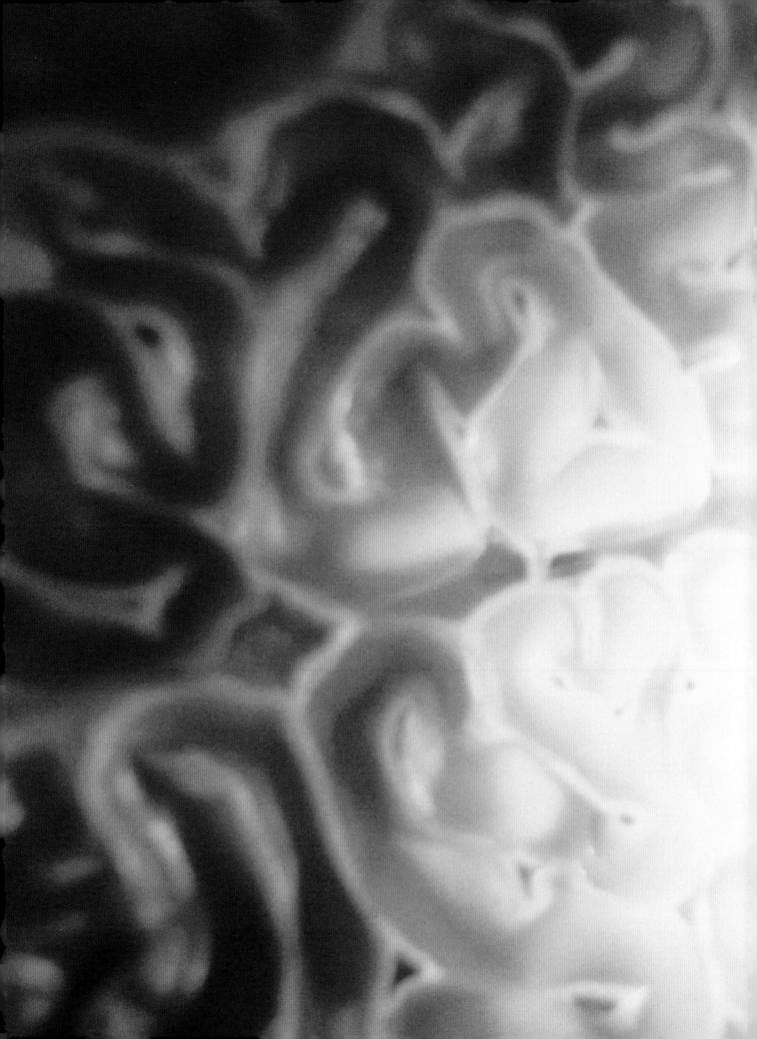

BRAIN & NERVOUS SYSTEM

6

The brain is the control centre that determines how every system in the body works, and the central nervous system is the circuitry that connects everything. Problems related to this complex network are often debilitating and difficult to diagnose.

Because nerves are present throughout the body, individual nervous system disorders may require different preventative approaches. Dizziness and headaches can result from correctable causes such as poor diet or stress. But many serious conditions such as Parkinson's and Huntington's disease have a genetic component and may be unpreventable.

Avoiding traumatic injuries such as concussion can prevent neurological disorders such as memory loss. Diet and exercise can help mitigate the symptoms of otherwise unpreventable disorders such as multiple sclerosis. And limiting exposure to radiation and chemical pesticides and pollutants can reduce the risk of some brain tumours.

Dizziness

Abnormal sensations of the body's physical relationship to space are called dizziness. These can be divided into four types. Vertigo is the sense that the body or the environment around it is moving (usually spinning). Presyncope is a feeling of light-headedness. Disequilibrium is a sense of imbalance. Other dizziness is described as vague or floating, and is often accompanied by a headache and abdominal pain or nausea. Dizziness is usually benign and temporary, but can also recur. It becomes more common with age, affecting as many as 40 percent of people over the age of 40.

CAUSES

Vertigo is usually the result of a condition that affects the inner ear, such as labrynthitis or Menière's disease (pp.72–3). Benign positional vertigo, which is a sudden dizziness that occurs when the head changes position, is believed to be caused by calcium particles in the inner ear canals. Normally, these particles are distributed among the three ear canals, but with this condition they clump together and collect in one canal, irritating its nerves.

Presyncope often results from a drop in blood circulation to the brain, which can occur with conditions such as low blood pressure (pp.236–9), anxiety (pp.354–5), heart failure (pp.234–5) and coronary artery disease (pp.230–3).

Disequilibrium is often caused by neuromuscular problems, such as migraine headaches (pp.166–7) and stroke (pp.168–9).

Other types of dizziness can be caused by too much alcohol, double vision (pp.36–9), cataract surgery (pp.34–5), anaemia (pp.312–3), motion sickness, nausea, dehydration and psychiatric disturbances. Dizziness is also a side effect of many medications (see *Clinical Query* on p.163).

PREVENTION

Do not consume more than two alcoholic drinks a day, or less if a smaller amount causes light-headedness. Take plenty of water and other nonalcoholic drinks throughout the day to avoid dehydration. Treating upper respiratory infections and middle ear infections promptly may reduce the risk of developing labrynthitis.

DIAGNOSIS

Occasional bouts of mild dizziness may not need a diagnosis, but see a doctor if the dizziness is severe, seems to be related to taking a new medication recently, if there has been dizziness off and on for at least three weeks, if there is a loss of consciousness, or if there are other symptoms. To narrow down the possible causes, the doctor will probably ask how often the dizziness occurs, if there is light-headedness, a feeling of off-balance, or a spinning sensation, and if there are other symptoms such as hearing loss, ringing in the ears, vision problems or chest pain.

A balance test which involves walking in a straight line may be done to check for balance problems. Several other tests can help identify the cause of dizziness, including a blood pressure test to check for low blood pressure, and various heart tests to detect heart disease or abnormal heart rhythms. When stroke is suspected, imaging tests of the brain, such as magnetic resonance angiography and ultrasound, can show

WHO IS AT RISK?

The risk factors include:

- Over age 40
- Drinking alcohol
- Labrynthitis
- Menière's disease
- Motion sickness
- Anaemia
- Migraines
- Double vision
- Low blood pressure
- Heart disease and abnormal heartbeat
- Stroke
- Brain tumour

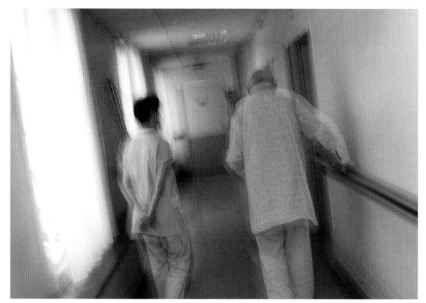

Dizziness is usually a benign, temporary condition that may not require treatment. Often, simple exercises done at home can relieve the symptoms of dizziness, and herbal remedies have shown promise in helping control the condition.

whether blood flow to the brain is adequate. Magnetic resonance imaging (MRI) of the brain may be done to check for a tumour.

TREATMENTS

Minor dizziness usually goes away on its own and requires no treatment, but when dizziness is recurrent, the treatments focus on the underlying cause. If dizziness is a side-effect of a medication, it may be possible to substitute another or use a lower dose. If dizziness is caused by an illness, such as heart disease or stroke, treating the illness can help control the dizziness.

• EPLEY MANOEUVRE This is a standard treatment for benign positional vertigo and is usually performed by a physical therapist or a doctor. The patient lies down, and the practitioner turns their head to one side and then the other. The purpose is to separate the calcium particles that have clumped together in the ear to cause the symptoms. In more than 90 percent of people with positional vertigo, the Epley manoeuvre provides immediate relief without medication. However, the vertigo may eventually recur, and the manoeuvre must be repeated.

• EXERCISE A simple exercise can be performed at home to relieve benign positional vertigo. First, sit on a bed and turn the head 45 degrees to the right. Now lie down on the left side and keep the head turned. Then sit up again and turn the head 45 degrees to the left. Next, lie on the right side, keeping the head facing left, then sit up again. Hold each position for 30 seconds. Do six to ten repetitions, three times a day.

• MEDICATION Various medicines can help relieve dizziness and related symptoms, including sedatives, antihistamines and anti-nausea medication.

• HERBAL REMEDIES *Ginkgo biloba* is widely used to relieve vertigo. A study published in the *Journal of Alternative and Complementary Medicine* in 2005 compared the effectiveness of ginkgo and vertigo-heel, a homeopathic treatment, in reducing vertigo in 170 people with heart disease. The study concluded that, after six weeks, measurements of vertigo diminished by an average of nearly half with either treatment.

• TRADITIONAL CHINESE MEDICINE A 2004 study of 167 patients at Daping Hospital, Third Military Medical University, Chongqing. China, found that patients with vertigo, headaches and ringing in the ears related to arteriosclerosis (pp.230–3) reported fewer symptoms and had better blood flow to the brain after taking conventional medicine and a Chinese remedy called *Yangxue gingnae* granule than patients who took only conventional medicine.

See also: *Low Blood Pressure, pp.236–9* • *Coronary Artery Disease, pp.230–3* • *Anxiety, pp.354–5*

Clinical Query

Am I taking a medication that can cause dizziness?

Many, if not most, common medications can cause dizziness in certain patients. These include high blood pressure medication, other cardiovascular drugs, psychiatric medication, anticonvulsants, sedatives and certain antibiotics. This type of dizziness is often mild and temporary, but if it is severe, tell your doctor right away.

Carpal Tunnel Syndrome

When the median nerve, which runs through a space in the wrist called the carpal tunnel, is compressed, the result is carpal tunnel syndrome. Symptoms include numbness, tingling, weakness, and pain in one or both wrists and hands. Carpal tunnel syndrome is most common among women.

CAUSES

Carpal tunnel syndrome may be caused by fluid retention and other forms of swelling that compress the median nerve as a result of pregnancy (pp.398–400), premenstrual syndrome (pp.386–7), menopause (pp.406–8), obesity (pp.348–9), rheumatoid arthritis (pp.136–9), diabetes (pp.338–41), high blood pressure (pp.236–9) or hypothyroidism (pp.344–7). Other conditions associated with carpal tunnel syndrome include kidney failure (pp.306–7), acromegaly (p.351), multiple myeloma (p.329), and recent tuberculosis (p.212).

Injury, trauma or pressure to the carpal tunnel area may result from repetitive wrist movement. People who spend long hours at a computer keyboard are among those at greatest risk.

PREVENTION

Prevent carpal tunnel syndrome by limiting the amount of time doing repetitive activities involving the wrist. When engaged in such activities, take frequent breaks. When typing, the wrist and hand should form a straight line, without bending at the wrist; a typing pad can help.

DIAGNOSIS

A doctor can diagnose carpal tunnel syndrome by tapping the wrist – pain or tingling in response is an indication of the syndrome. The doctor might also bend the wrist forward to see if there is any tingling, numbness, or weakness. Wrist X-rays may be used to rule out arthritis. Nerve tests that measure nerve impulse transmission may be used to confirm the diagnosis and evaluate nerve function.

TREATMENTS

When the cause is a condition such as rheumatoid arthritis, relieving the condition can often cure the carpal tunnel syndrome. When the cause is repetitive stress, the following treatments are used.

• **PHYSICAL ENVIRONMENT** Modify the work environment to reduce stress on the median nerve.

• **WRIST BRACES** These take pressure off the median nerve by keeping the wrist straight. Wrist braces are typically worn at night.

• **WARM COMPRESSES** Warm compresses applied several times a day can temporarily relieve wrist pain and improve range of motion.

• **MEDICATION** Nonsteroidal anti-inflammatory agents can temporar-

ily relieve pain and swelling. When these medications and wrist braces do not provide adequate relief, the next option is oral steroids or an injection of corticosteroid medication into the carpal tunnel space.

• **CHIROPRACTIC** Studies suggest that chiropractic (p.446–7) reduces symptoms, but there is insufficient scientific data to draw conclusions.

• **SURGERY** For half the people with carpal tunnel syndrome, the only treatment that yields permanent relief is surgery to cut the ligament pressing against the median nerve.

• **OTHER TREATMENTS** Ultrasound treatments, administered for several weeks, and yoga (p.476–9) both can lead to significant relief, although symptoms usually return. Vitamin B$_6$ supplements are controversial because scientific proof is lacking and supplementation may be harmful in high doses.

See also: *Obesity, pp.348–9 • High Blood Pressure, pp.236–9 • Yoga, pp.476–9*

See also: *Obesity, pp.348–9 • High Blood Pressure, pp.236–9 • Yoga, pp.476–9*

WHO IS AT RISK?

The risk factors include:

- Female
- Using a keyboard for many hours a day
- Using hand tools for many hours a day
- Racquetball and handball
- Pregnancy
- Menopause
- Conditions like obesity, diabetes, and rheumatoid arthritis

---

Sciatica

Pain that radiates from the lower back or buttock down one leg is sciatica; the leg may also feel numb or weak. The symptoms occur when there is pressure or damage to the sciatic nerve, which runs down the back of each leg and controls the muscles and provides sensation. It usually starts suddenly and goes away on its own within a few weeks.

CAUSES

Injury to the sciatic nerve can bring on sciatica, although often no cause is found. Injuries include motor vehicle accidents and hip fractures (p.143). Back disorders such as a slipped disc and bone disorders such as osteoporosis (pp.146–7) and osteoarthritis (pp.136–9) can compress the sciatic nerve. Other causes include nerve damage from diabetes (pp.338–41) or Lyme disease (pp.326–7), and the narrowing of the bone surrounding the spine, called spinal stenosis, which occurs with age. In rare cases, sciatica is due to a serious condition such as a tumour or blood clot near the sciatic nerve.

PREVENTION

When lifting heavy objects, bend at the knees to prevent back injury. Prevent osteoporosis by getting plenty of calcium and vitamin D, lower the risk of diabetes by maintaining normal weight and exercising regularly, and guard against Lyme disease by using tick repellent when outdoors in tick-prone areas. Avoid sitting or lying on the back for prolonged periods to minimize pressure on the sciatic nerve.

DIAGNOSIS

There is no need for a doctor's diagnosis if sciatica is mild and lasts just a few days. However, see a doctor if the pain persists, is severe, or getting worse and is accompanied by either loss of sensation or function, if there is a family history of cancer, or if you are younger than 20 or older than 55 and are having sciatica symptoms for the first time. A doctor can diagnose sciatica based on the symptoms, a physical examination and a medical history. Tests may be done to check for particular causes.

TREATMENTS

Treatments involve controlling the underlying cause, if there is one, as well as easing the symptoms. In general, therapies for low back pain (pp.132–3) may also relieve sciatica.

• MEDICATION Nonsteroidal anti-inflammatory agents, such as ibuprofen, can help relieve the pain. If they are not sufficient, the doctor may prescribe corticoteroids or narcotics, such as codeine or morphine. Injections of botulinum toxin (Botox) appear to be effective for people with long-lasting sciatica.

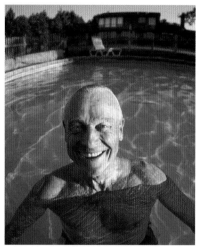

Although sciatica can limit physical activity, low-impact exercise such as swimming will not usually aggravate symptoms.

• HYDROTHERAPY A cold compress on the affected area, followed by a hot compress, can decrease pain.

• PHYSICAL ACTIVITY Even if sciatica is painful enough to limit physical activity, bed rest for longer than two days can make symptoms worse. It is better to walk or exercise as much as is tolerable.

See also: *Osteoporosis, pp.146–7 • Diabetes, pp.338–41 • Back Pain, pp.132–3*

WHO IS AT RISK?

The risk factors include:

• Most common in people over 20 and becomes more common with old age

• Injury to the spine or pelvis

• Bone disorders such as osteoarthritis and osteoporosis

• Medical conditions such as diabetes, Lyme disease and cancer

Headaches

There are several types of headache, each distinguished by location, severity and pattern of occurrence. Nearly everyone has had a tension headache, the most common type, which feels like a band tightening around the forehead. Another type is a migraine, a severe attack of throbbing pain that begins on one side of the head, is accompanied by other symptoms such as nausea and sensitivity to light and sound, and lasts anywhere from four hours to three days.

Other types include sinus and cluster headaches. Some experience more than one type of headache at the same time. In general, headaches are more common in women.

CAUSES

Tension headaches and migraines are believed to result from a similar underlying mechanism related to serotonin, a neurotransmitter that relays pain message. An imbalance leads to overstimulation of the trigeminal nerve, which relays sensory and motor impulses through the face. These abnormalities cause blood vessels in the area to constrict, adding to the symptoms. However, the particular triggers and underlying risk factors for each type of headache are different.

Headaches can also be a symptom of common illnesses, such as flu, as well as brain disorders such as aneurysm, meningitis (p.180) or tumour (p.196–7). The sudden onset of an unusual, very severe headache may signal a life-threatening event such as stroke (pp.168–9) or bleeding in the brain.

Tension Headaches

If these occur less than once a month, they can be triggered by stress, fatigue or anger. Other causes include caffeine withdrawal, holding the head and neck in the same position for an extended period (when working at a computer, for example), sleeping in an awkward position and lack of sleep. Chronic tension headaches, which occur daily, are often caused by depression or other ongoing emotional difficulties.

Migraine

If both parents suffer from migraines, there is a 75 percent chance their offspring will have them, compared to about a 20 percent chance in the general population. Many factors can trigger a migraine, although the mechanism is unclear. Common triggers are:
• Physical or emotional stress
• Tension headaches
• Bright lights
• Allergies
• Alcohol
• Caffeine

• Foods that contain tyramine, an amino acid, including aged cheese, smoked fish, and red wine
• Other foods, including chocolate, nuts, peanut butter, bananas and pickled foods
• Smoking or exposure to tobacco smoke
• Hormonal fluctuations before menstruation
• Oral contraceptives

Sinus Headaches

Headaches around the sinus cavities above and below the eyes may occur because of a temporary inflammation or infection of the sinuses (pp.58–60) or as the result of a rapid change in barometric pressure. Recurrent sinus headaches may be confused with some types of migraine and may have other causes.

Cluster Headaches

Cluster headaches, in which pain is usually concentrated on one side around an eye, get their name because they tend to strike in clusters of several headaches in a day. The cause is unknown, but they are most common in spring and autumn, and are often triggered by alcohol, even in small amounts. Unlike other headaches, cluster headaches are most common in men.

PREVENTION

Reduce the effects of stress with proven relaxation techniques such as yoga (pp.476–9), meditation (pp.514–19) and deep breathing. Do not smoke and avoid exposure to secondhand smoke. Do not have more than two alcoholic drinks a day (the equivalent of 340 ml/12 fl. oz beer, 150 ml/5 fl.oz wine, or 50 ml/1.5 fl.oz distilled spirits). When working at a computer, take frequent breaks to stretch the neck and upper body. Exercising daily can improve sleep and reducing stress.

DIAGNOSIS

A doctor can probably diagnose the type of headache based on the symptoms. To get this information, the doctor may ask the patient to describe how the headache feels, which areas of the head are painful, and when and how often the pain

On Call

If you want to give up coffee but do not want the headache of caffeine withdrawal, taper off slowly. First, determine how much caffeine you usually consume from all sources, including tea, cola and chocolate, as well as coffee itself, and then gradually reduce over several weeks.

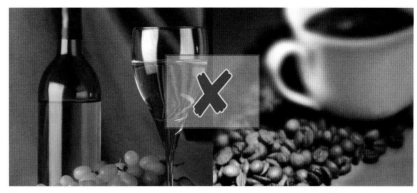

Headaches have many common triggers, including alcohol, coffee, smoking, stress, and allergies. Moderating intake of substances that can lead to headaches, and adopting techniques for managing stress, can greatly reduce the occurrence of headaches.

occurs. The doctor may also ask them to keep a headache diary for several weeks to identify possible triggers. If the doctor suspects the underlying cause is sinusitis or a potentially serious condition such as an aneurysm, imaging tests may be performed, including a CT scan and MRI of the brain, and an X-ray or CT scan of the sinuses.

TREATMENTS

Home remedies are often sufficient to relieve mild to moderate headache pain, including ice packs or hot compresses applied to the affected area, massaging the head and neck, pain relievers such as ibuprofen or paracetamol, and rest.

• **MEDICATION** Chronic tension headaches can often be controlled with antidepressants such as amitriptyline in low doses. Preventative medicine for migraines is taken daily to reduce the occurrence in people who suffer from more than two per month. These medicines include tricyclic antidepressants, beta-blockers, and antiseizure drugs, as well as supplements of vitamin B$_2$ and magnesium. Abortive medications are taken to relieve migraine symptoms, and includes

triptans (such as sumatriptan and zolmitriptan), ergotamine tartrate, lidocaine nose drops and muscle relaxants. Other medication, including lithium and verapamil, may be used to prevent cluster headaches.

• **BIOFEEDBACK** This therapy (pp.504–7) is a helpful adjunct to medication for preventing and relieving migraines.

• **CHIROPRACTIC** Manual manipulation by a chiropractor (pp.446–7) may help relieve the pain of chronic tension headaches.

• **SUPPLEMENTS** Feverfew preparations made from dry leaves appear more effective than other preparations of the herb in helping to prevent migraine. A clinical trial published in the journal *Neurology* in 2005 found that supplements of coenzyme Q$_{10}$ were better than placebo in preventing migraine attacks in 42 migraine sufferers.

• **MIND–BODY THERAPIES** Guided imagery (pp.520–2) may help control migraines and chronic tension headaches and hypnosis (pp.508–13) may help control chronic tension headaches.

See also: *Brain Tumours, pp.196–7 • Sinusitis, pp.58–60 • Yoga, pp.476–9*

Stroke

Normally, a steady flow of blood nourishes the brain with oxygen and nutrients. But when that flow is slowed or stopped, such as when a blood vessel to the brain is injured, it causes a stroke. This is a medical emergency. Without sufficient blood, brain cells die, potentially taking with them the ability to speak, feel, move or carry out other functions. Each year, 15 million people around the world suffer strokes and 5 million are left permanently disabled.

CAUSES

At least 80 percent of strokes are ischaemic, occurring when a blood vessel becomes blocked. The process usually starts with atherosclerosis (pp.230–1), in which cholesterol and other debris accumulate inside a blood vessel, narrowing the vessel and staunching the flow of blood. The slowdown sets the stage for a blood clot to form, which can then completely block the vessel. A blood clot can also form elsewhere, and then break away and lodge in the narrowed blood vessel.

Most of the remaining 15 to 20 percent of strokes are of the haemorrhagic type – they begin with the rupture of a blood vessel in the brain, which causes blood to gush into the brain, compressing blood vessels and ultimately impeding the normal flow of blood. Many haemorrhagic strokes are caused by aneurysms, bubbles in blood vessels that cause weak spots in the vessels' walls.

The main risk factor for both types of stroke is high blood pressure (pp.236–9).

PREVENTION

A diet that is rich in fruit, vegetables and fish, and low in saturated fats can help reduce blood pressure and LDL cholesterol. Eating fish such as light tuna, salmon and pollock, which are high in omega-3 fatty acids (pp.252–3), lowers the risk of stroke. Magnesium, potassium, and calcium from foods (but not supplements), as well as orange juice, may reduce the risk of ischaemic strokes.

Do not smoke. Drinking alcohol in any amount appears to increase the risk of haemorrhagic stroke, and heavy alcohol consumption can lead to ischaemic stroke. However, one or two drinks a day may lower the risk of ischaemic stroke.

Regular exercise can lower the risk of stroke in several ways: controlling weight, lowering blood pressure and making blood less likely to clot. It can also help reduce psychosocial stress, a risk factor for high blood pressure. Aim for about an hour of brisk walking or other moderate exercise on most days.

WHO IS AT RISK?

The risk factors include:

- Age 55 and older
- High blood pressure
- High LDL cholesterol
- Heart arrhythmia
- Obesity
- Diabetes
- Smoking
- More than two alcoholic drinks a day
- Diet high in salt and saturated fats
- Family history of stroke
- Head trauma
- For women, hormone therapy for menopause or birth control

Medication may be necessary to control conditions that can lead to stroke, including high blood pressure, high LDL cholesterol and heart arrhythmia. Drugs such as aspirin, which thin the blood, can also lower the risk of stroke in some people.

DIAGNOSIS

Stroke symptoms come on suddenly and include:

- Numbness or weakness in the face, an arm, or a leg, especially on one side of the body
- Trouble seeing
- Confusion, difficulty speaking
- Dizziness
- Loss of balance or coordination
- Severe, sudden headache with no apparent cause

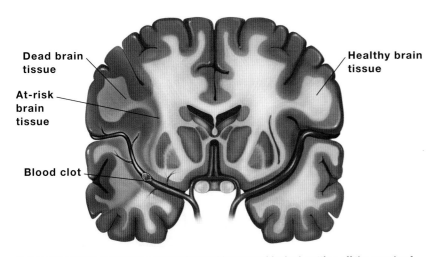

Ischaemic strokes occur when a blood vessel becomes blocked, cutting off the supply of nutrients and oxygen to a portion of the brain. Without a sufficient supply of blood, brain cells begin to die, and that can impair functions such as walking, talking or seeing.

Go to a hospital immediately. The doctor will ask about the symptoms and when they occurred, and will take a medical history. A physical examination should include checking for carotid bruits – abnormal sounds made by blood flowing through a narrowed carotid artery in the neck. A neurological examination will test brain functions such as memory, hearing, vision and speech to provide clues to the area of the brain that has been affected. Imaging tests, such as CT, computed angiography, MRI and Doppler ultrasound, can determine whether the stroke is ischaemic or haemorrhagic.

TREATMENTS

Ischaemic and haemorrhagic strokes have different treatments. For both types, rehabilitation is often necessary to help regain functions that were weakened. Rehabilitation may include speech and language therapy, physical therapy and occupational therapy to help with everyday activities such as eating, bathing and dressing.

Ischaemic Stroke

• MEDICATION The first phase of treatment, which must begin within the first three hours after the onset of symptoms, is thrombolytic therapy, which is medication given intravenously to dissolve blood clots. The main thrombolytic medication is recombinant tissue plasminogen activator (tPA). The second phase of treatment is intravenous anticoagulant medication, which prevents new blood clots from forming. A day or more after a stroke has occurred, oral medications such as aspirin and warfarin may be used for several months to prevent clots.

• SURGERY If there is a significant narrowing of a carotid artery, which supplies blood to the brain, a surgical procedure called carotid endarterectomy opens the blocked artery and cleans out the plaque and other debris. In another procedure, called carotid artery stenting, the surgeon places a prosthetic device called a stent into a narrowed artery to prop it open.

• MAGNETIC THERAPY In a clinical trial of 26 patients published in the journal *Neurology* in 2005, magnet therapy (p.572) was used in conjunction with conventional treatments. Special magnets placed over the head daily for ten days hastened recovery from ischaemic stroke.

Haemorrhagic Stroke

• COILING The goal is to prevent further haemorrhaging. To treat aneurysm there is a procedure called coiling, in which a catheter with a ball-shaped coil at one end is threaded into a large artery in the arm or groin to the site of the aneurysm and released, causing the blood in the aneurysm to clot.

• SURGERY Excess blood is removed from the brain and the ruptured blood vessel is clamped to prevent further bleeding.

See also: *High Blood Pressure, pp.236–9* • *Omega-3 Fatty Acids, pp.252–3* • *Magnet Therapy, p.572*

Clinical Query

What is a transient ischaemic attack (IT)?

It is a stroke that lasts only a few minutes. It occurs when the blood supply to part of the brain is briefly interrupted. Symptoms are similar to those of stroke but usually disappear within an hour, although they may persist for up to 24 hours. TIAs are often warning signs that a person is at risk for a more serious stroke. About one-third of those who have a TIA will have an acute stroke some time in the future.

SLEEP DISORDERS

Most adults need six to eight hours of sleep at night to be refreshed and alert during the day. If they do not get enough sleep or the sleep is interrupted, they may have a sleep disorder. About half of all adults suffer from insomnia, the most common sleep disorder, which is difficulty falling or staying asleep. Other sleep disorders include parasomnias, or abnormal behaviours during sleep, such as night terrors, which affect young children.

Night terrors differ from nightmares in that they do not occur during dreams. Children having night terrors may sit up, scream, and show other signs of terror while sleeping. Though frightening, the condition is not dangerous and children usually outgrow it.

CAUSES

There are many causes of sleep disorders.

• ENVIRONMENTAL FACTORS Fly ing to a different time zone can trigger a bout of insomnia that lasts for several days or weeks by re-setting the biological clock, the area of the hypothalamus in the brain that governs the sleep–wake cycle. Shift work – working at night and trying to sleep during the day – can also disrupt the biological clock. Smoking can cause insomnia because the nicotine in cigarette smoke is a stimulant. Other environmental factors include too much light or noise in the bedroom, and an uncomfortable mattress.

• AGE A sleep–wake cycle that has not fully matured is believed to increase the risk of night terrors in young children. Insomnia becomes more common in middle age because the architecture of sleep changes. Less time is spent in deep sleep, increasing the odds of waking up. It also takes longer to fall asleep, although the reason is unclear.

• PSYCHOSOCIAL FACTORS Stress that leaves the mind racing at night can cause acute insomnia, which usually lasts a month or less. Worry, grief, and anticipating a significant event can also temporarily disrupt sleep. Psychological distress increases the risk of night terrors in children. Fatigue and family history also increase the odds that a child will have night terrors.

• BEHAVIOURAL FACTORS Many habits can contribute to insomnia by adding stress or by making people feel stimulated when they should be unwinding. These can include doing work in the bedroom, engaging in upsetting conversations just before bedtime, and exercising within three hours of going to bed. Napping in the afternoon can keep people from feeling tired at night, making it hard to fall asleep.

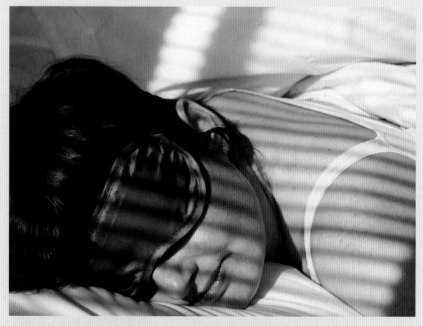

Sleep disorders can result from a number of health conditions such as depression, stress, and hormonal disorders including an overactive thyroid. Conditions that cause sex hormone levels to fluctuate, such as menstruation, pregnancy, and menopause, can also lead to disruptions in a healthy sleep cycle.

• **NUTRITION** Several foods, drinks and nutrients can interfere with a good night's sleep. Caffeine, a stimulant found mainly in coffee, tea, chocolate and colas, can keep people awake when consumed in the afternoon or evening. Alcohol, although it is a depressant, can cause people to wake up in the middle of the night when the depressant effect wears off.

• **HEALTH CONDITIONS** Chronic insomnia may be a symptom of several illnesses, including narcolepsy, a neurological disorder in which sleep–wake cycles are abnormal and a person feels sleepy during the day and awake at night. Other causes of insomnia include depression (pp.364–5), gastroesophogeal reflux disease (pp.264–5), overactive thyroid (pp.344–7), heart failure (pp.234–5), cancer, asthma (pp.206–9), kidney disease (p.308), Alzheimer's disease (pp.178–9), and sleep apnoea (pp.214–15). The incidence of insomnia rises when sex hormones are in a state of flux, such as just before and during menstruation (pp.384–5), during pregnancy (pp.398–400) and around the time of menopause (pp.406–8).

• **MEDICATION** Many medications contain stimulants that can cause people to have difficulty falling asleep at night, including some selective serotonin reuptake inhibitors taken for depression, thyroid medicines, oral contraceptives and decongestants. If someone has been taking sleeping pills, tapering off may cause insomnia to return.

PREVENTION

Making sure a child gets enough sleep and minimizing stress may help prevent night terrors. Behavioural and dietary changes can help reduce the incidence of insomnia.

• Go to bed and wake up at the same time each day. Following a consistent schedule helps keep the biological clock running smoothly.
• Do not work in the bedroom.
• Do not consume caffeinated drinks in the afternoon or evening. If there is still trouble falling asleep, cut back on caffeine earlier in the day, too.
• Do not smoke.
• Do not consume more than two alcoholic drinks a day. Avoid any alcohol during the few hours before bedtime.
• Exercise daily. Exercising increases the odds of a good night's sleep because it helps to control stress. However do not exercise during the three hours before bedtime, as this may energize the body too much to sleep.
• Keep the bedroom dark and quiet when sleeping.
• Be comfortable: Wear loose-fitting pyjamas, keep the temperature moderate (not too hot or cold), and replace the mattress if it is sagging or lumpy.

DIAGNOSIS

A doctor can diagnose a sleep disorder by doing a physical examination and asking questions about sleep problems and their pattern. The examination can help detect underlying health conditions that can cause insomnia.

Clinical Query

How can I minimize jet lag?

To help reset your biological clock to the time zone of your destination, when you get there, spend as much time as possible outdoors in the morning and afternoon. Take a melatonin supplement before bedtime. Avoid caffeine and limit your alcohol consumption.

If the doctor suspects an underlying condition, they may do other tests, such as blood tests for thyroid hormones and an electrocardiogram, or they may refer the case to a specialist. If depression is a possible cause, the doctor may make a referral to a psychologist. Night terrors can be diagnosed based on the symptoms described by the patient.

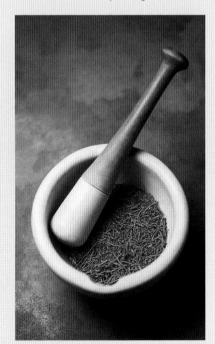

Supplements of valerian root, a herbal sedative, can help alleviate insomnia by reducing the time it takes to fall asleep.

TREATMENTS

There is no treatment for night terrors. Treating insomnia depends on the cause. If an underlying disorder, such as sleep apnoea or narcolepsy, is causing it, treating the disorder can often alleviate the insomnia. Otherwise, the first line of treatment is to establish good 'sleep hygiene' by following the strategies listed under Prevention. Various integrative approaches may also help.

• **MEDICATION** Sedatives, antianxiety medication and mild tranquilizers can treat insomnia for a few weeks. Most of these medications lose their effectiveness when taken for longer periods, and may cause negative side effects such as daytime drowsiness.

• **MELATONIN** This hormone helps regulate the biological clock. It is normally produced by the pineal gland in the brain in response to darkness and stimulates sleep, although levels decline with age.

healing hope I tend to be a light sleeper, and with my new job I have to travel a lot. I had the worst time getting used to sleeping in hotel beds, not to mention the jet lag. I ended up sleepy all the time and could barely keep my focus when it came to sitting through meetings. I knew my job might be in jeopardy if I didn't find a solution.

Then a colleague recommended valerian root supplements to help me fall asleep. I've been taking them for a few months now, and even though I'm not crazy about the way it smells, I feel much more rested overall and I never wake up groggy.

Jennifer L.

Melatonin supplements can help shorten the duration of jet lag, particularly when travelling east, and may help people with insomnia fall asleep faster.

• **VALERIAN** Pills, teas and tinctures made from the roots of valerian (*Valeriana officinalis*), a perennial herb native to North America, Europe and Asia, have sedative properties. Valerian is effective for reducing the time it takes to fall asleep, especially when taken nightly over a period of four weeks.

• **NUTRITION** Foods such as milk, turkey and certain other types of meats, cheese and pumpkin seeds contain a compound called L-tryptophan, an amino acid that helps induce sleep by leading to the production of melatonin.

• **COGNITIVE-BEHAVIOURAL THERAPY** This type of psychological therapy, which aims to resolve emotional conflicts by changing how a person thinks and behaves, helps people fall asleep faster and sleep more soundly, according to a review of the scientific literature published in the *Journal of Advanced Nursing* in 2005. The study found this type of therapy is more effective than various individual techniques, including relaxation therapy.

• **OTHER THERAPIES** There are several alternative approaches that may be helpful with inducing sleep, although the scientific evidence is still preliminary: aromatherapy (pp.548–9) with essential oils of chamomile and lavender, acupressure (p.472), yoga (pp.476–9), tai chi (p.450), hypnosis (pp.508–11), acupuncture (pp.464–5), listening to music and meditation (pp.514–19).

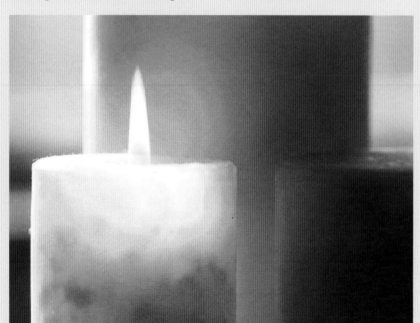

Aromatherapy with essential oils of lavender and chamomile may help encourage falling asleep. Other therapies that may help are acupressure, hypnosis, yoga and tai chi, although the scientific evidence for the effectiveness of these approaches is uncertain.

See also: *Depression, pp.364–5* • *Hypnosis, pp.508–13* • *Yoga, pp.476–9*

Tremors

The most common involuntary movement disorder is tremors. They may affect one or both sides of the body, and the incidence increases with age.

CAUSES

There are five types of tremors, each with different causes.

• RESTING TREMORS An arm or a leg shakes when a person is sitting or at rest. It can be caused by Parkinson's disease (p.181), lithium, antipsychotic drugs, and poisoning by heavy metals such as copper.

• POSTURAL TREMORS These occur when a person extends their hand. They can be due to alcoholism, an overactive thyroid (pp.344–7), Parkinson's disease or post-traumatic stress (pp.356–7).

• KINETIC OR INTENTION TREMORS These follow a purposeful movement, such as touching a finger to the nose or ringing a doorbell. The cause is believed to be damage to the cerebellum – the part of the brain that coordinates movement – from alcoholism, stroke (pp.168–9), multiple sclerosis (pp.182–3), or anticonvulsant or sedative medications.

• TASK-SPECIFIC TREMORS These occur with a specific task – for example, a shaking hand when a person writes. The cause is unclear.

• PSYCHOGENIC TREMORS These diminish or stop when a person is distracted, suggesting a psychological cause. People with psychogenic tremors often have psychological or psychosomatic illnesses.

PREVENTION

Fatigue, stress and caffeine can lead to tremors or make tremors more noticeable. Drink no more than two alcoholic beverages a day (one drink equals 340 ml/12 fl. oz beer, 150 ml/5 fl.oz wine, or 50 ml/1.5 fl.oz distilled spirits), exercise regularly and do not smoke. Avoid caffeine and get plenty of sleep to prevent or lessen tremors.

DIAGNOSIS

A doctor can diagnose tremors based on symptoms and health history. Blood tests are done when overactive thyroid is suspected. For resting or postural tremor, a neurological evaluation may be used to check for Parkinson's disease. Brain imaging may be done to look for signs of injury in kinetic tremors.

TREATMENTS

Treating disorders such as Parkinson's disease and overactive thyroid can eliminate the tremors. If medication is the cause, eliminate the medicine, reduce its dosage, or switch to a similar medicine.

• MEDICATION Several drugs are used to treat tremors, including anticonvulsants, blood pressure medication such as propranolol, antiseizure medicine such as primidone and tranquillizers.

• SURGERY When medicine is insufficient, surgery on the thalamus, a brain structure involved with tremor, may reduce symptoms. Deep brain stimulation involves implanting an electrical device in the chest with a wire to the thalamus, sending an electric current that blocks the nerve impulses that cause tremors. Thalamotomy is surgery in the brain that cuts the thalamus to reduce tremor-causing impulses.

• NEUROTOXINS Botulinum toxin type A, a derivative of botulism (a toxic bacteria) was found to improve voice tremor in a 2004 study published in *Archives of Neurology*. In the study, the toxin, injected into the vocal cords, led to improvement within an average of two days that lasted at least seven weeks.

• HYPNOSIS Combined with medication, self-hypnosis (pp.508–13) can be useful in the treatment of tremors related to Parkinson's.

See also: *Parkinson's Disease, p.181* • *Stroke, pp.168–9* • *Hypnotherapy, pp.508-11*

WHO IS AT RISK?

The risk factors include:
• Alcohol abuse
• Caffeine
• Stress
• Overactive thyroid
• Parkinson's disease
• Multiple sclerosis
• Sedatives and anticonvulsants
• Toxic metals

Concussion

Confusion, dizziness or loss of consciousness following a head injury are signs of concussion, a mild brain injury. Other symptoms include short-term memory loss, headaches and nausea. Most people with mild concussions recover completely within a few minutes to several hours. However, some people have symptoms such as headaches, dizziness and insomnia for months. Severe or repeated concussions can cause permanent brain damage, such as dementia pugilistica, a condition often seen in boxers.

CAUSES

A forceful blow to the head from a motor vehicle collision, sports injury, fall or other accident can cause concussion.

PREVENTION

Take precautions against head injuries: wear seat belts when riding in motor vehicles, and helmets

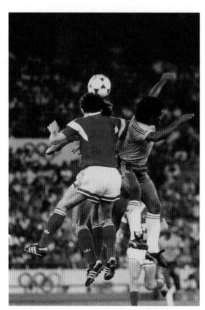

Special care should be taken after even minor concussions, because in some cases a second blow could be fatal.

when participating in activities such as bicycling, in-line skating, skiing and hockey. Do not participate in sports when you are ill or very tired. In addition, avoid mood-altering drugs and excess alcohol consumption, because these increase the likelihood of falls and other accidents.

DIAGNOSIS

There may be a concussion if a blow to the head is followed by:
• Loss of consciousness
• Confusion
• Headache
• Dizziness
• Nausea or vomiting
• Short-term memory loss
Anyone who has received a head injury should see a doctor. The doctor can diagnose concussion by conducting a thorough physical and neurological examination and evaluating the symptoms. The examination may include testing reflexes and memory for impairment. The doctor will probably ask about drug and alcohol use.

WHO IS AT RISK?
The risk factors include:
• Motor vehicle collision
• Contact sports such as hockey, football and boxing
• High-speed activities such as skiing, bicycling, and in-line skating
• Falls
• Drug or alcohol abuse

If the neurological examination is abnormal or if the symptoms are severe, the doctor may ask for a CT scan of the head to check for bleeding in the brain or other injuries that need emergency treatment.

TREATMENTS

A severe concussion with bleeding in the brain needs to be treated in a hospital, but most concussions are mild enough to be treated at home (after a visit to the doctor) with bed rest or reduced activity for a period of time prescribed by the doctor. Someone should stay with the patient for about 24 hours in case the symptoms get worse.

Bruises on the scalp caused by the head trauma can be treated to reduce the swelling with ice compresses for about 30 minutes every two to four hours over the first 24 hours.

See also: *Memory Loss, pp.178–9 • Headaches, pp.166–7 • Nausea, pp.274–5*

Shingles

Clusters of burning, itching blisters, typically on one side of the chest or back, are the signs of shingles – a reactivation of varicella-zoster, the virus that causes chickenpox. Shingles only affects people who have had chickenpox. Shingles can be very painful and the symptoms can linger for weeks or longer.

CAUSES

After a chickenpox infection, the virus lies dormant, probably in the nervous system. When it is reactivated, it courses through the nerves. The virus can become reactivated for several reasons. Immunity is believed to decline as people get older, and shingles is most common in people aged 50 and older. People whose immune systems are suppressed because of cancer or HIV are also at risk. Stress may play a role, as well.

PREVENTION

The chickenpox vaccine may reduce the risk of developing shingles. But if someone has had chickenpox, there is no sure way to prevent shingles. Tai chi, the exercise system used in Traditional Chinese Medicine (pp.446–7), may strengthen the immune system against varicella-zoster. A clinical trial published in the journal *Psychosomatic Medicine* in 2003 looked at a group of 36 adults aged 60 and older who had impaired health and were at risk for developing shingles. The half who received tai chi instruction had a stronger immune response to the virus than the control group.

DIAGNOSIS

A doctor can diagnose shingles based on the symptoms and whether the patient has had chickenpox. A blood test or a tissue culture of a blister may reveal signs of activated varicella-zoster virus.

TREATMENTS

The rash and pain usually go away on their own in three to five weeks. Cleaning the blisters once or twice a day can prevent infection. Go to an eye doctor immediately if you develop a blister near an eye; without prompt treatment it can cause permanent eye damage.

• **MEDICATION** Antiviral medications such as acyclovir, with or without corticosteroids, when given within 24 hours after symptoms appear, can reduce the severity and duration of shingles. They may also reduce the risk of complications, such as postherpetic neuralgia, which is ongoing pain caused by nerve damage at the sites of the blisters which lasts for three or more months.

Anti-inflammatory drugs, pain relief and antihistamines can reduce pain and itching. Applying a cream made of capzasin to the rash may prevent postherpetic neural-gia. Topical anaesthetics such as lidocaine can also decrease pain. Antidepressants may be prescribed to relieve postherpetic neuralgia.

• **VACCINATION** An experimental vaccine against herpes zoster reduced the incidence of shingles by 51 percent and, in those who did get shingles, reduced the severity by 61 percent in a clinical trial published in the *New England Journal of Medicine* in 2005. The vaccine reduced the incidence of postherpetic neuralgia by 66 percent.

• **HYDROTHERAPY** Pain and itching can be eased with cool, wet compresses, as well as oatmeal baths.

• **TENS** Transcutaneous electrical nerve stimulation therapy (p.443) can help relieve pain from shingles.

• **LIGHT THERAPY** A study published in the journal *Experimental Molecular Pathology* in 2005 reported that shingles lesions that were first treated with a chlorinated solution of red liquid and then exposed to ultraviolet-A light began to heal within 24 hours.

See also: *Traditional Chinese Medicine, pp.446–50 • TENS, p.443 • Blisters, p.98*

WHO IS AT RISK?

The risk factors include:

• Chickenpox
• Age 50 and older
• Cancer, particularly if you are undergoing radiation or chemotherapy
• HIV

Epilepsy & Seizures

Temporary episodes of convulsions, muscle spasms and loss of consciousness are examples of seizures, which are abnormal electrical activity in the brain. Having two or more seizures is a sign of epilepsy, a chronic neurological disorder that usually starts either in childhood or in old age. With epilepsy, neurons signal one another too rapidly.

Neurons normally signal one another 80 times per second, but during an epileptic seizure they signal as many as 500 times per second. There are many types of epilepsy, each affecting different parts of the brain and with variations in level of consciousness and symptoms.

CAUSES

Epilepsy can be caused by infections, brain trauma and neurological abnormalities such as cerebral palsy. A family history of epilepsy increases the risk. For half of people with epilepsy, however, the cause is unknown. The triggers of epileptic seizures include stress, lack of sleep, smoking, and alcohol consumption.

There are numerous factors underlying onset of seizures:
- High temperatures (in children)
- Metabolic disorders such as diabetes (pp.338–41)
- Nutritional deficiencies

- Birth defects
- Brain trauma
- Brain tumours (pp.196–7)
- Neurological disorders such as Alzheimer's disease (pp.178–9) and stroke (pp.168–9)
- Infections such as meningitis (p.180)
- Recreational and some prescription drugs
- Alcohol abuse

PREVENTION

Protect against head injuries by wearing seat belts in motor vehicles, and helmets during physical sporting activities such as bicycling and hockey to reduce the risk of trauma-related seizures. People who have epilepsy should avoid smoking and excessive alcohol consumption, establish healthy sleeping patterns, and manage stress to help prevent the occurence of seizures. Proven stress-reduction techniques include guided imagery (pp.520–2), yoga (pp.476–9) and meditation (pp.514–19).

Traumatic brain injury can result from a blow to the head, causing the brain to impact the inside of the skull, which in some cases leads to non-epileptic seizures. Taking precautions to protect the head during sporting activities greatly reduces the risk of this type of injury.

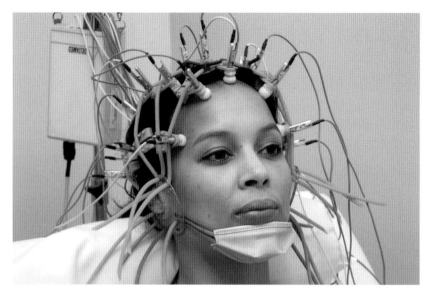

The EEG uses a collection of electrodes to record electrical activity from different parts of the brain, which can help doctors identify abnormal patterns. Specific patterns can indicate the presence and location of the abnormal activity in epilepsy patients.

DIAGNOSIS

Epilepsy is diagnosed on the basis of several tests and the symptoms that characterize the seizures. An electroencephalograph (EEG) is a test that measures electrical activity in the brain. It can help identify the presence and sometimes the location of abnormal brain electricity through a series of electrodes attached to the scalp. Blood tests, tests of liver and kidney function, and analysis of cerebrospinal fluid can identify infections and other reversible causes of seizures. Brain imaging tests, such as a CT scan or an MRI, may be used to look for evidence of brain damage.

TREATMENTS

Seizures that are caused by a treatable disorder, such as an infection, may be stopped when the disorder is treated. Otherwise, treatment focuses on preventing seizures.

• **MEDICATION** Anticonvulsant drugs such as phenytoin, carbamazepine and valproate are first-line treatments for preventing seizures. The medication may be used individually or in combination.

• **VAGUS NERVE STIMULATION** When medication does not control seizures adequately, vagus nerve stimulation is an option. An electrical device is implanted beneath the skin in the chest to send regular electrical pulses to the vagus nerve, which controls involuntary movement. This electrical stimulation can reduce the incidence and severity of seizures. Vagus nerve stimulation is reserved for patients over the age of 12 with partial onset seizures – those that begin in a limited area of the brain.

• **SURGERY** When less invasive treatments do not work, doctors consider surgery to remove abnormal parts of either the temporal lobes of the brain or the cortex that are generating seizures.

• **YOGA** As an adjunct to anti-seizure medication, yoga may further reduce the number of seizures, possibly by reducing stress.

• **NUTRITION** A ketogenic diet, which is low in carbohydrates and derives as much as 80 percent of calories from fat, is often prescribed to reduce the frequency of seizures in children. The goal of the diet is to stimulate the body to produce ketones, which cause the body to burn fat instead of glucose. Doctors are unsure why the diet works. However, the diet only works in children, and there have been no clinical trials scientifically testing its effectiveness.

• **SUPPLEMENTS** Melatonin, a hormone that helps promote sleep, may reduce insomnia, a side effect of epilepsy. Vitamin E supplements may reduce the frequency of seizures in people with epilepsy. Omega-3 fatty acids (pp.252–3) can help limit the number and severity of seizures.

See also: *Diabetes, pp.338–41* • *Alzheimer's Disease, pp.178–9* • *Meditation, pp.514–19*

MEMORY IMPAIRMENTS

Around age 50, the brain undergoes changes that can affect memory, such as a drop in serotonin and dopamine – neurotransmitters involved in memory processing. Although occasional forgetfulness is normal, significant memory problems – regularly missing appointments or forgetting how to cook a meal – can be signs of a memory impairment such as Alzheimer's disease or other dementias.

Alzheimer's is a progressive loss of memory and other intellectual functions and is the most common type of dementia. It begins with short-term memory loss and progresses until the ability to care for oneself and recognize loved ones is impaired. Mild cognitive impairment also affects memory and related functions but is less severe than Alzheimer's disease.

CAUSES

Dementia and mild cognitive impairment become more common with age. These disorders also have the same risk factors as cardiovascular disease. In addition, Alzheimer's disease and other dementias, as well as other memory problems, have their own set of causes.

Alzheimer's Disease

Genes play a role in Alzheimer's. A gene called ApoE4 increases the risk of developing the disorder. Mutations of three other genes (presenilin 1, presenilin 2 and the amyloid precursor protein gene) cause early-onset familial Alzheimer's disease, a rare form of the disease that starts as early as age 40.

Other Dementias

A wide range of conditions can cause brain damage that ultimately leads to dementia: stroke (pp.168–9), Parkinson's disease (p.181), alcoholism (pp.358–60), HIV/AIDS (pp.316–17), Huntington's disease (p.193) and traumatic brain injury.

Other Memory Problems

Many illnesses not normally associated with memory loss can impair the ability to learn and remember, including depression, diabetes and thyroid dysfunction. Stress and inadequate amounts of sleep are also significant causes of memory impairment. Fortunately, treating these illnesses and finding ways to reduce stress and get sufficient amounts of sleep usually helps restore some or all of the lost memory function.

Memory impairment can also be a side-effect of several medications, including sleeping pills, some painkillers, and cimetidine, a medication that decreases stomach acid production. Discontinuing these drugs or switching to other medications in their class usually reverses the memory loss.

PREVENTION

Memory disorders are easier to prevent than they are to treat. Regular exercise may decrease the risk of memory loss by helping to prevent cardiovascular disease (pp.234–5), one cause of memory problems.

Mental exercise in the form of formal education and learning

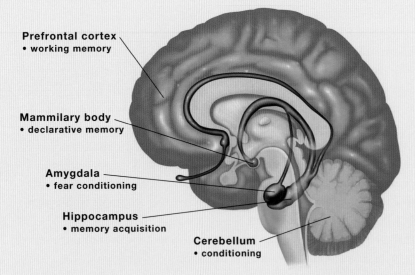

Prefrontal cortex
• working memory

Mammilary body
• declarative memory

Amygdala
• fear conditioning

Hippocampus
• memory acquisition

Cerebellum
• conditioning

Memory impairment can be caused by a number of conditions. Deep structures in the brain are responsible for processing short-term and long-term memory, and either type of memory can be affected differently by conditions such as Alzheimer's disease.

new things can preserve memory function. Even among people with Alzheimer's disease, those with the most education had the slowest rate of cognitive decline in studies done at Columbia University in New York and Rush University Medical Center in Chicago.

Vitamin C and E supplements (pp.532–41) may reduce the risk of developing Alzheimer's disease when taken in combination. High dietary intake of vitamin E has also been associated with a decreased risk of developing Alzheimer's. But research on these vitamins as prevention is inconclusive.

Human studies suggest eating foods that are high in omega-3 fatty acids (pp.252–3) and other healthy unsaturated fats may also protect against Alzheimer's disease.

Stress-reduction techniques, such as a regular exercise regimen, meditation (pp.514–19), progressive muscle relaxation (pp.474–5) and guided imagery (pp.520–2), can improve memory and help prevent memory problems.

DIAGNOSIS

The first step is to have a checkup to see if the cause is a treatable condition that affects memory. If not, the doctor may refer to a specialist in memory testing. Memory testing involves paper-and-pencil tests that assess a person's ability to remember specific things such as words, shapes and patterns, as well as how well they pay attention, plan and solve problems. These tests can identify specific areas of weakness in memory and related cognitive functions. The findings can help determine whether the difficulties

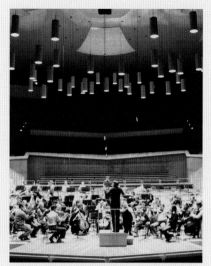

Listening to classical music has been shown to help people with Alzheimer's improve their ability to pay attention.

are characteristic of dementia or mild cognitive impairment.

If a memory disorder is suspected, other tests may be done, including an electroencephalogram to measure electrical activity in the brain, magnetic resonance imaging or CT scanning to check for abnormalities in the brain, and genetic testing for one of the gene mutations or variants associated with Alzheimer's disease.

TREATMENTS

There is no cure for Alzheimer's disease and most other types of dementia, including mild cognitive impairment, but several medications and integrative strategies can improve the symptoms.

• **MEDICATION** Several prescription drugs, including donepezil, rivastigmine and memantine, can bring about moderate, temporary improvement in memory and other symptoms of Alzheimer's disease and mild cognitive impairment. Donepezil was found to reduce the probability of mild

cognitive impairment progressing to Alzheimer's disease in a study published in the *New England Journal of Medicine* in 2005.

• **GINKGO BILOBA** Extracts from the nuts and leaves of the ginkgo tree are about as beneficial as the memory drugs in bringing about short-term improvement of memory problems related to Alzheimer's disease.

• **THERAPEUTIC TOUCH** This therapy (p.563) has helped reduce restlessness and other symptoms in people with Alzheimer's disease, according to a study published in the journal *Alternative Therapy in Health and Medicine* in 2005.

• **TENS** Transcutaneous electrical nerve stimulation (p.443), which uses electrical impulses from a portable generator to stimulate nerves, increased memory and verbal fluency of people with Alzheimer's disease in several studies, and improved mood and self-efficacy in people with mild cognitive impairment in a study published in the journal *Neurorehabilitation and Neural Repair* in 2004.

• **MUSIC** Listening to classical music helped people with Alzheimer's disease temporarily improve their ability to pay attention in a study published in *Experimental Ageing Research* in 2005.

• **AYURVEDA** Brahmi (*Bacopa monniera*) is an herbal preparation used in Ayurveda (pp.451–4) which seems to improve the ability to learn and remember information, although more research is needed.

See also: *Stroke, pp.168–9 • Parkinson's Disease, p.181 • TENS, p.443 • Ayurveda, pp.451–4*

Meningitis

This inflammation of the meninges, the membranes that line the brain and spinal cord, can be caused by a viral, fungal, or bacterial infection. Viral meningitis is usually mild and goes away without treatment, but bacterial and fungal meningitis are more serious and can be fatal.

CAUSES

Viral meningitis, the most common form of the disease, is caused by a class of viruses called enteroviruses, which are spread by coughing and sneezing or by water contaminated by sewage. Viral meningitis infections usually occur in winter and mainly affect people under the age of 30.

Meningococcal bacteria most commonly cause bacterial meningitis, but other causes are *Streptococcus pneumoniae*, *Haemophilus influenzae* and the tuberculosis bacteria. The bacteria generally originate in an infection elsewhere in the body and then migrate through the bloodstream to the brain. Bacterial meningitis is most common in children under the age of 5. The symptoms can emerge within hours of infection and may progress rapidly to loss of consciousness and death.

Fungal meningitis most often occurs in people with immune deficiencies. Bacterial and fungal meningitis are medical emergencies that require prompt diagnosis and treatment.

PREVENTION

The same precautions that can help prevent colds and flu, such as washing hands frequently and avoiding infected people, can also help protect against viral meningitis. Vaccination against *Haemophilus influenzae* can prevent bacterial meningitis caused by that bacterium. The vaccine does not guard against the many other bacterial causes of meningitis, but antibiotics can prevent infection in people who have been exposed.

DIAGNOSIS

Symptoms of all types of meningitis are similar: headache, fever and a stiff neck, often accompanied by sensitivity to light, nausea, vomiting, drowsiness and confusion. Contact a doctor immediately if someone has these symptoms.

Meningitis is diagnosed by drawing fluid from the spine. The fluid is then examined in a laboratory to see if viruses, fungi or bacteria are present and, if so, to identify what type they are.

TREATMENTS

Bacterial and fungal meningitis must be treated immediately with large doses of intravenous antibiotics. There is no medicine that can cure or speed up recovery from viral meningitis. This form of the disease usually goes away on its own in about a week. However, because all types of meningitis can cause severe exhaustion and pain, comfort care to relieve the symptoms can help ease recovery.

See also: *Bone fractures, p.143* • *Fever, p.318* • *Nausea & Vomiting, pp.274–5*

WHO IS AT RISK?

The risk factors include:

- Bacterial meningitis mainly affects children under the age of 5
- Viral meningitis affects mainly people under age 30
- Exposure to tuberculosis
- Skull fractures
- Exposure to pesticides

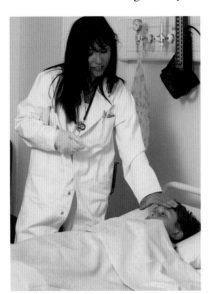

Bacterial meningitis can be life-threatening and should be treated immediately with intravenous antibiotics.

Parkinson's Disease

Parkinson's disease is a progressive, neurological disorder that occurs when the neurons that produce dopamine in an area of the brain called the substantia nigra die or deteriorate. Normal movement is smooth and fluid in part because of adequate levels of dopamine (a chemical that transmits nerve impulses) in the brain. The result is a constellation of abnormal movements, including tremors, rigidity, shuffling, slow gait and loss of balance.

Depression, muffled speech, sleep disorders and a frozen facial expression are other symptoms. The disease most often affects people over 60, but it can also occur in younger adults. Men are affected 50 percent more frequently than women.

CAUSES

While the cause of Parkinson's is generally unknown, there are several environmental risk factors, including exposure to pesticides and herbicides, living in a rural environment, drinking well water, and proximity to industrial plants or quarries. Parkinson's can be induced by the use of illicit drugs laced with toxic chemicals.

There may also be a genetic component: people with a parent or sibling who developed Parkinson's disease in their 40s or 50s are at increased risk.

PREVENTION

There is no known way to prevent Parkinson's disease other than avoidance of the known toxins mentioned above.

DIAGNOSIS

A doctor can make a diagnosis based on the symptoms. Blood tests and brain imaging may be done to rule out neurological illnesses such as Creutzfeldt–Jakob disease (pp.188–9) and autoimmune diseases.

TREATMENTS

There is no cure. The goal of treatment is to relieve the symptoms.

• **MEDICINE** The mainstay of treatment is medicines that either replace dopamine, such as levdopa (L-dopa), or function like dopamine, such as bromocriptine and pergolide. Selegiline may protect neurons and delay the need for L-dopa early in the course of the disease. These drugs reduce tremors, rigidity and other symptoms. Medication, such as carbidopa, may be given along with L-dopa to reduce its side-effects, which include nausea, vomiting, low blood pressure and hallucinations. Catechol-o-methyl-transferase inhibitors may be prescribed to increase the effectiveness of L-dopa.

• **SURGERY** One procedure involves implanting electrodes in the brain and stimulating targeted areas with electric impulses. Another destroys areas of the brain responsible for symptoms. Experiments with implanting stem cells into the brain may generate healthy new brain cells and possibly cure the disease.

• **SUPPLEMENTS** A multi-centre clinical trial published in *Archives of Neurology* in 2002 found that supplements of coenzyme Q_{10} slowed the early progression of Parkinson's. Coenzyme Q_{10} is made from a chemical found in the mito-chondria and is lacking in people with Parkinson's.

• **ALEXANDER TECHNIQUE** This therapy (pp.488–9) reduces the disability associated with Parkinson's.

• **NEUROMUSCULAR MASSAGE** A pilot study of 32 patients, published in the *Journal of the American Osteopathic Association* in 2005, found that neuromuscular massage (p.471) improved motor control in people with Parkinson's.

See also: *Neuromuscular Massage, p.471 • Alexander Technique, pp.488–9 • Creutzfeldt–Jakob Disease, pp.188–9*

WHO IS AT RISK?

The risk factors include:

• Over 60 years of age

• Male

• Family history of Parkinson's disease

Multiple Sclerosis

A broad spectrum of neurological symptoms, ranging from a mild tingling or numbness in the limbs to disabling vision loss and paralysis, can signal multiple sclerosis, one of the most common central nervous system diseases. It can also profoundly impair cognition. It affects more than 2,500,000 people around the world, twice as many women as men, and usually strikes between the ages of 20 and 40.

There are four forms of the disease. Relapsing–remitting is the most common form, in which attacks are separated by periods of partial or total recovery. Benign multiple sclerosis consists of one or two mild episodes and little or no disability. Secondary–progressive begins with relapses and periods of remitting, but then becomes steadily worse. Progressive multiple sclerosis gets progressively worse from the start.

CAUSES

Multiple sclerosis occurs when myelin, the sheath that protects the nerves cells and helps transmit nerve impulses, becomes damaged. The cause of this damage appears to be an abnormal attack from the immune system. It is not known what causes this autoimmune reaction, but experts think a virus may be a trigger. There may be a genetic predisposition, because it runs in families and certain genetic markers have been found only in people with multiple sclerosis.

Other factors also appear to be involved. One is environment – the farther from the equator, the more cases there are. The disease is more common in northern North America and Europe, and southern Australia and New Zealand than it is in tropical areas. Temperature extremes can trigger symptoms in people with multiple sclerosis, as can stress and fatigue.

PREVENTION

There is no known way to prevent multiple sclerosis, but the frequency of attacks may be reduced by getting plenty of rest and controlling stress with measures such as regular exercise, guided imagery (pp.520–2), meditation (pp.514–19) and yoga (pp.576–9).

DIAGNOSIS

Doctors diagnose multiple sclerosis based on the symptoms, a medical examination and medical tests that rule out other disorders that can cause similar symptoms. The symptoms of multiple sclerosis vary from person to person, but they include:

- Weakness of one or more extremities
- Paralysis
- Tremors
- Spasms
- Abnormal gait
- Facial pain
- Loss of vision or double vision
- Dizziness
- Urinary abnormalities
- Fatigue
- Slurred speech
- Depression

The medical examination consists of tests of neurological functions, such as sensation, vision and eye movement. Imaging tests, such as an MRI scan of the brain and spine, can show the destruction of myelin around neurons. Examination of the fluid surrounding the brain and spinal cord (cerebrospinal fluid) may help in the diagnosis as well.

TREATMENTS

There is no cure for multiple sclerosis, but medication and other treatments can help relieve symptoms and prevent recurrences. The kind of treatment depends on the type of multiple sclerosis and the symptoms.

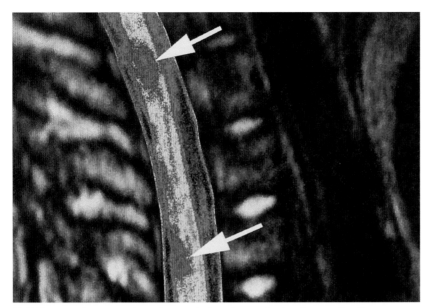

Multiple sclerosis occurs when plaques destroy the myelin sheaths covering the nerves, impairing their ability to function properly. An MRI scan can reveal damage (pink, arrowed) to the spinal cord caused by multiple sclerosis. The healthy nerve tissue is in yellow.

• **MEDICATION** Medicines that suppress the immune system are used to prevent relapses in relapsing–remitting multiple sclerosis. These medications, which are taken by injection several times a week, include interferon and glatiramer acetate. Mitoxantrone, a drug used in cancer chemotherapy that suppresses some immune system cells, is also used to treat the relapsing–remitting and secondary progressive types of multiple sclerosis.

Corticosteroids are given intravenously during relapses to relieve the symptoms and possibly shorten their duration. Other medication is prescribed for specific symptoms, such as muscle spasticity, seizures, bladder dysfunction and depression. Aspirin may help with fatigue. In a clinical trial of 30 patients published in 2005 in *Neurology*, patients who took 1,300 mg a day of aspirin reported less fatigue than patients who took a placebo.

• **EXERCISE** Regular exercise helps people with multiple sclerosis improve muscle strength and mobility, as well as mood. No particular exercises have been found to be superior to others.

• **PHYSICAL, SPEECH, AND OCCUPATIONAL THERAPY** Physical therapy can help improve muscle strength and mobility. Occupational therapy can improve everyday functioning. Speech therapy can help improve slurred speech.

• **MASSAGE** This can relieve anxiety and depression, and improve social functioning in people with multiple sclerosis.

• **MUSIC** Music therapy was shown to lead to a significant reduction in anxiety and depression and an increase in self-esteem in a clinical trial of 20 patients published in the *Journal of Music Therapy* in 2004.

• **SUPPLEMENTS** Preliminary research suggests that vitamin D supplements may help reduce the frequency of attacks, but the findings need to be confirmed by larger studies. Preliminary studies also suggest cannabinoids (compounds derived from the active agents in marijuana; cannabinoids are also produced naturally by the body) may help reduce subjective symptoms of spasticity.

See also: *Guided Imagery, pp.520–2 • Yoga, pp.476–9 • Tremors, p.173*

healing hope My multiple sclerosis symptoms were getting worse. I had to walk with a cane and I started having urinary incontinence. Then I heard about a strange therapy – bee stings. Some participants in an online multiple sclerosis support group said they were having themselves stung a few times a week, and that now they felt less pain and other symptoms. They admitted that the stings hurt, but they said the results were worth it.

So I talked with my doctor. She said bee sting therapy had been around for years, but she warned me that there was very little research on how – or how well – it worked. She also reminded me that bee stings themselves could cause a deadly allergic reaction (although I knew I wasn't allergic). She said she could refer me to a beekeeper who was knowledgeable.

That was six months ago. Now I get bee sting therapy twice a week by putting a bee on each leg. It's really helped me. I still have incontinence, but I feel more stable when I'm walking. *Gina B.*

Peripheral Nerve Disorders

The peripheral nervous system is the extensive network of nerves that allows the brain and spinal cord to communicate with the rest of the body. Peripheral nerve disorders, also known as peripheral neuropathies, occur when one or more of these nerves are damaged. There are more than 100 types of peripheral nerve disorders, each with different symptoms.

CAUSES

Because there are many types of peripheral nerve disorders, there are also many causes. Diabetes (pp.338–41) is the most common cause of chronic peripheral neuropathy in developed countries, while leprosy is most common in third world nations.

- Trauma from accidents, injuries and repetitive stress can tear, compress or completely sever peripheral nerves. Carpal tunnel syndrome (p.164) is the most common repetitive stress cause of neuropathy.
- Systemic diseases can damage nerves by interfering with the body's use of nutrients, disposal of waste products or other vital functions. Diabetes is one of the most common causes of peripheral nerve disorders, and 60 to 70 percent of diabetics have some nerve damage. Other causes are autoimmune diseases such as lupus (pp.324–5) and rheumatoid arthritis (pp.136–9), kidney disease (p.308), thyroid disorders (pp.344–7) and various cancers. Benign tumours of the nervous system, such as neuromas, can squeeze peripheral nerves, causing damage.
- Infections that directly attack the nerves, causing acute peripheral neuropathies, include shingles (p.175), Epstein–Barr virus (p.319), herpes simplex (pp.392–3), HIV (pp.316–7) and Lyme disease. Late stages of syphilis (pp.424–5) can also cause neuropathy.
- Autoimmune diseases cause inflammation, which can damage nerve fibres. One such autoimmune disease is Guillain-Barré syndrome, which usually develops days or weeks after an infection like influenza or diarrhoea. In some cases, pregnancy, minor surgery, or, in extremely rare events, vaccinations can lead to Guillain–Barré. It can cause numbness and weakness in the arms and legs which may progress to paralysis.
- Deficiencies of vitamins E, B_1 (thiamin), B_3 (niacin), B_6, and B_{12} can starve nerves of essential

WHO IS AT RISK?

The risk factors include:

- Trauma
- Diseases such as diabetes, kidney disease, and auto-immune diseases
- Tumours
- Lyme disease and shingles
- Deficiencies of vitamin E and vitamins B_1, B_3, B_6, and B_{12}
- Alcoholism
- Exposure to toxic substances
- Side-effects of medications such as anticonvulsants and some anti-cancer drugs

Guard against trauma by wearing seat belts when riding in motor vehicles and using helmets when engaged in activities such as roller blading, hockey, and skiing.

nutrients. Alcoholism can cause thiamin deficiency. Toxicity from overdoses of vitamins such as B_6 can also cause neuropathy.

• Toxic substances, such as lead, mercury and arsenic, can cause peripheral nerve damage.

• Long-term use of some anti-cancer drugs, anticonvulsants and antiviral medicines, can cause nerve damage.

• Inherited conditions can cause some peripheral nerve disorders. The most common are a group of conditions called Charcot–Marie–Tooth disease. People with the disease inherit mutations in some of the genes that oversee the formation of neurons or myelin, the protective layer of fatty tissue around neurons that speeds communication of nerve impulses.

In some cases, no cause can be identified, and these are referred to as idiopathic neuropathies.

PREVENTION

Keeping blood sugar levels under tight control is the first line of defence for people with diabetes. The Diabetes Control and

Clinical Query

Once peripheral nerves are damaged, can they regenerate?

Yes, if the cause of the nerve damage can be identified and then minimized or removed. Prompt treatment of wounds, a good diet, quitting smoking and regular exercise, may promote nerve regeneration.

Complications Trial Research Group found that those who maintained low blood sugar levels cut their risk of diabetic neuropathy by 60 percent. The highest rate of neuropathy occurs in diabetics who have had the disease for 25 years or longer and in men.

Foot problems are the most common results of peripheral neuropathy in people with diabetes, because the nerves to the feet are among the longest in the body. Losing sensation in the feet may lead to the development of wounds or sores that fail to heal and can become infected. Such infections can spread to the bone and may, in some cases, necessitate limb amputation. It is estimated that nearly half of the limb amputations among diabetics could be avoided with improved foot care, including a daily inspection for any injuries or sores.

Reduce the risk of developing diabetes by exercising regularly, maintaining a normal weight, and eating a healthy, balanced diet. Guard against trauma from injuries and accidents by wearing seat belts when riding in motor vehicles and using helmets when engaged in activities such as roller blading, hockey and skiing. Avoid exposure to toxic chemicals and metals. Take precautions against Lyme disease by using tick repellent when outdoors in areas with the tick-borne illness. Avoid excess alcohol consumption (more than two drinks a day for men and one for women). Do not smoke, because smoking constricts blood vessels that feed peripheral nerves.

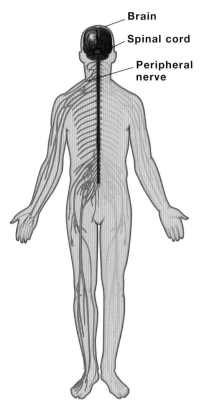

The central nervous system (CNS) is made up of the brain and the spinal cord. The peripheral nervous system transmits signals from the body to the CNS.

DIAGNOSIS

A doctor can diagnose peripheral nerve disorders based on a medical history as well as the symptoms and their pattern of occurrence. Depending on the cause, symptoms can include numbness, tingling, pricking sensations, sensitivity to touch, muscle weakness, burning pain, muscle wasting, or even paralysis.

• **BLOOD TESTS** Diabetes, vitamin deficiencies and Lyme disease can be diagnosed using blood tests.

• **NERVE CONDUCTION TESTS** The speed of electrical communication between nerves is measured using a nerve conduction velocity test.

• **ELECTROMYOGRAPHY** The electrical activity in the muscles is measured by inserting fine-needle

On Call

The symptoms of Guillain–Barré syndrome can appear suddenly and quickly over the course of a day and may require immediate treatment in an emergency room. It may result in paralysis and, in some cases, may even be fatal. The symptoms include:

- Weakness or tingling that may start in the feet and legs and spread to the upper body
- Pain in the entire body
- Trouble breathing
- Trouble with eye or facial movement, or speaking, chewing, or swallowing
- Paralysis of legs, arms, face, and respiratory muscles
- Problems with bladder or bowel control
- Very slow heart rate or low blood pressure

electrodes into the muscle. Electromyography can be used to differentiate between muscle and nerve disorders. Other tests can be used to check muscle strength.

• **BIOPSY** A nerve biopsy, in which a small piece of nerve tissue is removed and analysed in a laboratory, is sometimes needed to make a definitive diagnosis.

A skin biopsy can detect damage to smaller nerve fibres. Because it has fewer side-effects, it is sometimes performed instead of a nerve biopsy.

• **OTHER TESTS** A spinal tap can be used to detect any abnormal antibodies in the cerebrospinal fluid. A doctor may also request additional tests, including imaging exams such as CT scans and MRIs.

• **MONITOR DIABETES SYMPTOMS** People with diabetes should have their feet checked at least once a year by a professional for signs of peripheral neuropathy. Symptoms usually begin in the feet and legs before moving to the hands and arms, and are often worse at night.

TREATMENTS

The treatment of peripheral nerve disorders depends on their cause. If it is an underlying illness, such as Lyme disease or diabetes, the first step is to control that illness. The goal of other treatments is to reduce the symptoms.

• **MEDICATION** For mild pain, analgesics such as ibuprofen may be sufficient. For severe pain, narcotic pain relief, which can be habit-forming, or injections or topical patches with local anesthetics such as lidocaine may be needed. Antiepileptic medications, such as phenytoin and gabapentin, and tricyclic antidepressants can also help reduce pain.

• **ANTIOXIDANT SUPPLEMENTS** Acetyl-L-carnitine, in 1,000 mg doses, alleviated pain and stimulated nerve fibre regeneration in people with diabetic neuropathy, according to the results of two yearlong clinical trials published in *Diabetes Care* in 2005. The supplements may also relieve peripheral neuropathy induced by chemotherapy. Alpha-lipoic acid supplements dramatically reduce pain, burning and other symptoms.

• **EVENING PRIMROSE OIL** This essential oil may relieve peripheral neuropathy caused by diabetes, but more research is needed to confirm its effectiveness.

• **AUTOIMMUNE DISEASE TREATMENTS** Plasmapheresis, or plasma exchange, helps shorten the duration of Guillain–Barré syndrome by removing antibodies that may contribute to the abnormal autoimmune process causing the disorder. With this treatment, blood is withdrawn and its liquid component (plasma) is separated out and replaced with fresh frozen plasma. Immunoglobulin treatment, in which substances are given intravenously to suppress abnormal immune system activity, speeds recovery from Guillain–Barré syndrome as effectively as plasma exchange. Combining the two treatments is not superior to using only one of them.

• **EXERCISE** A regular exercise regimen may help improve muscle strength in people with peripheral nerve disorders. Resistance exercise of the affected muscles appears especially effective.

• **TENS** Transcutaneous electrical nerve stimulation (p.443) may reduce pain from peripheral neuropathy.

• **SURGERY** In some cases, surgery may be recommended to remove tumours, or to loosen ligaments and tendons that are pressing on or otherwise interfering with nerves.

• **MEDICAL DEVICES** Hand and foot braces can stabilize weak muscles and relieve pain by taking pressure off the nerves. For people with pain or loss of sensation in the feet, orthopedic shoes can make walking easier and help prevent further nerve damage to the feet.

See also: *Shingles, p.175 • Diabetes, pp.338–41 • Lyme Disease, pp.326–7*

Bell's Palsy

Pain around one ear and muscle weakness on one side of the face can be early signs of Bell's palsy, an inflammation and swelling of the seventh cranial nerve, which runs along each side of the face and controls most of the muscles. The inflammation causes weakness or paralysis on the affected side of the face, making eating, drinking and completely closing the mouth very difficult.

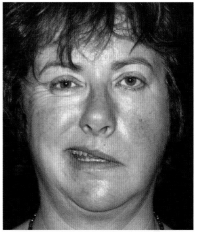

Bell's palsy affects a nerve on one side of the face, often causing paralysis and making it difficult to eat or close the mouth.

Most people recover from Bell's palsy completely, although the process can take several weeks or months. The incidence of this condition varies worldwide, with the greatest number of cases reported in Japan and the fewest in Sweden.

CAUSES

The usual cause of the inflammation characteristic of Bell's palsy is believed (but not universally accepted) to be a herpes virus – either the one that causes cold sores (pp.82–3) or the one that causes chickenpox. Lyme disease (pp.326–7) may also cause Bell's palsy. Women who are pregnant and people with diabetes, the flu or a cold are at increased risk for developing the condition.

PREVENTION

There is no known way to prevent Bell's palsy.

DIAGNOSIS

A doctor can usually diagnose Bell's palsy based on the symptoms and a physical examination that looks specifically for muscle weakness on one side of the face,

including in some cases nerve problems. The doctor may also test for Lyme disease if the patient has had a risk of exposure. Symptoms of Bell's palsy include:
- Pain around one ear
- Sensitivity to sound in the ear on the affected side
- Weak muscles on one side of the face
- Difficulty smiling or grimacing
- Loss of sense of taste
- Drooping or stiffness on one side of the face
- Difficulty closing one eye
- Difficulty closing the mouth on one side
- Drooling
- Facial paralysis

TREATMENTS

Treatments aim to reduce the symptoms and hasten recovery.

WHO IS AT RISK?

The risk factors include:
- A cold or flu
- Diabetes
- Lyme disease
- Pregnancy

- **MEDICATION** Drugs such as acyclovir, which fight herpes viruses, may shorten the duration of the disease. High-dose corticosteroids can decrease the time it takes to make a full recovery.
- **EYE PROTECTION** This is important to prevent corneal abrasions when the lid is unable to close. If a patient is unable to close one eye, artificial tears may be needed to prevent dry eye (p.33).
- **ACUPUNCTURE** This therapy may be done with or without moxibustion (pp.464–5) to speed recovery. Acupuncture may help prevent nerve damage, as well.
- **HYPERBARIC OXYGEN THERAPY** This treatment (p.579), in which the patient is exposed to concentrated oxygen levels, may also hasten recovery.

See also: *Lyme Disease, pp.326–7* • *Acupuncture, pp.464–5* • *Dry Eye, p.33*

Creutzfeldt–Jakob Disease

In people with Creutzfeldt–Jakob disease, a wide range of symptoms comes on suddenly: personality changes such as aggressiveness, hallucinations, difficulty walking, sleepiness, dementia (pp.178–9), and depression (pp.364–5). The muscles jerk and go rigid. This is a rare, fatal condition in which nerves and brain tissue deteriorate, leaving sponge-like holes in the brain.

This disease belongs to a family of transmissible brain disorders called spongiform encephalopathy. About one in one million people around the world contracts Creutzfeldt–Jakob, mainly in middle age. Death usually occurs within a year.

CAUSES

The disease is believed to be caused by a prion, which is a type of protein. Harmless prions exist naturally in the human body, but infectious ones behave like viruses and bacteria and cause disease. The most common form of Creutzfeldt–Jakob disease is sporadic, with no known risk factor. With sporadic disease, it is possible that normal prions in the body somehow turn infectious. Another 5 to 10 percent of cases are caused by mutations in a particular gene that is responsible for normal prion production.

About 1 percent of cases develop as a result of exposure to nervous system tissue that is infected with a prion-causing illness. One mode of exposure is having a medical procedure that involves the nervous system, such as grafts of brain tissue, cornea transplants and injections of growth hormone.

Another mode of exposure is eating beef from cows infected with bovine spongiform encephalopathy, or BSE (see Clinical Query), which is believed to cause a variant of Creutzfeldt–Jakob. First identified in 1984, nearly all of the 140 cases diagnosed have occurred in the United Kingdom, with a handful of others in Ireland, Italy, Canada, and the United States.

PREVENTION

Avoiding contact with infected nervous system tissue can reduce the risk of contracting Cruetzfeldt–Jakob disease. Many countries

> ## WHO IS AT RISK?
> **The risk factors include:**
> - Age 60 and older
> - Family history
> - Medical procedures that involve the nervous system
> - Eating beef from cows infected with bovine spongiform encephalopathy (BSE)

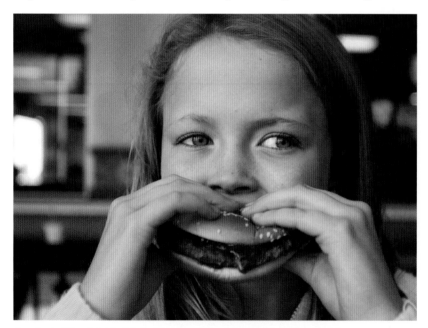

A variant of Creutzfeldt–Jakob disease can be contracted by eating beef from cows infected with BSE, also called mad cow disease. Many countries around the world test for BSE and keep infected beef away from the human food supply.

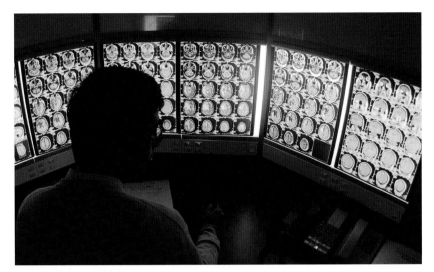

No specific test can definitively diagnose Creutzfeldt–Jakob disease, but brain imaging techniques, such as a CT scan, may be used to help in the diagnosis by ruling out brain tumours and other conditions that have similar symptoms.

reduce cell death from infectious prions. Several other medications are under investigation.

• **COUNSELLING** Some form of counselling may help control aggressive or agitated behaviour in people with Creutzfeldt–Jakob disease and offer support to family members.

See also: *Depression, p. 364–5* • *Dementia, pp.178–9* • *Meningitis, p.180* • *Immunizations, pp.314–15*

around the world routinely test cattle for bovine spongiform encephalopathy to prevent infected meat from entering the human food supply. To reduce the likelihood of transmission through medical procedures, pharmaceutical companies no longer use growth hormone from cadavers, which can be infected; instead, they now use genetically engineered growth hormone.

DIAGNOSIS

There are no diagnostic tests specifically for Creutzfeldt–Jakob disease. Doctors make a diagnosis by testing for treatable brain diseases that can cause similar symptoms, such as encephalitis and meningitis, and by detecting some signs of Creutzfeldt–Jakob. An electroencephalogram (EEG), which measures the brain's electrical activity, can reveal a pattern of electrical activity that is common in people with Creutzfeldt–Jakob disease. A spinal tap is done to examine the

spinal fluid for signs of infection, tumours, and other neurological disorders. A CT scan of the brain can rule out a brain tumour and an MRI can reveal patterns of brain deterioration that can suggest Creutzfeldt–Jakob disease.

TREATMENTS

There is no therapy to slow or reverse the course of the disease, but medication and other treatments can help temporarily relieve symptoms. Nursing care is often needed when patients become bedridden.

• **MEDICATION** Anti-epileptic drugs such as valproate are prescribed to reduce muscle spasms. Sedatives and antipsychotic medications may be used to control aggressive behaviour. Opiates can relieve extreme pain. Flupirtine maleate, an analgesic, reduced the progression of dementia in a clinical trial of 28 Creutzfeldt–Jakob patients published in the journal *Neurology* in 2004. In laboratory experiments, the drug was found to

Clinical Query

What is mad cow disease?

It is a neurological disease, more properly known as bovine spongiform encephalopathy (BSE), that occurs in cattle and is believed to cause a variant of Creutzfeldt–Jakob disease in humans who eat beef from infected animals.

Since 1984, when the first Creutzfeldt–Jakob variant was identified in the United Kingdom, more than 181,376 cattle infected with BSE have been identified and destroyed in the UK. More than 3,000 infected cattle have been reported in other countries throughout Europe, as well as in Israel, Japan, Canada and the United States. BSE is spread by feeding calves rendered bone and meat from cattle, a practice that has now been banned by most countries.

Preventative measures include routine testing of cattle for BSE eliminating infected cattle from the human food chain. Since the introduction of preventive measures in the United Kingdom in 1992, the incidence of BSE there has declined dramatically.

Amyotrophic Lateral Sclerosis

To move a muscle, the brain sends signals to motor neurons in the spinal cord that tell the muscle to move. Amyotrophic lateral sclerosis (ALS) is the deterioration of motor neurons that convey these signals, resulting in a loss of muscle function. At first, muscles in the hands, arms, and legs feel weak. The hands and feet twitch.

Speaking and eventually breathing become difficult, and paralysis occurs in the final stages, although thinking and other cognitive functions remain intact. Death usually occurs within five years of the onset of symptoms. This rare, progressive disorder is also known as Lou Gehrig's disease, after a famous baseball player whose life was cut short by it.

CAUSES

Although the exact cause of ALS is unknown, about 10 percent of cases run in families. Mutations in the superoxide dismutase gene are associated with the condition. Superoxide dismutase neutralizes free radicals, substances that damage cells. Experts believe several other, as-yet unidentified, genes are also involved in ALS. A genetic test can detect mutations in the superoxide dismutase gene.

PREVENTION

A study of 957,740 adults published in the *Annals of Neurology* in 2005 found that those who took vitamin E supplements (pp.532–41) regularly had a lower-than-average risk of dying of ALS over a 16-year period, suggesting that the supplement may help prevent the disease.

DIAGNOSIS

ALS is difficult to diagnose because early symptoms are similar to some other illnesses, including thyroid disorders (pp.344–7) and toxic exposures. Doctors do a neurological examination and several tests:

- Electromyography to measure electrical activity in the muscles
- Blood and urine tests to measure levels of thyroid and parathyroid hormone levels, as well as heavy metal content, to rule out thyroid illness and toxic exposures
- Imaging tests, including myelography, X-rays, and MRI, to detect abnormalities of the spine
- Lumbar puncture to examine cerebrospinal fluid for signs of infection, tumours, multiple sclerosis and other illnesses.

TREATMENTS

There is no cure. Treatment aims to relieve the symptoms. Canes, walkers and special utensils can make it easier for people to walk, eat and take care of themselves.

- **MEDICATION** Riluzole is the only medication found to prolong life in people with Lou Gehrig's disease. This drug is primarily aimed at relieving symptoms and preventing complications. It extends survival by about two months. It also helps prolong the time patients are able to breathe on their own. Other substances, such as human growth factors, are currently being studied as a way of treating for Lou Gehrig's disease.
- **SUPPLEMENTS** Creatine supplements, derived from a substance used by muscles, may delay the progression of symptoms when used with conventional treatments for Lou Gehrig's disease. Many doctors also recommend taking vitamins C and E, which are antioxidants that may help neutralize free radicals, a potential factor in the disease. There is evidence that vitamin E prolongs life in patients, but no such evidence for vitamin C.
- **EXERCISE** Endurance exercises involving the limbs and trunk, performed for 15 minutes twice a day, can reduce spasticity.

See also: *Thyroid Diseases, pp.344–7* • *Nutritional Supplements, pp.532–41*

WHO IS AT RISK?

The risk factors include:

- Age 50 and over
- Family history

Trigeminal Neuralgia

Doctors consider trigeminal neuralgia to be among the most painful medical disorders. A piercing pain like an electric shock strikes the scalp, forehead, nose, jaw and gums – areas served by the trigeminal nerve, the major sensory nerve in the face. The pain usually occurs on one side of the head, but it sometimes affects both sides. Attacks of pain last for a few seconds and often come in clusters, although months or years can pass between them.

WHO IS AT RISK?

The risk factors include:

- Age 50 and older
- Female
- Multiple sclerosis
- *Herpes zoster* infection
- Tumours

They can be prompted by ordinary activities, such as brushing the teeth, washing, shaving, eating or drinking. Trigeminal neuralgia, also called *tic douloureaux*, is most common in women ages 50 and older. The condition in a young person is often a sign of multiple sclerosis (pp.182–3).

CAUSES

This neuralgia occurs when the trigeminal nerve becomes inflamed or compressed. Sometimes the cause is pressure from a nearby artery. Other causes are nerve damage from multiple sclerosis and, in rare cases, infection with herpes zoster (p.175), the virus that causes chickenpox, or any tumour that compresses the trigeminal nerve roots.

PREVENTION

There is no known way to prevent trigeminal neuralgia.

DIAGNOSIS

Doctors can diagnose trigeminal neuralgia based on the symptoms and by ruling out other disorders that can cause these or similar symptoms, such as sinusitis (pp.58–60) or a toothache. Magnetic resonance imaging (MRI) may be used to check for brain tumours (p.196), abnormalities of blood vessels and signs of multiple sclerosis.

TREATMENTS

Medication and sometimes surgery are used to treat trigeminal neuralgia. Other treatments, such as acupuncture (pp.464–5), chiropractic (pp.446–7), and hypnosis (pp.508–13), are used by many patients, but their effectiveness for trigeminal neuralgia is unproven.

• **MEDICATION** The first line of treatment is anti-seizure medicine, such as carbamazepine, oxcarbazepine, gabapentin or phenytoin. If these drugs do not work, doctors sometimes prescribe baclofen, which relieves muscle spasms, and tricyclic antidepressants.

• **SURGERY** If medicine does not offer relief, surgery may be recommended. There are several surgical procedures, but it is often unclear which one is best for which patient.

An exception is microvascular decompression, which is performed when blood vessels compress the trigeminal nerve. With this operation, the blood vessels are removed and the nerve is encased in a protective material. Other forms of surgery, such as percutaneous radiofrequency ablation, aim to deaden the pain fibres around the trigeminal nerve. Overall, they have a success rate of 85 percent, but 25 percent of patients have symptoms that recur within one to five years.

See also: *Acupuncture, pp.464–5 • Brain Tumours, p.196–7 • Hypnotherapy, pp.508–13*

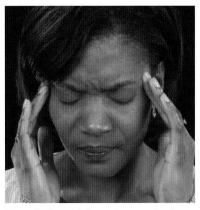

Trigeminal neuralgia produces a piercing pain in the areas served by the trigeminal nerve, the major sensory nerve in the face.

Myasthenia Gravis

Unusual muscle weakness that develops after a period of activity is the hallmark of myasthenia gravis. The muscles most often affected are those that control facial expressions, eye movement, chewing and swallowing, as well as those in the arms and legs. Other symptoms include shortness of breath, double vision, the head drooping to the side and slurred speech. One key feature of this disorder is muscle weakness without a loss of sensation.

WHO IS AT RISK?

The risk factors include:
- Women under age 40
- Men over age 60
- A mother with the condition can cause temporary myasthenia gravis in newborns

Myasthenia gravis is most common in women under age 40 and men over age 60, but it can affect children and adults of all ages. Although usually a chronic disease, it does not necessarily shorten the lifespan when properly treated.

CAUSES

This is an autoimmune disease in which the immune system attacks the neuromuscular junction, the place where neurons transmit messages to muscles. Immune system antibodies block, change or destroy receptors on the muscles for acetylcholine, a neurotransmitter that neurons release to signal muscles to contract. The cause of this attack is unknown. One theory is that it involves the thymus, a gland that helps the immune system develop, and which is abnormal in adults with myasthenia gravis.

Myasthenic crisis is a life-threatening breathing problem sometimes caused by the disease, and can be triggered by fever, infection, an adverse reaction to medication or emotional stress.

PREVENTION

There is no known way to prevent myasthenia gravis.

DIAGNOSIS

Doctors diagnose myasthenia gravis based on symptoms, a medical history, and a physical evaluation, including an assessment of muscle strength and abnormal eye movements which give clues to muscle weakness. Several tests may be done, including:
- Electromyogram to measure the electrical transmission from neurons
- Nerve conduction study, which can cause muscle fatigue in people myasthenia gravis
- Blood test for acetylcholine antibodies, which are abnormally high in approximately 90 percent of people with myasthenia gravis
- Edrophonium, which increases the action of acetylcholine; muscles become stronger for a while in people with myasthenia gravis, but not in people who do not have the disease
- CT scan to detect abnormalities of the thymus.

TREATMENTS

Treatment is aimed at reducing the symptoms.
- **MEDICATION** Immunosuppressive drugs, such as prednisone and cyclosporine, reduce the attack on acetylcholine receptors to improve muscle strength. Other drugs, such as neostigmine and pyridostigmine, do the same by reducing acetylcholine breakdown.
- **BLOOD TREATMENTS** Plasmapheresis removes abnormal antibodies. High-dose immunoglobulin is an infusion of donated blood containing normal antibodies. Both are used for myasthenic crisis.
- **SURGERY** Removing the thymus (thymectomy) provides long-term reduction of symptoms in 70 percent of patients, even curing the disease in some, although patients often experience some worsening of symptoms just after the operation.
- **LIFESTYLE CHANGES** Scheduling naps during the day and avoiding over-exertion can reduce episodes of muscle weakness.

See also: *Fever, p.318* • *Double Vision, pp.36–9*

Huntington's Disease

This incurable brain disease is a genetic disorder. Because it is present in different degrees in the gene pool of each population, its incidence varies widely throughout the world. It affects between one and nine people out of every 10,000 in Europe, 10 in 10,000 in the United States, and 70 in 10,000 in the Lake Maracaibo region of Venezuela.

Huntington's disease often begins with mood changes, such as unusual irritability, passivity or anger. As the disease progresses, it causes uncontrollable jerking, grimacing and other movements, as well as difficulty with learning, memory, decision-making and other cognitive functions. The symptoms usually begin in people ages 35 to 50, although a rare juvenile form starts before age 20. Death usually occurs within 15 years of the onset of symptoms.

CAUSES
Huntington's disease is caused by a single gene mutation. The mutation is an abnormal repetition of a sequence of chemicals in DNA called bases. The flawed gene causes neurons to die in the basal ganglia, the part of the brain that controls coordinated movement and other functions, as well as in the cortex, which controls rational thinking, memory and other cognitive functions. The greater the number of abnormal repetitions, the earlier the disease appears and the more severe it is.

People with one or both parents who have Huntington's disease have a 50 percent chance of inheriting a flawed gene, and those who do inherit the gene are certain to develop the disease. In rare cases, people develop Huntington's disease even without a family history. Experts believe these cases are caused by mutations that develop spontaneously in the Huntington's disease gene in the father's sperm.

PREVENTION
Genetic testing can determine if an individual with a family history of the disease has a flawed copy of the Huntington's disease gene. The only way people with a flawed gene can absolutely prevent it from being passed down to future generations is by not having any children.

DIAGNOSIS
A neurologist can diagnose Huntington's disease based on a neurological examination, symptoms, and a family medical history. The neurological examination includes tests of hearing, strength, coordination, reflexes, and balance, and observations of involuntary movements. The doctor also looks for abnormalities in the ability of the eyes to track moving objects, a symptom of the disease. An imaging test, such as CT scanning or magnetic resonance imaging (MRI), is usually used to check for abnormalities in the brain that are characteristic of the disease.

TREATMENTS
There is no cure for Huntington's disease, but several medications can help to relieve some of the physical, emotional and psychiatric symptoms.

• MEDICATION Antipsychotic drugs, such as clonazepam and haloperidol, can help reduce involuntary movements, hallucinations, delusions and bouts of violence. Antidepressants can help control depression, plus sedatives for anxiety and lithium for mood swings. Rivastigmine, a medication used for Alzheimer's disease (page 178–9), leads to a slight improvement in cognitive and motor symptoms.

• SUPPLEMENTS Preliminary evidence suggests pure ethyl-EPA, one of the two main ingredients in omega-3 fish oils (pp.252–3), may help reverse brain changes typical of Huntington's disease.

See also: *Alzheimer's Disease, pp.178–9* • *Depression, pp.364–5* • *Anxiety, pp.354–5*

WHO IS AT RISK?
The risk factors include:
• Family history
• Age 35 to 50

Tourette's Syndrome

This complex neurological disorder causes tics, or sudden, repetitive, and involuntary movements, such as blinking, grimacing, and head- or shoulder-jerking, as well as vocalizations of odd sounds and, sometimes, inappropriate words. Symptoms usually begin in childhood, peak in the early teenage years, and may diminish during adulthood.

Named for George Gilles de la Tourette, the French doctor who first described it in 1885, the condition affects about 2 to 3 percent of people and is four to five times as common in boys as in girls. Tourette's syndrome often occurs along with other disorders, especially attention-deficit hyperactivity disorder (pp.362–3) and obsessive-compulsive disorder (pp.354-5).

CAUSES

The condition runs in families and is believed to be genetic. An article in *Science* in 2005 described the gene, SLITRK1, on chromosome 13, as associated with some forms of Tourette's syndrome. The gene affects the cortex and basal ganglia, the areas of the brain believed responsible for the symptoms of Tourette's syndrome.

Abnormalities of neurotransmitters such as dopamine and serotonin also appear to be involved in the syndrome.

There is growing evidence that a strep throat infection (pp.56–7) increases the risk of developing neurological disorders such as Tourette's syndrome and obsessive-compulsive disorder. A study

published in the journal *Paediatrics* in 2005 found that children with such disorders were twice as likely to have had recent streptococcal infections than their healthy peers.

PREVENTION

There is no known way to prevent Tourette's syndrome. However, excitement, anxiety or fatigue may exacerbate tics. Some physical situations may trigger them as well, for instance, a too-tight collar may cause a neck-related tick such as neck-stretching, or hearing another person clearing the throat may result in the mimicking of those sounds.

DIAGNOSIS

Most commonly, one of the earliest signs of Tourette's syndrome is a facial tic. Other types of tics, such as shoulder-shrugging or throat-clearing, may then follow. Contrary to what many people believe, only a small percentage of people with the condition utter socially inappropriate or obscene words. Symptoms generally first appear during childhood, between the ages of seven and ten.

No laboratory tests exist to

diagnose Tourette's. A physical examination, which may include a CT scan, MRI, EEG, or certain blood tests, should be done to rule out any other possible causes. It is possible for other conditions to occur along with Tourette's, including obsessive-compulsive disorder, attention-deficit hyperactivity disorder, anger control problems, depression (pp.364–5), anxiety (pp.354-5), sleep problems (pp.170-2) and poor social skills.

Tics may be classified as either simple or complex. Simple tics involve only a few muscle groups

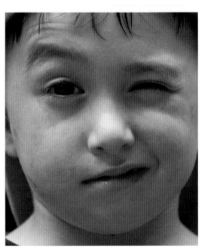

Tourette's syndrome can cause involuntary movements and facial expressions such as blinking and grimacing.

My son had just started third grade when I noticed he'd developed a facial tic. At first, I blamed it on the stress of school, but it got worse. He started thrusting his arm out suddenly, over and over, and clearing his throat constantly. When his teacher called me in for a meeting and explained that his behaviour was disrupting the class, I knew I had to do something.

It didn't take long for his paediatrician to diagnose Tourette's. I was appalled and frightened at first. But since then, he's been on a few different medications, and the tics are now under control to some extent. We've also started seeing a family counsellor, and that's helping us figure out how to cope with the day-to-day problems we're facing. *Laura H.*

and are characterized by sudden, brief, repetitive movements, such as eye-blinking, shoulder-shrugging, or head-jerking. Complex tics involve several muscle groups with a distinct, coordinated pattern of movement that may even look like it is being done with a purpose in mind. These complex tics may include throat-clearing, sniffing, grunting or barking.

Although tics are considered involuntary, in some cases an urge or sensation, called a premonitory urge, precedes the tic.

Doctors can usually diagnose Tourette's syndrome based on the symptoms and their pattern:

- Several motor tics and one or more vocal tics
- Tics that occur several times a day on most days
- No more than three months without symptoms during the past year
- Symptoms begin when the patient is younger than 18 years old

TREATMENTS

Mild tics may not require any treatment at all. Behavioural and medical treatments can help reduce tics and other symptoms, such as attention, concentration and learning difficulties.

- **BEHAVIOURAL THERAPY** A form of therapy called habit reversal can help reduce tics by making people with the condition aware of the sensory experience associated with a particular tic and then teaching them to substitute a more socially acceptable action. The approach has been found successful in adults but unproven in children.
- **MEDICATION** Antipsychotics such as haloperidol and pimozide, and antihypertensives such as clonidine, are given for tics, but can cause severe side-effects, including tardive dyskinesia, a movement disorder with persistent, repetitive, and involuntary movements of the lower face and mouth.

Other medications are used to treat associated disorders, such as selective serotonin reuptake inhibitors such as fluvoxamine and fluoxetine, for obsessive-compulsive disorder. Benzodiazepines may be prescribed for short-term relief of anxiety in children who also have attention-deficit hyperactivity disorder.

For Tourette's patients who have mild symptoms, medication may not be recommended. Some of the medication can cause severe side-effects, such as weight gain, liver toxicity and diabetes (pp.338–41). Other medication is under investigation, including ondansetron, an anti-nausea medicine often given with chemotherapy, a nicotine patch, and a cannabinoid patch.

- **ACUPUNCTURE** This Traditional Chinese Medicine (pp.464–5) reduced Tourette's syndrome symptoms enough for 73 percent of children to stop using medication, in a study of 156 patients in China published in 1996 in the *Journal of Traditional Chinese Medicine*. A large clinical trial is still needed to confirm the effectiveness of acupuncture for the condition.
- **BOTULIN INJECTIONS** The bacterial toxin that causes botulism, botulin, has been injected into the muscles to paralyze them enough to stop the tics. In a study of 30 patients in Italy, botulin injections decreased or even stopped vocal tics in 93 percent of patients and also decreased the urge to do so.
- **PSYCHOTHERAPY** Although Tourette's syndrome is not due to any psychological problems, counselling can help a person living with condition learn how to cope with the disorder and the social and emotional problems that may accompany it.
- **RELAXATION METHODS** Various relaxation methods and biofeedback (pp.504–7) may help relieve stress that may be aggravating tics.

See also: *Attention-Deficit Hyperactivity Disorder, pp.362–3* • *Obsessive-Compulsive Disorder, pp.354–5* • *Strep Throat, pp.56–7*

Brain Tumours

Any cluster of abnormal cells within the skull is a brain tumour. The tumour can be benign, which means it will not spread to other tissues and organs, or it can be cancerous – capable of spreading. Although benign tumours in other parts of the body are usually harmless, benign brain tumours can interfere with brain functions such as vision, hearing, and memory by pressing against brain tissue.

Benign and cancerous brain tumours have similar symptoms – most commonly, recurrent headaches that are especially painful when lying down. Other symptoms vary depending on where the tumours are located, but can include nausea, dizziness, difficulty seeing or hearing, behaviour changes and trouble concentrating. Most brain tumours occur in adults between the ages of 40 and 70 and in children ages 3 to 12.

CAUSES

Most cancerous brain tumours have spread from another cancer site. The cause of most primary brain tumours – those that originate in the brain – is unknown. Radiation treatment to the head for leukaemia increases the risk of developing brain tumours. Pesticides, including the chemicals used in flea and tick repellents, have been associated with brain tumours, although they are not proven causes.

It is unclear whether mobile telephones, which emit electromagnetic waves, increase the risk of brain cancer. A study of more than 1,500 people done by the National Cancer Institute in the United States in 1998 found a slightly increased incidence of gliomas, the most common cancerous brain tumours in adults, among mobile users. But smaller studies, including one by Swedish researchers in 1999, found no increased risk. Other studies are under way. Older mobiles, which are more powerful than the models used today, may have a stronger correlation with brain tumours.

Other risk factors for brain tumours are epilepsy; some rare inherited disorders, such as neurofibromatosis, von Hippel–Lindau syndrome and Turcot's syndrome; and having parents with cancers of the nervous system, colon or salivary glands.

PREVENTION

Minimizing exposure to radiation, lead and chemical pollutants such as pesticides may reduce the risk of developing brain tumours. A study published in *Epidemiology* in 2002 found that taking a multivitamin during pregnancy reduced the risk of children developing neuroblas-

WHO IS AT RISK?

The risk factors include:

- Adults age 40 to 70 and children age 3 to 12
- Males have a higher overall risk of brain tumours, but women are more prone to meningiomas, the most common benign brain tumours
- Radiation treatment for leukaemia
- Epilepsy
- History of cancer of the breast or lung
- A parent with cancer of the nervous system, colon or salivary glands
- Rare inherited disorders, such as neurofibromatosis, von Hippel-Lindau syndrome and Turcot's syndrome

toma, a childhood brain cancer, by 30 to 40 percent.

DIAGNOSIS

A neurologist can diagnose a brain tumour on the basis of the symptoms and by conducting a neurological examination, which includes tests of reflexes, coordination, sensation and muscle strength. Several other tests may be used. A CT or MRI scan of the brain can reveal the presence and location of abnormal tissue. A lumbar puncture may be done to examine cerebrospinal fluid for cancer cells. If a tumour is found, cerebral angiography, an X-ray of the blood vessels in the brain, may be done to get more detail on its size and location.

A biopsy of the abnormal tissue is taken and analysed in a laboratory to identify the type of tumour and whether it is benign or cancerous. The biopsy can be performed by inserting a needle into the brain to withdraw tissue while also performing a CT or MRI, or by testing a sample of the tumour that has been removed during surgery. If the tumour is cancerous, it will be identified by grade or severity (see *On Call* below).

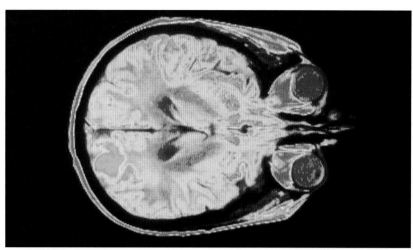

A neurologist can diagnose a brain tumour with a CT scan or magnetic resonance imaging (MRI) scan. The MRI image above shows a bright blue colour where brain cancer has metastasized in the occipital lobe, near the back of the skull (left side of the image).

TREATMENTS

The treatments used depend on whether the tumour is benign or cancerous, and many other factors, including its grade and location.

• SURGERY Cancerous and benign brain tumours that are accessible

enough to be excised without significant risk to healthy brain tissue are surgically removed. Various surgical techniques are used, depending on the tumour's location, size and other factors. Craniotomy removes a tumour through an opening in the skull. Stereotactic surgery is the more precise removal of tumours deep inside the brain under the guidance of CT scanning. Gamma knife radiosurgery uses high doses of radiation to destroy brain tumours without cutting.

• RADIATION This therapy may be used alone or with surgery to destroy cancer cells in the brain, using X-rays or other forms of radiation. External radiation uses a machine to direct beams of X-rays or other radiation energy into the body. Internal radiation involves injecting or implanting radioactive substances in and around a tumour. Either type of radiation may be used for adults, but only external radiation is used for children.

• CHEMOTHERAPY Medication to kill, or stop the division of, cancer cells may be used following sur-

gery. It may be given by injection or pills, infused into the spinal column, or implanted into brain tumour site in the form of a dissolving wafer.

• MEDICATION Anticonvulsant medication is sometimes needed to control seizures caused by a brain tumour. Anti-neoplastons, experimental medicines derived from amino acids and other compounds in the human body, appear effective in treating gliomas, according to pilot studies at the Burzynski Research Institute in Houston, Texas.

• SUPPLEMENTS Melatonin supplements, derived from a hormone that regulates the body's biological clock, may increase survival in people with glioblastomas, when combined with conventional radiation therapy.

• AROMATHERAPY MASSAGE This therapy induces relaxation and may reduce anxiety in people with malignant brain tumours.

See also: *Epilepsy & Seizures, pp.176–7* • *Headaches, pp.166–7* • *Aromatherapy, pp.548–9*

On Call

Cancerous brain tumours are categorized, or graded, according to appearance of the cancer cells, which indicates how fast they are likely to grow and spread.

- Grade I: The cancer cells look similar to normal cells and therefore are unlikely to spread. It may be possible to remove the entire tumour with surgery.
- Grade II: The tumour grows slowly and may spread to nearby tissue.
- Grade III: The cancer cells look very different from normal cells. They grow quickly and are likely to spread.
- Grade IV: The tumour grows aggressively and is difficult to treat.

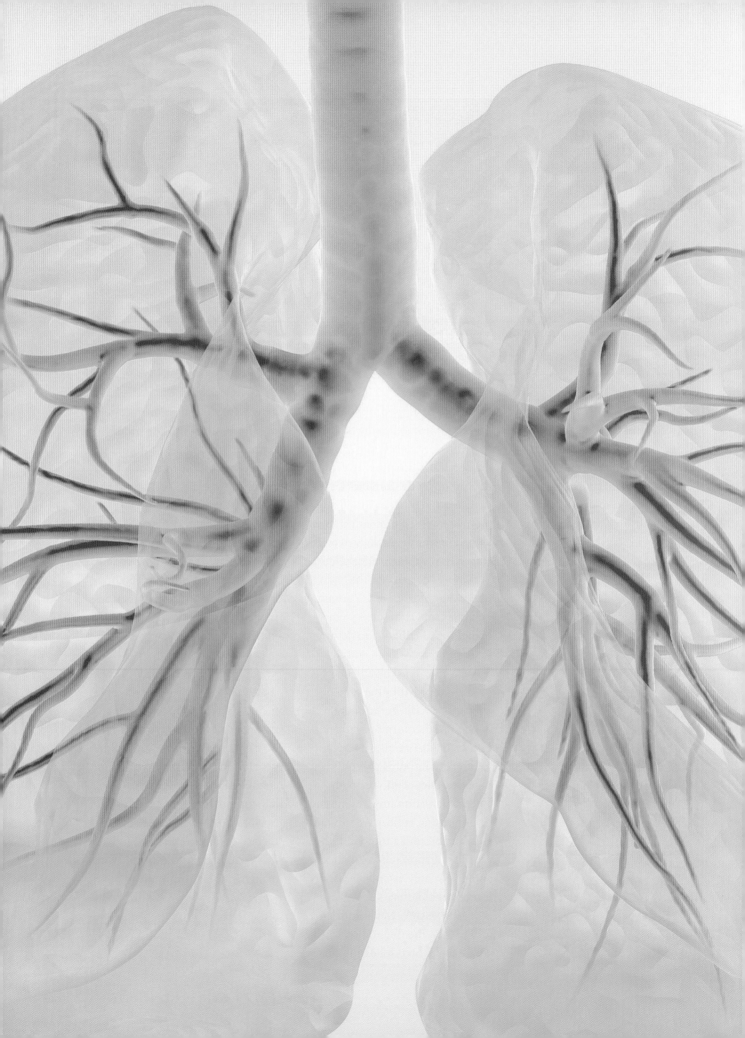

7 RESPIRATORY SYSTEM

The lungs are spongy, expandable organs protected by the rib cage that infuse the blood with oxygen as we breathe. When these organs lose their flexibility or ability to oxygenate blood, the result is usually a serious or life-threatening illness. Conditions such as emphysema and occupational lung disease destroy the tiny air sacs, called alveoli, where blood cells take on oxygen. Bacterial and viral infections that cause pneumonia and bronchitis can lead to inflammation that permanently obstructs the narrow airways deep within the lungs.

Many respiratory disorders can be prevented by minimizing exposure to harmful substances. Conditions that are either chronic or unpreventable, such as asthma and cystic fibrosis, respond to alternative treatments such as acupuncture and herbal medicines.

Chronic Obstructive
Pulmonary Disease

When air flow in the lungs is limited and breathing is difficult, the condition is chronic obstructive pulmonary disease, or COPD. It is due to chronic bronchitis, emphysema, or sometimes the two diseases together.

CAUSES

Smoking is the leading cause of COPD. It can damage the lungs in two ways: by destroying the alveoli, or air sacs, in emphysema; or by scarring the lining of the bronchial tubes in bronchitis.

With emphysema, longterm smoking destroys the air sacs in the lungs by damaging their delicate walls. In these air sacs, carbon dioxide from the blood is exchanged with oxygen from the air. Once destroyed, the damage is permanent and the air sacs cannot transfer oxygen to the bloodstream as efficiently. This creates shortness of breath and the lungs become less flexible, making it difficult to exhale.

With bronchitis, repeated irritation and infections inflame the lining of the bronchial tubes, limiting air flow to and from the lungs. The lining becomes scarred and an excessive amount of thick mucus is produced. It becomes a vicious cycle as the lining of the bronchial tubes become more thickened and scarred, resulting in more mucus. This creates a hospitable environment for bacterial infection, which leads to more irritation of the lining of the bronchial tubes.

In very rare cases, COPD is due to an enzyme deficiency of the protein alpha1-antitrypsin (AAT). This deficiency is suspected when COPD develops in a person younger than age 40 or in a non-smoker.

PREVENTION

Not smoking is the best way to prevent COPD. Patients who have COPD should get an annual flu innoculation as well as the pneumo-coccal vaccination to prevent complications that can occur with respiratory infections.

DIAGNOSIS

Symptoms may take years to develop, often starting with a morning cough that produces clear sputum. Shortness of breath with exertion may follow. Physical activity becomes more difficult and shortness of breath may occur without exercise. Fatigue, weakness and weight loss result. The cough may be accompanied by wheezing and thickening phlegm.

A doctor may listen for any wheezes and other sounds with a stethoscope, and notice the chest moves less than normal during

WHO IS AT RISK?

The risk factors include:
- Smoking
- Second-hand smoke
- History of childhood respiratory infections
- Family history of COPD
- Exposure to industrial pollutants

breathing, while the neck and shoulder muscles try to compensate. Chest X-rays and CT scans may be carried out. Pulmonary function tests can measure airflow obstruction. A blood test can show whether an AAT deficiency is responsible for COPD.

TREATMENTS

COPD cannot be cured, but treatments aim to slow down the progression of the disease and ease the symptoms.

• SMOKING CESSATION Smoking must be stopped (pp.216–17) so that the lungs are not further damaged. A five-year study of 5,887 middle-aged people with early COPD, done by the Lung Health Study Research Group in the United States, found that quitting smoking decreased the death rate from COPD by 46 percent.

• MEDICATION Bronchodilators help dilate the airways and are available as inhalers, such as albuterol or formoterol, and oral medications, such as theophylline. A combination may be required for effective treatment.

When bronchodilators fail to relieve symptoms, steroids may be used to help reduce lung inflammation. Using an inhaler has the fewest side-effects, but if COPD becomes serious, it may be necessary to give intravenous or oral steroids. Unfortunately, not all patients will respond to steroids.

Antibiotics may be needed to treat a bacterial infection. Antiviral medicines can be prescribed if the patient has influenza.

• SUPPLEMENTAL OXYGEN COPD can lower the amount of oxygen in the blood and some patients

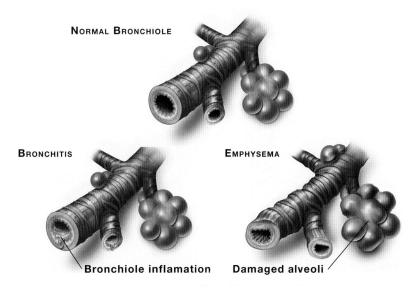

NORMAL BRONCHIOLE

BRONCHITIS

EMPHYSEMA

Bronchiole inflamation

Damaged alveoli

COPD can result from two separate conditions. Chronic bronchitis, which is an inflammation of the bronchiole lining, limits air flow to and from the lungs. Emphysema is caused by damage to air sacs and collapse of the bronchioles, causing shortness of breath.

Clinical Query

I have COPD and I keep losing weight. My doctor says it's because the effort it takes just to breathe is burning up a lot of calories. What can I do?

Some COPD patients need as much as ten times more calories than normal. In fact, more than 30 percent of people with COPD suffer from malnutrition, and that increases their risk of infection. You may want to consult a registered dietitian to discuss whether you would benefit from nutritional supplements (pp.532–41). You definitely need to eat a healthy diet, with plenty of fruits, vegetables and fibre. Be sure to drink six to eight glasses of fluids a day to stay hydrated and help thin mucus secretions. Avoid caffeine and alcohol, because they can dehydrate you.

may need supplemental oxygen therapy. Oxygen should never be used while smoking because of the risk of fire.

• PHYSICAL THERAPY Percussing or clapping the front and back of the lung area is used to help patients with cystic fibrosis (p.218) and other lung disorders cough up phlegm trapped deep within the lungs. This may also help some patients with COPD.

• SURGERY Damaged portions of the lungs may be removed in lung volume reduction surgery, so that the remaining lung can expand normally. However, this procedure will not help all patients and may, in fact, worsen the condition for some. Another option when COPD becomes severe, also appropriate only for certain patients, is lung transplantation.

• PULMONARY REHABILITATION These programmes are multi-faceted and will help educate patients about their condition. They usually provide exercise training,

instruction on breathing techniques, and psychosocial support with others who have the same condition. The most crucial component of such programmes, according to research, is exercise training. The programmes do relieve shortness of breath and fatigue, and also improve the patient's control over the disease.

• YOGA This practice (pp.476–9) may help relieve some of the shortness of breath associated with COPD.

• ACUPRESSURE This complementary therapy (p.472), which is designed to help patients relax, has also been found to relieve shortness of breath.

• AAT REPLACEMENT THERAPY People with the type of emphysema caused by the deficiency of the alpha1-antitrypsin (AAT) protein will need life-long AAT replacement therapy.

See also: *Smoking Cessation, pp.216–17* • *Cystic Fibrosis, p.218* • *Acupressure, p.472*

Pneumonia

There are more than 50 kinds of pneumonia. Some are very mild, but pneumonia is also a leading cause of death around the world, especially for the very old, very young and those who are already quite sick. It is not uncommon to develop reactive airways and have symptoms typical of asthma for a period of time after the infection is cured.

CAUSES

There are many causes of pneumonia: bacteria, viruses, mycoplasma (tiny organisms similar to bacteria) and even inhaled substances such as foods and moulds. Bacterial pneumonia is the most common type among adults and is often the most serious. Viruses cause about half of pneumonia cases in all age groups, and the majority of pneumonia cases in young children under school age. Viral cases are usually milder. Mycoplasma is responsible for about 20 percent of all pneumonia cases but, again, is usually mild. Pneumonia can also be caused by inhaling food, liquid, gases, dust or fungal spores. It may also follow influenza or a common cold.

Pneumonia is sometimes classified by where or how it was acquired. Hospital-acquired (nosocomial) pneumonia is just that – acquired in a hospital or similar environment, such as a nursing home. Patients in intensive care units, on mechanical ventilators, or with compromised immune systems are especially vulnerable, and this type of pneumonia can be dangerous for the elderly, young children and patients with COPD (pp.200–1) or HIV/AIDS (pp.316–17). Community-acquired pneumonia is spread through school, work or other places in the community. Aspiration pneumonia refers to the type caused by foreign matter that is aspirated, or inhaled, into the lungs, often after vomiting. Pneumonia caused by opportunistic organisms is dangerous for those with compromised immune systems, such as AIDS patients, and those on chemotherapy or corticosteroids.

Pneumonia can potentially

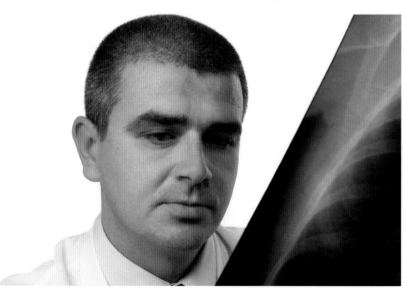

Pneumonia is an inflammation of the lungs that is usually caused by a virus or bacteria. A doctor may order a chest X-ray to verify a diagnosis of pneumonia after listening to the lungs with a stethoscope.

be fatal within 24 hours for the elderly, and people with chronic heart and lung disease. It can cause a number of complications. Bacteraemia occurs when the infection spreads from the lungs into the bloodstream and then travels to other organs in the body. The pleura, or lining around the lungs and inside the chest wall, may become filled with fluid – a condition called pleural effusion. An abscess, or pus, may form in the area of the lung with pneumonia. It may be treated with antibiotics or with surgery.

PREVENTION

The pneumococcal pneumonia vaccine will prevent most cases caused by *Streptococcus pneumoniae*. Anyone over age 65 or in a high-risk group should be vaccinated. The flu vaccine, which must be administered each year, will help prevent influenza, which can lead to pneumonia in vulnerable populations. The Hib vaccine for children protects again pneumonia caused by *Haemophilus influenzae* type b.

Avoiding smoking – and smokers – will help the lungs fight off infections. Frequent hand-washing also decreases exposure to germs that can cause disease. A healthy diet and adequate rest can help the immune system fight off infection. Wearing a mask when cleaning any areas that are dusty or mouldy can prevent pneumonia that results from inhaling these substances.

Patients who are hospitalized after surgery, especially abdominal surgery or an injury, are at higher risk of pneumonia because

coughing and deep breathing are painful. They will benefit from respiratory therapy, which helps clear secretions.

DIAGNOSIS

The symptoms of pneumonia can vary according to the type. With bacterial pneumonia, the individual may experience chills, high temperature, sweating, chest pain, and a productive cough with thick greenish or yellow phlegm, although the elderly and chronically ill may have milder symptoms and even a lower-than-normal temperature. Viral pneumonia is typically characterized by a dry cough, headache, temperature, muscle pain and fatigue, and eventually shortness of breath. The cough may produce small amounts of white phlegm. The pneumonia caused by mycoplasma may result in symptoms similar to either bacterial or viral pneumonia, but they are usually milder and more like a case of the flu.

A doctor can hear abnormal breathing sounds such as rales (bubbling or crackling noises) and rhonchi (rumblings) when listening to the lungs with a stethoscope. A chest X-ray often shows the areas in the lungs affected by pneumonia; in some cases, a CT scan is needed. Bloodwork can reveal if white blood cell counts are elevated, which may indicate a bacterial infection. Tests will be done to ensure there is enough oxygen in the blood. Cultures of sputum or blood may be taken to diagnose the organism causing the disease; bronchoscopy may be used to collect a specimen.

TREATMENTS

The various treatments for pneumonia depend on what is causing the inflammation. The success of these treatments depends on the age and health of the patient.

• **MEDICATION** Antibiotics are effective only in treating pneumonia caused by bacteria or mycoplasma infections. Many cases can be treated at home with an oral antibiotic, but sometimes hospitalization and intravenous antibiotics, along with supplemental oxygen, are needed. New antibiotic-resistant strains of pneumonia are developing, which are more difficult to treat because they reduce the effectiveness of current antibiotics.

Serious cases of viral pneumonia may be treated with antiviral drugs. Most patients with viral pneumonia, however, will recover in one to three weeks, even without medication.

• **SELF-TREATMENT** Drinking plenty of fluids helps loosen phlegm. Getting enough rest helps the body fight infection. Paracetomol or aspirin can lower temp-erature, although aspirin should not be given to children.

See also: *Chronic Obstructive Pulmonary Disease, pp.200–01* • *HIV/AIDS, pp.316–17* • *Smoking Cessation, pp.216–17*

CAUTION

If you feel worse after the cold or the flu, or you have symptoms such as a fever of 39°C (102°F) or higher, along with a cough, shortness of breath, chest pain, chills, and sweats, see your doctor.

Pleurisy

The double layer of thin membranes that line the chest wall and surround the lungs is called the pleura. When these membranes become inflamed, the condition is known as pleurisy. It is characterized by sharp pain in the chest, which is often made worse by deep breathing.

CAUSES

Normally, the two layers of pleura are smooth and rub against one another with little friction. But various diseases and conditions can irritate the pleura, resulting in inflammation. It then becomes painful for the pleura to move when breathing. The causes of this irritation include respiratory infections such as pneumonia (pp.202–3) and tuberculosis (p.212), viral infections such as influenza, autoimmune diseases such as systemic lupus erythematosus (pp.324–5) and rheumatoid arthritis (pp.136–9), injury to the chest, cancers (pp.412–15), exposure to asbestos, and pulmonary embolism (pp.210–11).

PREVENTION

Some cases can be prevented by getting prompt treatment for respiratory infections. It may also be helpful to get regular immunizations against influenza and pneumonia. Adopting healthy habits, such as frequent hand-washing, can help prevent infections.

DIAGNOSIS

If your chest hurts when you breathe or the pain gets worse from taking deep breaths or coughing, see a doctor. The pain may also extend to the shoulder. Other symptoms may include a temperature, chills, shortness of breath, a dry cough and general malaise. If the condition is severe, cyanosis (bluish skin colour) may result from lack of oxygen.

Sometimes the chest pain disappears even though the condition has got worse. This occurs when a large amount of fluid, called pleural effusion, accumulates between the pleura. The fluid cushions the pleura and relieves the pain, but it can lead to collapsed lungs and additional infection.

Pleurisy is easily diagnosed because the distinctive sound made by the pleura rubbing together can be heard with a stethoscope. Identifying the underlying cause may require X-rays, CT scans, ultra-sounds, blood tests, thoracentesis (in which fluid is withdrawn with a needle from the pleural lining), and pleural biopsy (in which a small sample of tissue is collected from the pleura with a needle to determine the specific cause of the condition).

TREATMENTS

Treatment for pleurisy depends on the specific cause.

- **MEDICATION** Antibiotics may be prescribed to treat pleurisy caused by a bacterial infection. Viral infections do not respond to antibiotics, although some drugs are used for influenza type A. Nonsteroidal anti-inflammatory (NSAID) drugs may control pain. Corticosteroids can be used when pleurisy results from an autoimmune disease.
- **BREATHING TECHNIQUES** Deep breathing and even coughing will help prevent complications such as lung collapse and pneumonia. Holding a pillow against the painful area of the chest may make it hurt less to cough. Another option is to wrap the chest with a wide, nonadhesive bandage, as long as it does not inhibit the expansion of the chest while breathing.
- **THORACENTESIS** This procedure is used to remove fluid, which is checked for infection. A large amount of fluid may be drained through a chest tube over several days in hospital.

See also: *Pneumonia, pp.202–3 • Tuberculosis, p.212 • Lupus, pp.324–5*

WHO IS AT RISK?

The risk factors include:

- Respiratory infection
- Autoimmune disease
- Exposure to dangerous inhalants, such as asbestos
- Lung cancer

Respiratory Syncytial Virus

This common and highly contagious virus infects the lungs and lower respiratory tract. Respiratory syncytial virus (RSV) occurs seasonally, peaking in the winter months. Most children have had a bout by the age of three, and most will have only minor cold-like symptoms. But in some infants and children, the illness needs hospitalization and can be fatal.

CAUSES
RSV spreads via coughs or sneezes. It enters the body through the nose, eyes or mouth. It can survive for half an hour on the hands, and up to several hours or longer on used tissues and surfaces such as work surfaces, playpens and toys, making it highly contagious.

PREVENTION
Washing hands before holding or touching a child will help prevent the spread of RSV. Drinking glasses should not be shared. Work surfaces, toys and other areas should be kept clean. Anyone with

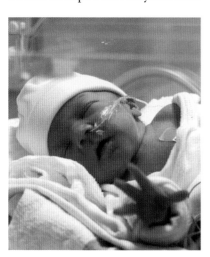

RSV is usually a mild condition, but hospitalization may be needed for some high-risk children if the condition worsens.

a cold or high temperature should avoid close contact with an infant. Even kisses can spread the virus.

Keep infants and young children away from crowds during outbreaks of RSV, which are most common from late autumn to spring. Smoking should not be allowed around infants and children, because it increases their susceptibility to all respiratory infections.

Monthly injections of palivizumab, an expensive medication with antibodies against RSV, can be given to children at high risk of life-threatening complications.

DIAGNOSIS
Anyone with cold symptoms may be infected with RSV. Seek medical treatment for symptoms such as difficult or rapid breathing, wheezing, bluish or greyish skin colour, a worsening cough, or high temperature. Infants at high risk of RSV who have cold symptoms should see a doctor.

Nasal secretions can be tested for RSV. Chest X-rays can reveal complications such as pneumonia (pp.202–3) and bronchiolitis (inflammation of the small airways in the lungs).

WHO IS AT RISK?
The risk factors include:
- Premature infants
- Children and infants with chronic heart and lung disease
- Children with compromised immune systems
- Children exposed to second-hand smoke
- Adults with congestive heart failure or COPD
- Age 75 and over

TREATMENTS
Plenty of fluids, acetaminophen, extra rest and sitting up will all help. Over-the-counter saline drops are safe, and mucus can be suctioned with a bulb syringe. Aspirin should not be given to a child if influenza is present, because of the risk of Reye's syndrome, a potentially fatal illness.

• MEDICATION Because RSV is a virus, antibiotics are prescribed only for secondary bacterial infection. Bronchodilators may help open airways. Antiviral medication such as ribavirin is given in high-risk cases, but its effectiveness is controversial.

• HOSPITALIZATION In some cases, hospitalization may be required to provide oxygen, humidified air, intravenous fluids and, rarely, a ventilator or breathing machine.

See also: *Pneumonia, pp. 202–3 • Smoking Cessation, pp.216–17 • Congestive Heart Failure, pp.234–5*

Asthma

Wheezing, shortness of breath, chest tightness and episodes of night-time or early morning coughing are all signs of asthma, the most common chronic disease in children. Asthma affects many adults as well. It cannot be cured, although some children do seem to 'grow out of it'. Asthma can be fatal – more than 180,000 people die from asthma worldwide each year – but it can be managed so that it does not interfere with work, school or physical activities.

CAUSES

The airways in the lungs resemble a tree, and are sometimes even referred to as the bronchial tree. As they branch out, they get smaller. In a person with asthma, the linings of these airways are inflamed or swollen, making them extra sensitive to substances such as dust mites or animal hairs that normally do not cause problems. When exposure to one of these triggers occurs, an asthma attack results, and it becomes difficult for air to move through the airways. The muscles around them go into spasms and tighten. Inflammation of the lining of the airways worsens and the airways narrow. Mucus is produced and further clogs the already swollen airways.

These attacks may occur only occasionally or several times a day, depending on the severity of the disease. They may last from minutes to days. For some, asthma is an occasional inconvenience; for others, it can be deadly.

Unlike COPD (pp.200–1), airflow restriction in asthma is temporary during an attack. It can be reversed and return to normal. If left untreated, however, severe asthma can lead to a permanent narrowing of the airways.

What causes asthma to develop in the first place is still a mystery, but what can trigger an asthma attack makes for a long list. For many, it is inhaled allergens such as dust mites, pet hairs, cockroach allergens, pollens and moulds (both indoor and outdoor variet-ies). Exercise is a common trigger, but the asthma can be easily con-trolled by treatment with inhalers before starting an activity.

Other triggers include respiratory infections such as a cold, cold air, tobacco smoke, air pollution, scented products, sulfites in wine and dried fruits, stress, aspirin and non-steroidal anti-inflammatory medications (NSAIDS), fumes from burning wood or gas, and food or drug allergies.

Gastro-oesophageal reflux disease (GORD, pp.264–5) some-times accompanies asthma, but whether the reflux triggers an attack or having asthma encourages the presence of GORD is not known, and may vary from case to case.

Occupational asthma results from exposure to various substances in the workplace, such as wood dust, grain dust, animal hairs, fungi and chemicals.

PREVENTION

Asthma as a condition cannot be prevented, but the attacks often can. The first step is identifying what sets off an attack and then eliminating the trigger. Some-times that can involve difficult decisions, such as when the family pet is the culprit.

No one with asthma should smoke, and no one should smoke around an asthmatic person. That

CAUTION

A severe asthma attack can be fatal. Seek emergency treatment right away if the person having the attack has these symptoms:
- Blue skin colour
- Extreme difficulty breathing
- Confusion and lethargy
- Loss of consciousness
- Rapid pulse rate

means no smoking in the house or the family car. Even smoking elsewhere can bring in smoke on clothes and in hair.

To eliminate other triggers, put mattresses and pillowcases in allergy-proof casings to protect against dust mite exposure. Reduce clutter and keep stuffed animals out of bedrooms. Do not use pillows, duvets or comforters that contain down or feathers. Do not use scented detergents, fabric softeners or cleaning products in the home. Repair water leaks promptly and keep humidity indoors low (between 35 and 50 percent) to discourage the growth of mould. If pets are a trigger, keep them out of the bedroom of anyone with asthma and outside the house as much as possible. Bathe pets weekly and vacuum frequently. Keep the kitchen clean and remove crumbs of food to prevent cockroach infestation. Use roach traps or gel poisons, if necessary, to get rid of the pests.

Long-acting medication such as inhaled steroids are actually prescribed to prevent, rather than to treat, asthma attacks, and should be taken regularly, even if no symptoms are present.

Immunotherapy, a series of injections to reduce the allergic reaction to certain substances, may also decrease asthma attacks triggered by those allergens, and could potentially reduce the need for medication.

DIAGNOSIS

Although wheezing – a whistling or squeaky sound during breathing – is one of the classic signs of asthma, not everyone wheezes during an attack. For some, the major symptom is a dry, persistent cough that is often worse at night or early in the morning, and interferes with sleep. That night-time cough may be the only symptom for some, especially children. Others may also experience chest tightness, shortness of breath, fast or noisy breathing, or the feeling that it is impossible to get enough air.

A doctor will listen to the lungs with a stethoscope but may not hear any abnormal sounds unless an asthma attack is occurring. That is why a test using a spirometer is usually done to diagnose asthma. The patient simply takes deep breaths and blows out hard and fast into a mouthpiece connected to a spirometer. This device measures three important values in diagnosing asthma: vital capacity, the largest amount of air that can be inhaled and exhaled; peak expiratory flow rate or peak flow rate, the fastest speed at which air can be blown out of the lungs; and forced expiratory volume, the largest amount of air that can be exhaled in one second. People who have asthma cannot blow out as much air or as quickly. After the test, the patient is given a short-acting bronchodilator to open up the airways, and then will repeat the test to see if taking the medication improves the results. If it does, asthma is the likely diagnosis.

If someone has asthma symptoms but the spirometry readings are normal, a bronchial challenge

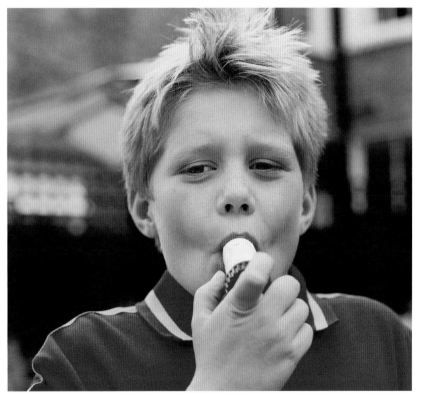

For people with mild or occasional asthma symptoms, an inhaler may be the only treatment needed. For chronic asthma, however, inhalers offer quick relief, but they should not be used as a substitute for the long-term medication that keeps the condition under control.

test may be done. A substance that narrows the airways is given before the spirometry.

Some people, especially children younger than five, simply cannot use a spirometer. A trial of asthma medication may be tried to see if it improves symptoms.

To rule out other lung conditions with similar symptoms, additional tests may be done, including chest and sinus X-rays, a complete blood count, CT scans, GORD assessment and a sputum examination. Arterial blood gases can be checked to ensure there is adequate oxygen in the blood.

Allergy tests can identify what substances cause allergies.

TREATMENTS

Asthma cannot be cured, but it can be managed so that the number and severity of attacks is lessened. Medication for asthma uses a two-pronged approach. There are long-acting medications that reduce inflammation and open airways. These must

healing hope I've had asthma since childhood, but it's got worse. My doctor blamed it on all the stress at my job. It seemed like I was pulling out my albuterol inhaler all the time. Then I took a yoga class, thinking it might help me relax. Well, it's helping my asthma. I'm still taking my medication – a steroid inhaler and a long-term bronchodilator. But I'm using the albuterol much less often for attacks.   *Marcel B.*

be taken regularly, even if no symptoms are present. Then there are short-acting bronchodilators that are used when an asthma attack begins. Many of these are dispensed by an inhaler, so that the medicine is breathed directly into the lungs. A machine called a nebulizer is available for people who cannot use an inhaler; it delivers the medicine in a fine mist.

It is also important to develop an overall plan for treating asthma and to establish what to do in case of an asthma attack, especially with children.

• SHORT-ACTING MEDICATION Bronchodilators, known as beta-2 agonists, are quick-relief medications taken during an asthma

attack. Bronchodilators open the airways, and these drugs work quickly but for only a short time. Inhalers such as albuterol fall into this class. For people with mild, occasional symptoms, a short-acting bronchodilator may be the only treatment needed.

• LONG-ACTING MEDICATION This medication must be taken regularly to prevent attacks, and it works by either reducing inflammation in the airways or acting as a bronchodilator to open the airways. But it cannot treat an attack in progress. Inhaled corticosteroids reduce inflammation and have fewer side-effects when taken in an inhaler. That way the medication goes straight to the lungs, where it can work. Long-acting beta-2 agonists are bronchodilators, and are sometimes combined with inhaled corticosteroids. The long-acting forms are useful to prevent symptoms during the night. Other long-acting medicines include leukotriene modifiers, such as montelukast and zafirlukast, which are taken in pill form. They work by reducing the impact of leukotrienes – substances that cause inflammation in the airways. They may be used alone or with inhaled steroids, but the safety of montelukast beyond six

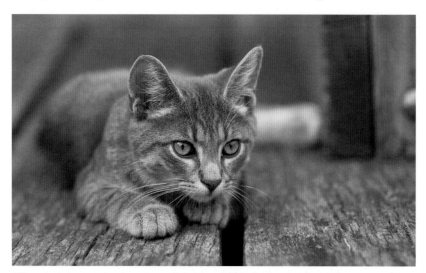

Although the cause of asthma is not yet well understood, many of the common triggers, such as pet hair, are well-known. Keeping pets bathed, brushed and away from bedding can help minimize the risk of inhaling pet hair and triggering an attack.

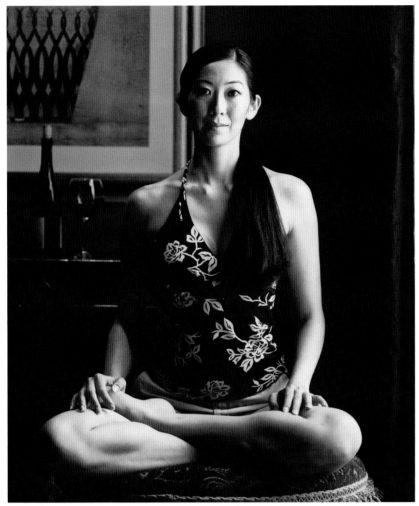

Yoga can be a useful treatment for helping control asthma. By practising breathing exercises and relaxation techniques, patients can learn to better control and reduce stress, which is a common asthma trigger.

peak flow may warn of an impending attack before symptoms appear.

• **YOGA** Taking a yoga (pp.476–9) class at least once a week is a useful secondary treatment for asthma, because it teaches breathing exercises and relaxation techniques, improving lung function and reducing levels of stress hormones in the body.

• **HERBAL THERAPY** Boswellia (*Boswellia serrata*), an Ayurvedic (pp.451–4) herb, taken in 300 to 400 mg doses three times a day, has been used to treat asthma.

• **SUPPLEMENTS** Up to of 100 mcg a day (only 10 to 50 mcg a day for children, depending on age) of supplemental selenium, a trace mineral found in soil, water and some foods, may be helpful in cases of chronic asthma. Omega-3 fatty acids (pp.252–3) also reduce occurrence of exercise-induced asthma in children. Omega-3 fatty acids are also proven leukotriene modifiers that can help decrease inflammation in the airways.

See also: *Chronic Obstructive Pulmonary Disease, pp.200–1 • Gastroesphogeal Reflux Disease, pp.264–5 • Ayurveda, pp.451–4*

On Call

Sometimes exercise triggers an asthma attack, but because physical activity is so important to good health, it is crucial to find ways to prevent symptoms during exercise. A doctor can work out a plan that may include using a short-term bronchodilator before activity. Remember to pace activity and to stop before symptoms of an attack become severe.

months of use has not been studied. Cromolyn and nedocromil, generally used for mild but persistent asthma, are another type of long-acting medication.

• **ORAL AND INTRAVENOUS CORTICOSTEROIDS** Drugs such as prednisone may be prescribed for use over a short duration to get asthma under control, or longer periods for severe cases of the disorder. However, long-term side-effects of the drug can include cataracts, thinning of bones, muscle weakness, decreased resistance to infections, high blood pressure, thinning of the skin, and inhibition of growth.

• **PEAK-FLOW METER** This simple device can be used at home to measure daily air flow rates, which are compared against the peak rate of airflow when asthma is under control. A deep breath is taken and then blown out as hard as possible into the plastic mouthpiece of the meter. Peak flow is usually measured every morning. By keeping track of the flow number every day, the person with asthma can record how well the disease is being controlled. In addition, changes in

Pulmonary Embolism

The platelets in blood enable it to clot in response to an injury. But sometimes the platelets clump together with red blood cells and fibrin, a protein, to form a blood clot (called a thrombus) even when there has been no injury. If this thrombus breaks off and travels through the heart to an artery in the lung, eventually blocking that artery, it becomes a pulmonary embolism.

Anyone experiencing a sudden shortness of breath, chest pain and a cough with bloody sputum should get immediate medical attention, because about 10 percent of these cases can prove fatal within an hour.

CAUSES

Blood clots can form in any vein in the body, but 90 percent of the ones that lead to trouble are located in the deep veins of the legs or pelvis, a condition known as deep vein thrombosis (DVT). However, some cases of pulmonary embolism may originate in the veins of the arm, the right side of the heart, or at the tip of a catheter placed in a vein.

When a clot ends up in the lungs, it may lodge in an artery and damage the heart, which can cause pulmonary hypertension (too much pressure in the blood vessels supplying the lungs), or even result in death.

It is believed that around half the people who develop pulmonary embolism have an inherited tendency to form blood clots. Clots are more likely to form during extended periods of inactivity or bed rest. Even some people who must remain still for a long trip in a car, train or plane are at higher risk because the blood flow is restricted under such circumstances. Surgery or trauma can injure a vein, making a clot more likely as well.

In rare cases, it is not a blood clot that causes the pulmonary embolism, but an air bubble, a clump of fat, or piece of a tumour or other tissue that has broken loose and entered the bloodstream.

PREVENTION

Avoiding prolonged periods of bed rest or inactivity is crucial to preventing thromboses; that is why patients are encouraged to walk soon after surgery or during any extended illness. Pulmonary embolism is the third leading cause of death among hospital patients. Compression stockings (tight garments worn on the legs) may help promote circulation. A pneumatic compression device massages the veins in the leg and helps surgical patients, especially after a hip replacement.

WHO IS AT RISK?

The risk factors include:

- Family history of blood clots
- Over 60
- Long period of inactivity or bed rest
- Overweight or obese
- Sitting for extended periods, for example on a plane or car trip
- Pregnancy, childbirth, and six weeks post-natal
- Birth control or hormone replacement pills
- Some cancer treatments, such as tamoxifen or raloxifene for breast cancer in menopausal women
- High blood pressure
- Varicose veins
- Smoking

Low doses of anticoagulants or blood thinners such as heparin or warfarin provide protection for high-risk patients.

Losing weight may help prevent both DVT and pulmonary embolism. A 2005 study done at St. Joseph Mercy Oakland Hospital in Pontiac, Michigan, of more than 700 million hospital records across the United States found that obesity (pp.348–9) was a risk factor, especially for people under 40.

When travelling by car or plane, be sure to take a break and walk every hour or two. Quitting smoking can also reduce the chance of developing blood clots.

DIAGNOSIS

A doctor will start by reviewing a patient's medical history and symptoms. Chest X-rays can rule out conditions with similar symptoms. An electrocardiogram or ECG measures the pulse and the electrical activity of the heart. A special blood test can reveal the amount of D-dimer in the body. D-dimer is a by-product of clot formation that may be elevated if blood clots are present. Blood tests can also reveal some inherited disorders that cause clotting and measure the amount of oxygen and carbon dioxide in the blood. A test called a ventilation/perfusion scan uses inhaled and injected radioactive substances to track and measure the air and blood flow in the lungs. However, a more sensitive and faster test is a spiral (or helical) CT scan, which can generate three-dimensional images of the pulmonary arteries in fewer than 20 seconds.

Other tests are used to check for DVT. A blood clot in the deep veins of the leg may cause redness, swelling or tenderness. Duplex venous ultrasonography uses sound waves to measure blood flow in the veins and identify clots. Less popular is venography, which uses injected contrast dye and a catheter to look for DVT. An MRI, because of high expense, is usually reserved only for pregnant women and others who cannot have contrast dyes.

TREATMENTS

Treatment depends on the severity of the pulmonary embolism.

• **THROMBOLYTIC THERAPY** 'Clot-busting' drugs such as strepto-kinase or tissue plasminogen activator (TPA) are used to break up and dissolve blood clots, and are given to people who are at high risk of death or serious complications from clots. These drugs cannot be administered to anyone who has had surgery in

the previous two weeks or has suffered a recent stroke, is pregnant or has any bleeding disorder.

• **MEDICATION** Anticoagulants, or blood-thinners, may be given over a period of several months. Heparin can be injected under the skin at home without close monitoring of how thinned the blood has become.

• **PREVENTATIVE DEVICES** Pneumatic compression and compression stockings can improve blood flow and help keep new clots from forming. These stockings can also help prevent some of the complications once a blood clot in the legs is diagnosed.

• **ACTIVITY** Avoiding long periods of bed rest and inactivity is key to good circulation and the prevention of future clots.

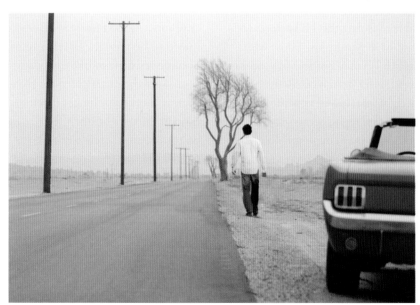

A pulmonary embolism can occur when a blood clot foms after long periods of inactivity. When travelling by car or plane, be sure to take a break to stretch or walk around every hour or two to keep blood from pooling in the deep veins of the legs.

See also: *Obesity, pp. 348–9 • Venous Disorders, pp.240–2 • High Blood Pressure, pp.236–9*

Tuberculosis

Each year nearly two million people around the world die of tuberculosis (TB). About ten million new cases are diagnosed annually, and more strains of TB are becoming resistant to the drugs used for treatment. Up to one-third of the world's population may be infected with the bacterium that causes TB, although most will never develop the active stage of the disease.

CAUSES

Tuberculosis is caused by a specific airborne bacterium (*Mycobacterium tuberculosis*) that generally infects the lungs; it can take several exposures over time for infection to occur. When someone with active TB coughs, sneezes or speaks, the bacteria are released into the air, where they can survive for hours. Other people will inhale these bacteria, but for most, their immune system will protect them. Some will become infected, but only 10 percent or fewer will develop the active stage of the disease, perhaps years later when their immune system weakens due to age, illness or other conditions. They are not contagious until that happens. Some, such as AIDS patients, will develop the disease sooner because their immune system cannot fight the disease.

PREVENTION

Adequate ventilation and the use of ultraviolet light to kill airborne bacteria may help prevent the spread of the TB in crowded places such as hospitals and clinics. Drugs such as isoniazid can prevent the disease from becoming active in those with TB infection. A vaccine called BCG is used for high-risk populations in underdeveloped areas, but its use and effectiveness remain controversial.

Anyone diagnosed with TB should remain in isolation for the first week or two of treatment, until coughing stops and the danger of contagion is greatly reduced.

DIAGNOSIS

Anyone exposed to TB should seek immediate medical treatment. People whose immune system is able to isolate the TB bacteria will not have symptoms. Those with active TB may not feel sick, or they may suffer from a persistent cough, weight loss, loss of appetite, temperatures, night sweats, tiredness and they may cough up blood.

A skin test can show whether the infection is present in the body. However, chest X-rays, and cultures and microscopic examination of sputum are still needed to confirm that the disease is active.

TREATMENTS

Today, antibiotics can effectively treat most cases of TB. Multi-drug

WHO IS AT RISK?

The risk factors include:

- HIV/AIDS
- Impaired immune system
- Elderly and very young
- IV drug use
- Poverty and homelessness
- Residents of long-term care facilities
- Healthcare workers and prison guards
- Malnutrition

resistant TB is harder to treat because the bacteria cannot be killed by several of the drugs usually prescribed. This type of TB is dangerous and can spread easily. It is most commonly seen in strains in Asia and Africa.

- **MEDICATION** A combination of antibiotics is used to treat TB infection because the bacteria may become resistant to one medication. Antibiotics are given for six to nine months or longer. Even though the patient often feels better after just a few weeks, it is crucial that treatment continues in order to completely eradicate the disease. Directly observed therapy, in which a healthcare worker supervises the taking of the drugs, can shorten the duration of treatment by ensuring that treatment is being maintained.

See also: *HIV/AIDS pp.316–17* • *Fever, p.318*

Bronchiectasis

An infection or injury can damage the walls of the airways in the lungs. Mucus accumulates and thickens until the lungs have difficulty clearing it. The airways get stretched out and scarred. More mucus is collected, and the vicious cycle known as bronchiectasis begins.

CAUSES

Cystic fibrosis (p.218) is a major culprit, as are pneumonia (pp.202–3), tuberculosis (p.212), fungal infections, immunodeficiency disorders such as AIDS (316–17), conditions that affect the cilia, or a tumour. Even an injury such as inhaling food or a foreign object can later show up as bronchiectasis, as it can take years for the condition to appear. In some cases, individuals are born with the condition.

PREVENTION

Prompt treatment of lung infections is the first line of defense. Immunizations against measles,

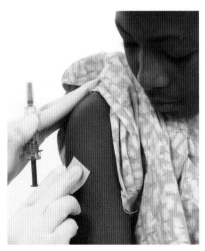

Immunizations can help prevent lung infections that can develop into bronchiectasis, a disease caused by scarring of the lungs.

influenza, pneumonia, whooping cough, and other infections may help. Preventing the accidental inhalation of small objects may prevent bronchiectasis from developing. Smoking and being around smokers should be avoided.

DIAGNOSIS

Symptoms are often similar to those of other lung disorders, including a chronic cough that worsens when lying on the side, and which may produce blood or foul-smelling phlegm. Shortness of breath, chest pain or pleurisy, wheezing, bluish skin, weight loss, fatigue, pallor and bad breath may also be present.

No specific test exists for bronchiectasis, so a doctor must rule out other disorders. Chest X-rays can reveal scarring or infection of the airway walls. A CT scan can provide a more detailed look. Blood tests can show the presence of infection. A sputum culture analysed in a lab can identify bacteria, fungi or tuberculosis.

Pulmonary function tests measure how well the lungs work and how much damage has been done. Other tests such as a sweat test for cystic fibrosis or a skin test for tuberculosis will check for possible

underlying causes. In some cases, a fiberoptic bronchoscopy will be done, under local anaesthesia, using a bronchoscope to look at the airways and collect mucus samples.

TREATMENTS

Treatment depends on the underlying cause. The condition cannot be cured, but it can be managed.

• MEDICATION Antibiotics are given for respiratory infection. Bronchodilators, administered from an inhaler or a nebulizer, open airways. Corticosteroids can reduce inflammation. Mucus thinners and expectorants loosen mucus, but avoid cough suppressants because they prevent mucus from being expelled.

• PHYSICAL THERAPY A technique, called chest percussion, is also used to treat cystic fibrosis and helps to loosen mucus so it can be coughed up more easily. The hands or a special device called a mechanical percussor are used to pound on the chest and back.

See also: *HIV/AIDS, pp.316–7 • Pneumonia, pp.202–3 • Tuberculosis, p.212*

WHO IS AT RISK?

The risk factors include:

- Lung infections
- Cystic fibrosis
- Pneumonia
- Immunodeficiency disorders
- Inhaling food or foreign objects

Sleep Apnoea

The Greek word *apnoea* means 'without breath'. Sleep apnoea is a condition in which breathing stops repeatedly during sleep for at least ten seconds. These brief pauses may occur as often as 20 or 30 times an hour, and they interrupt normal sleep patterns and decreasing the amount of oxygen in the blood, causing the brain to send a wake-up signal so that breathing starts again.

Although loud snoring is frequently associated with sleep apnoea, not everyone who snores has apnoea, and not everyone with apnoea snores. Those who suffer from it may sound as if they are gasping for air or choking during their sleep, or they may snort when they resume breathing after a pause. They are often unaware of the problem, but they feel excessively sleepy during the day, even after 'a good night's sleep'. That is because rapid eye movement (REM) sleep, the restorative stage of sleep, has been disturbed by frequent awakenings.

If left untreated, moderate or severe sleep apnoea can lead to cardiovascular disease (pp.234–5), stroke (pp.168–9), high blood pressure (pp.236–9), complications with surgery and medications, and even increase the death rate from heart attack and stroke. People with sleep apnoea are anywhere from two to five times more likely to have road accidents.

The condition is twice as common in men as in women: 4 percent of middle-aged men and 2 percent of middle-aged women suffer from sleep apnoea, but some 80 percent of them may not realize that they do.

CAUSES

The most common cause of apnoea is airway obstruction, and this type is called obstructive sleep apnoea. Muscles in the back of the throat that support the soft palate, uvula, tonsils and tongue relax too much to keep the throat open. In other cases, airflow into the lungs is blocked by a naturally narrow airway, enlarged tonsils, nasal obstruction, or an abnormally shaped palate or tongue. Although 40 percent of people with sleep apnoea are not, being overweight or obese can also block the airway because of an increased amount of tissue around the neck and throat.

Much less common is central sleep apnoea, in which the brain fails to send signals to the muscles of the diaphragm to breathe, or the muscles do not receive the message. It may be caused by a stroke, brain tumour (pp.196–7),

spinal injury, or neuromuscular disorder such as ALS (p.190). In some cases, the apnoea is due to both a failure of signal being sent and received.

PREVENTION

Reducing the risk factors may help prevent sleep apnoea or even treat mild cases. Losing as little as 10 percent of body weight may reduce the severity of sleep apnoea by more than 50 percent.

Avoiding alcohol and sedatives such as sleeping pills, muscle relaxants, and some antihistamines before bedtime is crucial. Over-the-counter and herbal remedies may also have sedative side-effects which can encourage apnoea.

Sleeping on the side instead of the back also helps keep the airway open. To discourage rolling over onto the back, sew half a tennis ball into the back of a t-shirt or pyjama top near the neck and the other half in the mid-back area; or put a tennis ball in a tube sock and pin it to the back of nightwear.

Allergies and nasal congestion should be treated to keep airways clear, but use non-sedating anti-histamines and decongestants or nasal sprays to avoid over-relaxing the muscles of the neck and throat.

Cigarettes should be avoided; smoking makes the swelling in the upper airway worse.

DIAGNOSIS

Symptoms may include morning headaches, frequent night-time urination, difficulty concentrating, forgetfulness, poor judgement, irritability, changes in mood or behaviour, anxiety and depression. Children may have hyperactive behaviour and even be diagnosed with ADHD.

Nocturnal polysomnography, usually done overnight in a hospital or centre that specializes in sleep disorders, measures heart rate, breathing patterns and brain waves while the patient sleeps to diagnose apnoea conclusively and rule out other sleep disorders, such as insomnia (pp.170–2) and narcolepsy. An oximeter, which uses light to measures oxygen levels in the blood during sleep, can be used at home. Other tests may include an echocardiogram to examine heart function, thyroid tests, and X-rays or CT scans to look for blockages.

TREATMENTS

There is no cure for apnoea, but controlling symptoms can reduce the risk of the heart and blood pressure problems that can result from the condition. Treatment depends on the type of sleep apnoea and its severity, and may require a combination of therapies. To treat central sleep apnoea, it is necessary to treat the underlying cause.

• MEDICATION Drugs such as acetazolamide and theophylline may be prescribed to help stimulate breathing during sleep.

• CONTINUOUS POSITIVE AIRWAY PRESSURE (CPAP) This device uses air pressure to keep the airways open. A mask connected to an air hose is worn over the nose. The air pressure from an air blower keeps the airway open. It is the most common and most effective treatment, but some patients find it uncomfortable to use.

• DENTAL APPLIANCES Fitted by a dentist, these change the position of the jaw and tongue so that the airway stays open. This approach is not always as effective as using a CPAP device.

• SURGERY A uvulopalatopharyngoplasty, or UPPP, removes excess tissue at the back of the throat that may be blocking the airway. Laser-assisted uvulopalatoplasty (LAUP) uses a laser to trim the palate to help ease snoring (pp.62–3), but it has not yet been proven to help sleep apnoea. A tonsillectomy and adenoidectomy can remove enlarged tonsils and adenoids (lymphatic tissue at the back of the nose), and is 90 percent successful in treating children who suffer from sleep apnoea. Other procedures can remove a blockage in the nose or upper throat. If all other treatments have failed for severe apnoea, a tracheostomy makes an opening in the trachea so air can detour around the blocked airway.

See also: Cardiovascular Disease, pp.234–5 • High Blood Pressure, pp.236–9 • Snoring, pp.62–3

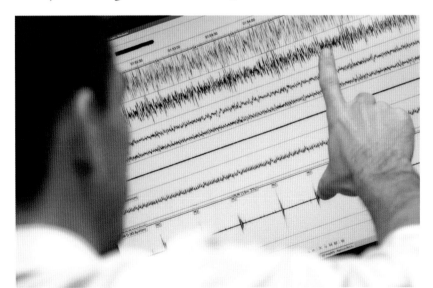

Polysomnography can be performed in a hospital or a centre that specializes in treating sleep disorders. Sleep apnoea can be diagnosed using polysomnography to measure such things as heart rate, breathing patterns and brain waves while a patient is sleeping.

SMOKING CESSATION

Kicking the smoking habit can save lives and money, and prevent health problems. But it is a tough habit to break. Nicotine, the drug in cigarettes, is physically addictive – just as addictive as cocaine and heroin and more so than alcohol. Withdrawal can cause cravings for tobacco, irritability, anxiety, poor concentration, restlessness, headache, drowsiness and stomach upset. In addition, smoking is often associated with emotional and social situations, so smoking also becomes an emotional habit.

REASONS TO QUIT

It is estimated that, on average, each cigarette smoked takes seven minutes off one's lifespan. Smoking is the leading preventable cause of death and is estimated to have killed some 100 million people worldwide in the last 100 years. It is responsible for almost 90 percent of lung cancer (pp.222–3) cases and is a risk factor for cancers of the oesophagus, larynx, kidney, pancreas and cervix. It increases the risk of heart disease, stroke and high blood pressure, and it is the major cause of COPD (pp.200–1). It worsens other lung conditions, such as asthma (pp.208–9). In pregnancy, smoking can cause premature delivery and low birth weight.

Today, smoking is becoming socially unacceptable. Many workplaces are smoke-free; restaurants and other public places are adopting smoke-free policies as well.

HOW TO QUIT

Despite the addictiveness of smoking, it is certainly not impossible to quit. Most people who stop smoking for three months are able to quit permanently.

Clinical Query

I'm so afraid I'll gain weight if I quit smoking. What can I do to avoid that?

A 2.25–4.5 kg (5–10 lb) weight gain carries far fewer health risks than continuing to smoke, but many people still do not want to risk putting on the additional weight. Quitting does not cause weight gain by itself, but many people snack constantly to deal with the irritability and loss of something to do with their hands and mouth.

Substitute exercise for smoking. Exercise will help prevent weight gain – and may even reduce your craving for a cigarette. If you must snack, choose vegetable sticks or other healthy foods.

- **CUT DOWN** Start reducing the daily number of cigarettes smoked.
- **QUIT DATE** Choose a date to quit and announce it to friends and family. Ask for their support.
- **CLEAN** Get rid of ash-trays, and anything that smells like smoke.
- **SMOKING TRIGGERS** Figure out the times that it is the most tempting to smoke. If possible, avoid the settings and the activities that trigger the urge for a cigarette.
- **NEW HABITS** Find different things to do as substitutes for smoking. Take a walk; smoking relieves stress, and exercise can too. Keep a supply of sugar-free hard sweets or sunflower seeds for oral gratification. Play with a paperclip or marble to keep restless hands occupied.

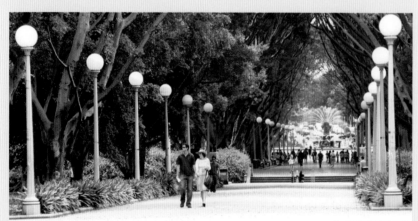

Choose new behaviours to substitute for smoking. Take a deep breath – of fresh air instead of nicotine – when the urge for a cigarette strikes. Take a walk; people often smoke because they are stressed and exercise can relieve stress.

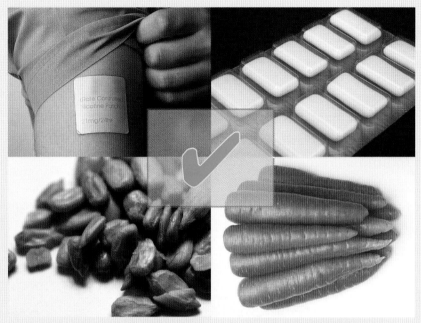

The nicotine patch or gum can help curb cravings by providing measured doses of nicotine while a smoker quits. Also, it can be helpful to have a supply of healthy snack foods available to satisfy oral gratification, such as celery, carrots or sunflower seeds.

Smoking cessation programmes are offered by hospitals, health departments, community centres, workplaces and other organizations. Such programmes help smokers deal with habit patterns, as well as social support from peers who are trying to make the same change.

• **ACUPUNCTURE** Studies have shown that acupuncture is effective in helping people to quit if they are strongly self-motivated. However, placebo, or fake, acupuncture, works almost as well.

• **HYPNOSIS** No studies have proven the effectiveness of hypnotherapy in smoking cessation, but it may benefit certain individuals.

Nicotine Replacement Therapy
Although 5 to 16 percent of people can quit smoking for at least six months without any type of medicine, one-quarter to one-third of smokers who use either nicotine replacement therapy or bupriopion can remain smoke-free for more than six months, and combining the two therapies may be more effective than either alone. Some prescription anti-depressants should not be used by anyone with a history of seizures or high blood pressure (pp.236–9). Nicotine replacement therapy is more effective when combined with a behavioural modification programme.

• **PATCH** The patch is often non-prescription and provides a steady dose of nicotine that is absorbed through the skin. It is available in varying strengths so that the dosage can be gradually decreased. Skin irritation can be a problem because of the adhesive tape.

• **GUM** Available without a prescription, chewing gum releases nicotine into the lining of the mouth. This product has the most flexibility in nicotine dosing and provides some of the oral gratification of smoking. It is not an option for people who cannot chew gum because of dental work, dentures or temporomandibular joint disorder (pp.84–5), and it can cause stomach upset, hiccups, throat irritation and flatulence.

• **NASAL SPRAY** Available by prescription only, this product may not be an option for people with nasal or sinus conditions such as allergies and asthma. Nasal spray is not recommended for young smokers.

• **INHALER** Also available only by prescription, the nicotine inhaler looks like a cigarette holder and releases nicotine into the mouth, not the lungs. It can cause throat and mouth irritation and coughing, and is not recommended for anyone with a bronchial problem.

AFTER QUITTING
A smoker's body begins to change soon after the last cigarette. Twenty minutes after quitting, blood pressure and pulse rate fall while the body temperature of the hands and feet increases. Eight hours later, oxygen and carbon monoxide levels in the blood are normal again. Just 24 hours later, the risk of a heart attack is reduced. And 48 hours later, nerve endings damaged by smoking will start to grow again, and the ability to smell and taste improves. One year later, the risk for coronary heart disease is half of that of a smoker's. Fifteen years after quitting, the risk of death for smoking-related conditions is almost the same as that for people who have never smoked.

See also: *Lung Cancer, pp.222–3 • Asthma, pp.206–9 • Chronic Obstructive Pulmonary Disease, pp.200–1*

Cystic Fibrosis

This inherited disease damages the lungs, pancreas and other organs. The defective gene that causes it is responsible for regulating the movement of sodium chloride (salt) in and out of cells. When this transport breaks down, thick, sticky secretions are produced in the lungs, digestive tract and reproductive system, and extra salt is released in the sweat. This change in the consistency of secretions can result in lung infections, respiratory failure, nutritional deficiencies and infertility. It may lead to diabetes (pp.338–41) and cirrhosis of the liver (pp.282–3).

CAUSES

Cystic fibrosis is a recessively inherited condition: both parents must carry the defective gene for a child to be born with the disease. Three to 10 percent of Caucasians are carriers, and many do not realize it.

PREVENTION

There is no way to prevent cystic fibrosis. A DNA test can sometimes reveal the presence of the defective gene. Prenatal tests can also be done to check for cystic fibrosis.

DIAGNOSIS

Early symptoms include no bowel movements in the first 24 to 48 hours of life, bulky and greasy stools, salty skin, frequent respiratory infections, coughing or wheezing, weight loss, failure to grow or delayed growth, diarrhoea and fatigue. Most children with cystic fibrosis are diagnosed by age 3.

The sweat chloride test is the standard for diagnosing cystic fibrosis. The salt content of a sample of sweat is measured, although it is sometimes difficult to collect enough sweat from an infant.

Other tests for the condition may include faecal fat test, upper GI and small bowel X-rays, and measuring pancreatic function.

TREATMENTS

Cystic fibrosis cannot be cured. Treatment is aimed at controlling symptoms and preventing life-threatening complications, such as pneumonia (pp.202–3), bronchitis (p.200), bronchiectasis (p.213), pneumothorax (p.219), bleeding from the lungs and nutritional deficiencies.

• **POSTURAL DRAINAGE AND CHEST PERCUSSION** These techniques are used to clear mucus from the lungs. Lying down with the head over the side of a bed lets gravity help dislodge mucus. Vigorous clapping on the back and chest also helps remove mucus. Families receive special instructions in how to perform these manoeuvres.

• **MEDICATION** Antibiotics can treat the frequent respiratory infections. Inhaled bronchodilators such as albuterol can open airways and mucus-thinning drugs can improve lung function. Pain relief from ibuprofen may slow lung deterioration.

• **SUPPLEMENTS** Pancreatic enzymes and vitamin supplements, especially A, D, E and K, can be given to aid digestion. Fish oil supplementation may also offer some benefits.

• **DIET** Because patients with cystic fibrosis do not absorb nutrients well, a high-calorie, nutritious diet is recommended. Drinking plenty of liquids can help thin mucus.

• **ACUPUNCTURE** This Traditional Chinese Medicine (pp.446–50) can decrease the amount of pain experienced by cystic fibrosis patients without causing any side effects or complications.

• **TRANSPLANT** Some patients with life-threatening complications or resistance to antibiotics may benefit from lung or combined heart–lung transplants.

See also: *Diabetes, pp.338–41* • *Pneumonia, pp.202–3* • *Pneumothorax, p.219*

WHO IS AT RISK?

The risk factors include:

- Caucasian, especially of northern and central European descent
- Family history

Pneumothorax

When air enters the pleura, the double layer of thin membranes that line the chest wall and surround the lungs, the condition is called a pneumothorax. It is a problem because one or both of the lungs may collapse as a result.

CAUSES

The cause of a pneumothorax depends on the type. It is believed that a rupture of a bleb or bulla, an air- or fluid-filled sac in the lung, is responsible for a spontaneous, or primary, pneumothorax – although the cause is sometimes unknown. This type is most common in tall, thin men under age 40. Family history and cigarette smoking may be factors in developing primary pneumothorax. It may occur while diving or travelling in a plane, when the air pressure changes.

Secondary spontaneous pneumothorax occurs as a complication of pulmonary diseases.

Traumatic pneumothorax is a condition caused by an injury to the chest or upper body, such as a gunshot or a blunt blow, as an injury sustained in a car accident. It is also one of the leading, though very rare, complications of acupuncture.

Any of these causes may lead to tension pneumothorax – the most dangerous type. This condition occurs when tissues around the pleura allow air to enter but not to exit, creating so much pressure that the lung collapses and the heart may not be able to pump effectively because the pressure prevents the veins from filling the heart with blood. Shock may occur, and the patient may die if they are not given immediate treatment.

PREVENTION

There are few ways to prevent a pneumothorax. The risk may be reduced by quitting smoking and keeping lung diseases such as asthma (pp.206–9) under control.

DIAGNOSIS

Pneumothorax may be suspected when an individual suffers from sudden, sharp chest pain that gets worse with deep breathing or coughing, along with symptoms such as shortness of breath, tightness in the chest, rapid heart rate, fatigue and bluish skin colour. Anxiety, stress and low blood pressure may also be present.

A doctor may listen to the chest with a stethoscope to identify the lack of breath sounds, which indicates a collapsed lung. Percussing, or tapping, the chest also produces abnormal sounds. Chest X-rays can show the extent of the damage, and blood tests can measure levels of oxygen and carbon dioxide.

WHO IS AT RISK?

The risk factors include:

Primary pneumothorax

- Male
- Tall and thin
- 20 to 40 years old
- Family history
- Smoking

Secondary pneumothorax

- Underlying chronic pulmonary disease, such as COPD

Traumatic pneumothorax

- Injury to the chest

TREATMENTS

Treatment depends on the size and type of pneumothorax. A small pneumothorax may result in mild shortness of breath and will resolve on its own after several days with no specific therapy other than watchful waiting. A larger pneumothorax may take several weeks for the air in the pleura to be absorbed. About half of patients with pneumothorax will have another one.

• SURGERY A chest tube, inserted through an incision in the chest wall and attached to a suction device, can remove air from the pleura, allowing the lung to expand. In some cases, surgery is required to repair an underlying cause and prevent relapse.

See also: *Asthma, pp.206–9 • Smoking Cessation, pp.216–17 • Acupuncture, pp.464–5*

Occupational Lung Disease

Years of inhaling asbestos fibres, coal dust, silica and the dusts from textiles such as cotton, flax, hemp or sisal – even moulds from bird droppings or hot baths – can damage the lungs, causing occupational lung disease. It can lead to respiratory failure, failure of the right side of the heart and pulmonary hypertension (excessive pressure in the lungs). Black lung, a disease affecting coal miners, is one of the most well-known of the conditions, but the most common form of the disease is occupational asthma.

CAUSES

Breathing various toxins over time will result in inflammation or swelling of the alveoli (air sacs), and the interstitium, their supporting structures in the lungs. Repeated inflammation results in scarring, making the lungs less flexible and the air sacs no longer efficient at transferring oxygen into the blood.

Occupational Asthma

The most common occupational lung disease, this type of asthma results from exposure to irritants in the workplace. It can also exacerbate existing cases of asthma.

Occupational Lung Cancer

The most frequent cancer resulting from occupational exposure is lung cancer, and some 10 percent of cancer of the lung, trachea and bronchus, is caused by toxins in the workplace. Worldwide, 20 to 30 percent of men and 5 to 20 percent of women of working age have been exposed to carcinogenic agents at work.

Asbestosis

Construction and industrial workers exposed to asbestos, once used for insulation, may develop asbestosis. It may progressively worsen and can be fatal.

Mesothelioma

Asbestos exposure also causes this rare and incurable cancer of the chest lining. The risk is particularly increased in individuals who are exposed and also smoke.

Byssinosis

Also called brown or cotton worker's lung, byssinosis results from inhaling dust from hemp, flax or cotton processing. Thousands of textile workers have been affected by this disease which involves obstruction of the small airways. It is common in developing countries, but less so in industrialized nations.

Coal Workers' Pneumoconiosis

More familiarly known as black lung disease, this condition is caused by inhaling coal dust, which eventually becomes embedded in the lungs and hardens the tissues. It affects almost 3 percent of all coal miners, and 0.2 percent have the most severe form of the disease.

Silicosis

This condition is caused by inhaling silica, a common and naturally occurring crystal. Workers in mines, foundries, blasting operations and stone, clay and glass manufacturing may be exposed. Silicosis increases the risk for developing active tuberculosis.

Hypersensitivity Pneumonitis

Fungus spores from mouldy hay, bird droppings, or other organic dusts cause this condition, which is the result of inflammation of the air sacs of the lungs that eventually leads to the development of fibrous scar tissue.

WHO IS AT RISK?

The risk factors include:
- Smoking
- Years of exposure

Professions at increased risk include:
- Coal miners
- Textile workers
- Sand-blasters
- Construction workers
- Foundry workers
- Quarry workers
- Glass manufacturer workers

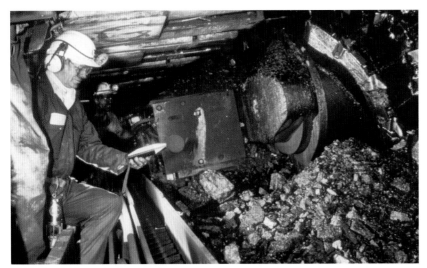

Occupational lung diseases are often caused by years of exposure to substances that can destroy delicate lung tissues. Inhaling toxins such as coal dust or asbestos can destroy air sacs and block airways in the lungs, causing permanent damage.

Popcorn Workers Lung Disease

Exposure to diacetyl, an ingredient released from the artificial butter flavouring used in microwave popcorn, has caused chronic coughs and shortness of breath, along with bronchitis and asthma.

World Trade Center Lung Disease

Workers exposed to a variety of material during and after the collapse of the World Trade Center developed a persistent cough and other respiratory systems. Cement dust may be at least partly responsible for injury to the airways.

PREVENTION

Wearing a mask, respirator or other protection can help reduce the amount of inhaled toxins. Annual chest X-rays of workers at risk can identify disease in its early stages. It may be necessary to change jobs.

Because smoking either increases the risk for many types of occupational lung disease or can worsen symptoms, it is important not to smoke.

DIAGNOSIS

Shortness of breath, either at rest or with exercise, and a chronic cough are the major symptoms of all types of occupational lung disease. In some cases, there may be chest pain, a tight feeling in the chest or wheezing. As occupational lung disease becomes more severe, any type of activity becomes difficult, if not impossible, to do.

A doctor will take a medical history to evaluate any exposure to toxins in the workplace or as a result of hobbies or other activities. For example, individuals may have been exposed to asbestos fibres on the clothes their spouses wore home from work.

Listening to the lungs with a stethoscope may reveal abnormal breathing sounds. Other tests that may be needed include chest X-ray, CT scan of the chest, pulmonary function tests, measurements of blood oxygen levels, bronchoscopy, and, rarely, surgical lung biopsy.

TREATMENTS

There is no cure for occupational lung disease, but the symptoms can be treated. First, however, exposure to the offending toxin must be stopped immediately to keep the disease from progressing.

• OXYGEN Supplemental oxygen may alleviate symptoms.

• CHEST PHYSICAL THERAPY Techniques such as postural drainage (where a specific body posture helps clear fluid from the lungs), chest percussion (tapping) and vibration can remove phlegm from the lungs.

• MEDICATION Cortiscosteroids may be prescribed for severe cases of lung disease, but they do have the potential to cause both uncomfortable and serious short and long-term side effects. Antibiotics for respiratory infections are given when needed. These drugs, taken either orally or by inhaler, can improve airflow.

• LUNG TRANSPLANT In some advanced and severe cases, the only option may be a lung transplant.

• SMOKING CESSATION Because smoking aggravates any kind of lung disease, it is crucial to stop (pp.216–17).

• EXERCISE Physical activity and breathing exercises may help. Many patient education programmes are available for patients with chronic lung disease.

• SUPPORT GROUPS It may be helpful to join a support group to share experiences with others and to learn more about treatments and lifestyle changes.

See also: *Asthma, pp.206–9* • *Smoking Cessation, pp.216–17*

Lung Cancer

When the lungs are exposed to a cancer-causing substance, abnormal cells may develop and eventually lead to a malignant, or cancerous, tumour. Lung cancer is the leading cause of death from cancer among both men and women, and the most common type of cancer in the world.

CAUSES

Smoking causes nearly 90 percent of cases of lung cancer in men and about 80 percent of such cases in women. Cigarette smoke contains more than 4,000 different substances, many of which are carcinogenic and damaging to the tissues in the lungs. The risk of lung cancer increases with the length of time an individual smokes, the number of cigarettes smoked in a day, the age the smoker started, and how deeply the smoker inhales.

The second leading cause of lung cancer in North America and many parts of Europe is radon, an invisible and odourless radioactive gas found in the soil beneath many homes.

Another major cause is exposure to cancer-causing, or carcinogenic substances in the workplace, such as asbestos, various kinds of industrial dust, radiation and arsenic. Workers who are around these substances and who also smoke greatly increase their risk.

Second-hand smoke can cause lung cancer, and air pollution also contributes to the risk. Tuberculosis can lead to lung cancer in some cases, but rarely does.

PREVENTION

Not smoking is the single most effective way to prevent lung cancer. Reducing the number of cigarettes smoked a day can lower the risk somewhat. A heavy smoker (15 or more cigarettes a day) who cuts that by half can lower the risk of developing lung cancer by 25 percent, but that risk is still higher than it is for a lifelong light smoker (one to 14 cigarettes a day), or someone who has quit. Also, avoid second-hand smoke as much as possible.

WHO IS AT RISK?

The risk factors include:
- Smoking and second-hand smoke
- Exposure to radon
- Exposure to carcinogenic substances
- Tuberculosis
- Air pollution
- Age 45 or older

Radon levels in homes can be checked and repairs made to reduce levels. If you are exposed to carcinogens at work, take steps to reduce that exposure. Wearing a mask, respirator or other protection can help reduce the amount of inhaled toxins.

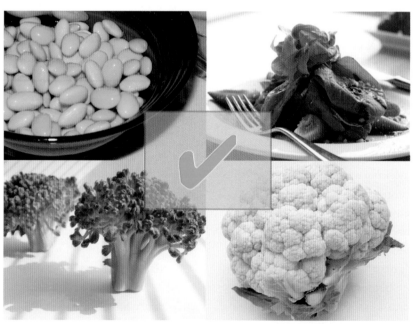

The risk of lung cancer may be lower for people with a diet rich in foods like soy and spinach that contain compounds called phytoestrogens. Foods such as broccoli and cauliflower may slow the growth of cancer cells in people who already have the disease.

A healthy diet may play a role in protecting against developing lung cancer. Foods high in compounds called phyto-oestrogens – which include soy products, grains, carrots, spinach, broccoli, and other fruits and vegetables – may reduce the risk of lung cancer somewhat in smokers and even more so in non-smokers. Isothiocyanates, a group of compounds found in cruciferous vegetables such as broccoli, cabbage and cauliflower, may help slow the development of existing cases of lung cancer.

DIAGNOSIS

Lung cancer may not cause any symptoms in the early stages. As the disease becomes more advanced, symptoms may begin to appear. Such symptoms include a worsening cough, hoarseness, coughing up blood, weight loss, reduced appetite, shortness of breath, raised temperature for no apparent reason, wheezing, recurring bouts of bronchitis (p.200) or pneumonia (pp.202–3), and constant chest or upper back pain. Other symptoms can include weakness, difficulty swallowing, nail abnormalities and facial swelling.

Researchers are seeking better screening tools to identify lung cancer in its earlier stages, which could result in better cure rates of the disease. Unfortunately, chest X-rays and lab tests of sputum have failed to effectively identify lung cancer in the earliest stages. A large study is currently under way to examine the usefulness of CT scans, which remain controversial because they result in many false positives, causing patients unnecessary worry, biopsies and even surgery.

When a doctor suspects lung cancer, cases are usually far enough advanced to show up on a chest X-ray. A CT scan may show additional detail. A sample of sputum can be examined microscopically for cancer cells to establish a positive diagnosis once the disease is advanced, or a sample of lung tissue may be necessary. CT scans of the head and abdomen and a bone marrow biopsy can show whether the cancer has spread to other tissues of the body.

TREATMENTS

Treatment depends on the type of cancer, its location in the lungs, and how advanced it is. Unfortunately, the general outlook for patients with lung cancer is grim, with only a 13 percent survival rate after five years. Lung cancer can spread to other organs, including the brain, liver, adrenal glands, spinal cord and bones, especially in cases of small cell carcinoma (see *On Call*).

• SURGERY Depending on the size and location of the cancer tumour, it may be removed surgically. In some cases, a lobe or the entire lung may have to be removed. If the cancer is the result of small cell carcinoma or if the disease has spread beyond the tissues of the lungs, surgery is not an option.

• RADIATION THERAPY High-energy X-rays can be used to kill cancer cells. Using a machine called a linear particle accelerator, specially focused beams of radiation are targeted directly at the tumours. Radiation can be used before surgery to shrink tumours before they are removed or after surgery to kill any cancer cells left behind. It can also be used to reduce the severity of symptoms, even though it may not improve the overall survival rate.

• CHEMOTHERAPY Anticancer drugs can be administered by injection, by catheter or in pills. These drugs may be given after surgery to destroy remaining cells or used instead of surgery when an operation is not possible, such as in cases of small cell carcinoma. For some patients, a combination of radiation therapy and chemotherapy is used, which may ultimately have a more powerful effect on the cancer than either treatment alone.

• PALLIATIVE CARE Supplemental oxygen therapy and bronchodilators that widen the airways can help relieve symptoms like shortness of breath. Painkillers such as morphine can reduce the pain.

See also: *Smoking Cessation, pp.216–17 • Pneumonia, pp.202–3*

On Call

Lung cancer is classified into two main types: small cell and non-small cell. Small cell is sometimes called oat cell because of its oatmeal-like appearance. It grows faster but responds better to chemotherapy. Non-small cell includes subtypes of adenocarcinoma, squamous cell carcinoma, and large cell carcinoma. Each of these three subtypes responds differently to treatment.

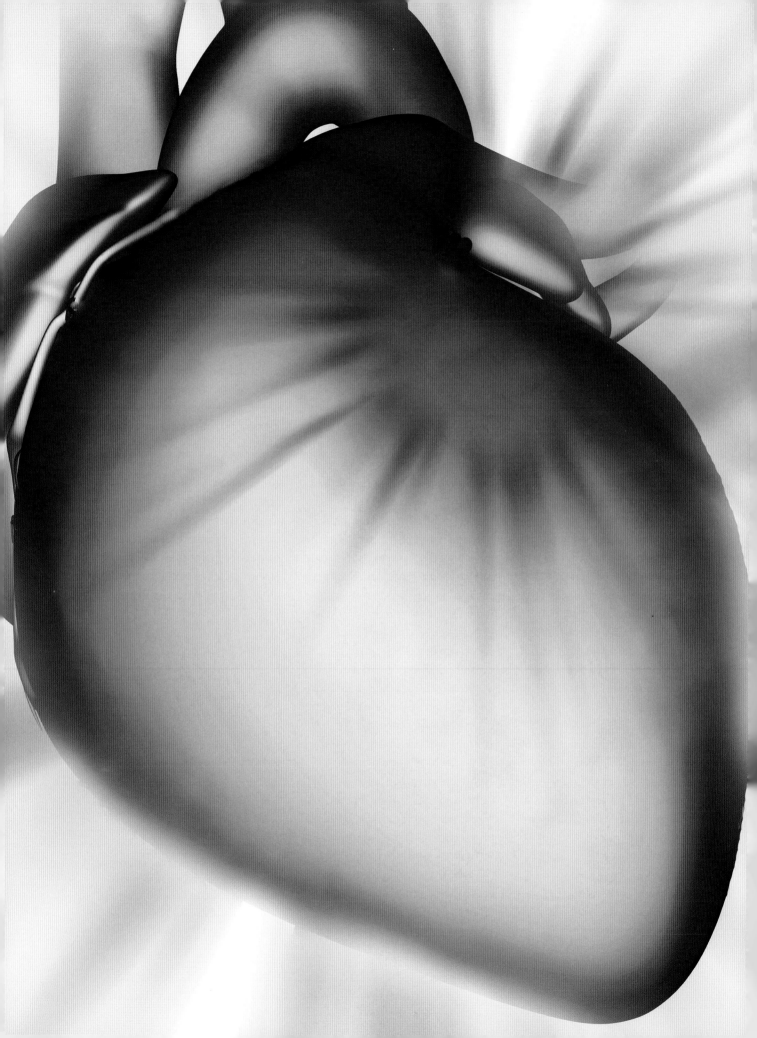

HEART & BLOOD VESSELS

8

The fist-sized heart forces the equivalent of 7,570 litres (2,000 gallons) of blood through 96,560 km (60,000 miles) of arteries and vessels every day. Acting as a pump, the heart beats 60 to 100 times a minute, but electrical impulses power the heart and control the rhythm of the heartbeat.

An erratic electrical signal can cause a life-threatening arrhythmia. The accumulation of fatty deposits in the arteries can lead to atherosclerosis and heart attack. High blood pressure from diet and a sedentary lifestyle can lead to heart attack and other conditions.

Together, regular exercise and a low-cholesterol, low-fat and low-salt diet can prevent many types of heart disease. Today, new medicines and procedures can treat many more diseases of the heart and blood vessels than ever before.

Arrhythmias

The heart beats about 100,000 times a day, more than 2.5 billion times over a 80-year life span, at a normal rate of 60 to 100 beats a minute. This fist-sized organ is powered by electrical impulses that control the rhythm of the heartbeats. Problems with that electrical system result in arrhythmias – heartbeats that are too fast, too slow or irregular. These arrhythmias can vary from harmless to fatal. Palpitations occur when arrhythmias are experienced as a pounding sensation, or as an extra or sometimes skipped beat.

WHO IS AT RISK?

The risk factors include:

- Inherited heart conditions
- Coronary artery disease
- Thyroid disorders
- Certain drugs and supplements that can increase heart rate
- High blood pressure
- Obesity
- Diabetes
- Obstructive sleep apnoea
- Electrolyte imbalance
- High alcohol consumption
- Smoking

CAUSES

A heartbeat, which takes about a second, has two parts: the upper chambers, or atria, of the heart contract to push blood through the tricuspid and mitral valves into the two lower chambers, or ventricles. Then the ventricles contract, sending blood through the pulmonary valve to the lungs (to pick up oxygen) or through the aortic valve or the body (to deliver oxygen).

The electrical impulse to start the heartbeat is sent from the sinus node, which is the heart's natural pacemaker. Other nodes in the heart have different jobs. Arrhythmias can develop when the blood supply to the heart is reduced or when heart tissue has been damaged from such conditions as coronary artery disease (pp.230–33), cardiomyopathy (pp.246–7) or valvular heart disease (pp.248–50).

The different types of arrhythmias are described by where they start in the heart (either in the atria or the ventricles) and by the change in speed. Tachycardia is a heartbeat faster than 100 beats a minute, while bradycardia is less than 60 beats a minute. However, a fast heartbeat during exercise is normal, and athletes may have a slow resting heart rate because their hearts are extremely efficient.

Atrial Ectopic Beats

These are extra heartbeats caused by electrical impulses in the atria. They occur more frequently in people with lung disorders and in older people. Coffee, tea, alcohol, excessive smoking and some cold, allergy and asthma medication may cause them or make them worse. They usually do not produce any symptoms and can occur in healthy people. If they occur due to electrolyte abnormalities in the blood or ischaemia (p.230), the underlying cause should be treated.

Atrial Fibrillation

An extremely common disorder, atrial fibrillation means the heartbeat is too fast and is also irregular, usually in the range of 150 to 180 beats per minute. The disorder may not be immediately dangerous, but can lead to other arrhythmias, chronic fatigue and congestive heart failure, and increases the risk of stroke by 500 percent.

Ventricular Ectopic Beats

Extra heartbeats caused by an electrical impulse in the ventricles are ventricular ectopic beats. The condition may feel like a strong or skipped beat and may result from stress, caffeine, alcohol, medication that stimulates the heart (such as pseudoephedrine), coronary artery disease, heart attack, heart failure and heart valve disorders. It may not be dangerous unless heart disease is present, when it may lead to ventricular tachycardia or ventricular fibrillation (p.227).

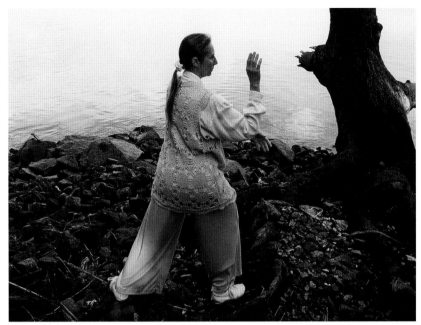

A healthy lifestyle that includes regular exercise and a diet low in salt and fat can keep weight in check and help prevent arrhythmias. Relaxation techniques such as yoga or tai chi help reduce stress, which is a risk factor for certain kinds of arrhythmia.

it. Follow treatment plans for conditions such as arteriosclerosis (p.230), high blood pressure (pp.236–9), heart valve problems, high cholesterol, diabetes (pp.338–41), and thyroid disease (pp.344–7). Avoid medication, supplements and herbal remedies that can increase the heart rate, such as pseudoephedrine in cold remedies.

DIAGNOSIS

Most people have experienced what feels like a skipped heartbeat or a fluttering feeling in the chest. These are probably not serious. But when there is shortness of breath, wheezing, weakness, dizziness, lightheadedness, fainting, and chest pain or discomfort, seek immediate medical attention.

Various tests can monitor the heart's rhythm. An electrocardiogram (ECG) uses sensors, or electrodes, that measure the timing and length of each phase in the heartbeat. A Holter monitor is a portable ECG that is worn for 24 hours or longer to measure the heart rhythm during daily activities. An event recorder is a similar

Ventricular Tachycardia

This condition is an extremely fast heartbeat. It is usually caused by other types of heart disease, although it can affect healthy people. Prompt treatment is required, because it can lead to life-threatening ventricular fibrillation.

Ventricular Fibrillation

This is the most deadly of the arrhythmias, responsible for sudden cardiac death or cardiac arrest. About half the deaths from heart problems are due to ventricular fibrillation. The heartbeat becomes rapid and chaotic, causing the ventricles to spasm and the heart to pump blood ineffectively.

Ventricular fibrillation may be caused by a heart attack, but it is not the same thing. It can occur without warning and requires immediate emergency treatment or death will result, because there is no effective circulation in the body.

Heart Block

With this condition, electrical impulses in the upper chambers are not transmitted correctly to the lower chambers, resulting in a heartbeat that is too slow, and causing oxygen deprivation in the body.

PREVENTION

Although it is not possible to prevent all arrhythmias, it is possible to reduce the risk for the heart conditions that can cause many of them. Get regular exercise, eat a low-sugar and low-salt diet with plenty of vegetables and fruit, maintain a healthy weight, do not smoke and avoid second-hand smoke. Omega-3 fatty acid supplements (pp.252–3) can reduce the risk of heart disease. Limit coffee to fewer than four cups and alcohol to two drinks a day, or eliminate them completely. Learn how to avoid or reduce stress and to use relaxation techniques to deal with

CAUTION

Get immediate emergency help if you faint or have shortness of breath, chest pain, unusual sweating, dizziness or lightheadedness. Call your doctor if you experience palpitations or frequent extra heartbeats and have risk factors for heart disease, your palpitations change in nature, or your pulse is more than 100 beats a minute without exercise, anxiety or fever.

device, but it only records heart activity when the patient has symptoms, and the patient must activate it when palpitations are felt.

An echocardiogram uses sound waves to create images of the heart's structures and movements. The tilt-table test uses a tilted table to gauge the body's reaction to changes in position. In an electrophysiology study, electrode catheters are inserted into veins and threaded into the heart to measure electrical impulses. The ability of the heart to pump can be measured in a test known as radionuclide ventriculography, or first pass technique, or multiple-gated acquisition scanning. Cardiac catheterization and coronary angiography use a catheter threaded through blood vessels to collect tissue samples of the heart, measure pressure, or diagnose different types of heart disease.

A treadmill test is used to take an ECG reading of the heart before, during and after physical activity, as a patient walks on a treadmill. Blood tests may also be needed to check levels of oxygen and cardiac enzymes in the blood.

TREATMENTS

Emergency treatment is required for serious arrhythmias, such as ventricular fibrillation, which can be fatal within minutes. Cardiopulmonary resuscitation (CPR) can be performed, but the best choice is to use an external defibrillator to provide an electric shock through the chest. Anti-arrhythmic medicines may be given intravenously.

For other arrhythmias, or once the emergency has passed, it is important to determine the underlying condition that is responsible for the heart rhythm problem, such as thyroid disease or arteriosclerosis, and then treat it.

• LIFESTYLE CHANGES Follow the strategies outlined in the Prevention section to prevent heart disease that can lead to arrhythmias.

• RELAXATION TECHNIQUES If it is determined that palpitations are not caused by a serious arrhythmia, reducing stress and anxiety may help. Breathing exercises, deep relaxation (tensing and then relaxing each muscle group in the body), yoga (pp.476–9), tai chi (p.456), and other techniques may keep stress at bay.

• MEDICATION Several drugs, including beta-blockers and certain calcium channel-blockers, can control the fast heart rate caused by atrial fibrillation. Anticoagulants are prescribed to prevent strokes in patients with atrial fibrillation. Antiarrythmic drugs are used less often than in the past because of severe side-effects, but they can help regulate the heart's rhythm.

• ELECTRONIC DEVICES A small device called a pacemaker can be implanted in the chest to send electrical charges to the heart when the heart rate slows down too much. Another device, an implantable cardioverter/defibrillator (ICD), can treat too-rapid heartbeats, which are more likely to be fatal. The ICD is implanted surgically in the chest and monitors the heart rate, sending a small electrical shock when the heart rhythm changes.

• ABLATION In this procedure, a catheter threaded through the veins and into the heart uses radiofrequency energy to destroy the abnormal heart muscle cells that are causing arrhythmias. In some cases, a permanent pacemaker will be required after the procedure.

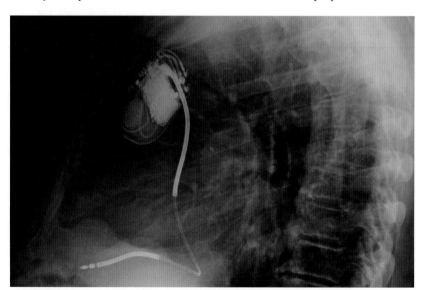

Conditions that cause arrhythmia can sometimes damage the heart's ability to generate electrical impulses. An artificial pacemaker, such as in the X-ray above, is an implantable electronic device that is used to regulate electrical activity in the heart.

See also: *Coronary Artery Disease, pp.230–3* • *Cardiomyopathy, pp.246–7* • *Diabetes, pp.338–41*

Aneurysm

A weak area in the wall of an artery that has ballooned out is called an aneurysm. It has the potential to rupture, which can lead to death if it is not treated immediately. Aneurysms may occur in any artery, but common locations are the aorta – the major artery from the heart to the rest of the body – as well as the brain, leg, intestine and splenic artery (the artery going into the spleen). Three-quarters of aortic aneurysms occur in the abdominal area of the aorta and one-fourth in the chest, or thoracic area.

CAUSES

Atherosclerosis (p.230), the accumulation of fatty deposits in arteries, is the most common cause of aortic aneurysms and the most likely culprit in older people. High blood pressure and cigarette smoking increase the risk of developing an aneurysm. However, some aneurysms are congenital – the person is born with the condition.

Less frequently, aneurysms may result from an injury (often from a fall or a car accident), inflammatory diseases of the aorta, hereditary connective-tissue disorders such as Marfan's syndrome, and even some infectious diseases such as syphilis (pp.424–5). Pregnancy (pp.398–400) may be the cause of a splenic artery aneurysm.

PREVENTION

Some aneurysms can be prevented. Control high blood pressure and the risk factors for coronary heart disease: eat a low-fat and low-cholesterol diet, avoid excess fat or sweets, maintain a healthy weight, exercise regularly and do not smoke.

DIAGNOSIS

If the aneurysm is near the skin's surface, it may be seen as a throbbing mass. Otherwise, aneurysms often have no symptoms until they rupture, and then they can cause excruciating pain. With an aortic abdominal aneurysm, it may be a deep, penetrating pain in the back or lower abdomen. With a thoracic aortic aneurysm, the pain may begin high in the back and radiate down and into the abdomen and even into the chest and arms. Abdominal and thoracic aneurysms are potentially life-threatening, and if they rupture can cause rapid blood loss and death.

Most aneurysms are diagnosed by accident during a routine examination or imaging procedure for another reason. Aneurysms may show up on ultrasonography, which uses ultrasound waves to create images, a CT scan using injected a radiopaque dye, X-rays or an MRI.

WHO IS AT RISK?

The risk factors for aortic aneurysm include:
- Male
- Age 50 to 80
- High blood pressure
- Atherosclerosis
- Family history of aneurysm
- Smoking

The risk factors for splenic artery aneurysm include:
- Pregnancy

TREATMENTS

A small aortic aneurysm less than 5 cm (2 in) across will rarely rupture and so is usually not treated. It may be checked regularly for any changes. Aneurysms larger than 6 cm (2.5 in) across are candidates for surgical repair.

- SURGERY Repairing a ruptured aortc aneurysm usually involves a synthetic graft to replace the damaged section of the artery. In the newer endovascular surgery, a synthetic graft inside a stent (a metal cylinder) attached to the tip of a catheter is inserted through an artery in the leg. Emergency surgery to repair a rupture, or threatened rupture, of an aortic aneurysm carries a 50 percent risk of death, but without surgery, the ruptured aneurysm is always fatal.

See also: *Atherosclerosis, pp.230–1* • *Pregnancy, pp.398–400* • *High Blood Pressure, pp.236–9*

CORONARY HEART DISEASE

Heart disease kills more than seven million people a year worldwide. The leading cause of death in many western countries, it is becoming a problem in developing nations as well. Smoking, high-fat diets and a sedentary lifestyle are major factors that are contributing to this.

CAUSES

Coronary heart disease starts with changes in the arteries that may lead to a heart attack. The progression is described below.

Arteriosclerosis

Commonly known as hardening of the arteries, this is a condition involving changes in the blood vessels that usually occur with age. The arteries become thick and stiff, losing their elasticity and eventually restricting blood flow throughout the body.

The terms arteriosclerosis and atherosclerosis are sometimes used interchangeably, although atherosclerosis is one type of arteriosclerosis. Atherosclosis occurs when the arteries thicken due to the accumulation of fatty deposits, or plaque, and other substances, including calcium. These deposits may block the arteries and cause a heart attack. Symptoms usually occur after the artery is more than 70 percent blocked.

Ischaemia

When an adequate supply of blood – and the oxygen it carries – fails to reach an organ such as the heart, the resulting condition is called ischaemia. The most common cause is arteriosclerosis.

Angina

The specific type of chest pain or discomfort caused by insufficient blood flow through the vessels of the heart is angina. It is most commonly caused by atherosclerosis. Other conditions can also cause angina, including spasm of the coronary arteries.

Heart Attack

During a heart attack, one or more of the coronary arteries (vessels that transport blood and oxygen to the heart) becomes blocked, usually due to a clot in an artery already narrowed by atherosclerosis. The clot, or thrombus, starts to form when a piece of plaque breaks off. When blood and oxygen cannot reach the heart muscle for a long enough period of time, the cells in that area die. That weakens the heart, and can result in congestive heart failure (pp.234–5), heart arrhythmias (pp.226–8) or even death.

PREVENTION

Up to 80 percent of the cases of coronary heart disease could be prevented if people ate a healthier diet, exercised more and stopped smoking, according to the World Health Organization (WHO).

• SMOKING Smoking more than doubles the risk of developing coronary artery disease, and doubles or even triples the risk of

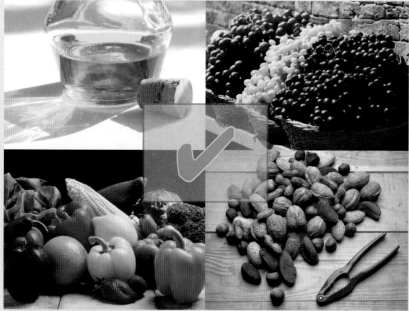

The Mediterranean diet, which includes large amounts of fruit, vegetables, nuts, olive oil and lower amounts of refined sugar may reduce the risk of developing arteriosclerosis because antioxidants in those foods prevent the build-up of fatty deposits on artery walls.

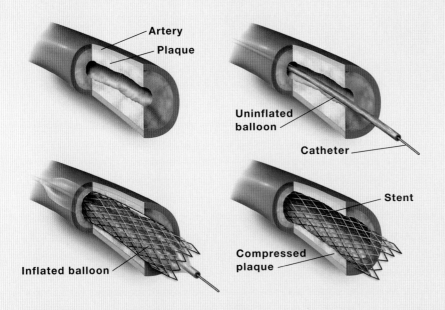

Atherosclerosis occurs when arteries become clogged with fatty deposits called plaque, restricting the free flow of blood through the blood vessels. Angioplasty is a procedure to open clogged arteries using a small balloon threaded into the arteries and inflated to compress the palque and restore blood flow.

dying from it. It is considered the most important risk factor that can be changed (pp.216–17). Even secondhand smoke can increase the risk of heart disease.

• NUTRITION A number of simple dietary approaches can lower the risk of developing coronary disease. Limit sodium intake to 2,000 mg or less a day and eat plenty of fruit and vegetables to decrease the risk of developing high blood pressure and limit the amount of refined sugar. Reduce the amount of fat in the diet to no more than 25 to 35 percent of daily calories. Transfats and saturated fats may be the most harmful when it comes to heart health; they are found in meats, dairy products, and artificially hydrogenated vegetable oils. Healthy fats, such as monounsaturated fats, are found in olive and rapeseed oils. Polyunsaturated fats are found in omega-3 oils (pp.252–3), which are in deep-sea fatty fish such as

salmon and tuna. Omega-6 fats are found in sunflower, safflower, corn and soy oils. Five servings of fruit and vegetables a day will ensure an adequate intake of fibre, vitamins C and E, and phytochemicals. The Mediterranean diet, which includes large amounts of fruit, vegetables, nuts and olive oil, reduces the risk of developing atherosclerosis because antioxidants in those foods prevent the build-up of fatty deposits on artery walls.

• ALCOHOL One or two drinks a day (but not more) may lower the chances of developing heart disease in men over 40 and post-menopausal women.

• EXERCISE Just 30 minutes of physical activity, such as walking, five days a week can cut the risk of heart disease by lowering cholesterol levels and controlling blood pressure. Talk to a doctor before starting an exercise programme.

• WEIGHT CONTROL The waist-to-

hip ratio may be the most accurate way to determine the risk of heart attack for the overweight and obese. The higher the number, the higher the risk.

• BLOOD PRESSURE CONTROL One study found that relatively small increases in blood pressure doubled the risk of developing coronary heart disease in people ages 40 to 69. The study, funded by the British Heart Foundation and the Medical Reseach Council, analysed data from 61 observational studies worldwide of blood pressure and mortality, covering one million adults, and was published in *The Lancet* in 2002.

• DIABETES CONTROL Keep blood sugar levels under control to prevent damage to arteries that can lead to heart disease.

DIAGNOSIS

Risk factors, family history, and symptoms will determine which specific diagnostic tests are needed for each patient. Blood tests will check blood sugar and cholesterol levels. An electrocardiogram (ECG) reveals the rate and

On Call

The average French diet is higher in saturated fat than the typical diet in any other European country, yet the death rate in France from heart disease is low. This is known as the 'French paradox'. It is speculated that the antioxidants in red wine, or in the high amount of fruit and vegetables that are also part of the diet, offer some protection.

regularity of the heartbeat and shows evidence of old damage to the heart as well as changes that indicate current problems. An echocardiogram uses sound waves to make an image of the heart, providing more detail than a chest X-ray, which is used sometimes as well. An exercise stress test shows how well the heart handles exercise: ECG and blood-pressure readings are taken before, during, and after physical activity such as walking on a treadmill.

Cardiac catheterization and coronary angiography are procedures that use a thin, flexible tube passed through an artery in the groin or arm to the arteries around the heart. Instruments on the end of the tube can provide information on the pressure and blood flow in the heart, get blood samples from the heart, and look at the arteries of the heart by X-ray. In coronary angiography, a special dye is injected into the coronary arteries that illuminates the blood flow on X-ray film. A nuclear heart scan uses radioactive tracers to show any damage to the heart and blood vessels. Electron beam computed tomography measures the calcium build-up in the coronary arteries.

TREATMENTS

For patients with arteriosclerosis, angina and ischaemia, treatment is aimed at relieving the symptoms with the goal of preventing a heart attack.

Arteriosclerosis

The strategies listed under Prevention are also the first line of treatment for this condition.

• **MEDICATION** Cholesterol-lowering medication can help prevent the build-up of plaque in the arteries. Anticoagulants prevent clots from forming in the arteries, which could lead to heart attack. Aspirin and other anti-platelet medications also help prevent clots by stopping platelets in the blood from clumping together. ACE inhibitors help control blood pressure and reduce the heart's workload. Beta-blockers have much the same results by slowing the heart rate and lowering blood pressure. Calcium channel-blockers control blood pressure by relaxing blood vessels. Nitroglycerine tablets prevent or relieve angina. Long-acting nitrates must be used over an extended period to help open up the arteries to the heart.

• **SUPPLEMENTS** Omega-3 fatty acids, found in fish, may help reduce cholesterol and prevent arteriosclerosis. The best source for these fats is eating two to

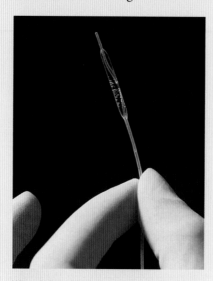

When inflated inside an artery, a slim, cigar-shaped angioplasty balloon widens the channel through which blood flows.

three servings a week of fatty fish, such as salmon, tuna or sardines. Advice on which supplements should be taken for preventing heart disease vary. Health officials in the United States recommend 1.6 g (0.6 oz) a day for men and 1.1 g (0.03 oz) for women; Health Canada and the British Nutrition Task Force recommend getting 0.5 percent of one's daily calories from omega-3s.

Supplements of folic acid, usually 1 mg a day, can lower high levels of homocysteine, an amino acid that may play a role in heart disease. Foods high in folic acid include citrus fruits, tomatoes, vegetables and grain products.

Taking 25–50 g (1–1.5 oz) of soy protein a day may help lower high cholesterol. In premenopausal women, 400 mg of soy milk a day may reduce cholesterol.

The fibre in oatmeal, called beta-glucans, has been found to lower cholesterol, but it takes several servings a day to be effective.

Taking 1–3 g (0.03–0.1 oz) of niacin a day may treat atherosclerosis and lower cholesterol, but discuss it first with a healthcare professional because there is a risk of liver enzyme abnormalities, flushing of the face and potential drug interactions, especially with increased dosages.

Psyllium taken two or three times a day, for a total dose of 10–20 g (0.3–0.4 oz), can lower cholesterol. It may also lower blood sugar levels and intensify the effect of any laxatives.

• **YOGA** This form of exercise (pp.476–9) may lower such risk factors as high blood pressure,

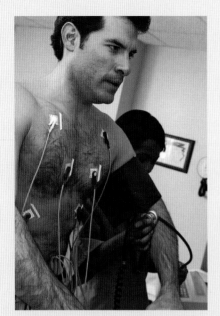

A stress test measures blood pressure and electrical activity in the heart, and can help doctors diagnose heart disease by assessing how the heart handles exercise.

cholesterol and blood sugar levels. It may also help the heart work more efficiently and decrease chest pain. It is not known if yoga is superior to other types of exercise, but it may be helpful when used in conjunction with medication that lowers blood pressure and cholesterol. Remember to check with a healthcare professional before beginning any exercise programme.

Heart Attack

A heart attack is considered a medical emergency. Half the deaths caused by a heart attack happen in the first three or four hours. Earlier treatment improves the chances of survival. Treatment of a heart attack is aimed at limiting damage to the heart as well as preventing future attacks.

• **ASPIRIN** Anyone who suspects they are having a heart attack should chew up an aspirin tablet (as long as they are not allergic to aspirin), which helps to prevent any further clotting.

• **OXYGEN** Supplemental oxygen is given in an effort to prevent further damage to the heart muscle.

• **THROMBOLYTIC THERAPY** These clot-busting drugs may be given within six hours to help dissolve the blood clot. They increase the risk of bleeding so cannot be given to people who have certain conditions, such as bleeding in the digestive tract, severe high blood pressure, a recent stroke or surgery during the month before the heart attack.

• **ANGIOPLASTY** This procedure may be done immediately to clear the blockage from the arteries. A thin, flexible catheter tipped with a balloon is inserted into an artery until it reaches the obstruction. Then the balloon tip is inflated, clearing the blockage. In most cases, a stent may be inserted into the artery to keep the plaque from developing again in that location. Angioplasty can also be used to treat arteriosclerosis before a heart attack occurs.

• **SURGERY** Coronary artery bypass surgery uses arteries or veins from elsewhere in the body to create a detour, or bypass, around the blocked arteries.

• **CARDIAC REHABILITATION** This is a team approach in which doctors, nurses, physical and occupational therapists, exercise specialists, dietitians and psychologists work with patients after a heart attack, heart surgery or other treatment for heart disease. Education, counselling and training are provided to help patients understand heart disease and how to reduce their risk of future heart problems, while learning to cope with lifestyle changes and the depression that sometimes accompanies heart attack. Exercise training is individualized to help patients exercise safely, improve muscle strength and increase stamina.

• **CHELATION** This therapy (pp.576–7) involves the use of chemicals that bind with metal ions to remove toxins from the blood, and has proven effective in treating cases of lead poisoning. A large-scale clinical trial is currently under way in the United States to examine whether chelation could be effective in removing plaques.

See also: *Congestitive Heart Failure, pp.234–5 • Arrhythmias, pp.226–8 • Chelation, pp.576–7*

CAUTION

The symptoms of a heart attack can range from none – called a silent heart attack – to excruciating. Some people who experience mild pain for several hours may be unsure of the cause and delay getting help. Here is what to watch for:

• Chest pain, ranging from mild discomfort to a squeezing pressure
• Pain or discomfort in the upper body, such as one or both arms, the back, neck, jaw or stomach
• Shortness of breath, which may or may not be accompanied by chest pain
• Cold sweat or profuse sweating
• Nausea or vomiting (indigestion may be suspected)
• Lightheadedness, dizziness or fainting
• Anxiety or feelings of dread

Congestive Heart Failure

Although the term congestive heart failure may suggest the heart stops beating, it actually means the heart has lost the ability to pump blood efficiently and, as a result, blood backs up within the organs of the body. Heart failure can affect the left side of the heart, the right side, or both.

With failure on the right side of the heart, a condition known as cor pulmonale, fluid often accumulates in the body, especially in the lower extremities such as the feet, ankles and legs, resulting in peripheral oedema (pp.244–5). Failure of the left chambers of the heart may cause fluid to build up in the lungs, causing pulmonary congestion and oedema.

CAUSES

Any kind of heart disease, defect or damage to the heart's tissues may result in congestive heart failure, but coronary artery disease (pp.230–3), which includes angina and heart attack, is the leading cause of this disease. High blood pressure (pp.236–9) and diabetes (pp.338–41) are also major causes. Other diseases and conditions that can lead to congestive heart failure include cardiomyopathy (pp.246–7), diseases of the heart valves (pp.248–50), arrhythmias (pp.226–8), congenital heart disease (pp.256–8), radiation and chemotherapy for cancer, thyroid disorders (pp.344–7), alcohol abuse, HIV/AIDS, and the use of cocaine and other illegal drugs.

PREVENTION

The best way to avoid congestive heart failure is by preventing the conditions that can lead to it. Anyone already diagnosed with coronary artery disease, high blood pressure, other heart conditions or diabetes should follow their prescribed treatment plans.

Lifestyle changes can also help. Do not smoke. Individuals who are overweight or obese should lose weight (pp.348–9). Follow dietary guidelines: reduce the intake of fat and sugar, and/or carbohydrates, and stick to a low-sodium diet, if recommended. Exercise and stay – or become – active. Take all prescribed medication as directed by a doctor.

DIAGNOSIS

Shortness of breath, even during rest, along with fatigue and oedema (pp.244–5), are the classic signs of heart failure. A medical history, physical examination and various tests will rule out other conditions with the same symptoms. Abnormal sounds in the heart and lungs may be detected with a stethoscope.

The most important test in diagnosing heart failure is the echo-cardiogram, which uses sound waves to provide a measurement of how well the heart pumps; this is called the ejection fraction (EF). A healthy heart should have an EF of 50 to 60 percent or higher; people with heart failure usually have an EF of 40 percent or lower. People with diastolic dysfunction may have a normal EF, even though the heart has a problem filling with blood. (Diastolic dysfunction occurs when the ventricles of the heart become relatively stiff, making it difficult for them to fill with blood between heart beats.)

Cardiac catheterization involves passing a thin, flexible tube through an artery and injecting a special dye that is visible using X-rays. This procedure, called coronary angiography, enables doctors to visualize the coronary arteries and the blood flow of the heart muscle.

An electrocardiogram (ECG)

WHO IS AT RISK?

The risk factors include:
- Over age 65
- High blood pressure
- History of heart attack
- History of heart murmur
- Damaged heart valves
- Enlarged heart
- Family history of enlarged heart
- Diabetes

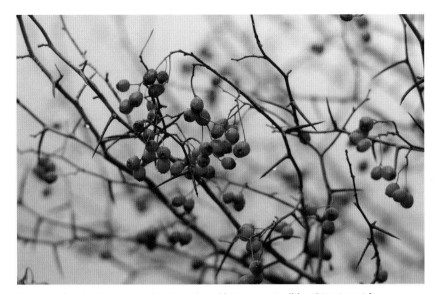

Hawthorn is a herbal remedy that has a long history as a traditional treatment for mild to moderate congestive heart failure. This remedy should only be used under the supervision of a doctor to avoid dangerous interactions with other drugs.

measures the rate and regularity of the heartbeat. A chest X-ray shows whether the heart is enlarged or if there is fluid in the lungs. A Holter monitor functions like a portable ECG and is usually worn for 24 hours; it helps diagnose problems of heart rhythm than can lead to heart failure. A cardiac blood pool scan uses a radioactive dye injected into a vein to show how well the heart is pumping blood. An exercise stress test reveals how the heart works during physical activity.

The newest blood test measures the level of a hormone called B-type natriuretic peptide, or BNP, that is elevated with heart failure. Blood tests may also be done to rule out thyroid problems (pp.344–5), as they can be a cause of heart failure.

TREATMENTS

Congestive heart failure cannot be cured unless it results from a treatable condition, such as thyroid disease. Treatment is aimed at re-ducing the symptoms and prevent-ing progression of the damage.

• DIET A low-sodium diet may be necessary to keep blood pressure under control and prevent fluid from accumulating in the body. A low-fat diet will help prevent blocked arteries. Fluids and potas-sium intake may also be restricted.

• MEDICATION Numerous drugs can aid the heart's function and reduce symptoms. Diuretics will help remove excess fluid that ac-cumulates in the lungs, feet and legs and relieve symptoms. ACE inhibitors and beta-blockers both lower blood pressure and work in different ways to reduce the strain on the heart and extend life span. Digoxin, used less and less frequently because it does not prolong life, enables the heart to beat with more force.

• HERBAL REMEDIES Hawthorn (*Crataegus oxyacantha*), a member of the flowering rose shrub fam-ily, has been used for thousands of years to treat mild to moderate con-gestive heart failure. Two to three doses a day, for a total of 160–900 mg (depending on the strength of the preparation), is recommended. A doctor must be consulted before using and adjusting dosages, as hawthorn may increase the effects of digoxin and some hypertension drugs to dangerous levels.

• EXERCISE Because exertion often worsens the shortness of breath that accompanies congestive heart failure, patients may limit their activity – which lowers their fitness levels and creates a vicious cycle. A doctor-supervised exercise programme has been shown to improve the health of those with mild to moderate heart failure.

• OXYGEN Supplemental oxygen therapy may be given if the level of oxygen in the blood falls.

• COUNSELLING Psychological interventions, such as cognitive-behavioural therapy (p.355) or other types of counselling, help reduce the depression common in patients with heart failure.

• SURGERY If heart failure becomes severe, a mechanical heart pump may be considered to help the heart pump. In some cases, a heart transplant is the only option.

See also: *Peripheral Oedema, p. 244–5* • *High Blood Pressure, pp.236–9* • *Obesity, pp.348–9*

CAUTION

If you have congestive heart failure, be sure to weigh yourself every day. Call your doctor immediately if you notice a sud-den weight gain, which could indicate a build-up of fluid.

High & Low Blood Pressure

The heart pumps the equivalent of 7,570 litres (2,000 gallons) of blood each day through 96,560 km (60,000 miles) of arteries, veins and capillaries. It does this with about the same force that a human hand squeezes a tennis ball. That force – called blood pressure – can vary greatly. Some of these variations are natural. For example, blood pressure is usually lowest at night during sleep and highest in the morning; lower at rest and higher during activity.

Variations that fall outside the normal range can be dangerous. High blood pressure, also known as hypertension, has become increasingly common in industrialized nations around the world, and the complications can be serious: heart attack and heart failure, stroke, damage to the blood vessels, aneurysm, kidney failure, brain damage and loss of vision. Low blood pressure, also known as hypotension, can harm the body when blood pressure falls so low that the brain does not receive enough oxygen.

CAUSES
In many cases, the cause of blood pressure that is too high or too low is not diagnosable.

High Blood Pressure
There are two types of high blood pressure: essential (sometimes also called primary) and secondary. Essential hypertension, by far the most common type, is diagnosed when the cause of the high blood pressure cannot be identified.

It may be influenced by genetics. Other factors that can contribute to high blood pressure include obesity, a sedentary lifestyle, smoking, a high-salt diet and heavy drinking. Emotional factors, such as stress, anxiety and depression, and environmental factors such as cold weather, may also play a role.

Spouses of people with high blood pressure have a much higher risk for it, as well – probably due to the fact that they share the same diet and lifestyle.

Secondary hypertension is a form of the condition that has an identifiable cause. One of the most common causes is kidney disease or damage. The kidneys regulate removal of salt and water from the body, which plays a role in controlling blood pressure. Other conditions that may be responsible for secondary hypertension are hormonal disorders such as Cushing's syndrome (pp.342–3) and hyperthyroidism (p.350), certain drugs such as birth-control pills and appetite

WHO IS AT RISK?
The risk factors for high blood pressure include:
- Family history of high blood pressure
- Advancing age
- High-salt diet
- Environmental factors such as cold weather
- Smoking
- Kidney disorders
- Hormonal disorders
- Birth-control pills
- Certain medications, such as appetite suppressants
- Arteriosclerosis
- Obesity
- Sedentary lifestyle
- Alcohol abuse
- Stress
- Diabetes

The risk factors for low blood pressure include:
- Uncontrolled bleeding
- Severe allergic reaction
- Severe infection
- Heart problems
- Hormonal disorders
- Pregnancy
- Some medications, such as tricyclic antidepressants and beta-blockers
- Dehydration

suppressants, and arteriosclerosis (p.230), because the resulting stiff arteries can no longer dilate and this elevates blood pressure.

Stress often gets blamed for causing high blood pressure, but the increase is usually temporary and blood pressure returns to normal when a person is calm again. For example, blood pressure is sometimes higher at the doctor's because of the stress involved.

Low Blood Pressure

Sudden and extreme drops in blood pressure can cause dizziness and fainting, and may be caused by uncontrolled bleeding, severe infections or life-threatening allergic reactions. Some medication, such as tricyclic antidepressants, beta-blockers, narcotics and those taken for Parkinson's disease (p.181), may lower blood pressure. Other causes include pregnancy, heart arrhythmias (pp.226–7), heart disease (pp.230–3), endocrine disorders and dehydration. It can also occur when taking medication for hypertension, which sometimes can end up reducing the blood pressure too much.

A condition that is known as postural, or orthostatic, hypotension occurs when systolic pressure falls drastically when a person stands up from a sitting or prone position. Postprandial hypotension, more common in older people, is a drop in blood pressure after eating a meal.

Prevention

Lifestyle changes can prevent problems with blood pressure. Hypertension is twice as common in obese people, and losing weight may be the only treatment needed to reduce blood pressure to a safe level. A reduction in weight of just 4.5 kg (10 lbs) can be effective. Exercise can aid in weight loss while strengthening the heart. Reduce salt intake to less than 2,000 mg a day. Watch out for hidden sources of sodium, such as MSG and baking soda. Cut the amount of alcohol to two drinks or less a day. Quit smoking. Eat more fruit, vegetables and fibre. Cut down on caffeine – fewer than four cups of coffee a day is the maximum.

Clinical Query

My doctor always tells me two numbers when he takes my blood pressure. What do the numbers mean?

When a blood-pressure reading is taken, two kinds of blood pressure are measured, and the numbers are written one over the other. The top number, the systolic, measures the amount of pressure when the heart pumps blood through the arteries. The bottom number, the diastolic, measures the amount of pressure in the arteries when the heart rests between beats.

Keeping properly hydrated is important in the prevention of low blood pressure.

DIAGNOSIS

Blood pressure is usually measured with a sphygmomanometer, which consists of an inflatable soft rubber cuff and a meter. It is important that the arm used for testing blood pressure be relaxed and held at about the same level as the heart. Other devices can measure blood pressure, and home blood-pressure kits are available. In some cases, a 24-hour blood-pressure monitor, which is portable and battery-operated, is needed to provide blood-pressure readings over a longer period. A reading lower than 120 over 80 is now considered the healthiest blood pressure. (See Clinical Query above for information on what blood-pressure readings mean.)

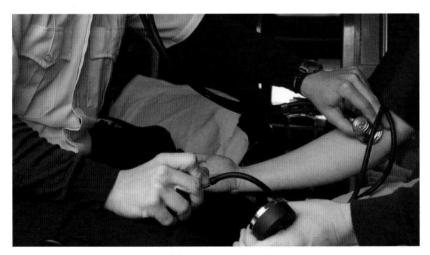

Blood pressure is measured by two numbers, which represent the pressure inside the arteries when the heart is beating and at rest. To measure blood pressure, an inflatable cuff is wrapped around the upper arm. While the cuff is slowly deflated, the doctor listens to the sound of the pulse in an artery in the arm with a stethoscope.

High blood pressure is sometimes called 'the silent killer' because it rarely causes any overt symptoms but can seriously damage organs such as the heart, the kidneys and the brain, and can harm the vision as well, while contributing to the risk of heart attack and stroke. It is often detected by a routine blood-pressure check at the doctor's surgery, although a large number of cases go undiagnosed.

To confirm a diagnosis of high blood pressure, readings should be repeated several times. Hypertension is considered to be 140 systolic or higher or 90 diastolic or higher. A condition called pre-hypertension is diagnosed when blood pressure falls between 130 and 139 systolic or between 80 and 89 diastolic. Because this condition frequently progresses to high blood pressure, lifestyle changes are recommended.

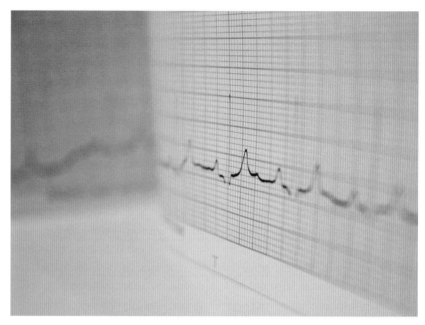

A patient who is diagnosed with high blood pressure may need tests to check for organ damage. Electrocardiography (above) or echocardiography can check for damage to the heart muscle by measuring its rhythm and electrical activity.

CAUTION

Malignant hypertension, which is considered a medical emergency, occurs when blood pressure is at least 210 systolic over 120 diastolic. If you have a severe headache with high blood pressure, get medical treatment immediately. If you know your blood pressure is high because you have a monitor at home, call your doctor if you also experience excessive tiredness, confusion, vision changes, crushing chest pain, nausea and vomiting, shortness of breath, significant sweating, blood in the urine, nosebleed, irregular heartbeat, or noise or buzzing in the ears.

If secondary hypertension is suspected, additional tests will be done to find the underlying cause. Tests include blood tests, urinalysis, X-rays of the kidneys, electrocardiogram (ECG), or echocardiogram. An ophthalmoscope is often used to check the blood vessels in the retina for any changes brought about by high blood pressure.

Low blood pressure is sometimes said to be a measurement lower than 90 systolic or 60 diastolic. However, many doctors do not worry about low blood pressure unless it causes symptoms.

Special tests can also help identify low blood pressure. The Valsalva manoeuvre is done to check how blood pressure responds after taking several deep breaths and forcing the air out through a closed mouth. The tilt-table test uses a tilted table to gauge the body's reaction to changes in position.

TREATMENTS

Weight loss, exercise and changes in diet may be necessary to treat blood-pressure abnormalities.

High Blood Pressure

Treatment for high blood pressure may have to continue for the rest of the patient's life, with regular monitoring and occasional adjustments.

• MEDICATION A number of medications, collectively called anti-hypertensives, lower blood pressure by various methods, and sometimes a combination of them will be needed for effective control. Diuretics cause blood vessels to dilate and help the kidneys remove excess water and salt, reducing the volume of fluid in the body. Beta-blockers and other adrenergic blockers prevent vessels from constricting, while ACE inhibitors, calcium channel-blockers, and direct vasodilators dilate the blood vessels.

• **DIET** Diuretics prescribed for blood pressure abnormalities may remove potassium from the body, so potassium supplements may be needed, or potassium-rich foods should be added to the diet. These include bananas, cantaloupe, grapefruit, oranges, tomato or prune juice, honeydew melon, prunes, molasses and potatoes.

• **SUPPLEMENTS** The omega-3 fatty acids (pp.252–3) found in fish or fish oil supplements may lower blood pressure slightly, but may also increase the risk of bleeding. Eat fish, such as mackerel, lake trout, herring, sardines, albacore tuna and salmon at least twice a week.

• **YOGA** While yoga (pp.476–9) may help control high blood pressure, it may not be any more effective than other forms of exercise. Anyone with high blood pressure should avoid inverted yoga positions, such as headstands and shoulder stands.

• **QI GONG** This Traditional Chinese Medicine (pp.446–50) technique has shown some benefit to people suffering from high blood pressure, when used in combination with medication. One form involves daily meditation, combined with sounds and movements.

• **ACUPUNCTURE** This Chinese technique (pp.464–5) may help lower blood pressure, although more research is needed.

• **MEDITATION** Transcendental meditation (p.519) was found to lower blood pressure nearly twice as much as progressive muscle relaxation, in a study of 200 African-American men and women published in 2005 in the *American Journal of Hypertension.* Systolic pressure went down an average of 10.7 points and diastolic 6.4 points in those who practised transcendental meditation.

Low Blood Pressure

In many cases, low blood pressure does not require any treatment.

• **MEDICATION** Pyridostigmine is sometimes prescribed to raise blood pressure without adversely affecting the pressure when sitting or lying down.

• **DIET** An increased salt intake or additional caffeine may raise the blood pressure. Check with a doctor before making either change. Cut out alcohol, because it can have a dehydrating effect. Drink more water to prevent dehydration and increase blood volume, which can result in higher blood pressure. To counteract postprandial hypotension, eat small meals several times a day and limit the intake of high-carbohydrate foods. Coffee or tea with meals can stimulate blood pressure, as well.

• **SUPPLEMENTS** Anaemia, caused by a lack of vitamin B_{12} and folic acid, can lead to low blood pressure. Supplements may be needed.

• **COMPRESSION STOCKINGS** Elastic stockings used to treat varicose veins and chronic venous insufficiency (pp.240–2) can aid the circulation in the legs and help normalize blood pressure.

• **LIFESTYLE CHANGES** Sleeping with several pillows to elevate the head at night can help reduce the risk of feeling dizzy when getting up. If suffering from postural hypotension, be sure to stand up slowly. If dizzy when standing up, cross the thighs in a scissors style and then squeeze, or place one foot up on a chair and lean forward to stimulate blood flow from the legs to the heart.

See also: *Arrhythmias, pp.226–8 • Traditional Chinese Medicine, pp.446–7 • Omega-3 Fatty Acids, pp.252–3*

healing hope

I hated the thought of having to take pills for my blood pressure, which had been creeping up over the years but finally reached 140/90. That's when my doctor gave me an ultimatum: get that blood pressure down or I'm writing you a prescription.

My wife and I started walking 30 minutes every day and I watched how much salt I was eating. We took the salt shaker off the table and found recipes that used different spices. We also started eating fish at least twice a week and made sure to get plenty of vegetables and fruits. I learned to substitute carrot sticks for crisps – it wasn't easy! But the hardest thing was probably walking into the transcendental meditation class. I felt pretty silly at first, but then I found I liked the way it made me feel getting rid of all the stress and feeling more relaxed.

After several months, I'd lost 7 kg (15 lbs) and my blood pressure went down to 125/80. It's still close to the borderline, according to my doctor, but I'm working hard to keep it at a safe level.
                                                                    Amos K.

Venous Disorders

Arteries carry oxygen-enriched blood away from the left side of the heart out to the body, while veins bring blood, now depleted of oxygen, back to the right side of the heart. Veins must fight the pull of gravity; muscles in the feet and legs help by squeezing the veins to force the blood upwards, while one-way valves in the veins keep blood from flowing backwards.

These veins can develop problems, such as chronic venous insufficiency and deep vein thrombosis. The first is the failure of the veins to push blood upwards adequately, which causes blood to pool in the legs. This condition is rarely life-threatening. Deep vein thrombosis, however, is the development of a blood clot inside the deep veins, away from the surface of the skin. These clots can break off and travel elsewhere in the body, and may even pass through the heart and lodge in the lungs – causing a potentially fatal condition known as pulmonary embolism (pp.210–11).

CAUSES

Chronic venous insufficiency can cause deep vein thrombosis, while having a blood clot can stretch the veins and result in chronic venous insufficiency.

Chronic Venous Insufficiency

Walking keeps the leg muscles squeezing the veins and the blood moving, but prolonged sitting or standing allows the blood to pool, raising the blood pressure in those veins. The veins stretch and lose their elasticity over time, until the valves can no longer work properly. Veins close to the surface that swell and become inflamed are known as varicose veins and can be seen through the skin.

Deep Vein Thrombosis

Blood clots are more likely to form when someone is inactive; that is why most cases occur in hospitalized patients. Prolonged sitting or bed rest enables blood to accumulate in the veins, encouraging the formation of blood clots. Surgery, especially hip, knee and gynaecological procedures, increases the risk of deep vein thrombosis because of trauma or injury to the vessels and slowed blood circulation. The same is true of fractures and childbirth within the last six months. Taking oestrogen and birth-control pills also raises the risk because oestrogen increases the blood's tendency to clot. The clots usually develop in the pelvis, thigh or calf, although they may be found in the arms, chest or other parts of body.

WHO IS AT RISK?

The risk factors for chronic venous insufficiency include:

- Family history of varicose veins
- Overweight
- Lack of exercise
- Smoking
- Pregnancy
- Age 50 and older
- Standing or sitting for long periods of time

The risk factors for deep vein thrombosis include:

- Over age 60
- Prolonged inactivity, such as sitting or bed rest
- Recent surgery or injury
- Fractures
- Childbirth within the last six months
- Oestrogen or birth-control pills
- History of polycythaemia vera
- Cancerous tumour
- Inherited or acquired blood-clotting problems
- Obesity
- History of heart attack, stroke or congestive heart failure
- Inflammatory bowel disease

PREVENTION

Activity is the best prevention for all venous disorders. Avoid sitting, standing or lying down for long periods of time. Stop at least every two hours on long car trips to get out and stretch and walk for a few minutes. On long plane trips, stand up and move if possible, or flex and extend the ankles about 10 times every 30 minutes. While standing for long periods, flex the leg muscles to help the veins work more efficiently. When sitting or lying down, elevate the feet above the level of the heart.

For patients who are hospitalized or in a long-term care facility, elastic stockings can be worn to help maintain proper circulation in the legs. Pneumatic devices mimic the action of the calf muscles with an electric pump that squeezes the plastic stocking in a rhythmic pattern to help the blood circulate. Anticoagulants to slow down the blood's clotting time may be prescribed for people at high risk for thrombosis or for surgical patients. Getting up and walking is encouraged as soon as possible for patients who have had surgery or are hospitalized.

DIAGNOSIS

An accumulation of fluid in the legs and ankles, or oedema (pp.244–5) is the major symptom of chronic venous insufficiency. Walking may cause pain and the legs may feel heavy, tired, restless or achy, while the calves feel tight. The skin may turn a brownish colour because plasma is leaking out of the veins. Varicose veins, a rash called stasis dermatitis, and sores or ulcers may develop on the legs.

With deep vein thrombosis, typically only one leg is affected. Symptoms can include pain, tenderness, swelling, increased warmth and often redness in that leg. About half the people who have deep vein thrombosis will not have any symptoms at all.

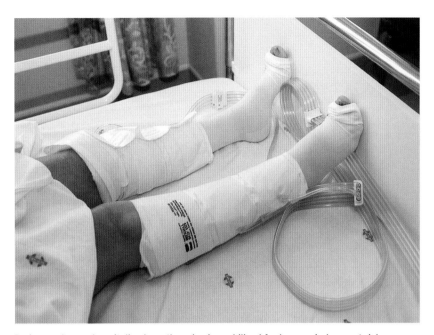

Patients who are hospitalized or otherwise immobilized for long periods are at risk of developing deep vein thrombosis. Pneumatic stockings can help circulate the blood, mimicking the action of the lower leg muscles by squeezing the legs in a rhythmic pattern.

Many of the same tests are used to diagnose both conditions. Blood pressure in the legs may be measured. A duplex ultrasound test shows images of the structure of the veins, as well as how fast the blood moves through them and any blood clots. In venography, a special dye may be injected so that the veins, and sometimes blood clots, show up on X-ray. Blood tests can check for both inherited and acquired causes of hypercoagulability, or increased blood-clotting tendency.

If someone has deep vein thrombosis or a history of blood clots, and is experiencing chest pain, shortness of breath, fainting or loss of consciousness, they should go to hospital or call for emergency help immediately.

TREATMENTS

Although some of the same things prevent both chronic venous insufficiency or deep vein thrombosis,

the treatments are very different.

Chronic Venous Insufficiency

Exercise is an important component of any treatment programme.

• **COMPRESSION STOCKINGS** These elastic stockings squeeze the veins and prevent blood from flowing backward. If chronic venous insufficiency is a long-term problem, they may have to be worn every day.

• **SUPPLEMENTS** Horse chestnut (*Aesculus hippocastanum*) seed extract is a popular treatment in Europe. It is recommended that a standardized product containing 50–75 mg of escin (the therapeutic substance contained in horse chestnut seed extract) be taken every 12 hours, which may mean the total dose of extract is 300 mg twice a day. Pycnogenol, a patented trade name for a water extract of the bark of the French maritime pine

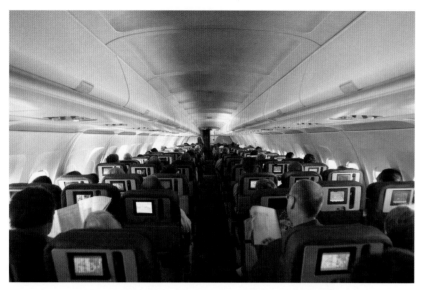

Deep vein thrombosis, a condition with potentially dangerous complications, can occur when blood clots form in the deep veins of the legs. To reduce the risk of developing clots, keep blood circulating properly by avoiding long periods of inactivity. On long flights, for example, periodically stand and walk around the cabin.

blood-thinners needs regular blood tests to monitor the clotting factor; this measurement, called INR, should be between 2 and 3.

• NON-SURGICAL PROCEDURES Thrombolysis is a procedure in which clot-dissolving drugs are injected through a catheter into the clot. This approach may be used to dissolve large clots. The procedure is rare, though, because it has a higher risk for bleeding complications and stroke than does blood-thinning, or anti-coagulant, medication.

• SURGERY Although rarely used, a surgical procedure called venous thrombectomy can remove the deep vein clot. Another procedure involves insertion of a vena cava filter, which can be surgically inserted into the vena cava, the large vein returning blood from the abdomen. This filter prevents clots that have dislodged from reaching the lungs and the heart.

See also: *Oedema, pp. 244–5* • *Pulmonary Embolism, pp.210–11*

tree (*Pinus pinaster*), is another potential treatment. Two doses are taken a day, for a total of 100–360 mg for one to two months, with or after meals because of the potential for problems of stomach discomfort. This supplement can interfere with chemotherapy agents and immunosuppressant drugs. As always, the use of these supplements should be discussed with a health care professional.

• NON-SURGICAL PROCEDURES In the procedure known as sclerotherapy, a chemical is injected into the affected insufficient veins that scars them from the inside so they no longer are able to fill up with blood. As a result, blood flow is diverted through other, more efficient veins.

• SURGERY In vein-stripping, the primary superficial vein, the saphenous vein, which is close to the surface of the skin, is removed. Another procedure, sometimes done separately or with vein-

stripping, is small incision avulsion, in which varicose veins are removed through tiny incisions.

Deep Vein Thrombosis

Treatment for deep vein thrombosis is important to prevent complications such as pulmonary embolism (pp.210–11).

• MEDICATION The most common way to treat deep vein thrombosis is through the use of prescription medications known as blood-thinners. They do not actually thin the blood, but increase the amount of time it takes for the blood to clot. Heparin is the intravenous form of the drug and is given while the patient is hospitalized. A more recent breakthrough is low molecular-weight heparin, which can be given by injection once or twice a day and does not require hospitalization. Warfarin is the oral form of an anticoagulant, given in pill form. Patients taking

On Call

Make sure your compression stockings fit properly and are not worn out. If they bunch up or are tighter at the top near the knee than at the ankle, they will not work and, in fact, could cause more damage than if you do not wear them at all. Some doctors advise owning seven pairs – one for each day of the week – so they can be alternated and will last longer.

Raynaud's Disease

When exposed to cold temperatures or intense emotion, people with Raynaud's disease suffer from attacks of cold fingers or toes, along with colour changes and pain. The condition is much more serious than simply having cold hands and feet.

CAUSES

The body's normal response to cold is to reduce blood flow to the extremities by narrowing the small arteries near the skin's surface. In people with Raynaud's disease, that response is exaggerated, drastically decreasing blood in the fingers or toes, ears, lips or tip of the nose. Eventually, small arteries to the extremities may thicken, cutting down the blood supply even more.

Primary Raynaud's disease has no underlying cause, and is the most common form. Secondary Raynaud's, or Raynaud's phenomenon, results from another disease, especially connective tissue or autoimmune diseases such as scleroderma (p.332), lupus (pp.324–5), rheumatoid arthritis (pp.136–9) and Sjogren's syndrome. Other conditions include Buerger's disease, atherosclerosis (pp.230–3) and carpal tunnel syndrome (p.164). Raynaud's phenomenon can also occur after injuries, repetitive trauma, or medications, such as beta-blockers and ergot preparations.

PREVENTION

While there is no known way to prevent Reynaud's disease, there are ways to prevent the attacks that characterize it. Smokers should quit (pp.216–17), because nicotine constricts the blood vessels. Avoid all cold temperatures, including air-conditioning. Put on a hat to prevent heat loss. Wear socks and mittens to bed. Use gloves when handling cold food. Other aids include insulated glasses for cold drinks and chemical warmers worn in mittens, shoes or pockets. Exercise promotes overall well-being, but discuss it first with a doctor.

DIAGNOSIS

During an attack, which can last a minute to as long as hours, the skin in the affected body parts turns white as arteries spasm, then turn blue from lack of blood, and finally red, as blood returns. Cold and numbness occur first, followed by tingling and throbbing.

To diagnose Raynaud's, a doctor may use a cold-simulation test, using cold water or air to induce an attack. To determine whether Raynaud's is primary or secondary, the capillaries in the nailfolds may be examined under a microscope, a test called a nailfold capillaroscopy.

TREATMENTS

Treating the underlying cause of secondary Raynaud's is crucial. Once an attack begins, warm the hands or feet by running warm water over them, soaking them in a bowl of warm – never hot – water, or holding them under the armpits.

• **MEDICATION** Prescription drugs, such as calcium-channel blockers and alpha-blockers, may bring relief by either dilating small blood vessels or acting against the hormone that constricts blood vessels.

• **RELAXATION** Techniques such as biofeedback (pp.504–7) can help avoid attacks triggered by stress or strong emotions. Autogenic training, a self-relaxation procedure, has been found to be effective at reducing symptoms.

• **ACUPUNCTURE** This Traditional Chinese Medicine (pp.446–50) has been shown to reduce the frequency of attacks by 63 percent in a study done during the winter at Hannover Medical School in Germany and published in the *Journal of Internal Medicine* in 1997.

See also: *Lupus, pp. 324–5 • Arthritis, pp.136–9 • Biofeedback, pp.504–7*

WHO IS AT RISK?

The risk factors include:

- Cigarette smoking
- Female
- Age 15 to 40
- Living in a cold climate or cold weather
- Autoimmune diseases such as scleroderma, lupus and rheumatoid arthritis
- Stress

Oedema

An excessive amount of fluid can develop in several locations around the body; the condition is called oedema. One of the most common types of oedema is the painless accumulation of fluid in the ankles, feet and legs, which is sometimes called peripheral oedema. A more dangerous type is pulmonary oedema – a build-up of fluid in the lungs – which can be a sign of a serious condition, for example congestive heart failure.

CAUSES

Numerous conditions and diseases can lead to oedema. Some are serious and even life-threatening; others are not. Congestive heart failure (pp.234–5) is one of the most dangerous. Failure of the left side of the heart can cause fluid in the lungs. Excess fluid can accumulate in the legs as the right side of the heart also starts to fail as well. Chronic lung conditions such as COPD (pp.200–1), and failure of the kidneys or liver can also result in peripheral oedema.

Other conditions that cause oedema include a blood clot, leg infections (either current or a history of one), chronic venous insufficiency (pp.240–2), varicose veins, burns (even sunburn, pp.108–9), thyroid disease (pp.344–7), insect bites or stings (pp.96–7), or starvation or malnutrition. Certain medications may cause leg and ankle swelling, including calcium channel-blockers for high blood pressure, steroids, nonsteroidal anti-inflammatory drugs and antidepressants.

Standing or sitting for long periods of time, especially in hot weather, can result in oedema. Pregnancy, can also cause oedema because of a potentially serious condition known as pre-eclampsia (pp.398–400), or because the uterus may put pressure on the vena cava, the major blood vessel that returns blood from the legs to the heart.

PREVENTION

The best way to prevent oedema is to prevent its cause. That means getting treatment for any diseases or conditions that result in oedema, such as congestive heart failure, high blood pressure and coronary artery disease. Do not smoke, as this contributes to both lung and heart disease, which can cause oedema.

Exercise can improve blood circulation by helping the veins in the legs work more efficiently. Support stockings can also help. When lying down, elevate legs above the level of the heart, unless this causes or worsens shortness of breath. Eat a low-salt diet, because salty foods cause the body to retain fluid. Lose weight if necessary.

When planning a long trip, be sure to drink plenty of fluid, get up and walk around or rotate the ankles and stretch the calves at least once an hour, and do not wear clothing that fits tightly around the waist. People at high risk for oedema may need low-molecular weight heparin (an anticoagulant) given

CAUTION

Get emergency help immediately if you suddenly feel short of breath or have chest pain. Call your doctor if your weight increases by 0.9–1.4 kg (2–3 lbs) in one day, your urine output decreases, you have liver disease and notice swelling in your legs or abdomen, your swollen leg or foot is red or feels warm, you run a temperature, or you are pregnant and have a sudden increase in swelling.

before taking a plane flight.

Proper care of the skin is important in a patient with oedema, because any cuts, scrapes or burns heal more slowly and are more likely to get infected. Avoid exposure to pressure, injury and extreme temperatures. When resting or sleeping use a pressure-reducing mattress, lamb's wool pad or flotation ring.

DIAGNOSIS

Oedema may be classified as pitting or non-pitting. With pitting oedema, when a finger is pressed against a swollen area for five seconds, a dent or pit is left behind that slowly fills in. With non-pitting oedema, no indentation or pit is seen.

Pulmonary oedema (fluid in the lungs) can cause shortness of breath, difficulty breathing when lying flat, waking up at night with a feeling of breathlessness, more shortness of breath than

healing hope I thought swollen ankles were just part of getting older, but the sight of them alarmed my doctor. She immediately ordered several tests. She also told me to follow a low-salt diet, get some elastic stocking – and start exercising, even though I told her my legs ached.

Turned out varicose veins were causing the fluid to accumulate in my ankles. So far, I'm keeping it under control by wearing elastic stockings and walking every day. I've lost weight, and my ankles have slimmed down as well.   Wilma H.

normal during physical activity, and sometimes, significant weight gain. It can be a life-threatening condition and needs prompt medical attention. If severe symptoms develop suddenly, such as pink or blood-streaked sputum, trouble breathing, and blueish or greyish tint to the skin, emergency treatment is needed.

A number of tests may be required to try to pinpoint the cause of the oedema. These may include an electrocardiogram (ECG), transesophageal echocardiography (TEE), echocardiography, cardiac catheterization, X-rays, kidney and liver function tests, urinalysis and blood tests.

TREATMENTS

If the underlying cause of the oedema is diagnosed, it should be treated.

• **DIET** Reduce the amount of salt in the diet to help prevent and treat oedema. Controlling fluid intake and avoiding alcohol may be important as well. Measuring fluid intake and output may be required, alongside weighing daily.

• **MEDICATION** Diuretics may be prescribed to help the body get rid of excess fluid. Other medication treats the underlying causes, such as high blood pressure, congestive heart failure or coronary artery disease.

• **HERBAL MEDICINE** Horsetail (*Equisetum* type) has been used in Europe as a diuretic to treat oedema and is generally considered safe when taken for short periods. With more than 25 varieties of the plant, however, standardization of dosages can be difficult.

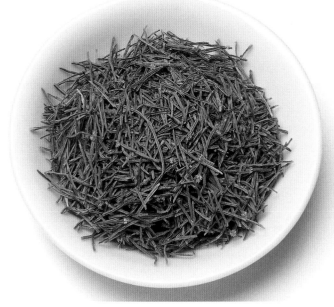

Along with prescription diuretics, there are many herbal extracts that may have diuretic properties. An extract made from a member of a group of herbs called horsetail is one of the most well-known.

See also: *Congestive Heart Failure, pp.234–5* • *Thyroid Disease, pp.344–7* • *Venous Disorders, pp.240–2*

Cardiomyopathy

The word cardiomyopathy means 'disease of the heart muscle'. The condition may progress to heart failure, and the risk of sudden death from a blood clot or irregular heart rhythm is increased, especially because cardiomyopathy sometimes goes undiagnosed. It is the most common cause of sudden cardiac death in people under the age of 30 and the most common reason a heart transplant is needed.

CAUSES

There are three major types of cardiomyopathy, each with their own set of causes.

Dilated Cardiomyopathy

The most common, dilated cardiomyopathy, is more frequent in people aged 20 to 60 and is three times more likely to occur in men. One or more of the ventricles enlarges and fails to pump enough blood. This occurs when heart muscle has been replaced by scar tissue because of reduced blood flow from coronary artery disease or viral infection that results in an acute inflammation of the heart muscle.

Other causes include a bacterial infection, long-standing and poorly controlled diabetes or thyroid disease, some chemotherapy drugs, antidepressants, and abuse of alcohol or cocaine. In rare cases, it results from pregnancy or connective tissue disease such as rheumatoid arthritis.

Blood clots are a risk because they are more likely to form when blood moves slowly, as it does through an enlarged heart.

Hypertrophic Cardiomyopathy

It is estimated that one in 500 people may have hypertrophic cardiomyopathy, although many

do not realize it. More than half the people with it have a family history of the condition. It can be present at birth or acquired later in life. It involves an abnormal thickening and arrangement of the cells of the heart muscle, often the left ventricle, which is the major pumping chamber. As the muscle thickens and later stiffens, the heart loses its ability to pump blood as well as it should.

Hypertrophic cardiomyopathy has caused the sudden death of several athletes due to ventricular fibrillation, a type of arrhythmia (irregular heart rhythm), during physical activity. Anyone with a close relative who has suffered

WHO IS AT RISK?

The risk factors include:
Dilated cardiomyopathy
- Age 20 to 60
- Male
- Coronary artery disease
- Viral infection
- Poorly controlled diabetes or thyroid disease
- Alcohol or cocaine abuse
- Antidepressants
- Some chemotherapy drugs

Hypertrophic cardiomyopathy
- Age 20 to 40
- Family history of hypertrophic cardiomyopathy

Restrictive cardiomyopathy
- Advancing age

healing hope Before I could play basketball in school, I had to get a physical. After my doctor listened to my heart, he looked worried.

After I had an ECG and the more tests, it turned out I have something called hypertrophic cardiomyopathy. It means my heart is enlarged and it could start beating too fast, which can be dangerous. I was taking some pills to keep my heartbeat regular, but they weren't working very well. So last year, I had something like a pacemaker put in my chest, called an implantable cardioverter defibrillator. It shocks my heart to get it back to beating normally when it needs to.

I felt it once when I was exercising and it does feel weird – and scary. But it's also a good feeling, because it's keeping me alive.   *David S.*

from sudden cardiac death should talk to a physician about the possibility they may have hypertrophic cardiomyopathy.

Restrictive Cardiomyopathy

Much less common than other types, restrictive cardiomyopathy results in a heart muscle that is rigid and less elastic, making it difficult for the heart to relax and fill with blood between beats. It occurs more often in older people. The cause may be unknown or may result from the deposit of abnormal proteins, called amyloid, in the heart.

PREVENTION

Take steps to prevent coronary artery disease and high blood pressure. Eat a low-fat, low-cholesterol diet and limit salt intake. Make sure to include plenty of vegetables and fruit in the diet. Exercise for 30 minutes a day, five days a week. Do not smoke, and avoid second-hand smoke. Do not abuse alcohol or cocaine.

Anyone with a family history of cardiomyopathy may want to discuss further measures and screening tests with a doctor. Unfortunately, many cases of cardiomyopathy cannot be prevented.

DIAGNOSIS

Symptoms are similar to those of congestive heart failure (pp.234–5): shortness of breath, chest pain, fatigue, irregular heart rhythm, fluid accumulation in the legs or abdomen and dizziness, lightheadedness, and fainting during exercise.

Several tests may be needed to diagnose cardiomyopathy. Abnormal heart sounds and irregular

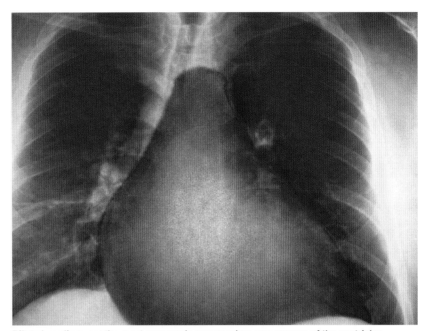

Dilated cardiomyopathy most commonly occurs when one or more of the ventricles of the heart becomes enlarged because of scarring due to coronary artery disease or a viral infection. Many people with the condition do not realize they have it.

heartbeats may be heard with a stethoscope. Imaging tests may include a chest X-ray and an echocardiogram. An electrocardiogram (ECG) measures electrical impulses in the heart. Cardiac catheterization can take a biopsy of the heart for analysis, although this is not usually helpful in planning treatment or revealing the cause. A number of blood tests may be done to rule out systemic diseases.

TREATMENTS

Treatment depends on the type of cardiomyopathy, but the aim is always to prevent heart failure, blood clots and arrhythmia.

• MEDICATION Anti-clotting drugs can help prevent blood clots. Anti-arryhthmic drugs can help correct irregular heartbeats, although sometimes a pacemaker is needed. Vasodilators relax the arteries and lessen the strain on the left ventricle, lowering blood pressure.

A beta-blocker or a calcium channel-blocker is usually prescribed for hypertrophic cardiomyopathy. Angiotensin-converting enzyme inhibitors are key drugs in preventing and treating heart failure.

• CARDIAC DEVICES In some cases, a pacemaker must be implanted surgically to ensure that the heart beats. For those at risk of sudden death from an arrhythmia, a cardioverter/defibrillator (ICD) can regulate too-rapid heartbeats. It is surgically implanted in the chest wall and monitors the heart rate, sending a small electrical shock when the heart rhythm changes.

• SURGERY Surgery can be considered to correct the thickened wall in patients with hypertrophic cardiomyopathy. In some cases, a heart transplant is the only option.

See also: *Congestive Heart Failure, pp.234–5 • Diabetes, pp.338–41 • Thyroid Disease, pp.344–7*

Valvular Heart Disease

The four valves in the heart – aortic, mitral, pulmonary, and tricuspid – act like one-way swinging doors. Two of the valves (the tricuspid and mitral) let blood in; the other two let blood out. Sometimes these valves fail. If a valve leaks so that blood flows in the opposite direction from normal, the condition is called regurgitation (or sometimes 'incompetence' or 'insufficiency'). If the valve does not open enough and partially blocks the blood flow, it is called stenosis, and if it fails to close properly because it moves abnormally, the valve is prolapsed.

CAUSES

Some people are born with congenital valve disorders, while others develop problems later.

Mitral Valve Prolapse

Sometimes called a floppy mitral valve, this condition occurs when the mitral valve separating the left upper chamber (atrium) from the left lower chamber (ventricle) billows out and fails to close correctly when the left ventricle contracts. If it is severe enough to allow blood to leak into the atrium, the condition is mitral valve prolapse with mitral regurgitation (see below).

Although 2 to 5 percent of people have mitral valve prolapse, it is usually harmless and may not even need treatment. Causes can vary; it may be congenital or the result of Marfan's syndrome, a hereditary condition.

Mitral Valve Regurgitation

Mitral valve regurgitation occurs when the mitral valve leaks blood back into the left atrium. When the leakage is severe, it may cause fluid to accumulate in the lungs due to heart failure, or result in potentially fatal arrhythmias (pp.226–8).

Rheumatic fever, a complication of untreated strep throat, was once the major cause, but that is becoming rare in developed nations where antibiotics are used for strep throat. A more common culprit is heart attack, as a result of either dilatation of the heart or damage to the valve structure itself. Other possible causes are endocarditis (p.259), mitral valve prolapse (see above), high blood pressure (pp.236–9), left ventricular enlargement, congenital heart defects, cardiac tumours, and myxomatous degeneration, a connective tissue disorder.

Tricuspid Valve Regurgitation

Blood flows backward into the right atrium from the right ventricle in people with this condition. Enlargement of the right ventricle is the most common cause, often due to emphysema (p.199), pulmonary hypertension or narrowing of the pulmonary valve. Damage to the valve may result from rheumatic fever, endocarditis, use of the diet drug fenfluramine, birth defects, injury or myxomatous degeneration.

Tricuspid Valve Stenosis

In people with this relatively rare condition, the tricuspid valve fails

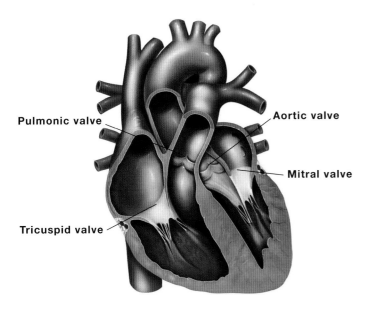

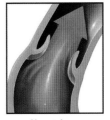 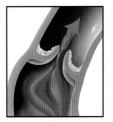

Normal open · **Stenosis**

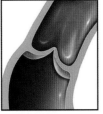 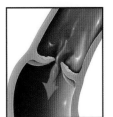

Normal closed · **Regurgitant**

The heart's four valves prevent blood from flowing in the wrong direction as the heart pumps and relaxes. Disorders that affect the valves either cause the valves to close improperly – allowing blood to leak – or to fail to open enough to allow blood to flow freely.

to open as wide as it should and prevents enough blood from entering the right ventricle. The valve has become stiff or developed scar tissue, usually due to medication or rheumatic fever.

Aortic Stenosis

This condition occurs when the aortic valve either narrows or becomes obstructed, blocking blood from flowing from the left ventricle to the aorta, the large artery that travels from the heart. It can cause sudden death from sharp drops in blood pressure. Aortic stenosis may be associated with bleeding in the gastrointestinal tract in the elderly.

A number of health problems can result in aortic stenosis; a common one is rheumatic fever. In some cases, aortic stenosis develops from a birth defect called bicuspid aortic valve, where the aortic valve has only two flaps, instead of three. This condition may not

cause any symptoms for years, but if discovered, should be checked with regular echocardiograms.

Aortic stenosis sometimes shows up after age 60 due to calcification and scarring of the valve. Diabetes, high cholesterol and coronary artery disease are risk factors.

PREVENTION

Many cases of valvular heart disease cannot be prevented, although the widespread use of antibiotics to treat strep throat has drastically decreased the incidence of rheumatic fever. Preventing coronary artery disease, keeping high blood pressure and diabetes under control, and not smoking further reduce the risks.

DIAGNOSIS

Symptoms can vary from none at all to dizziness, fainting, debilitating shortness of breath and chest pain, along with heart palpitations, ultimately leading to death.

Listening with a stethoscope reveals the sounds that are distinctive to the various valvular disorders. A heart murmur is the sound made by blood moving through the heart, either in an abnormal direction, or with abnormal flow in the normal direction.

Mitral valve prolapse creates a characteristic clicking sound, sometimes followed by a murmur. The character of the murmur and its location help determine the valvular problem. With some valvular disorders, there is a vibration or movement of the heart that can be felt with a hand on the chest, and pulses may be

CAUTION

Anyone who has had a replacement valve fitted or who has a valvular disease should take antibiotics as a preventative measure before certain dental, medical or surgical procedures.

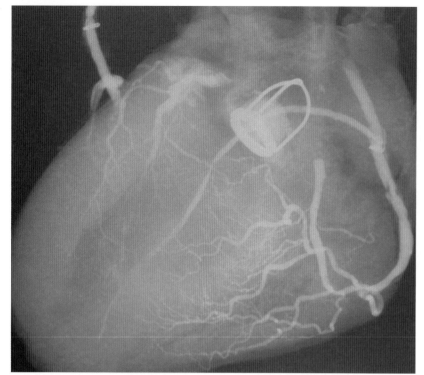

When the heart's valves fail to work properly, heart valve replacement surgery may be needed to prevent hear failure. In this procedure, a mechanical valve (seen above) is implanted in place of the failing valve.

abnormal. Abnormal breath sounds may be heard in the lungs if heart failure has occurred.

Various imaging techniques, such as echocardiogram (which uses ultrasound waves) can create images of the heart, the faulty valve and how much blood is leaking. There are two different ultrasound approaches: transthoracic is done with a probe on the chest wall, and transesophageal uses a probe placed in the oesophagus, requiring sedation. Chest X-rays, colour Doppler echocardiogram, MRI and CT scans, and radionuclide scans may also be done. Additional tests may include a cardiac catheterization.

TREATMENTS

Treatment can range from monitoring to surgery to replace a diseased valve.

• **MEDICATION** Antibiotics can treat and prevent bacterial infections. If congestive heart failure (pp.234–5) develops, it can be treated with a variety of medication. Anticoagulant or antiplatelets, both considered blood-thinners, can help prevent blood clots from forming and reduce the risk of stroke.

• **SURGERY** Repair or replacement of the diseased valve may be necessary. Mitral valves, especially, may be candidates for repair rather than replacement. When valves are replaced, either mechanical or biological valves are used. Mechanical valves, made of plastic and metal, last a long time but increase the risk of blood clots and require the use of anticoagulants, also called blood-thinners. Blood tests must be done regularly to check clotting factors, and the use of blood-thinners does increase the risk of a bleeding stroke. Biological valves, made with tissue from animals (usually pigs) or human cadaver donors, have a low risk of blood clots but wear out and may need eventual replacement, usually after about ten years.

• **NON-SURGICAL PROCEDURES** Balloon valvuloplasty uses a balloon-tipped catheter that is inflated when placed across the valve. It is used with children and with the elderly who are too frail for surgery.

See also: *Arrhythmias, pp.226–8* • *High Blood Pressure, pp.236–9* • *Congestive Heart Disease, pp.234–5*

healing hope

Just walking up the stairs made me short of breath. One day I had such severe chest pain, I thought it was a heart attack. But I got a surprise in the emergency room after they did an echocardiogram. My aortic valve was calcified and scarred, they said. They called it aortic stenosis and explained how this valve was blocking the blood from leaving my aorta.

The cardiologist recommended valve replacement surgery. Even though I am close to 70, I plan to live a long, long time, so I opted for the mechanical valve that is less likely to wear out.

It's been great. I'm back to doing everything I did before: fishing, camping, playing football with my grandson. I do have to get my blood checked once a month. But it's a small price to pay. *Mike D.*

Pericarditis

The pericardium is a thin, two-layered, sac-like membrane surrounding the heart that keeps it in place and protects it from infections. An inflammation, from infection or irritation, of this membrane is pericarditis. It may be acute (starting suddenly and with quite noticeable pain) or chronic (developing slowly without obvious symptoms). It can also be mild or life-threatening.

WHO IS AT RISK?

The risk factors include:

- Viral, bacterial or fungal infections
- History of pericarditis
- Systemic diseases such as lupus
- Tuberculosis
- Injury to the chest

CAUSES

One of the most common causes of acute pericarditis is a viral infection. The condition can also result from tuberculosis (p.212), a bacterial infection, or even an infection caused by parasites or fungi. The list of other causes is long: heart disorders such as a heart attack or myocarditis, autoimmune disorders, rheumatic fever, cancer, leukaemia, kidney failure, hypothyroidism, medication such as anticoagulants, penicillin and phenytoin, or even injuries to the chest. It is not unusual for the cause to be unknown, especially in chronic pericarditis.

PREVENTION

It may not be possible to prevent most cases. Respiratory infections should be treated promptly to prevent complications.

DIAGNOSIS

The chest pain from an inflamed pericardium may feel like a heart attack: sharp and stabbing pain radiating to the neck, shoulder, back or abdomen. Sometimes it may be dull and achy. Sitting up and leaning forward may relieve the pain, but deep breathing and lying flat intensify it. Breathing may hurt so much the patient may hold their chest when breathing. A dry cough, swelling of the ankles, feet, and legs, anxiety, fatigue, temperature and shortness of breath may accompany the condition.

Do not ignore symptoms. Complications include constrictive pericarditis, in which the pericardium permanently thickens and scars, causing it to shrink and contract, which sometimes leads to heart failure. Another serious complication is cardiac tamponade, which results when excess fluid forms in the pericardium and puts pressure on the heart so it does not fill properly.

A doctor listening with a stethoscope will hear the distinctive sounds of a pericardial rub, a scratchy sound not heard in a normal heart. Fluid in the pericardial sac may show up on a chest X-ray, but an echocardiogram, MRI or CT scan are much more sensitive. Ninety percent of patients with acute pericarditis will have an abnormal ECG somewhat similar to that of someone having a heart attack. (Laboratory tests will rule out a heart attack.)

TREATMENTS

Mild cases may get better on their own. Otherwise, treatment is aimed at the underlying cause.

- **MEDICATION** Analgesics relieve pain associated with pericarditis, while NSAIDs such as aspirin and ibuprofen, or corticosteroids if necessary, reduce inflammation. If infection is the cause, antibiotics or antifungal drugs may be prescribed.
- **SURGERY** Fluid can be removed in a procedure called pericardiocentesis. Surgery may also be done, but only if the fluid is rapidly accumulating or if symptoms suggest blood flow is being reduced to the body. Constrictive pericarditis, or chronic or recurrent cases, may require the surgical removal of part of the pericardium, known as a pericardiectomy.

See also: *Tuberculosis, p.212* • *Lupus, pp.324–5* • *Kidney Failure, pp.306–7*

OMEGA-3 SUPPLEMENTS

Omega-3 fatty acids are a type of unsaturated fats known as essential fatty acids because the body cannot synthesize them, so they must be derived from food. They help build cell membranes and the sheaths that encase the nerves, ensure that blood clots properly, and enable muscles to contract and relax. In recent years, research has shown that above and beyond their role in helping the body function normally, some omega-3s also have therapeutic properties. They can dramatically reduce the risk of heart disease and other serious illnesses, as well as relieve the symptoms of various conditions.

The two kinds of omega-3s associated with improved health are docosahexaenoic acid (DHA) and eicosapentaenoic acid (EPA). (The health benefits of alpha linolenic acid, ALA, another kind of omega-3, have not been established.) The best dietary source of DHA and EPA is fish, but are also available as supplements.

Diet and Omega-3s
Omega-3 fatty acids are found in fish, some vegetable oils (rapeseed oil and flaxseed oil), and walnuts. They are especially plentiful in fatty fish, such as salmon, tuna and sardines. Fish is the best food source of omega-3s – the human body cannot get enough of this nutrient from other dietary sources alone. Therapeutic benefits can be derived from eating fatty fish two or three times a week.

Government health recommendations on omega-3 fatty acid intake vary from country to country. The United States recommends 1.6 g (0.05 oz) a day for men and 1.1 g (0.03 oz) for women; Health Canada and the British Nutrition Task Force recommend getting 0.5 percent of daily calories from omega-3s.

Health Benefits
The therapeutic effects of omega-3s came to light after the 1960s, when it was discovered that people who ate a Mediterranean diet – which includes plenty of fish and monounsaturated vegetable oils such as olive oil and rapeseed oil

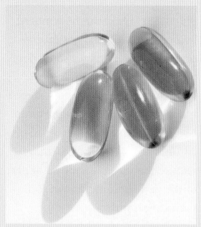
Omega-3s are found in fish such as salmon, as well as some nuts and seeds. They are also available as dietary supplements.

On Call
If you enjoy eating fish enough to have two to three servings a week, you can get the omega-3s you need from your diet. But not everyone likes that much fish, and it can be hard to get enough omega-3s from vegetable sources alone. Consider taking fish oil supplements, but not cod liver oil, which is not recommended as a source of omega-3s. Do not take too much; aim for about 0.03–1.1 g (1–2 oz) a day. Because omega-3s may thin the blood, large amounts can cause problems, especially for pregnant women and people on blood-thinning medication. Larger doses of fish oil are used to treat various problems, including high triglycerides and certain inflammatory conditions, but should only be taken under the guidance of a healthcare professional.

– had a lower incidence of heart disease and other illnesses. Much of the benefit was traced directly to omega-3s.

Specifically, omega-3s lower the levels of triglyceride (fats in the bloodstream) and low-density lipoproteins (LDLs), the 'bad' cholesterol that leads to the formation of fatty deposits in the arteries. High triglycerides and LDLs are both risk factors for cardiovascular disease. Omega-3s also prevent the blood from forming unnecessary clots, which, when they are lodged in blood vessels, can cause heart attacks and strokes. Omega-3s also have anti-inflammatory properties, which may help control the inflammation of plaques that result in the blockage of arteries.

• **CARDIOVASCULAR DISEASE** Numerous studies show that omega-3s reduce the risk of heart attacks, strokes and abnormal heart rhythms, which are a significant cause of heart attacks. In a large, ongoing study of thousands of American doctors conducted by researchers at

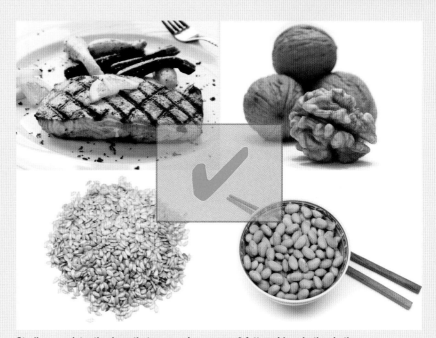

Studies consistently show that consuming omega-3 fatty acids, whether in the diet or by supplements, can help prevent or treat a variety of diseases such as stroke, hypertension, rheumatoid arthritis and heart disease.

Clinical Query

How can I balance the health benefits of eating fish against the health risks from mercury and other poisons found in most fish around the world?

There are many unknowns, but these guidelines can help minimize exposure to the pollutants found in fish.

• Choose fish that is rich in omega-3s but has low levels of mercury: sardines, canned light tuna, salmon, trout and pollock.

• Avoid fish with the highest levels of mercury: shark, swordfish, king mackerel, tilefish and albacore tuna.

• Eat wild fish. Fish caught in the wild have lower levels of pollutants in their bodies than farmed fish, which are raised with pesticides and other chemicals. (For example, farmed salmon is so pink because of added dye.)

Harvard University in the United States, those who ate fish at least once a week had a 52 percent lower risk of heart attack and 43 percent lower risk of stroke than those who ate it once a month or less. This study, known as the Physician's Health Study, found that men who ate fish as little as once a month were 43 percent less likely to have ischaemic strokes (strokes caused by blocked blood vessels leading to the brain) than men who ate fish less often. Similar results have been found for women. With regard to the cardiovascular benefits, it does not seem to matter whether the source of omega-3s is fish or fish oil supplements.

• **ASTHMA** Omega-3s can help prevent asthma attacks by reducing inflammation in the airways.

• **HYPERTENSION** Eating fish or taking omega-3 supplements has been shown to help lower blood

pressure in people with hypertension. It may also prevent the condition from developing.

• **RHEUMATOID ARTHRITIS** Taking omega-3 supplements can relieve joint pain and stiffness from rheumatoid arthritis by reducing inflammation. Some arthritis patients can reduce the number of pain medications they take, and in some cases discontinue them, when they take omega-3 supplements.

• **INFLAMMATORY BOWEL DISEASE** Large doses of omega-3 supplements can ease symptoms of Crohn's disease (pp.266–7), a chronic inflammation of the gastrointestinal tract. These supplements have also been shown to prevent recurrences of Crohn's disease following bowel surgery.

See also: *Asthma, pp.206–9 • Arthritis, pp.136–9 • Cardiovascular Disease, pp.234–5*

Peripheral Vascular Disease

When arteries in the legs becoming clogged or even totally blocked, usually from fatty deposits, the result is peripheral vascular disease. The condition can also occur in any artery outside the heart in which there are circulatory problems.

CAUSES

The major cause of peripheral vascular disease is atherosclerosis, which is the same accumulation of plaque (a sticky substance made of cholesterol, calcium, and fibrous tissue) that can clog the arteries leading to the heart and result in a heart attack. The arteries eventually narrow and stiffen as more plaque forms, which is why atherosclerosis has been called 'hardening of the arteries'.

The condition becomes more common with age, and it is made worse by smoking, which constricts the vessels, and by being over-weight, avoiding physical activity, and diabetes. In fact, smokers and diabetics have the greatest risk of suffering complications, such as gangrene (death of body tissue).

Anyone who has peripheral vascular disease due to plaque should

consider it a warning that the same process may be occurring in arteries leading to the heart and brain, increasing the risk for heart attack and stroke.

In some cases, peripheral vascular disease is the result of a blood clot in an artery, an injury, a tumour or cyst, abnormal growth of muscle in the wall of the artery, or an infection.

PREVENTION

Avoid the conditions that lead to atherosclerosis by following a low-fat, low-sugar diet. Stay active and exercise regularly – at least 30 minutes of walking three times a week. Lose weight, if necessary, with diet and exercise. If you have diabetes (pp.338–41) or high blood pressure (pp.236–9), keep these conditions under control. Perhaps most important, do not smoke.

DIAGNOSIS

Half the people with peripheral vascular disease have no symptoms, probably because about 70 percent of the artery must be blocked before symptoms appear. Somewhere between one-third and one-half of patients experience intermittent claudication, which is muscle pain or cramping, most often in the

WHO IS AT RISK?

The risk factors include:

- Male
- Personal or family history of heart disease or stroke
- High blood pressure
- High cholesterol or trigly-cerides
- High levels of homocysteine, an amino acid
- Kidney disease requiring dialysis
- Obesity
- Sedentary lifestyle

calves but sometimes in the arms, that is caused by the same amount of exercise each time. It disappears with a few minutes of rest.

For some, intermittent claudication is nothing more than a slight irritation, while for others, it is debilitating. Instead of pain, some people with peripheral vascular disease may have tightness, heaviness, cramping, weakness or numbness at the site of the clog. Pain when at rest is a sign of very severe disease.

Listening with a stethoscope may reveal arterial bruits – whooshing sounds that can be heard over the artery – potentially indicating a partial blockage. The pulse may be slower and the blood pressure lower in the lower limbs than elsewhere in the body. High cholesterol may be diagnosed with a blood test. Blocked or clogged arteries can show up on imaging

CAUTION

If you notice sores forming on your toes or feet that do not heal and turn dry, grey or black, see your doctor. You may have tissue that has died, causing a condition known as gangrene, which, if it progresses, may require amputation of the affected limb.

tests such as a Doppler ultrasound exam, an intravascular ultrasound (IVUS), an MRI scan, or an angiography of the arteries in the legs, also called an arteriography.

TREATMENTS

Treatment is aimed at relieving symptoms, improving circulation, and stopping the progression of the disease, as well as decreasing the risk of heart attack and stroke. If the disease is detected early enough, lifestyle changes may be sufficient to manage it. Otherwise, medication and, eventually, surgery may be required.

• SMOKING CESSATION This is the most important lifestyle change (pp.216–17) to make to lower the risk of complications and stop the

disease from getting worse.

• EXERCISE Although exercise such walking often brings on intermittent claudication, exercise will also make it better. Exercise works better than any medication. The key is to do it correctly: walk until the pain begins, then stop and rest. Once the pain subsides, start walking again. Continue this routine for 30 minutes a day, not counting rest periods, to encourage the development of new blood vessels in the affected areas.

• MEDICATION Various medication may be prescribed, such as aspirin and clopidogrel to reduce the chances of developing blood clots, statin drugs to lower blood cholesterol and anti-hypertensives to control high blood pressure.

• SURGERY Several procedures may help correct peripheral vascular disease when it becomes severe. Bypass surgery uses one of the body's own veins or an artificial vein to build a detour around the blocked section of artery, so that blood can reach all tissues. An endarterectomy involves removing the plaque stuck in the inner lining of the artery.

• NON-SURGICAL PROCEDURES Less invasive than surgery, in an angioplasty, a catheter is inserted into the artery and threaded to the area that is blocked. A balloon at the tip of the catheter inflates and deflates several times to push the plaque in the artery out of the way. In some cases, a tiny metal mesh tube called a stent is placed permanently to keep the artery open.

• DIET Follow a low-cholesterol, low-fat diet to prevent additional plaque from forming, and decrease salt intake if high blood pressure is a problem. Diabetics should follow diet guidelines to keep blood sugar levels under control.

• SUPPLEMENTS Taking 80 mg of *gingko biloba* once or twice a day may relieve intermittent claudication. Do not use an extract with gingkolic acid because of the risk for allergic reaction, and be sure to discontinue the supplement at least 36 hours before surgery. Discuss its use with a doctor, because gingko may affect insulin levels and increase bleeding, so caution must be exercised if any blood-thinners, including aspirin, are also being taken.

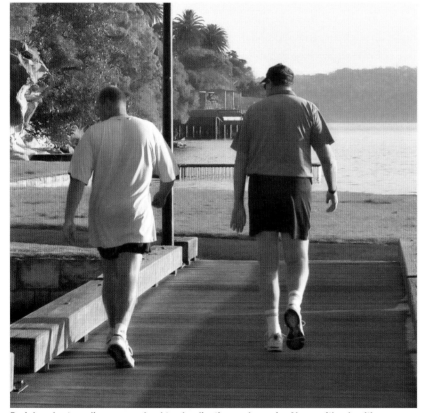

Peripheral artery disease can lead to claudication, or leg pain. Along with a healthy diet and not smoking, it is important to exercise. Begin by walking 30 to 40 minutes a day, resting when leg pain begins and resuming walking when pain subsides.

See also: *Diabetes, pp.338—41 • High Blood Pressure, pp.236–9 • Smoking Cessation, pp.216–17*

Congenital Heart Disease

The word congenital means present at birth. The heart is formed by the end of the second month of pregnancy, so any heart defect develops during the first two months in the womb. One in 120 babies will be born with some kind of congenital heart disease. It is the most common type of major birth defect.

CAUSES

There are many types of congenital heart defects, involving the heart itself, blood vessels, heart valves, and passages between the heart and blood vessels (as outlined below). What causes most of them is a mystery. Heredity or family history may be partly responsible. Babies with other birth defects, such as Down's syndrome, are more likely to also have congenital heart defects.

Having a viral infection during pregnancy, such as rubella (German measles), or taking certain prescription or over-the-counter medication, including accutane and lithium, may cause a problem with the heart's development. Certain risk factors – such as abusing alcohol or illegal drugs during pregnancy – may increase the chances of having a baby with congenital heart disease

Problems with the Development of the Heart

• HYPOPLASTIC LEFT HEART SYNDROME The left side of the heart, along with the aorta, aortic valve, left ventricle and mitral valve, fail to develop. Blood from the lungs flows through an atrial septal defect (see below), while the oxygen-enriched blood from the lungs flows to the aorta through a patent ductus arteriosus (p.257).

• SINGLE VENTRICLE The child is born with just one side of the heart.

Problems with the Blood Vessels

• TRANSPOSITION OF THE GREAT VESSELS The aorta and the pulmonary artery, or great vessels, are reversed, so that blood without oxygen is pumped to the body.

• TETRALOGY OF FALLOT This is a combination of four defects: ventricular septal defect, pulmonary valve stenosis, overriding aorta (the aorta is positioned incorrectly), and right ventricular hypertrophy (thickening).

• TRUNCUS ARTERIOSUS There is one large artery, the truncus, instead of the aorta and pulmonary artery being separate vessels.

• COARCTATION OF THE AORTA The aorta is narrowed, slowing down or even blocking blood flow to the body.

• TOTAL ANOMALOUS PULMONARY VENOUS CONNECTION One or more of the four pulmonary veins carrying oxygen-rich blood from the lungs is connected to the right side of the heart, instead of the left.

Problems with the Heart Valves

• AORTIC VALVE STENOSIS The aortic valve opening is too narrow,

healing hope We counted ten fingers and ten toes when Hannah was born, but we didn't realize that it was what we couldn't see that threatened her life: a condition called coarctation of the aorta, which was reducing the amount of blood to her body. I worried what I had done while pregnant to cause this, but the doctors reassured me it wasn't my fault.

Hannah had a procedure called balloon angioplasty to enlarge the aorta; she'll have surgery when she's older. We're just grateful medical science can help her. Laura H.

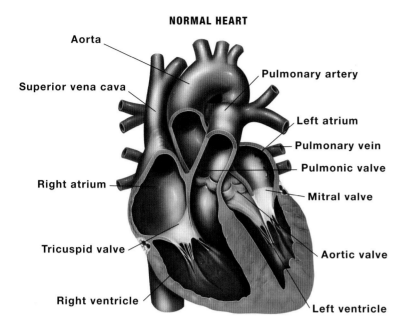

NORMAL HEART

Aorta

Superior vena cava

Pulmonary artery

Left atrium

Pulmonary vein

Pulmonic valve

Right atrium

Mitral valve

Tricuspid valve

Aortic valve

Right ventricle

Left ventricle

Congenital heart disease occurs when the heart fails to properly form during pregnancy. Conditions such as rubella infection or taking certain medication such as accutane and lithium can disrupt the correct development of the heart.

blocking blood flow. The most common cause is bicuspid aortic valve, which means the valve has only two, instead of the normal three flaps. Symptoms may not appear until middle age or older, when the valve narrows.

• PULMONARY VALVE ATRESIA The pulmonary valve has failed to form; instead, there is a solid piece of tissue, so blood cannot pass through to the lungs and become oxygenated.

• PULMONARY VALVE STENOSIS The pulmonary valve, which enables blood to pass through to the lungs, is too narrow, causing the heart to pump harder.

• TRICUSPID ATRESIA The tricuspid valve, between the upper and lower chambers on the right side of the heart, fails to form, so blood flow is blocked by tissue.

• EBSTEIN'S ANOMALY The tricuspid valve has formed abnormally and is incorrectly placed so that it

allows oxygen-poor blood to leak back into the heart, instead of going to the lungs. It may accompany atrial septal defect.

• SUBAORTIC STENOSIS The left ventricle, just below the aortic valve, is narrowed, slowing down blood flow.

Abnormal Passages in the Heart or Blood Vessels

• ATRIAL SEPTAL DEFECT The upper chambers of the heart, called atria, are separated by a wall. In this condition, a hole in the wall allows blood to leak from one chamber to the other.

• VENTRICULAR SEPTAL DEFECT The lower chambers of the heart, called the ventricles, are also separated by a wall. A hole in the wall allows blood to leak from one ventricle to the other.

• ATRIOVENTRICULAR CANAL DEFECT Sometimes called atrioventricular septal defect, this condition is

characterized by a large hole in the centre of the heart between the upper and lower chambers. Abnormal development of the tricuspid and mitral valves may also be present. These defects allow blood to flow abnormally inside the heart.

• PATENT DUCTUS ARTERIOSUS The ductus ateriosus is an open passage between the pulmonary artery and the aorta that generally closes soon after birth. But it fails to close in some children, especially those born prematurely.

• EISENMENGER'S COMPLEX This is a combination of defects that include ventricular septal defect (see below left), pulmonary high blood pressure, passage of blood from right to left side of the heart, an enlarged right ventricle, and sometimes the aorta being in the wrong position.

PREVENTION

Many cases of congenital heart disease cannot be prevented and are simply due to genetics or family history. No mother of a baby born with a heart defect should feel guilty that she did something wrong or failed to do something right during pregnancy.

However, pregnant women can take steps to avoid certain habits and exposures that can increase the risk of a variety of congenital defects. Do not drink alcohol and do not smoke. Avoid exposure to X-rays, unless they are a medical necessity. Talk to a doctor before taking any prescription medication, over-the-counter drugs, or even vitamins and herbal supplements. Vitamins are important during pregnancy, especially folic

On Call

The death rate after surgery for congenital heart defects was around 30 percent in the 1960s and 1970s; now it has dropped to around 5 percent.

acid, but too much of a good thing can be as dangerous as not enough.

DIAGNOSIS

Some congenital heart defects may be diagnosed during pregnancy with the use of ultrasound or within the first few months of a child's life. Other defects do not result in severe disability and may not be noticed until a child is older or, in some cases, after a person reaches adulthood.

Symptoms can include shortness of breath, rapid breathing, a blueish colour to the skin (called

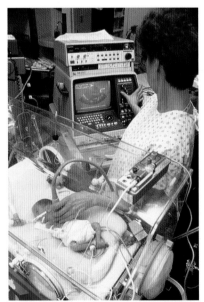

Babies born prematurely are at increased risk of having congenital heart defects because, before 37 weeks, the heart has not completely developed.

cyanosis) and delayed growth. A physician may hear abnormal sounds with a stethoscope in the heart or lungs.

The most commonly used test for diagnosing congenital heart disease is the echocardiogram, which uses sound waves to make images of the heart. It will show structural problems in the heart and how the heart is working. A foetal echocardiogram can be done during pregnancy, usually during the fifth month.

Other tests may include an electrocardiogram (ECG) that measures the heartbeat, a chest X-ray to show the heart and lungs, pulse oximetry to test the amount of oxygen in the blood, and cardiac catheterization, combined with X-rays and injection of a special dye, to show the blood flow in the heart and blood vessels.

TREATMENTS

Treatment depends on the type of congenital heart disease.

• MEDICATION Diuretics remove the build-up of excess fluid that may accumulate in the heart and body. ACE inhibitors relieve some of the workload on the heart. Beta-blockers lower blood pressure and slow the heart rate. Inotropes help the heart pump with more strength. Prostaglandin E1 keeps the ductus arteriosus open until surgery can correct the defect. Digoxin helps the heart pump with more force and helps keeps the heartbeat regulated.

• CATHETERIZATION Some corrective procedures can be done with cardiac catheterization, delaying the need for surgery until the

child is older or even indefinitely. For example, aortic stenosis can be treated by inserting a catheter in the child's groin through blood vessels to the heart. A balloon at the tip of the catheter may be inflated to stretch out too-narrow valves and blood vessels, such as those that characterize aortic stenosis. In some cases, the catheter can be used to repair holes in the interior wall of the heart or to close a patent ductus. The procedure is generally safer for infants and children. In other cases, surgery will have to be done when the child is older or reaches adulthood.

• SURGERY When medication and catheterization are not enough to repair the defect, open-heart surgery may be necessary. Unfortunately, some surgeries will have to be repeated as the child grows. Surgeries can close holes in the heart, using sutures or a patch; repair faulty valves; widen arteries or openings to valves; and put the aorta and pulmonary artery into the correct position.

• HEART TRANSPLANT A child whose heart has several defects that cannot be repaired may be a candidate for a heart transplant.

See also: *Diabetes, pp.338–41* • *Alcoholism, pp.358–60* • *Pregnancy, pp.398–400*

CAUTION

People born with a heart valve defect may need to take antibiotics before certain dental, medical and surgical procedures because they are at increased risk of endocarditis (p.259).

Endocarditis

The endocardium is the lining of the heart; the infection of either the endocardium or the heart valves is called endocarditis. Acute infective endocarditis starts suddenly and can become life-threatening in days, while subacute infective endocarditis develops over weeks or months.

CAUSES

A type of strep bacteria often found in the mouth causes about half of all cases of infective endocarditis. Dental treatment is the most common cause; these bacteria enter the bloodstream when a procedure such as a cleaning makes the gums bleed. Artificial or damaged heart valves, unlike normal valves, provide a sticky surface for the bacteria to adhere to, more easily allowing an infection that can result in endocarditis.

Some surgical and medical procedures, such as a colonoscopy and especially those involving the respiratory, urinary or intestinal tracts, may also release bacteria into the bloodstream that could cause endocarditis. IV drug users are also at risk, usually for the acute form.

PREVENTION

Always tell dentists and other healthcare providers if there are any congenital heart defects, heart valve abnormalities or artificial heart valves. Anyone with these conditions, with the exception of atrial septal defects, should take antibiotics before certain dental, surgical and medical procedures.

Practise good oral hygiene with daily brushing and flossing, and do not avoid regular visits to the dentist.

DIAGNOSIS

The acute form of endocarditis may start suddenly with a high fever of 39°C (102°F), along with a rapid heart rate, fatigue and possibly severe musculoskeletal pain. Damage to the heart valve from the infection can occur quickly and be extensive.

The subacute form may result in fatigue, a mild fever of 37–39°C (99–101°F), a moderately fast heart rate, weight loss, sweating and anaemia that lasts for weeks or months before the heart valves are damaged or an artery is blocked. Large blood clots may break off and cause a stroke (pp.168–9) or heart attack. Tiny blood clots may cause reddish spots in the skin and the whites of the eyes, and streaks of red under the fingernails.

Blood cultures can tell what bacteria is responsible for the infection. A transesophageal echocardiogram, using ultrasound to show the structure of the heart, can reveal endocarditis in more

WHO IS AT RISK?

The risk factors include:
- Artificial heart valve
- Damaged heart valves (by rheumatic fever, for example)
- Congenital heart disease
- Heart valve defects
- Hypertrophic cardiomyopathy
- History of infective endocarditis
- Male
- Over age 60
- IV drug users

than 90 percent of cases. Other tests may include a chest X-ray and blood tests.

TREATMENTS

Treatment often starts with hospitalization to confirm the diagnosis and give antibiotics intravenously. It is important to find the correct antibiotic to treat the specific infection. If not treated, endocarditis can be fatal.

- **MEDICATION** It may take six weeks of antibiotics given intravenously in high doses to cure endocarditis, depending upon the organism causing the infection.
- **SURGERY** Surgery to replace the damaged heart valve may be necessary, due to problems that either start suddenly or that develop slowly over time.

See also: *Stroke, pp.168–9 • Substance Abuse, pp.358–60 • Fever, p.318*

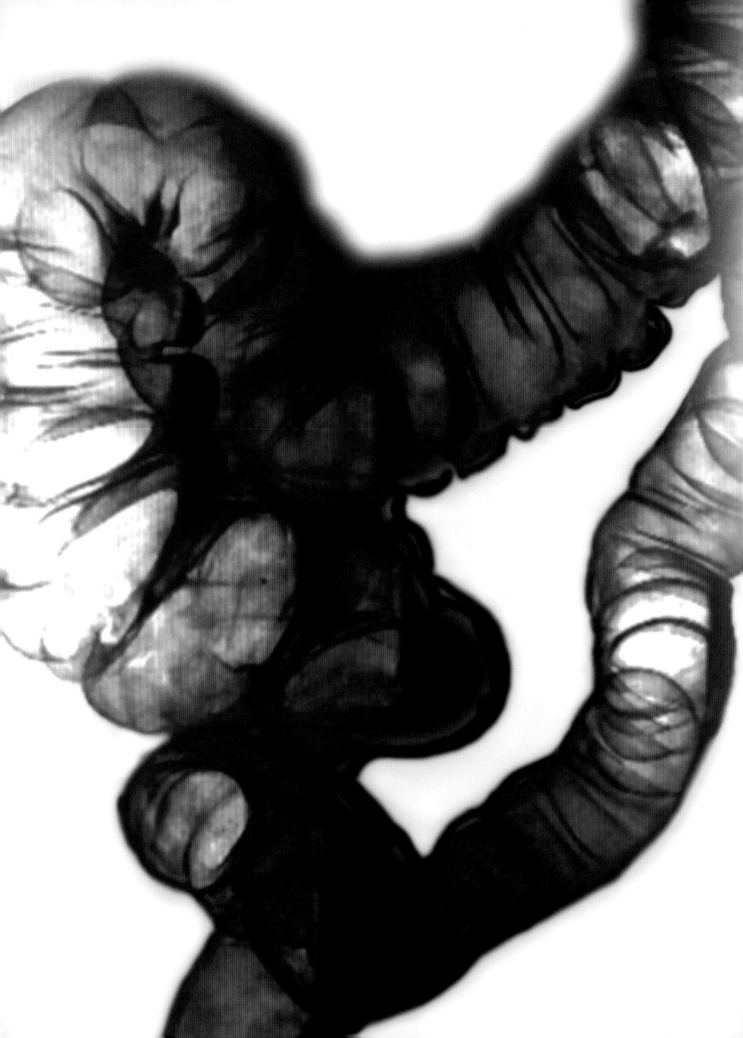

9 DIGESTIVE SYSTEM

Digestion converts food into nutrients that the body uses to burn as fuel and repair itself. Whenever the body is unable to break down food and process those nutrients properly, a variety of serious illnesses can occur. Food allergies are common when the immune system reacts to certain proteins in foods. More serious conditions, such as digestive cancers, occur after years of poor diet, cigarette smoking and heavy alcohol consumption.

Avoiding alcohol and cigarettes can help relieve digestive conditions and can lower the risk of cancer. Regular exercise and a high fibre diet will normally keep the digestive system working properly. Stress reduction techniques, such as yoga and meditation, and herbal supplements can also minimize disorders such as gastro-oesophageal reflux disease and constipation.

Food Allergies & Intolerance

Some people's immune systems over-react to ordinary foods. Responses range from hives, rashes, nausea and diarrhoea, to vomiting and shock. Food intolerance is a pharmacological reaction (like the side-effects of a drug) to chemicals in foods. Food allergy is an immune reaction to food proteins. True allergies can be triggered by even tiny amounts of allergen. The most common allergens are proteins in milk, eggs, peanuts, wheat, soy, shellfish and tree nuts.

WHO IS AT RISK?

The risk factors include:

- Allergies or family history of allergies
- Asthma
- Eczema
- Feeding formula to infants
- Children younger than 6

CAUSES

The antibody IgE (immuno-globulin C) triggers the release of chemicals called histamines. Even a trace of a trigger food may cause a histamine reaction. A child with seasonal allergies, asthma, or eczema is more likely to develop food sensitivity.

PREVENTION

Avoid triggers completely and learn to read food labels, because allergens may be present in a food but not obvious. Milk proteins may be listed as milk solids, whey or caseinate; egg as albumin. Some labels are inaccurate and some products contain unlisted ingredients. Ask restaurant servers about possible hidden ingredients. Educate school personnel, coaches and family members.

DIAGNOSIS

An allergist or immunologist can distinguish between food allergy and intolerance. Controlled food challenges are the primary diagnostic technique. Patients keep a detailed diary of what they eat, then one specific food is eliminated, and if symptoms are relieved, that food is gradually reintroduced to confirm the reaction. Skin-prick allergy testing and blood tests for specific IgE antibodies to food extracts and individual allergens are also helpful.

TREATMENTS

Avoiding allergens is the only treatment. Dietary control is crucial in children, because they are often unable to make their own food choices. If a problem food is ingested, get emergency help. Once shock sets in, it can progress rapidly.

- **EDUCATION** An allergist or immunologist can increase understanding of how to avoid trigger foods. This includes learning about ingredients in packaged foods.

- **PREPAREDNESS** Anyone who has ever gone into allergic shock must avoid even the tiniest amount of the trigger food. Severely allergic people should also carry injectable epinephrine (a drug that treats allergic shock) and wear a medical alert bracelet. Teach spouses, coworkers, teachers, and daycare providers how to inject epinephrine.

See also: Asthma, pp.206–9 • Nausea and Vomiting, pp.274–5 • Diarrhoea, p.268

healing hope It took time to figure out what was causing my stomach trouble. Finally, my doctor suggested an elimination diet. I kept a food diary where I wrote down absolutely everything I ate. It turned out I was allergic to albumin, a protein in egg whites. I had no idea how many foods have albumin in them! My dietitian gave me a list of packaged and processed foods that might contain eggs. Sometimes I take so long reading labels at the store that my little girl starts to fuss. But now I know an egg when I see one. I'm keeping an eye on my daughter, too, just in case she has inherited this allergy from me.   *Mariel M.*

Constipation

When bowel movements are small, hard and dry, this means that someone is constipated. Generally, fewer than three bowel movements a week indicate constipation. Constipation makes bowel movements difficult or painful, and can cause sluggishness and bloating.

CAUSES

Constipation can be caused by inadequate fibre or water in the diet, lack of exercise, irritable bowel syndrome (pp.270–1), pregnancy, ageing, travel, overuse of laxatives, and a suppression of the urge to move the bowels. Some pain relief, antacids, iron supplements, blood pressure medicines, antidepressants, anticonvulsants, antispasmodics and drugs used to treat Parkinson's disease (p.181) can cause constipation, as can a stroke (pp.168–9) or problems with the colon, rectum or intestines.

PREVENTION

Eat a high-fibre diet and drink eight glasses of fluids every day. Exercise regularly. Do not ignore the urge to have bowel movements, as this can lead to not recognizing those physical signals. Avoid overusing laxatives or enemas; they can be habit-forming and hamper the proper functioning of the colon.

DIAGNOSIS

If constipation is severe or long-lasting, or a rectal exam reveals soreness, blood or an obstruction, tests may be required. These might include blood tests or a colorectal transit study, which uses X-rays to reveal a special capsule as it moves through the colon. To rule out colorectal cancer (pp.288–95), tests may include a barium enema, which involves drinking a liquid that is visible on X-rays. Also, a flexible, lighted tube can be used for views of the rectum and lower colon (sigmoidoscopy), or the entire colon (colonoscopy).

TREATMENTS

A healthy diet, with plenty of fresh fruit and vegetables and whole grains, combined with regular daily exercise (which stimulates the bowels), may be all that is needed.
- **NUTRITION** Consume 20–35 g (0.7–1.25 oz) fibre each day, especially from beans, whole grains, bran, fresh and dried fruits and vegetables. Limit the amount of low-fibre foods such as ice cream, cheese and meat. Drink eight glasses daily of water, fruit and vegetable juices, and clear soups.
- **LAXATIVES** A doctor may advise short-term use of fibre supplements, stimulants, stool softeners, lubricants or saline solutions. Laxatives can interact with some medications, however, and prolonged use can make constipation worse.

- **SUPPLEMENTS** Psyllium seeds can be consumed with juice or protein drinks to stimulate bowel action. Ground flaxseed is also an excellent source of fibre.
- **ACUPUNCTURE** This Traditional Chinese Medicine (pp.464–5) can relieve chronic constipation.
- **TIBETAN MEDICINE** Padma lax, a Tibetan herbal formula (pp.460–1), can relieve constipation associated with irritable bowel syndrome (pp.270–1).
- **ABDOMINAL MASSAGE** This traditional therapy (pp.468–73) can be effective alternative to medication.

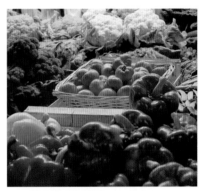

A high-fibre diet that includes fruit, vegetables and whole grains can stimulate the bowel and prevent constipation.

See also: *Irritable Bowel Syndrome, pp.270–1* • *Stroke, pp.168–9* • *Acupuncture, pp.464–5*

WHO IS AT RISK?
The risk factors include:
- Sedentary lifestyle
- Low-fibre, high-fat diet
- Recovering from illness or surgery
- Dehydration

Gastro-oesophogeal Reflux Disease

Persistent heartburn or acid regurgitation are signs of gastro-oesophogeal reflux disease (GORD). When the lower oesophageal sphincter muscle (the ring of muscle that acts like a valve between the oesophagus and the stomach) does not function normally, stomach acid can leak, or reflux, into the oesophagus. This causes the burning sensation of heartburn. Nighttime heartburn can disrupt sleep.

Some people can have GORD without heartburn. It may trigger chest pain, morning hoarseness, difficulty swallowing or a dry cough. Untreated, GORD can cause painful inflammation or scarring of the oesophagus, or lead to a condition called Barrett's oesophagus, abnormal changes in the cells that line the oesophagus, which increases the risk of oesophageal cancer (p.290).

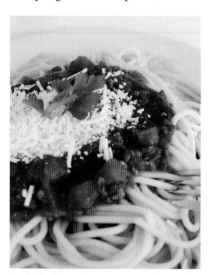

Avoid foods such as tomato sauce and chili, as well as fried or fatty foods, because they can trigger acid reflux.

CAUSES

Several conditions increase pressure on the lower oesophageal sphincter muscle, preventing it from effectively blocking acid from washing into the oesophagus. One is hiatus hernia (p.273), which causes the upper part of the stomach to protrude above the diaphragm (the wall of muscle that separates the stomach from the chest). Many people have hiatus hernia without GORD, however.

A major cause is excess weight, which increases pressure within the abdomen. For the same reason, as well as due to hormonal effects, pregnancy may contribute to the development of GORD.

Certain foods may cause GORD by irritating the oesophagus or relaxing the sphincter. Citrus fruit, chocolate, caffeinated drinks, fatty and fried foods, garlic, onions, mint, and tomato-based foods such as pasta sauce and chilli may cause heartburn. Drinking alcohol and smoking may also be contributing factors.

WHO IS AT RISK?

The risk factors include:
- Family history
- Obesity
- Smoking
- Anti-cholinergic broncho-dilator drugs (used to dilate the bronchial passages)
- Alcohol consumption
- Food allergies
- Asthma

GORD tends to run in families, suggesting a genetic component. It is also often found in people with asthma, although scientists are not sure how the two are linked.

PREVENTION

Help keep the contents of the stomach where they belong by remaining upright after eating for at least three to four hours, and by raising the head of the bed on bed-risers or 15 cm (6 in) blocks. Do not use piles of pillows, because they bend the body and increase intra-abdominal pressure. Wearing loose belts and clothing also reduces pressure that contributes to heartburn.

Avoid foods and drinks that seem to trigger heartburn. Do not eat large meals. Keep portion sizes moderate and eat frequent, smaller meals. Smokers should get help to stop (pp.216–17).

It is also important to reach and maintain a healthy weight (pp.348–9). People with a body–mass index (BMI) over the recommended range for their height are much more likely to develop GORD. (BMI is a ratio between weight and height used to evaluate whether a person is at an unhealthy weight.)

DIAGNOSIS

Anyone using antacids for more than two weeks should see a doctor, who can diagnose GORD by noting how often a patient has heartburn or acid regurgitation – when stomach acid rises into the mouth. Either symptom occurring twice a week or more is considered the threshold for GORD.

In asthma sufferers, a nighttime cough may be a sign of GORD. Symptoms such as hoarseness, laryngitis or sinusitis may also be signs. Damage to tooth enamel or dental erosion from regurgitated acid are signs a dentist may observe. In children and infants, ear pain sometimes indicates GORD.

A gastroenterologist should evaluate possible damage to the oesophagus if symptoms persist. The doctor may recommend tests to reveal problems such as inflammation (oesophagitis), hiatus hernia, narrowing of the oesophagus (stricture), or precancerous cell changes. Tests may include a barium swallow radiograph, in which the patient drinks a barium solution before an X-ray is taken. More detailed images are obtained using upper endoscopy. After the throat is numbed with a spray, a thin, flexible tube carrying a tiny camera, called an endoscope, is inserted. Ambula-

tory pH monitoring measures how often and how much acid rises into the oesophagus. For this test, the patient wears a tiny tube inserted in the oesophagus for 24 hours while going about their normal routine.

TREATMENTS

Lifestyle changes, as described above, and over-the-counter antacids are the first remedies for GORD.
• **MEDICATION** Many over-the-counter antacids use combinations of magnesium, calcium and aluminum salts to neutralize stomach acid. Foaming agents coat stomach contents to prevent reflux. Acid-blockers, available in prescription or over-the-counter strengths, interfere with acid production; these should only be taken for a few weeks at a time, unless under the direction of a healthcare professional. Prescription proton pump inhibitors are highly effective for heartburn and are sometimes taken in combination with acid-blockers. Prokinetics are drugs that strengthen the lower oesophageal sphincter muscle and help the stomach empty more quickly. A doctor may advise a combination of these medications.

A herbal extract preparation may be as effective as cisapride, a heartburn medication. The combination includes extracts of angelica (*Angelica archangelica*), chamomile (*Anthemis nobilis*), lemon balm (*Melissa officinalis*), liquorice (*Glycyrrhiza glabra*), milk thistle (*Silybum marianum*) and peppermint (*Mentha piperita*).
• **SURGERY** If symptoms do not improve over a long period of time, surgery may be the best option. Most surgery to control heart-

burn can be performed laparoscopically. The surgeon passes tiny instruments through a tube that is inserted through the abdomen. The laparoscope can also take tissue samples for biopsy. A procedure called fundoplication, which can be performed laparascopically, wraps the upper part of the stomach around the lower oesophageal sphincter muscle to strengthen it, and can also repair a hiatus hernia.

Two new endoscopic devices are used to treat GORD. One places stitches in the lower oesophageal sphincter muscle to strengthen it, and the other uses electrodes to make tiny cuts in the muscle. As these cuts heal, they create strong scar tissue. A new treatment uses an implant that supports the lower oesophageal sphincter muscle. Through the endoscope, the doctor injects a solution that thickens into a spongy mass, helping the muscle to block stomach acid reflux.
• **ACUPUNCTURE** More research is needed, but stimulation of an acupuncture point (pp.464–5) on the wrist may reduce relaxations of the lower oesophageal sphincter muscle, which can help keep stomach acid from rising into the oesophagus.

See also: *Oesophageal Cancer, p.290* • *Smoking Cessation, pp.216–17* • *Obesity, pp.348–9*

CAUTION

Although GORD can sometimes cause chest pain, it is crucial to have unexplained chest pain evaluated to rule out heart attack.

INFLAMMATORY BOWEL DISEASE

This is the general term for diseases that involve inflammation of the intestines. The two most common forms of IBD, or inflammatory bowel disease, are colitis and Crohn's disease. Colitis means irritation of the large intestine, or colon. Ulcerative colitis occurs when irritation of the top layer of the colon's lining is severe enough to produce ulcers or sores. In patients with Crohn's disease, inflammation and sometimes ulcers extend deep into the lining of the affected organ, usually the lower part of the small intestine, although it can appear anywhere within the digestive tract.

CAUSES

The most common theory is that a virus or bacteria triggers ongoing inflammation. People with IBD also tend to have abnormal immune systems, but it is unclear whether these are a cause or a result of the inflammation. Family history may play a role. Food allergies (p.262) may aggravate IBD symptoms or make underlying intestinal illnesses worse, but they do not cause the problem. Emotional stress or depression can make symptoms worse, but doctors do not know if they contribute to developing IBD. The condition is most common in people between the ages of 15 and 30 or between 50 and 70.

PREVENTION

Although IBD may not be preventable, symptoms can be prevented from getting worse. Periods of remission are common with IBD.

Current or former smokers have a higher risk of developing Crohn's disease, and people who smoke have more severe cases. Relieving stress or depression can help to reduce flare-ups once a person has been diagnosed with IBD.

DIAGNOSIS

Every case of IBD is unique in the severity of symptoms and intestinal damage. The symptoms of ulcerative colitis can range from mild cramping to severe abdominal pain and bloody diarrhoea. Fatigue, loss of appetite and weight loss are also possible. Inflammation in the colon may trigger problems in other areas of the body, in some cases leading to arthritis (pp.136–9), eye inflammation, liver disease, osteoporosis (pp.146–7), skin rashes, or anemia (pp.312–13).

Crohn's disease also causes pain, often in the lower right abdominal area, and diarrhoea. Rectal bleeding, weight loss and fever are also possible. Bleeding may be serious and persistent enough to cause anaemia or even require hospitalization. In affected children, the disease may cause delayed development and stunted growth because the inflammation interferes with the absorption of nutrients and protein. The most common complications of Crohn's disease are intestinal blockage caused by thickening of the intestinal walls, and the formation of abnormal ducts, called fistulas. Other complications include arthritis, skin problems, eye or mouth inflammation, kidney stones (pp.304–5), gallstones (pp.280–1) and liver problems.

Because the symptoms of both diseases can be very similar, a thorough physical examination and a series of tests may be required to confirm a diagnosis of colitis or Crohn's disease. Blood tests may reveal anaemia, which could indicate intestinal bleeding, or a high white blood cell count, which is a sign of inflammation. A stool test can detect bleeding or infection. A doctor may also do a colonoscopy or sigmoidoscopy, which offer direct views of the lining of the colon and small intestine. A

Clinical Query

How do I know if I am dehydrated?

General signs include thirst, less frequent urination, dry skin, fatigue, light-headedness and dark-coloured urine.

In children, the following signs require immediate medical attention: dry mouth and tongue, no tears when crying, dry nappies for three hours or more, high temperatures, listlessness or irritability, and skin that does not flatten when pinched and released.

barium enema X-ray of the colon can reveal ulcers or abnormalities.

TREATMENTS

Dietary changes, supplements (pp.532–41), and medications, or some combinations of these can be effective in helping relieve inflammatory bowel disease.

• NUTRITION Because inflamed intestines can hamper the body's ability to digest and absorb the nutrients in food, restoring and maintaining healthy nutrition is crucial. It is important to try to prevent malnutrition, as well as prevent the dehydration that can result from diarrhoea (p.268). Although no single diet works for everyone, a dietitian's guidance is important to help each individual adopt an appropriate eating plan. This may mean consuming more food or different types of food. In very severe cases, parenteral nutrition, or feeding through a vein while hospitalized, may be needed to allow the intestines to rest or provide extra short-term nutrition.

• SUPPLEMENTS A doctor or dietitian may recommend taking nutritional supplements such as fish oil, which combats inflammation, or probiotics, beneficial bacteria that live in the intestines. Nicotine is effective in relieving mild cases of ulcerative colitis, and may be prescribed as a patch or gum.

• MEDICATION The goals of drug therapy are to induce and maintain remission and to improve the quality of life of people with IBD. Anti-inflammatory medicines called 5-ASAs are usually prescribed first, and are taken either orally, or through a suppository or enema. Corticosteroids may be

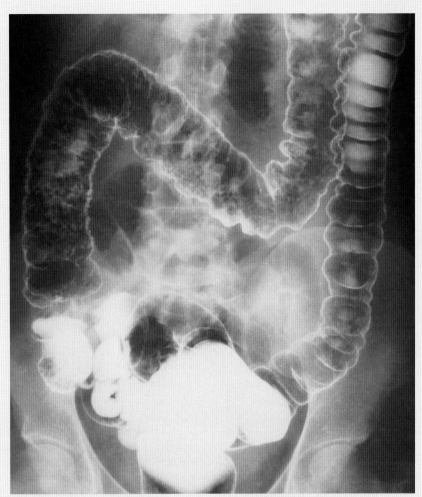

Ulcerative colitis, a condition in which ulcers attack the lining of the colon, can be diagnosed with X-ray images. In this image, the ascending colon (left) shows an abnormal, patchy pattern of mucus, an indication of ulcerative colitis.

used to control inflammation in people who do not respond to 5-ASA drugs. The third line of drug therapy is medication that suppress the immune system, which also help to control inflammation, although they increase patients' vulnerability to infection. Other drugs may be given to relieve pain, diarrhoea or infection.

• SURGERY Most people with ulcerative colitis will never need surgery, but in some severe cases, removal of the colon, called colectomy, may eventually be necessary to cure the disease. Following colectomy, an opening called a stoma

is created where waste can exit the body into a pouch. The majority of colectomy patients are then able to go on to live healthy, active lives. In patients with Crohn's disease, surgery to remove part or all of the intestine may be required to stop uncontrolled bleeding.

• ACUPUNCTURE This Traditional Chinese Medicine (pp.464–5) has been shown to provide additional benefit in mild to moderately active Crohn's disease.

See also: *Kidney Stones, pp.304–5* • *Food Allergies, p.262* • *Traditional Chinese Medicine, pp.446–50*

Diarrhoea

This is a common problem characterized by frequent, watery stools. It can be accompanied by abdominal pain, nausea and sometimes fever. It usually resolves in a day or two, and most bouts last less than four weeks, but some more serious cases can persist and be life-threatening. Prolonged diarrhoea can cause dehydration and also an imbalance of crucial electrolytes (minerals circulating in the blood that regulate potassium and sodium levels), which is particularly dangerous for children and the elderly.

CAUSES

Bacteria in contaminated food or water, parasites and viruses can cause diarrhoea. Other causes include food intolerance (p.262) and certain medications, particularly antibiotics and antacids. Chronic diarrhoea may signal problems such as inflammatory bowel disease (pp.266–7), irritable bowel syndrome (pp.270–1), or Coeliac disease (p.287).

PREVENTION

Wash produce, refrigerate it and eat it soon after it is bought to keep bacteria from growing. Disinfect surfaces used to prepare meats. When visiting areas that lack good hygiene, use no tap water or ice, buy no food from street vendors, and eat no raw fruit and vegetables, unpasteurized dairy products, or raw, rare or room-temperature meat or fish. Probiotic (bacteria that aid in digestion) supplements may help prevent antibiotic-related diarrhoea.

DIAGNOSIS

Because diarrhoea has many causes, a range of tests may be needed, including blood, hormone and stool analyses. Examination of the rectum and colon using a flexible tube called an endoscope (sigmoid-oscopy or colonoscopy) may be done, or the stomach and upper small intestine may be examined. Imaging tests such as barium X-rays or a CT scan may also be required.

TREATMENTS

Lots of fluids and a bland diet cure most cases of diarrhoea. For adults, anti-diarrhoeal medication may help, but avoid products that decrease bowel motility (movement) until a diagnosis is established.
- **FLUIDS** Water is crucial, but contains no electrolytes, so drink salted broth and fruit juices, or sports drinks. Give paediatric solutions that contain electrolytes to children.
- **NUTRITION** Start with the BRAT diet (bananas, rice, applesauce and toast), then gradually add bland foods such as boiled potatoes, crackers, carrots and skinless baked chicken. Avoid milk products for up to a week, because the bowel tends to lose the ability to digest lactose.

For infants, soy-based rather than dairy-based formulas may result in fewer episodes of diarrhoea.
- **MEDICATION** Over-the-counter medication may ease symptoms of viral diarrhoea but making bacteria-related diarrhoea worse by trapping bacteria in the intestines. A doctor can prescribe antibiotics.
- **SUPPLEMENTS** Psyllium, a plant seed that becomes gelatinous when wet, is common in bulk laxatives. It adds bulk to the stool and reduces their frequency.
- **TRADITIONAL CHINESE MEDICINE** Acupuncture (pp.464–5) and moxibustion (p.442) show promise in treating chronic diarrhoea.

See also: *Food Intolerance, p.262 • Inflammatory Bowel Disease, pp.266–7 • Irritable Bowel Syndrome, pp.270–1*

WHO IS AT RISK?

The risk factors include:
- Food- or water-borne bacterial infection
- Viral infection
- Antibiotics, blood pressure medication and antacids
- Inflammatory bowel disease
- Irritable bowel syndrome
- Coeliac disease
- Thyroid, adrenal and pancreatic disorders

Hepatitis

This is actually a family of viruses, some chronic and some acute. All can produce nausea, vomiting, loss of appetite, abdominal pain, jaundice, fatigue and diarrhoea. Dark, tea-coloured urine and joint pain are additional symptoms. Hepatitis A (HAV) causes an acute, flu-like illness lasting for weeks or months. Once it is gone, re-infection is impossible. Although most adults can fight off hepatitis B (HBV), in some it becomes chronic and may eventually cause cirrhosis, liver cancer or liver failure. Hepatitis C (HCV) persists in most cases; liver damage may appear years after infection.

HCV and hepatitis D (HDV) may be similarly life-threatening as other chronic hepatitis infections. HDV can only occur in conjunction with HBV, or be acquired after a person has had HBV for some time. Hepatitis G (or GBV-C) is a virus related to hepatitis C. Hepatitis G can lead to chronic infection in 15 to 30 percent of adults; long-term outcomes are not known.

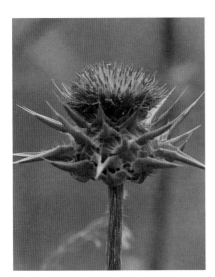

People with chronic hepatitis who take milk thistle (*Silybum marianus*) have seen improvement in liver tests.

CAUSES

HAV is spread by physical contact with objects or foods touched by an infected person who has not washed their hands after using the bathroom or changing nappies. It can also be transmitted through oral or anal sex, and is common in areas with poor sanitation.

HBV is spread by unprotected sex with, or sharing a razor or toothbrush with, an infected person; intravenous drug use; or exposure to infected body fluids. Infected mothers can pass it to their babies.

HCV is transmitted by an infected needle or other sharp object. People who received a blood transfusion or an organ transplant before July 1992, when a reliable test was developed, may have been infected.

HDV enters the body through unprotected sex with an infected partner, shared needles, and needle sticks in health care settings. It can be passed from an infected mother to her baby at birth.

TREATMENTS

Rest, nutrition and hydration are usually sufficient to treat hepatitis A.

• **MEDICATION** Chronic infections with HBV and HCV respond to drugs, particularly interferon, a genetically engineered protein that triggers healthy cells to fight infection.

• **HERBAL MEDICINE** People with chronic hepatitis who take milk thistle (*Silybum marianus*) have seen improvement in liver tests.

• **TRADITIONAL CHINESE MEDICINE** Anti-viral herbs are used extensively to treat liver disease in China, and they may effectively suppress HBV.

• **VACCINATION** Vaccinating all infants against HBV and treating those exposed in the womb with immunoglobin will substantially reduce their risk of developing HBV.

• **LIVER TRANSPLANT** When advanced hepatitis causes liver failure, a liver transplant may be the patient's only chance for survival.

See also: *Traditional Chinese Medicine, pp.446–50* • *Nausea and Vomiting, pp.274–5* • *Liver Cancer, p.389*

WHO IS AT RISK?

The risk factors include:

• Contact with contaminated food, water, or objects (HAV)
• Sexual transmission from an infected partner (HAV, HBV, HCV, HDV)
• Needle-sharing or a needle stick (HBV, HCV, HDV)
• Infected mother (HCV, HDV)

Irritable Bowel Syndrome

This is not a disease, but a disorder in the way the bowel functions. Irritable bowel syndrome, or IBS, produces a collection of symptoms, the most common of them being chronic abdominal pain, bloating, wind, alternating bouts of diarrhoea and constipation, and mucus in the stool. Some people with IBS also have other gastrointestinal symptoms such as wind, belching, heartburn, acid reflux, difficulty swallowing and nausea.

WHO IS AT RISK?

The risk factors include:

- Adolescence and early adulthood
- Female
- Emotional stress
- Family history of IBS

IBS is a very common condition that usually begins in late adolescence or early adulthood, often during periods of emotional stress, and more often among women. In most cases it is mild and does not significantly hamper quality of life. In a small percentage of people, however, it can cause serious discomfort or distress, with symptoms persistent and severe enough to interfere with self-esteem, social life and the ability to work or travel.

CAUSES

There is no anatomical cause or defect that fully explains IBS. However, researchers have found heightened intestinal sensitivity in some individuals that can increase the pain caused by normal amounts of wind, and abnormally strong bowel contractions that alter normal patterns of bowel movements, producing constipation, diarrhoea, or both.

Although the causes of IBS are not clear, triggers for the symptoms can often be identified. These triggers will vary from person to person. Many people are

reactive to emotional upset, diet, drugs or hormones, which may either trigger or aggravate their symptoms. Some people with IBS also have panic disorder or depression. However, emotional stress, conflict and periods of hormonal change such as premenstrual syndrome (pp.356–7) do not always coincide with symptoms. Eating will often trigger symptoms, but it remains unclear whether this is because of the specific food eaten or the actual process of eating, because chewing stimulates the colon.

PREVENTION

There is no known way to prevent IBS from starting, but there are many self-care measures that can help to control and minimize symptoms. Once diagnosed, learning to manage stress is an important factor in control, as is avoiding any particular food that seems to trigger symptoms.

DIAGNOSIS

It is important to see a doctor if there has been a persistent change in bowel habits or other signs of

IBS, so that more serious conditions of the colon can be ruled out, such as colitis, Crohn's disease (pp.266–7), and colon cancer (pp.288–95). For a formal diagnosis of IBS, abdominal pain and diarrhoea or constipation should be present at least 12 weeks and at least two of the following are also present: a change in frequency or consistency of stool; straining, urgency, or a feeling that the bowels do not empty completely; mucus in the stool; and abdominal bloating.

Because IBS usually involves no physical abnormalities of the colon, diagnosis often includes eliminating other conditions. To detect possible lactose intolerance, for example, a doctor may recommend eliminating all dairy products from the diet for several weeks to see if symptoms disappear.

The doctor will also do a rectal digital examination, a pelvic examination for women and take a stool culture. A sigmoidoscopy is also an important aid in diagnosis. In this test, a flexible tube is inserted into the lower part of the bowel, and the bowel is filled with air. This

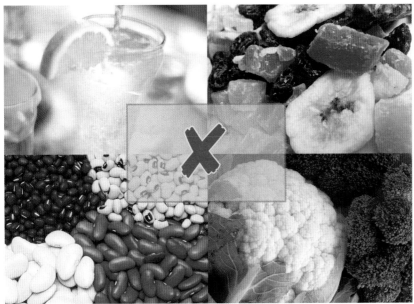

Irritable bowel syndrome is a disorder marked by a change in bowel function and is often caused by stress or diet. Avoiding certain foods, such as carbonated drinks, uncooked or dried fruit, beans, broccoli, cauliflower and raw vegetables, can minimize wind and bloating.

usually triggers spasm and pain in people who have IBS. A colonoscopy (examination of the entire colon), barium enema X-ray or biopsy of intestinal tissue may occasionally be needed, but only when less invasive studies have revealed some abnormality.

TREATMENTS

Changes in diet can help many people with IBS. Supplements (pp.532–41) or medication may also be needed to ease symptoms and relieve the discomfort.

• **NUTRITION** To curb bloating and flatulence, reduce the consumption of foods that cause wind, such as beans, cabbage, uncooked or dried fruit, raw vegetables, broccoli, cauliflower and carbonated drinks. Abdominal pain may be eased by sticking to a low-fat, high-protein diet.

• **FIBRE** Increasing dietary fibre with bran or a psyllium-based supplement can prevent constipation by adding bulk to stool. Small amounts of fibre can also help reduce diarrhoea associated with IBS by absorbing water and making stool more solid. Overuse of fibre supplements can lead to bloating and diarrhoea, however, so it is important to adjust the dose based on each individual's response.

• **SUPPLEMENTS** Peppermint oil, also known as an aromatic oil or carminative, has been shown to relax the muscle contractions that cause abdominal cramping. People with IBS may lack sufficient amounts of probiotics – beneficial bacteria that normally live in the intestine. Supplements containing these are believed to help ease many intestinal symptoms.

• **COUNSELLING AND HYPNOTHERAPY** Many forms of psychotherapy can provide relief from IBS. Cognitive or behavioural therapy, relaxation or biofeedback training (pp.504–7), and hypnotherapy (pp.508–13) have all been shown to help.

Individuals can benefit from one or a combination of these.

• **RELAXATION THERAPIES** Learning to deal with stress by achieving regular, deep relaxation through yoga (pp.476–9), massage (pp.468–73) or meditation (pp.514–19) can significantly reduce the frequency and intensity of IBS symptoms.

• **EXERCISE** Regular exercise relieves both anxiety and depression and also stimulates normal bowel contraction patterns.

• **MEDICATION** When IBS is accompanied by depression, antidepressant medication may be given. Tricylic antidepressants have the added benefit of calming the intestines. If pain and constipation are particular problems, SSRI antidepressants may be more effective. Some people with IBS need anticholinergic medicines, which affect the nerves that cause painful bowel spasms. Others may need occasional over-the-counter anti-diarrhoeal drugs. More powerful medication is available, but, because of its potential side-effects, it should be prescribed only by a gastroenterologist who specializes in IBS.

See also: *Crohn's Disease, p.266 • Colon Cancer, p.288 • Premenstrual Syndrome, pp.386–7*

On Call

If cramping or bloating occur most often after consuming dairy products, caffeine or sweets, the problem may not be IBS but a food intolerance to lactose (a milk sugar), caffeine or artificial sweeteners.

Gastroenteritis

This condition is usually caused by an infection or irritation of the stomach or intestines. Gastroenteritis often causes diarrhoea (p.268), nausea, vomiting, bloating and abdominal cramping. There are two primary forms: viral and bacterial. Viral gastroenteritis, or stomach flu, is the most common. It may persist up to a week and be accompanied by a fever, weakness and muscle aches. Bacterial gastroenteritis can last as briefly as 24 hours, until the body clears the infectious agent through vomiting and diarrhoea. Intestinal parasites can result in gastroenteritis that lasts much longer.

WHO IS AT RISK?

The risk factors include:

- Travel in areas with poor public hygiene
- Exposure to intestinal flu
- Foods prepared in unsanitary conditions
- Eating raw shellfish
- Camping and hiking

CAUSES

Viral gastroenteritis is spread by faecal contamination of food or water. A variety of viruses, chiefly rotavirus and the Norwalk virus, cause intestinal flu. Rotavirus is very common and is widespread in daycare centers and other group settings. The Norwalk virus is found in raw shellfish and salads, and is common in lakes and swimming-pools.

The most common cause of bacterial gastroenteritis is food or water contaminated by *E. coli*, *staphylococcus*, or salmonella. Bacteria like *staphylococcus* can also produce toxins in foods that are improperly cooled after cooking, such as custards and similar items in self-serve salad bars. These toxins may cause a form of gastroenteritis known as food poisoning.

PREVENTION

To prevent viral gastroenteritis, wash hands regularly, particularly after using the toilet or changing nappies. Disinfect shared children's toys. Avoid raw shellfish and prepare food hygienically: disinfect surfaces used to prepare meats and fish, and wash salad greens and vegetables. To deter bacterial gastroenteritis, when in areas where public hygiene is lax, avoid raw foods and foods prepared by street vendors, and drink purified water. Hikers and campers should carry purification tablets to clear parasites from drinking water. Probiotic supplements may help prevent acute viral gastroenteritis and some bacterial infections.

DIAGNOSIS

There is no specific test for most types of viral gastroenteritis. In some cases, a doctor may recommend a stool test for rotavirus.

TREATMENTS

Gastroenteritis normally resolves itself over time without specific treatment. Calming the digestive system and rehydrating are essential.

- **NUTRITION** While acute symptoms last, avoid eating. If you are vomiting, sip clear liquids or suck ice chips. Gradually reintroduce bland foods, such as bananas and rice, as symptoms subside. Avoid dairy products, caffeine and alcohol.

- **HYDRATION** Especially for infants, children, the elderly and people with compromised immune systems, it is critical to replace fluids lost to diarrhoea and vomiting. Be alert for symptoms of dehydration (see the Clinical Query on p.266). Give children oral electrolyte solutions. In severe cases, intravenous fluids and hospitalization may be required. Untreated severe dehydration is life-threatening.

- **SUPPLEMENTS** Boosting the beneficial bacteria that live in the intestines with probiotics may help relieve symptoms of acute viral gastroenteritis and some types of bacterial gastroenteritis.

See also: *Nutritional Supplements, pp.532–43 • Nausea and Vomiting, pp.274–5 • Fever, p.318*

Hiatus Hernia

A muscular wall called the diaphragm separates the oesophagus and the stomach. In hiatus hernia, the stomach bulges up into the chest through the opening in the diaphragm through which the oesophagus passes.

Most people with hiatus hernia have no symptoms and require no treatment. With a parasophageal hernia, however, the stomach squeezes up beside the oesophagus, in some cases causing strangulation in which the stomach's blood supply is cut off. Symptoms of hiatus hernia such as chest pain may be confused with heart attack.

CAUSES

There is no single cause of hiatus hernia, although a congenital weakness in the wall of the diaphragm may encourage a hernia to develop. An injury may contribute, as can increased pressure in the abdomen caused by pregnancy and delivery, or from straining during coughing or bowel movements. Smokers, overweight people and those over the age of 50 are more likely to develop hiatus hernia.

CAUTION

A strangulated hernia or obstruction is a medical emergency. Call the doctor immediately if you have been diagnosed with hiatus hernia and experience:
• Nausea and vomiting
• Inability to have a bowel movement
• Inability to pass wind

Hiatus hernia is often associated with heartburn and gastro-oesophageal reflux disease (GORD, pp.264–5), but one condition does not cause the other.

PREVENTION

Not smoking, maintaining a healthy weight, and a high fibre diet may prevent hiatus hernia. High-fibre foods reduce constipation (p.263) and minimize the strain of passing hard stools.

DIAGNOSIS

Hiatus hernia is usually diagnosed by a barium swallow X-ray, in which the patient drinks a barium solution before X-rays are taken, which reveals the structures of the upper digestive tract. More precise images of a hiatus hernia can be obtained through upper endoscopy. After the throat is numbed with an anaesthetic spray, a thin, flexible tube called an endoscope is inserted, carrying a tiny camera that relays images of the stomach and oesophagus to a computer monitor.

TREATMENTS

Symptoms of hiatus hernia may be relieved by several treatments for GERD (p.264–5). Over-the-counter antacids, herbal extracts

WHO IS AT RISK?

The risk factors include:
• Obesity
• Pregnancy and delivery
• Chronic constipation
• Chronic cough
• Abdominal injury

and prescription proton pump inhibitors may be effective. There is also evidence that acupuncture can help with symptoms of GORD.

An unusually large hernia or one that might become strangulated may require surgery. Most hiatus hernias can be repaired with laparascopy, in which a thin, flexible tube is passed through a small incision. Tiny instruments are passed through the tube to repair the hernia.

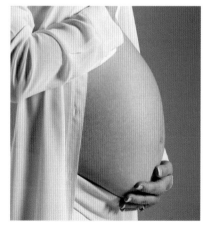

A hiatus hernia can be caused by increased pressure in the abdomen, which can result from pregnancy and delivery.

See also: *Constipation, p.263 • Gastro-oesophageal Reflux Disease, pp.264–5 • Obesity, pp.348–9*

Nausea & Vomiting

The unpleasant sensation of nausea, which is sometimes accompanied by feelings of clamminess or dizziness, is familiar to most people. Often, but not always, nausea leads to vomiting, when the contents of the stomach are expelled through the mouth.

CAUSES

There are many conditions that can cause nausea and vomiting. An ordinary problem in the stomach or intestines, such as overeating, indigestion, or food poisoning (p.262), often triggers the sensation of nausea or leads to vomiting. When nausea or vomiting happens regularly during the first trimester of pregnancy, it is called morning sickness.

Sometimes nausea is related to balance problems originating in the inner ear, which produce vertigo, seasickness or motion sickness. Intense pain, such as from a migraine headache, can cause nausea.

Certain smells or odours can cause the stomach to rebel, as can intense emotional stress. Nausea and vomiting can be side-effects of chemotherapy, gallbladder disease (pp.280–1) and various viruses.

Most of the time nausea and vomiting are self-limiting, but in some cases they may reflect a serious problem such as a heart attack, concussion or injury to the brain, bulimia, encephalitis, meningitis, a kidney or liver disorder, an intestinal blockage, appendicitis or a brain tumour.

PREVENTION

It may not be possible to prevent some episodes of nausea and vomiting. Avoid overeating and maintain a healthy, low-fat diet to keep the stomach more calm. Eating small meals throughout the day rather than three larger meals also helps prevent nausea, as does eating slowly and avoiding hard-to-digest foods. Sometimes nausea can be prevented by eating cold or room-temperature meals to avoid the smell of hot foods.

Proper food hygiene will help to prevent food poisoning, which is often caused by unwashed hands transferring faecal contamination to foods or beverages. Many intestinal viruses can also be avoided by regular hand-washing.

To help prevent morning sickness, a high-protein snack before bed and a few crackers first thing in the morning can help to settle the stomach.

DIAGNOSIS

When nausea begins shortly after a meal, it may indicate a peptic (gastric) ulcer or an emotional disorder such as bulimia. Food poisoning normally produces nausea and vomiting one to eight hours after the contaminated food or water is consumed – or longer in cases of some food-borne bacteria such as salmonella.

Because nausea and vomiting are symptoms, however, rather than a disease or condition to be diagnosed, no tests are required to confirm them. If nausea lasts more than a week or if pregnancy is possible, a doctor should be consulted to investigate any underlying cause.

TREATMENTS

Normally, nausea and vomiting will subside within six to twenty-four hours and can be treated successfully at home. Weathering the symptoms with comfort measures may be all that is needed.

• NUTRITION Clear or ice-cold sweetened liquids, such as soft drinks and fruit juice (other than

WHO IS AT RISK?

The risk factors include:
- Chemotherapy
- Pregnancy
- Viral infection
- Food poisoning
- Motion sickness
- High fever
- Overeating
- Alcohol binges
- Migraine headache
- Gallbladder disorders
- Intestinal blockage

citrus juices, which are too acidic) are more likely to stay down, particularly if taken slowly, in small sips. Small meals of light, bland foods, such as non-greasy crackers or plain bread, are less disturbing to an upset stomach; fried, greasy or sweet foods should be avoided. Eating slowly and smaller, more frequent meals is advised. Not mixing hot and cold foods also helps soothe the stomach. Resting after eating, either sitting or lying propped up, may prevent nausea from escalating. Brushing teeth right away is not advised, as the strong flavours in toothpaste may trigger nausea. If nausea has progressed to vomiting, solid food should be avoided while it lasts. It is best to temporarily stop taking oral medication that might irritate the stomach. Gradually increase the intake of clear liquids.

• MEDICATION Nonprescription drugs can help relieve nausea and vomiting, but should not be taken if food poisoning is suspected because vomiting is one way the body works to rid itself of the toxin. Products containing bismuth subsalicylate relieve nausea by coating the stomach lining. They are not appropriate for anyone who is allergic to aspirin, and should not be given to children who may have the flu or chicken pox, as this increases their risk of developing Reye's syndrome. Antihistamines help to control motion sickness by dulling the inner ear's sense of movement. They may cause drowsiness, which can affect the ability to drive or operate machinery. For nausea after surgery, aprepitant, a new class of drug, may be more effective than the drugs given traditionally.

• GINGER Powdered ginger, ginger tea or candied ginger may help prevent nausea. For morning sickness, it is safe to take ginger in amounts recommended by a doctor for up to five days, but some research indicates possible risk of damage to the foetus or miscarriage if too much is taken or if it is taken for a longer period. Ginger may reduce vomiting from motion sickness, but does not eliminate nausea. It may help to relieve nausea that often follows chemotherapy, but there are also effective prescription drugs for this purpose, so the use of ginger should be discussed with an oncologist (cancer specialist).

• ACUPRESSURE, ACUSTIMULATION, ACUPUNCTURE Mild nausea may be relieved by pressing firmly on a specific place, called the Neiguan point (P6), on the underside of the wrist. Acustimulation, which involves the mild electrical stimulation of pressure points using acupuncture needles or battery-powered appliances worn on the body, may also help to relieve nausea. Acupuncture (pp.464–5) is often used to relieve the nausea and vomiting associated with chemotherapy or anaesthesia.

• HYPNOSIS Although it is so far unproven, there is some scientific interest in whether the use of self-hypnosis or similar techniques, such as relaxation training or biofeedback (pp.504–7), can help alleviate nausea.

On Call

It is important to avoid dehydration by drinking at least six to eight glasses of water daily, but to prevent nausea it is best to drink between meals rather than while eating.

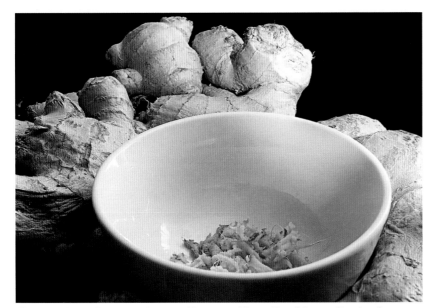

Ginger has been shown to reduce vomiting caused by motion sickness. Powdered ginger, ginger tea or candied ginger can help prevent nausea, but may not eliminate it. A doctor can advise you on taking ginger during pregnancy for morning sickness.

See also: *Food Poisoning, p.262* • *Gallbladder Disease, p.280–1* • *Acupuncture, p. 464–5*

Ulcer

Sores that develop on the walls of the stomach are gastric ulcers, and those on the upper part of the small intestine are duodenal ulcers. A gastric ulcer usually becomes more uncomfortable after eating or drinking. Duodenal ulcer pain improves while eating or drinking, but gets worse afterwards. Ulcer pain may be severe enough to awaken a sleeping person. Other symptoms include feeling full rapidly after eating, abdominal bloating, stomach pain, vomiting and weight loss.

WHO IS AT RISK?

The risk factors include:

- *H. pylori* infection
- Anti-inflammatory medications

CAUSES

Many ulcers are caused by infection with *Heliobacter pylori* bacteria. Other causes include long-term use of nonsteroidal anti-inflammatory drugs (NSAIDs) such as aspirin, ibuprofen, naproxen sodium, ketoprofen, and some prescription arthritis drugs.

PREVENTION

H. pylori infection is not easily prevented because it is prevalent, particularly in areas with poor hygiene. Most prevention strategies also aim to keep existing ulcers from getting worse. Quitting smoking helps (pp.216–17). Avoiding alcohol decreases the risk of developing ulcers and also reduces pain from existing ulcers. Although most people can take NSAIDs safely, a doctor can recommend additional medication to offset any irritation that may be caused by long-term use.

DIAGNOSIS

Endoscopy is the most current test for ulcers. A flexible, lighted tube is passed down the throat to the stomach and duodenum to relay images to a computer monitor. Tiny instruments are threaded through it to retrieve biopsy and culture samples. Alternatively, X-rays may be taken after the patient drinks a solution that highlights the stomach and duodenum on X-ray film.

Occasionally, an ulcer bleeds, breaks through the digestive tract wall, or obstructs food from leaving the stomach. Seek help immediately if blood or food eaten hours or days earlier is vomited, if dizziness or weakness is experienced, if there is blood in stools, if weight loss cannot be stopped, or if pain is spreading to the back.

TREATMENTS

Eliminating the *H. pylori* infection, healing the sores and avoiding digestive irritants are the focus here.

- **MEDICATION** *H. pylori* infection is treated with antibiotics taken for two to three weeks. Medication to reduce stomach acid is usually prescribed, and sometimes a coating agent, as well, to protect the ulcer until it heals.
- **NUTRITION** Some foods make ulcers worse in some people. It may be advisable to avoid spicy foods, coffee, tea, chocolate, meat extracts, black pepper, chilli powder, mustard seed and nutmeg.

See also: *Smoking Cessation, pp.216–17* • *Back Pain, pp.132–3*

---

healing hope I've always been a worrywart. My friends would always to say to me, "You'll get an ulcer if you keep that up." They were right. I did need to reduce my stress, and I did get an ulcer. I thought that meant I'd be stuck with a boring diet the rest of my life. But when I talked to my doctor, she suggested I undergo a few tests. It turned out I had a bacterial infection and all I needed was antibiotics, plus a little time to heal. I'm glad I saw my doctor, and especially glad I can still eat my grandmother's spicy meatballs. *Willam G.*

Gastritis

An acute or chronic inflammation of the stomach lining is called gastritis. Normally, it is mild enough to cause only minimal symptoms. These may vary, depending on the cause of the irritation. Some cases result from ulcers (p.276), which will cause more or worse symptoms. Abdominal upset or pain are the most common signs.

Gastritis may also cause belching, abdominal bloating, nausea and vomiting, or sensations of fullness or burning in the upper abdomen. In severe cases it may lead to serious bleeding, which can result in blood in vomit or stools.

CAUSES

The most common cause of chronic gastritis is infection with *Heliobacter pylori* bacteria, which is also the primary cause of ulcers. Other major causes of gastritis are drinking too much alcohol, smoking and long-term use of non-steroidal anti-inflammatory drugs (NSAIDs) such as aspirin and ibuprofen. Gastritis may also develop after severe stresses such as major surgery or injury, burns or serious infections. Other diseases, including Crohn's disease (pp.266–7), pernicious anaemia, autoimmune disorders and chronic bile reflux can cause gastritis. It may also be an after-effect of radiation treatment for cancer.

PREVENTION

Avoiding alcohol and smoking helps prevent gastritis. When taking anti-inflammatory medicines or corticosteroids over a long period, it is important to consult a doctor about ways to guard against stomach damage. A change in medication or additional medication to protect the stomach lining may be advised. Avoid foods that have proven to be irritating to the stomach. These may include fatty, spicy or very acidic foods or drinks.

DIAGNOSIS

A stool test will detect any blood in the stool, and various tests including breath tests, biopsies and cultures, can find *H. pylori* bacteria if it is present in the digestive tract. Blood tests may reveal low red blood cell counts, which may indicate anaemia caused by bleeding. An upper GI series of X-rays may be needed, along with endoscopic examination of the stomach. A thin, flexible tube with a light and camera on its tip is passed down the throat into the stomach to relay images to a monitor. Tissue specimens for culture or biopsy can also be retrieved using the endoscope.

TREATMENTS

Lifestyle and dietary changes can relieve gastritis, and medication may cure it. Giving up alcohol and quitting smoking are important steps in controlling gastritis, because both irritate the stomach and lead to further inflamation.

• **NUTRITION** Avoid fatty, spicy and acidic foods until healed.

• **MEDICATION** Drugs that reduce stomach acid or block its production may be prescribed. These may include antacids, H_2 blockers and proton pump inhibitors. If over-the-counter products are needed more than twice a week, a doctor should be consulted, who will also prescribe antibiotics for *H. pylori* infection. If this is the primary cause, it should heal quickly.

• **ACUPUNCTURE** This Traditional Chinese Medicine (pp.464–5) can help relieve gastritis.

See also: *Crohn's Disease, p.266* • *Traditional Chinese Medicine, pp.446–50* • *Acupuncture, pp.464–5*

WHO IS AT RISK?

The risk factors include:

• Over age 60
• Alcohol abuse
• Smoking
• Pernicious anaemia
• Lymph system diseases
• Radiation treatment
• Long-term NSAID use
• Digestive disorders
• Severe stress (surgery, head injury, respiratory or organ failure)

Haemorrhoids

Areas of widened or dilated veins in the rectum that sometimes become irritated or inflamed are called haemorrhoids, or piles. A person may have internal haemorrhoids, located inside the lower rectum, external haemorrhoids, which form under the skin around the anus, or both. Haemorrhoids may cause itching and bleeding with defecation that coats stool, streaks toilet tissue or drips into the toilet. Sometimes an internal haemorrhoid will protrude, or prolapse, through the anus. This may allow leaking of rectal contents.

Haemorrhoids usually cause only minor discomfort unless a blood clot forms inside one. This is called a thrombosed haemorrhoid, and it can produce severe pain, swelling and inflammation.

CAUSES

Whenever pressure in the veins of the rectum is increased, haemorrhoids may flare up and cause symptoms. Chronic constipation (p.263) contributes to problems with haemorrhoids because small, hard stools are much more difficult to pass. Straining repeatedly to have a bowel movement puts pressure on haemorrhoids, leading to irritation. Persistent diarrhoea (p.268) can also inflame existing haemorrhoids and lead to discomfort and bleeding, because of the repeated passing of loose stools. Over-zealous wiping or cleaning of the anal area is another source of irritation.

Pressure from prolonged sitting, pregnancy and anal intercourse is associated with haemorrhoid symptoms, as is advancing age, when the tissues that normally hold these veiny structures in place get thinner and grow more fragile. Any condition that increases the pressure in the body's venous system, for example cirrhosis (pp.282–3), can also result in haemorrhoids.

PREVENTION

Because hard stools are the main cause of haemorrhoids, prevention depends on combating constipation (p.263). Straining or pushing hard during a bowel movement increases pressure on rectal veins and irritates haemorrhoids. Ways of keeping stools soft and easy to pass include eating a diet rich in high-fibre foods and drinking more water and other non-dehydrating fluids (alcoholic and caffeinated beverages have a dehydrating effect). When the urge to have a bowel movement comes, it is important to go to the toilet without delay. Suppressing the urge can cause stools to dry and harden.

It is also important to exercise regularly to keep bowels moving. Exercise can help to prevent haemorrhoids by reducing rectal vein pressure in two ways. First, being more active reduces periods of prolonged sitting. Exercising for fitness also helps to reduce excess weight, which will reduce extra pressure on rectal veins.

DIAGNOSIS

Most people discover they have haemorrhoids without a visit to the doctor. Some haemorrhoids cause intense itching and others may bleed. Visible blood from haemorrhoids tends to be bright red because it is fresh, because it is caused by the passage of stool or other direct friction with the inflamed area. It is also possible for haemorrhoids to be a source of occult blood – that is, blood that is hidden in the stool. Because rectal bleeding can also signal more serious diseases, including colon cancer (pp.288–95), it is important to see a doctor.

A doctor can detect external haemorrhoids simply by looking at the area of the rectum. Internal haemorrhoids can often be found during a rectal examination using a lubricated glove, but this is not foolproof, because many internal haemorrhoids are too soft to be apparent to the touch. A small stool smear taken during a rectal examination will be chemically analysed to test for any occult bleeding.

To confirm haemorrhoids and detect or rule out other causes of rectal bleeding, a more thorough internal examination may be required. Using a thin, flexible tube equipped with a camera and a light on its end, called an endoscope, a doctor will examine the lining of the anus, lower intestine, or both, for any lesions or polyps. This procedure is called sigmoidoscopy. In older patients, at greater risk for colon cancer, the entire colon may need to be checked in a procedure called colonoscopy.

TREATMENTS

Dietary measures and soothing preparations help relieve most haemorrhoids, although surgical treatment is also available for severe cases.

• **NUTRITION** A high-fibre diet will help reduce haemorrhoid flare-ups. Approximately 25 g (1 oz) of fibre daily is recommended.

• **SUPPLEMENTS** Over-the-counter fibre supplements, made from psyllium or methylcellulose, can reduce bleeding episodes. When taking them, it is very important to increase water intake, or constipation will result.

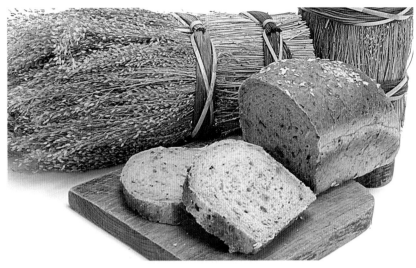

A high-fibre diet, including whole grains, can help reduce haemorrhoid flare-ups by increasing bowel motility (movement) and preventing hard stools. Straining to pass a hard stool increases the pressure on rectal blood vessels and irritates haemorrhoids.

• **MEDICATION** Pain-relieving creams, ointments, pads and suppositories are available without a prescription, as are stool softener capsules. A doctor can prescribe a hydocortisone suppository, but these should not be used for longer than a week unless directed, because of the potential for side-effects such as skin rash and inflammation.

• **SITZ BATHS** For a haemorrhoid that has thrombosed, or formed a blood clot, warm baths in sitz basins, a shallow basin that allows immersion of the pelvic and lower abdominal area, can relieve pain.

• **HYGIENE** Warm baths, rather than showers, are best for routine hygiene when treating haemorrhoids. Avoid using soap in the anal area, as it may increase irritation. Use moist paper towels or damp toilet paper after a bowel movement, rather than dry toilet paper.

• **COLD PACKS** Ice packs or cold compresses applied to the anal area help relieve swelling.

For very persistent or painful haemorrhoids, other procedures include the following.

• **BANDING** A doctor places tiny rubber bands around the internal haemorrhoid. This cuts off circulation and the haemorrhoid shrinks and falls off within a few days.

• **SCLEROTHERAPY** A chemical solution injected around the blood vessel shrinks the haemorrhoid.

• **COAGULATION** Various devices are used to remove internal haemorrhoids. A laser beam, an infrared light beam or an electric current can be used to destroy the excess tissue. Coagulation therapy has generally replaced cryosurgery (the application of extreme cold) for treating haemorrhoids.

• **SURGERY** For patients with severe haemorrhoids or for whom other treatments have failed, surgery may be needed. Although laser surgery has been promoted as less painful than scalpel procedures, there is no evidence to support these claims.

See also: *Constipation, p.263 • Cirrhosis, pp.282–3 • Diarrhoea, p.268*

GALLBLADDER DISORDERS

The gallbladder is part of the body's biliary system, which carries bile and other digestive enzymes from the liver, bladder and pancreas through a network of ducts into the small intestine. Bile is released from the gallbladder in response to food, particularly fats. When liquid bile hardens, gallstones may form and block the ducts. These can be as small as a grain of sand or as large as a golf ball. Most are made of cholesterol; the rest of bilirubin, a by-product of the breakdown of depleted red blood cells. Bilirubin stones are also called pigment stones.

A gallstone may block a duct leading to the pancreas, resulting in an extremely painful inflammation called pancreatitis (p.286).

More commonly, stones trap bile in the duct that leads out of the gallbladder, causing irritation and pressure, and possibly infection. Acute cholescystitis is a gallbladder attack that includes infection. It produces severe pain in the upper right part of the abdomen, often following a large or fatty meal, or sometimes during the night. Pain increases rapidly and may last from 30 minutes to several hours. Occasionally, nausea, vomiting and chest pain under the breastbone may also occur. Fever and chills, jaundice (yellowing of the skin and whites of the eyes), persistent pain and clay-coloured stools signal that the inflammation has reached dangerous levels. Serious damage to the gallbladder, or infections and damage in the liver or pancreas may result.

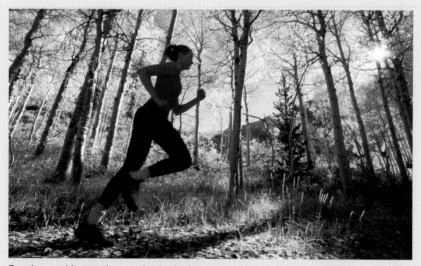

Regular aerobic exercise may lower the frequency of new gallstone formation because it helps regulate insulin and prevent weight-gain.

CAUSES

Gallstone formation is encouraged by conditions that either increase the amount of cholesterol in bile or hamper the gallbladder's ability to empty bile. Obesity (pp.348–9), or even moderately excess weight, does both, as can excess estrogen from pregnancy (pp.398–400), hormone replacement therapy (pp.406–8), or birth-control pills (pp.410–11). Women are at greater risk than men. Cholesterol-lowering drugs cause the liver to secrete extra cholesterol into the bile. Rapid weight loss causes the liver to secrete extra cholesterol, and fasting slows the emptying of the gallbladder. Alcohol consumption and cirrhosis (pp.282–3) also increase the risk.

Some ethnic groups (Native North Americans and Mexicans) have a genetic tendency toward excess cholesterol in the bile. People with diabetes (pp.338–41) often have high levels of triglyceride, another blood fat that increases the likelihood of gallstones.

Bilirubin, or pigment, stones may be related to cirrhosis of the liver, biliary tract infections, or to hereditary blood disorders such as sickle cell anaemia.

PREVENTION

It may not be possible to prevent some gallstones. Many people have undetected 'silent stones' that cause them no problems. In people who are genetically at risk, avoiding a high intake of refined sugars may be helpful. Soluble fibre such as psyllium, has been shown to help prevent gallstones caused by excess cholesterol. Regular aerobic exercise helps control hyperinsulinemia (excesses of insulin), which is associated with stone formation. In people who already have gallbladder disease symptoms, losing excess weight and reducing their intake of fatty foods may reduce discomfort or complications.

DIAGNOSIS

The most sensitive test for gallstones is ultrasound, which uses sound waves bounced off the gallbladder to reveal the presence and location of stones. A doctor may also need to do a CT scan, X-ray or MRI of the abdomen. Blood tests may reveal signs of infection, jaundice, pancreatitis or obstruction.

Another diagnostic tool is endoscopic retrograde cholangiopancreatography (ERCP), which is done using a flexible tube inserted down the throat, through the stomach, and into the small intestine. A dye is injected through the tube to identify the biliary ducts. A nuclear scan called cholescintigraphy, or HIDA, involves using an injected radioactive dye to diagnose obstructions or abnormal contractions of the gallbladder.

TREATMENTS

Although a healthy diet may help control symptoms, once gallstones cause pain, surgical removal may be the best solution.

• NUTRITION Eating unrefined carbohydrates, such as whole grains, rather than refined carbohydrates, may benefit people with gallbladder disease.

• EXERCISE Regular aerobic exer-

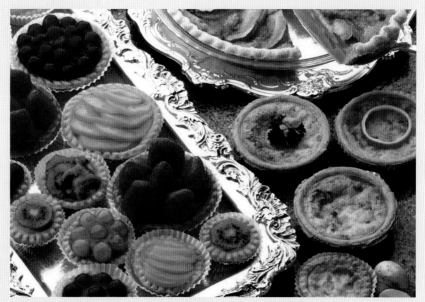

In people who are genetically at risk, avoiding a high intake of refined sugars, such as in desserts, may be helpful.

cise may lower the frequency of new gallstone formation because it helps regulate insulin and prevent excess weight.

• SURGERY The most common solution to gallbladder problems is to surgically remove the gallbladder. The intestines will work just as well after the surgery, although about 1 percent of patients develop chronic diarrhoea (p.268) afterwards. The gallbladder is most often removed with a laparascope, a tiny instrument with a miniature camera threaded through a very small incision in the abdomen. In some cases, due to obstructions or infection, surgery to open the abdomen may be required.

• MEDICATION Two treatments may be used for cholesterol stones only. One approach for people who cannot tolerate surgery due to a serious medical condition is long-term treatment (possibly lasting months or years) with drugs made from bile acid to dissolve the gallstones. A new, and still experimental, treat-

ment uses a drug injected directly into the gallbladder. It can dissolve some stones in one to three days, but carries risks of toxicity.

• HERBAL MEDICINE Evidence suggests that Oregon grape (*Berberis aquifolium*), bupleurum (*Bupleurum chinense*) and gold coin grass (*Lysimachia christinae hance*) may reduce gallbladder inflammation and relieve liver congestion. Other beneficial herbs are globe artichoke (*Cynara scolymus*), turmeric (*Curcuma longa*), white horehound (*Marrubium vulgare*), and soy products.

See also: *Pancreatitis, p.286* • *Cirrhosis, pp.282–3* • *Obesity, pp.348–9*

On Call

Because symptoms of heart problems can be confused with pain from a gallbladder condition, it is crucial to see your doctor for a definite diagnosis if you think you may have gallstones.

Cirrhosis

The liver plays a major role in digestion by producing more than a thousand enzymes, plus bile to help absorb fats. Disorders that damage the liver may weaken it or prevent it from functioning by blocking the flow of blood through the organ. One such disorder is cirrhosis. Although this is widely thought of as a disease of alcoholics, cirrhosis simply means scarring of the liver, and this has various causes.

Along with the kidneys, the liver is the principal site for the metabolism and elimination of all substances brought into the body. It fights infection by manufacturing substances that strengthen immunity, maintains blood sugar balance, regulates hormones and makes proteins that promote blood-clotting.

Cirrhosis may lead to complete loss of liver function, which is fatal. It may be difficult to detect in the early stages, and in some people, one or more complications of cirrhosis are the first sign of the disease. These may include fluid build-up in the legs and abdomen, unusual bruising or bleeding, vomiting of blood, jaundice (yellowing of the skin and the whites of the eyes), intense skin itching, gallstones (pp.280–1), unusual sensitivity to medication, insulin resistance and type 2 diabetes (pp.338–41), impotence, kidney problems, osteoporosis (pp.146–7), liver cancer (pp.288–295), mental confusion and coma.

WHO IS AT RISK?

The risk factors include:

- Alcoholism
- Female
- Infection with hepatitis B, C, D or E
- Untreated haemochromatosis
- Long-term exposure to toxic chemicals
- Medication, including steroids
- Family history of primary biliary cirrhosis

CAUSES

Cirrhosis is caused by a wide range of chronic liver diseases. The most common cause is alcoholism, although some people who drink far less than most alcoholics are also vulnerable, and women who drink are at much greater risk than men. Chronic viral hepatitis infection (p.269) may cause cirrhosis, as can autoimmune liver diseases or diseases of the bile ducts.

Some people have inherited conditions that lead to cirrhosis. Wilson's disease damages the liver's ability to process copper. Other diseases that produce scarring include primary biliary cirrhosis, which may be inherited and is much more common in women; and primary sclerosing cholantitis, a disease of the bile ducts that is associated with colitis (pp.266–7). Haemochromatosis (p.284), chronic exposure to environmental

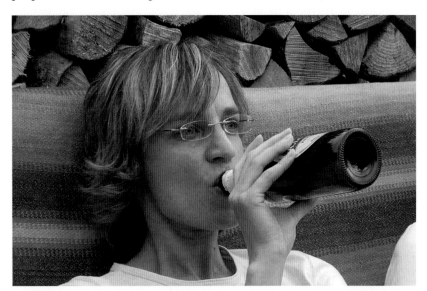
Alcoholism is the most common cause of cirrhosis, but some people who drink far less than most alcoholics can also develop the disease. Liver damage from cirrhosis cannot be reversed, but the progression of the disease can be stopped with proper treatment.

toxins, heart diseases that cause liver congestion and some parasitic infections may lead to cirrhosis. Although the liver can carry out some of its functions with limited damage, cirrhosis must be halted before it becomes life-threatening.

PREVENTION

The first defence against cirrhosis is to drink alcohol only in moderation, if at all. Moderate drinking is defined as no more than one drink a day for women, and no more than two drinks a day for men (one drink equals 340 ml/12 oz beer, 150 ml/ 5 oz wine, or 50 ml/1.5 oz distilled spirits). In women, as few as two or three drinks a day over more than a decade has been linked to cirrhosis, and in men, as few as three to four.

Avoiding infection with viral hepatitis is crucial for protecting the liver. Taking appropriate precautions when using toxic chemicals is important: adequate ventilation, protective clothing and following product directions carefully should reduce the risk of liver damage. Some medication can also be toxic, so it is necessary to follow label and physician's directions closely, and stay on schedule with recommended medical tests that check for early signs of cirrhosis.

DIAGNOSIS

A physical examination may reveal signs of cirrhosis, such as a hardened liver. Various scans may be used, including a CT scan, MRI or a scan that uses a radioactive substance to highlight the liver on X-rays. Another diagnostic option is a laparoscopic examination. This involves inserting a tube that carries

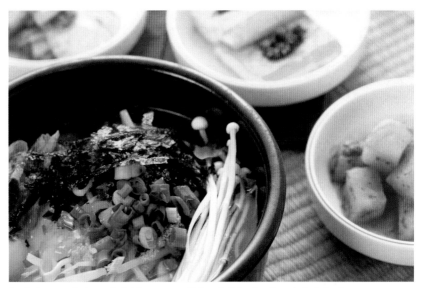

A wholesome, balanced diet is an essential part of the treatment of cirrhosis, alongside the elimination of alcohol. Poor nutrition is often a result of liver disease and not a cause.

a tiny camera through an abdominal incision to relay images of the liver to a computer monitor. A liver biopsy, performed by taking a small tissue sample with a needle, can confirm a diagnosis of cirrhosis.

TREATMENTS

Although most cirrhosis cannot be reversed to any significant degree, treatment can stop or delay its progression and reduce complications.

• NUTRITION Alcohol is toxic to the liver, and a liver damaged by cirrhosis from any cause cannot tolerate any amount of alcohol. A wholesome, balanced diet with adequate protein, fats and carbohydrates is an essential part of treatment. There is evidence that a healthy diet can actually help the liver grow some new cells. It is important to rely on wholesome foods rather than dietary supplements as sources of nutrition. Cirrhosis due to haemochromatosis, or iron overload, requires additional dietary limitations.

• HERBAL MEDICINE Studies have shown that milk thistle (*Silybum marianus*) may improve liver function in alcoholic cirrhosis, but there is concern over the accuracy of the research. The herb should not be taken without a doctor's advice.

• MEDICATION Various medications can slow the progress of cirrhosis, depending on the underlying cause. For cirrhosis caused by hepatitis, corticosteroids may be helpful. For cirrhosis patients with jaundice, supplemental fat-soluble vitamins may be needed. Medications that help expel copper are prescribed for patients with Wilson's disease.

• LIVER TRANSPLANT When advanced cirrhosis causes the liver to fail, a transplant may be the patient's only chance for survival. Success depends upon the patient's health and ability to withstand the procedure, and the availability of a suitable donor organ.

See also: *Gallstones, pp.280–1* • *Diabetes, pp.338–41* • *Hepatitis, p.269*

Haemochromatosis

Also known as iron overload, haemochromatosis is an inherited condition that causes the body to retain too much iron, which becomes concentrated in the liver. Many people have no symptoms, but others may develop fatigue, weakness, abdominal pain, joint pain, bronze or greyish discoloration of the skin, and impotence.

Haemochromatosis occurs when the intestines, which are responsible for the body's absorption of certain nutrients, are unable to keep out excess iron. If haemochromatosis is detected and treated early, individuals with the disorder can lead a normal life. Complications of untreated haemochromatosis include cirrhosis (pp.282–3), liver failure and liver cancer (pp.288–95), plus damage to other organs that may result in diabetes (pp.338–41), loss of body hair, heart problems, loss of libido, impotence and enlarged liver or spleen.

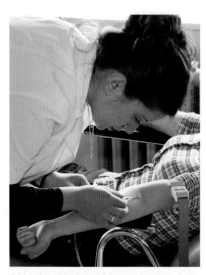

A blood test to detect iron overload can help diagnose haemochromatosis, a condition that can be managed if caught early.

PREVENTION

Haemochromatosis is not preventable. If a family history is known, however, early detection is crucial, because long-term complications can be prevented with ongoing treatment.

DIAGNOSIS

Blood tests to detect iron overload are used to screen for haemochromatosis. If repeated tests reveal persistently high iron levels, a test for the genetic mutation that causes the disease should be done. Some patients with alcoholic cirrhosis or chronic hepatitis (p.269) may also have haemochromatosis, which can be confirmed by a needle biopsy of the liver.

TREATMENTS

Removing excess iron, minimizing intake of iron, and preventing liver damage from other sources are the goals of treatment for haemochromatosis. As with any liver disease, alcohol is a liver toxin and should be avoided.

• NUTRITION Individuals with haemochromatosis should follow a well-balanced diet that is low in iron-rich foods. Red meats should

be limited and animal liver should not be consumed. Many cereal products are fortified with iron, so it is important to read product labels when making diet choices.

• PHLEBOTOMY Weekly blood letting, or phlebotomy treatment, may be needed for months or years until iron levels return to normal. The blood is removed from a vein by needle, as it would be for a diagnostic test. Once normal iron levels are achieved, maintenance treatments may continue every two to four months for life.

See also: *Cirrhosis, pp.282–3 • Liver Cancer, p.288–95 • Diabetes, pp.338–41*

WHO IS AT RISK?

The risk factors include:
• Family history

CAUTION

People with any form of liver disease should not take megadoses of vitamins or other nutritional supplements (pp.532–41) without first consulting a doctor. The liver must process every substance consumed, and a damaged liver may be too fragile for the concentrations present in many supplements. Further, actual ingredients and dosages often do not match what is listed on a product's label. This poses a special danger to people with liver disease.

Diverticulitis & Diverticulosis

Having diverticula – small pouches that bulge through weak areas in the walls of the large intestine (colon) – is called diverticulosis. When the diverticula become infected or inflamed, it is diverticulitis. Although most people are symptom-free, some develop complications, including bleeding, infections, perforations or tears, blockages and fistulas (abnormal tissue connections).

CAUSES

Constipation (p.263) may contribute to diverticulosis. Insufficient fibre in the diet causes smaller, harder stools that force the colon to contract harder, and this pressure creates bulges. Diverticulitis may result from stool or bacteria becoming caught in the diverticula. This causes severe pain in the lower abdomen and fever. Infection may create an abscess (a collection of pus), a serious complication. Rarely, peritonitis (perforation of the intestine) or bleeding is possible. Infection and bleeding do not usually occur together.

PREVENTION

Diverticular disease is less common in vegetarians. A diet high in fibre from fruit and vegetables and low in total fat and red meat, along with regular exercise, may help guard against diverticular disease.

DIAGNOSIS

Pain around the left side of the lower abdomen, fever, and altered bowel habits may indicate diverticulitis. A doctor will perform a physical, possibly including a digital rectal examination to detect tenderness or blood. A stool test for hidden bleeding and blood tests for infection may be done. X-rays, or sigmoidoscopy or colonoscopy (both of which give a direct view of the intestinal walls using a flexible, lighted tube) may be needed.

TREATMENTS

A healthy diet rich in fibre will help calm diverticular disease. Other treatments may also be necessary.

• NUTRITION Consuming 20–35 g (0.7–1.25 oz) of fibre daily may reduce symptoms if existing diverticula are causing pain. Fruit, vegetables and whole grains are the best sources of fibre, and eating more of them helps prevent complications. If diverticula are causing symptoms, avoid nuts, popcorn and sunflower, pumpkin, caraway and sesame seeds.

• MEDICATION Over-the-counter pain medication, such as paracetamol, relieves symptoms in most cases. Sometimes an attack of diverticulitis is very severe, requiring stronger pain medicine and, possibly, antibacterial drugs.

> ### CAUTION
>
> Peritonitis occurs when an infected diverticulum leaks from the intestine and its contents spill into the abdominal and pelvic cavities. It is life-threatening and requires emergency surgery. Sometimes an artery haemorrhages through a diverticulum's thinned wall. This requires emergency hospitalization, because blood loss can be sudden and severe. Normally, bleeding stops spontaneously, but in some cases part of the colon must be surgically removed.

• SURGERY About 25 percent of people with diverticulitis develop serious complications (see Caution above). Abscesses produce pus that must be drained through a needle by a radiologist or a surgeon. If infection spreads, it may be necessary to perform a temporary colostomy, in which the colon is brought to the surface of the skin and its contents collected in a pouch. Once the infection is treated, the affected part of the colon is removed and the colostomy opening is closed.

See also: *Constipation, p.263* • *Fever, p.318*

WHO IS AT RISK?

The risk factors include:
• Low-fibre, high-fat diet
• History of constipation

Pancreatitis

The pancreas secretes digestive juices into the small intestine, and produces insulin to regulate blood sugar. When it is inflamed, digestive enzymes leak into and attack the pancreas itself, causing bleeding, swelling and severe pain known as pancreatitis. The pain may begin gradually or suddenly in the centre of the upper abdomen, going through to the back, and worsen when eating. Pancreatitis also causes diarrhoea (p.268), nausea, vomiting (pp.274–5), fever, jaundice, shock, weight loss and symptoms of diabetes (pp.338–41).

Acute pancreatitis usually develops and subsides quickly, but in some cases leads to severe infection and bleeding. Chronic pancreatitis may destroy the pancreas, leading to malnutrition or, in rare cases, to pancreatic cancer (pp.288–95). It occurs most often in men.

CAUSES

Acute pancreatitis is most often caused by alcohol or gallstones (pp.280–1). When gallstones block the bile duct into the pancreas, enzymes build up in the organ. When pancreatitis results from alcohol abuse, an attack may occur hours or days after drinking. Chronic pancreatitis is normally due to years of excessive drinking. Less common causes include a build-up of fat or calcium in the blood; viruses such as mumps; medications such as oestrogens, sulphonamides, tetracycline, and thiazides; surgery or trauma to the pancreas; or heredity. In some cases the cause is unknown.

PREVENTION

The primary prevention is avoiding excess alcohol. Smoking stresses the body's ability to fight inflammation, so it is important to stop (pp.216–17).

DIAGNOSIS

Chronic and acute pancreatitis cause similar initial symptom. As the inflammation advances, many people develop malnutrition and weight loss. In late stages, signs of diabetes may appear.

Blood tests and imaging tests may be used to make a diagnosis. Ultrasonography creates sound-wave images of abdominal organs; a CT scan provides detail. Endoscopic retrograde cholangiopancretography (ERCP) may be done. It involves passing a flexible tube down the throat and into the small intestine; dye is injected to highlight the pancreatic ducts on X-rays.

TREATMENTS

Treatments range from pain relief to dietary changes to surgery.

WHO IS AT RISK?

The risk factors include:

- Alcohol abuse
- Gallbladder disease or gallstones
- Some medication
- High blood lipids
- High blood calcium
- Viral infections
- Family history
- Pancreatic cancer

• **NUTRITION** Many patients find high-fat foods difficult to digest. If pancreatitis results from gallstones, a low-fat diet is necessary. A pancreas prone to inflammation can be further damaged by alcohol.

• **MEDICATION** Acute pancreatitis may require hospitalization for pain relief and IV fluids. Antibiotics will be prescribed for any infection. A doctor may prescribe enzymes to compensate for those the pancreas cannot produce.

• **SURGERY** In severe cases, surgery may be necessary to drain abdominal fluid, open a blocked duct or remove part of the pancreas.

• **TRADITIONAL CHINESE MEDICINE** There may be potential benefit in Chinese herbal remedies (pp.446–50) for pancreatitis. However, there is insufficient evidence to recommend a particular herb.

See also: *Nausea and Vomiting, pp.274–5 • Diabetes, pp.338–41 • Pancreatic Cancer, p.288–95 • Smoking Cessation, pp.216-17*

Coeliac Disease

Also known as Coeliac sprue, Coeliac disease is an autoimmune disorder that hampers the body's ability to absorb nutrients. When people with Coeliac disease consume gluten, a protein found in wheat, rye, barley, oats and many packaged foods, the lining of the small intestine is damaged. This prevents proper absorption of nutrients and can cause malnutrition, producing widely varying symptoms.

Minimally, most adults with Coeliac disease experience diarrhoea and weight loss; 10 percent develop a painful, blistering rash called dermatitis herpetiformis. Children's symptoms include painful bloating and light-coloured, foul-smelling stools. Undiagnosed Coeliac disease may result in growth abnormalities, osteoporosis (pp.146–7), fluid retention, nerve damage, and iron deficiency anaemia, because iron is not absorbed well by the damaged bowel.

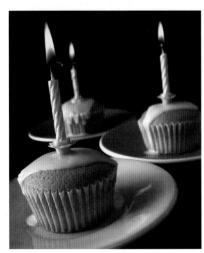

People with Coeliac disease should not consume gluten. It is possible, however, to make foods without gluten by substituting other ingredients.

CAUSES

The most likely cause is an inherited tendency triggered by exposure to gluten. Sufferers have higher than normal blood levels of certain autoantibodies, which are proteins that react to the body's own molecules or tissues. Other autoimmune diseases linked to Coeliac disease include type 1 diabetes (pp.338–41), thyroid disease (pp.344–7), lupus (pp.324–5), and rheumatoid arthritis (pp.136–9). Sometimes Coeliac disease first appears after surgery, pregnancy, childbirth, viral infection or severe stress.

PREVENTION

Coeliac disease cannot be prevented, but complications from it can be avoided if it is detected and treated early.

DIAGNOSIS

Coeliac disease may be confused with irritable bowel syndrome (pp.270–1), Crohn's disease (pp.266–7), diverticulitis (p.285) or chronic fatigue syndrome (pp.322–3). Before being tested, it is important to continue eating foods that contain gluten because eliminating gluten before the test may cause false negative results.

If blood tests suggest coeliac disease, a biopsy of the intestine can confirm the diagnosis. Using tiny instruments passed through an endoscope (a flexible tube inserted through the mouth and into the upper intestine), a doctor will remove a small tissue sample.

TREATMENTS

The only treatment for Coeliac disease is to stop consuming gluten. For most people, complete healing is possible on a gluten-free diet.

• **NUTRITION** Because gluten exists in many foods, it is crucial to follow a dietitian's guidance. A gluten-free diet is challenging, but education about product ingredients will help. There are also unexpected gluten hazards, such as adhesives on envelopes and stamps, soups, ice cream and hot dogs. The gluten-free diet must be followed strictly for life.

See also: *Osteoporosis, pp.146–7 • Lupus, pp.324–5 • Thyroid Disorders, pp. 344–7*

WHO IS AT RISK?

The risk factors include:
- First-degree relatives with Coeliac disease
- Type 1 diabetes
- Down's syndrome
- Thyroid diseases
- Lupus
- Rheumatoid arthritis

Digestive System Cancers

Cancer occurs when cells divide in an unregulated way. Benign tumours do not spread or invade surrounding tissues. In malignant tumours, cancer cells may break away and spread to other parts of the body (a process known as metastasis). Cancers that affect the digestive system include oesophageal, colorectal, stomach, liver, gallbladder and pancreatic.

CAUSES

Chronic irritation of the digestive tract, from infection, medication or environmental irritants, is often a trigger for digestive system cancers.

Oesophageal Cancer

Much oesophageal cancer is caused by long-term heavy consumption of alcohol. The same is true with the use of tobacco in any form, and the combination of long-term smoking and heavy drinking greatly increases risk. Another significant and increasing cause is chronic acid reflux, or GORD (pp.264–5), which can lead to a pre-malignant condition called Barrett's oesophagus. About 10 percent of people who have Barrett's oesophagus will develop oesophageal cancer.

Other causes include occupational exposure to high levels of silica dust, a component of sandstone and granite that is often found in brick, concrete and tiles; a diet deficient in fruit and vegetables and low in vitamins A, C, B$_1$ (riboflavin), beta-carotene and selenium; and being overweight, which increases the risk of GORD. Infection with *H. pylori*, a bacterium that causes gastric ulcer (p.276), increases the risk of developing oesophageal cancer risk, as does radiation therapy following a mastectomy (but not following a lumpectomy).

Colorectal Cancer

Benign tumours that develop on the lining of the rectum or colon are called polyps. Unless these are removed, they may progress to cancer. Although direct causes of colorectal cancer have not been identified, whatever increases the likelihood of developing these pre-cancerous polyps increases the risk of cancer.

Smoking greatly increases the incidence of colorectal polyps, as does heavy alcohol consumption. People who both smoke and drink are four times more likely to develop polyps. Diets high in red meat and saturated fat and low in fruit and vegetables have been linked to colon cancer. Obesity (pp.348–9) and a sedentary lifestyle are also believed to be contributors. Both diabetes (pp.338–41) and depression (pp.364–5) have been shown to increase the likelihood of colon

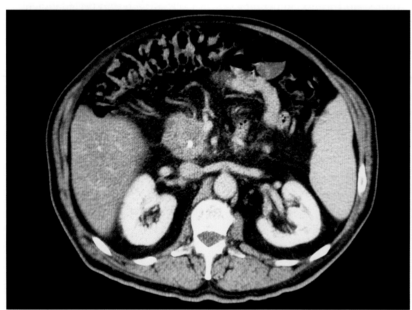

To diagnose a digestive system cancer, a CT scan or MRI may be used. This CT scan shows pancreatic cancer (white dot) in the head of the pancreas (grey, just left of centre). Many digestive system cancers have symptoms that are similar to other, less serious conditions, so it is important to have a doctor screen for possible malignancies.

WHO IS AT RISK?

The risk factors include:

Oesophageal cancer

- Excessive alcohol consumption
- Smoking
- GORD
- Barrett's oesophagus
- Silica dust exposure
- Overweight
- Deficiency of vitamins A, C, B$_1$, beta-carotene and selenium
- Radiation following mastectomy

Colorectal cancer

- Smoking
- Excessive alcohol consumption
- High-fat, low-fibre diet
- Obesity
- Diabetes
- Inflammatory bowel disease
- Over age 50

Stomach cancer

- Smoking
- *H. pylori* infection
- Diet high in salt, or smoked or nitrate-preserved foods
- Diet low in fruits and vegetables
- Chronic gastric irritation

Liver cancer

- Hepatitis A or B
- Excessive alcohol consumption
- Cirrhosis
- Anabolic steroids
- Exposure to toxic chemicals or aflatoxin
- Cancer elsewhere in the body

Gallbladder cancer

- Gallstones
- Women
- Smoking
- Overweight
- Exposure to toxic chemicals

Pancreatic cancer

- Family history of pancreatic cancer
- Family history of colorectal cancer

cancer. The chronic irritation of the colon associated with inflammatory bowel disease (pp.266–7) may also play a role.

Stomach Cancer

Chronic infection, such as with the *H. pylori* bacterium that causes gastric ulcers, and chronic irritation of the stomach lining are linked to stomach cancer. It is more common in older men. Diet plays an important role, particularly if too many salted or smoked foods and foods preserved with

nitrates are consumed, as well as too little fruit and vegetables. Smoking is strongly associated with stomach cancer, as is a family history of the disease.

Liver Cancer

The main causes of liver cancer are chronic liver diseases such as hepatitis B or C (p.269), haemochromatosis (p.284), or cirrhosis (pp.282–3). Malnutrition and excessive use of alcohol, which often go hand in hand, also play a role in this condition.

The liver filters, stores and metabolizes various substances that are taken into the body or that people are exposed to environmentally, so it is particularly vulnerable to toxins, which may increase the likelihood of developing cancer. Liver cancer can be caused by exposure to other substances, including anabolic steroids, vinyl chloride, thorium dioxide, arsenic or aflatoxin – a toxin produced by a fungus that infects wheat, peanuts, soybeans, corn and rice crops in Asia and Africa.

Metastatic tumours are those that have spread to the liver from another body organ, which may happen because the liver filters blood from all parts of the body.

Gallbladder Cancer

While the exact cause of gall-bladder cancer is not known, there is a prevailing theory. The gallbladder stores bile received from the liver. Because the liver metabolizes most substances taken into the body, when the gallbladder does not empty bile at a normal rate, its cells may be exposed to carcinogens for a longer period of time. Gallstones (pp.280–1) may slow bile emptying, although most people with gallstones never develop gallbladder cancer.

Smokers are at much higher risk for gallbladder cancer, as are women, because oestrogen causes more cholesterol (the main component of most gallstones) to be secreted in bile. Exposure to hazardous chemicals, particularly asbestos and azotoluene, also increase risk. People who are significantly overweight are more likely to develop

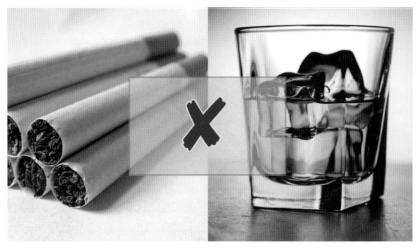

Smoking and heavy alcohol consumption have been linked to almost every type of digestive system cancer. Avoiding both is crucial to the defence against all the cancers listed in this section.

gallbladder cancer, as are those of Native North American, Alaskan or Hispanic ethnicity.

Pancreatic Cancer

The causes of pancreatic cancer are unknown, although some risk factors have been identified. People who have a family history of pancreatic or colon cancer are more vulnerable, as are those who have had multiple episodes of pancreatitis (p.286), a painful inflammation of the pancreas. People who have diabetes or who eat a high-fat diet are also more vulnerable, as are people who smoke or are exposed to toxic chemicals. However, most people with known risk factors do not develop the disease.

PREVENTION

Smoking and the heavy consumption of alcohol are both linked to almost every type of digestive system cancer. Avoiding both of these is crucial in the battle against all the cancers listed in this section.

Oesophageal Cancer

Quitting smoking not only reduces exposure to carcinogens in cigarette smoke, but also eliminates a major cause of GERD. Getting treatment for chronic heartburn is important to protect the oesophagus. A healthy diet rich in brightly colored fruits and vegetables, particularly those from the cabbage family such as broccoli, cauliflower and brussel sprouts, will also protect against cancer. Include cooked tomato products such as tomato sauce and tomato paste to increase dietary intake of the antioxidant lycopene. Selenium-rich foods such as fish, whole-grain breads, Brazil nuts and walnuts are important in preventing oesophageal cancer, but taking selenium supplements is not advisable because they can be toxic.

Recent research at the Fred Hutchinson Cancer Research Center in Seattle, Washington, USA, and published in 2005 in *The Lancet Oncology* suggests that people who have Barrett's

oesophagus and also take non-steroidal anti-inflammatory (NSAID) medication such as aspirin, ibuprofen, naproxen and some arthritis prescriptions have a much lower risk of the condition advancing to cancer.

Colorectal Cancer

A diet rich in phytochemicals from brightly coloured fruit, vegetables and legumes (beans), and low in animal fats is important. There is increasing evidence that calcium and folic acid can help keep the colon cancer-free. Achieving and maintaining a healthy weight and getting regular exercise may also lower the risk of colorectal cancer. Daily use of aspirin and other non-steroidal anti-inflammatory medicines may have a preventative effect.

Recent research done at the National Cancer Control Centre in Haifa, Israel, and published in the *Journal of the American Medical Association* in 2005 indicates that long-term use of a thyroid drug, L-thyroxine, also may help prevent colorectal cancer.

CAUTION

If you have been diagnosed with any type of cancer, bear in mind that taking large doses of antioxidant supplements is not recommended while you undergo chemotherapy or radiation therapy, because they may reduce the treatment's effectiveness. If you are considering taking supplements of any sort, discuss with your doctor what the best type and dosages are for you (pp.532–41).

Stomach Cancer

A diet rich in fruit and vegetables helps prevent stomach cancer. Avoid overindulging in smoked foods and foods preserved with nitrates. There is preliminary evidence that supplemental vitamin C (1,000 mg twice a day) and beta-carotene (300 mg once a day) may help prevent stomach cancer in those at high risk. An antibiotic treatment that destroys the *H. pylori* infection may also help.

Liver Cancer

Avoiding excessive alcohol consumption is important to protect the liver from cirrhosis. Moderate use is defined as no more than two drinks per day for men and one drink per day for women (one drink is equal to 340 ml/12 oz beer, 150 ml/5 oz wine, or 50 ml/1.5 oz distilled spirits). Hepatitis B (p.269) has been linked with liver cancer. Therefore, if syringes are used to inject medication or drugs, they must never be shared with another person. Using condoms during intercourse is advised in any non-monogamous relationship or when it is not known whether a sexual partner may have hepatitis. Children should be vaccinated against hepatitis B.

Gallbladder and Pancreatic Cancer

It may not be possible to prevent gallbladder or pancreatic cancer specifically, but it is wise to adopt the lifestyle measures that reduce cancer risk. These include eating a healthy low-fat diet that is rich in fruit, vegetables and whole grains, and losing excess weight. Not smoking and getting regular aerobic exercise are also very important preventative measures.

Diagnosis

Regular screening is often the way digestive system cancers are diagnosed. If there is a history of pancreatic or colorectal cancer in the family, a doctor can recommend an appropriate schedule for examinations that may detect it early.

Oesophageal Cancer

This form of cancer is not usually easily identified early on. Difficulty in swallowing may be the first sign that a tumour has narrowed the oesophagus (the tube that connects the throat to the stomach). Other signs of oesophogeal cancer may include unintended weight loss; pain in the throat, mid-chest or between the shoulder blades; and hoarseness, a chronic cough and the coughing up blood in the late stages.

When symptoms suggest the possibility of oesophageal cancer, diagnostic tests may include a chest X-ray; a barium swallow X-ray, which highlights the oesophagus on film after the patient drinks a special liquid; or an upper endoscopy, in which a thin, flexible tube instrument is used to light and view the oesophageal lining and retrieve tissue samples for biopsy.

If cancer is confirmed, one or more additional tests will be needed to determine its severity. These may include examination of the lungs with a bronchoscope, a CT scan, and endoscopic ultrasound, which uses sound waves to create images of the oesophagus and surrounding tissues. A positron emission tomography (PET) scan, which uses an injected trace amount of radioactive material to highlight cancerous areas, may also be done.

Colorectal Cancer

Many people experience no warning signs of colorectal cancer, but in some, symptoms may include a change in bowel habits or feeling that the bowel does not empty completely, blood in the stool, narrower-than-normal stools,

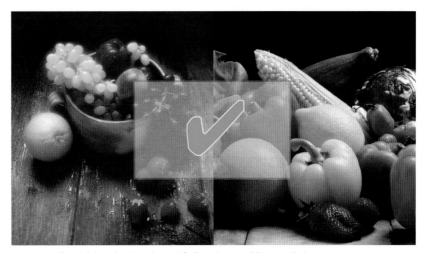

A healthy diet rich in brightly coloured fruit and vegetables may help prevent many cancers including oesophageal, colorectal and stomach cancer. Such foods contain antioxidants, which are substances that help rid the body of harmful toxins that can cause cancer.

frequent abdominal discomfort, unexplained weight loss and constant fatigue.

A physical examination, including a digital rectal exam, will be performed, and several tests that offer a view of the colon may be carried out. These include a barium enema, in which a chalky barium liquid that is visible on X-ray is introduced through the rectum; sigmoidoscopy, which uses a flexible lighted tube instrument to view the lower large intestine; or a colonoscopy. From the age of 50, it is recommended that all adults be screened for colon

cancer. Colonoscopy, which enables a doctor to view the entire large intestine, is the most effective screening method. If polyps are discovered, they can be removed or biopsied during the procedure.

Stomach Cancer

The symptoms of stomach, or gastric, cancer may mimic those of a variety of other digestive conditions, so it is important to see a doctor for evaluation. In its early stages, stomach cancer may cause indigestion and abdominal discomfort, a bloated feeling after eating, mild nausea, loss of

appetite and heartburn. In more advanced stages it may cause black stools due to bleeding from the stomach, vomiting, unexplained weight loss, jaundice, a build-up of fluid in the abdomen and difficulty swallowing.

In addition to a complete physical examination, a doctor will do blood chemistry studies including a complete blood count, which checks for levels of red blood cells, white blood cells, platelets and haemoglobin. An upper endoscopy, in which a doctor uses a thin, flexible lighted tube to view the oesophagus, stomach and upper small intestine, and take small tissue samples for biopsy, may also be done.

Liver Cancer

The symptoms of liver cancer are difficult to detect in the early stages, but as it progresses it may cause pain in the upper right side of the abdomen, abdominal bloating, loss of appetite, feelings of fullness, weakness or fatigue, nausea and vomiting, dark urine, extreme itching of the skin, jaundice and fever.

In addition to a complete physical examination, a doctor will do blood chemistry studies, including a complete blood count, which checks for levels of red blood cells, white blood cells, platelets and haemoglobin. Imaging tests such as ultrasound, CT scanning and MRI may be needed to look at the structure of the liver. If an abnormality is found, a biopsy may be performed by inserting a needle through the skin into the liver.

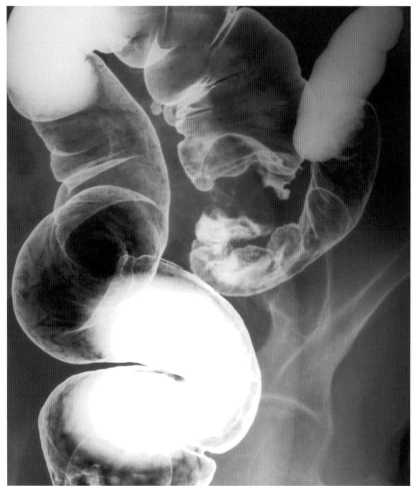

A barium-enema X-ray produces a detailed image of the colon, as in this 59-year-old patient who has cancer (white mass) of the sigmoid colon, which is at the end of the small intestine and start of the colon.

Gallbladder Cancer

Cancer of the gallbladder is a quite rare form of the disease. It usually produces few symptoms in the early stages, so it can be difficult to detect. Sometimes early gallbladder cancer is discovered when the gallbladder is removed to treat gallstones. When signs do appear, they may resemble those of many other illnesses. Such symptoms may include pain above the stomach, fever, nausea and vomiting, jaundice, unintended weight loss, bloating or lumps in the abdomen.

Clinical Query

Can antioxidant supplements help prevent digestive cancers?

Antioxidants may help protect cells from damage caused by unstable molecules called free radicals, which may cause cancer. Examples of antioxidants include beta-carotene, lycopene, selenium and vitamins C, E and A. Supplemental vitamin C and beta-carotene may help protect those at high risk for stomach cancer. Generally, however, it is best to get your antioxidants from a diet rich in fruit and vegetables, rather than by consuming high doses of supplements.

Anti-cancer properties are found in foods rich in antioxidant substances. Cruciferous vegetables such as cabbage, turnips and broccoli in particular, have high levels of a chemical called suforaphane, which suppresses the growth of the *H. pylori* bacteria, a known risk factor for stomach cancer.

Because the gallbladder is hidden behind the liver and is a relatively inaccessible organ, blood tests are the first tools for diagnosing gallbladder cancer. Elevated levels of bilirubin, certain enzymes, or tumour markers in the blood may indicate gallbladder cancer. Other tests include standard or endoscopic ultrasound, which uses sound waves to create images of the gallbladder. Other imaging techniques such as CT scans or MRI scans may also be needed.

A more specific diagnostic test for detecting gallbladder cancer is the endoscopic retrograde cholangiopancreatography (ERCP) diagnostic procedure, in which the intestinal tract is inflated with air and an endoscope is passed down the throat into the upper small intestine. A dye is injected through the scope that reveals obstructions of the bile ducts that may be caused by spreading gallbladder cancer. Laparoscopy uses a lighted instrument passed through a small abdominal incision to obtain images of the gallbladder and take tissue samples for biopsy and analysis.

Pancreatic Cancer

The symptoms of pancreatic cancer are usually vague, and easy to confuse with symptoms of other, less serious conditions. Such symptoms may include nausea, loss of appetite, unexplained weight loss, pain in the upper abdomen that may radiate through to the back, jaundice, dark-coloured urine, clay-coloured stools, weakness, dizziness, chills, muscle spasms and diarrhoea.

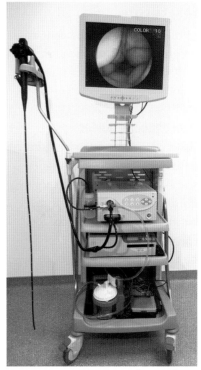

A colonoscopy, which uses a fibre-optic camera on the end of a flexible endoscope, is used to screen for colon cancer.

Blood, urine and stool samples will be taken to check for bilirubin, which may build up if the common bile duct near the pancreas is blocked by a tumour. This does not always occur with pancreatic cancer, however.

A CT scan and ultrasound scan will provide detailed views of the pancreas from various angles. In some cases an internal ultrasound, in which an endoscope with an ultrasound device on its tip is passed down the throat into the upper small intestine, may be performed. An ERCP also makes use of the endoscope to inject dye visible on X-rays into the pancreatic ducts. Another method of administering the dye is through percutaneous transhepatic cholangiography (PTC), in which it is injected using a thin needle.

TREATMENTS

In the past decade, tremendous progress has been made in the early detection and treatment of most cancers.

Oesophageal Cancer

Particularly for people who also have long-standing and progressive Barrett's oesophagus, surgery is usually recommended. It may be combined with radiation or chemotherapy, or both, depending on the stage to which the cancer has progressed.

• SURGERY The cancerous portion of the oesophagus and nearby lymph nodes are removed in oesophagectomy. In more advanced cases, it may be necessary to remove part of the stomach as well, in a procedure called oesophago-gastrectomy.

• RADIATION External radiation may be used, which is a procedure in which X-rays are sent into the oesophagus to kill the cancerous cells. In some cases of oesophageal cancer, tiny tubes containing radioactive material are implanted into the cancerous areas.

• CHEMOTHERAPY In this treatment, a combination of anti-cancer drugs is taken by mouth or injected into the veins. Chemotherapy is normally given in cycles, with periods between treatments to allow time for recovery.

• PHOTODYNAMIC THERAPY A light-sensitive drug which collects in cancer cells is injected, after which doctors will direct a laser light into the oesophagus through a special endoscope. Although normally used to control pain or relieve an obstruction, this type

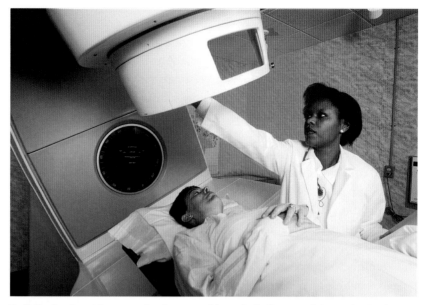

Radiation treatment for cancer involves a machine called a linear particle accelerator that uses high-energy X-rays to destroy tumours. This type of treatment focuses a specially shaped beam of radiation that targets only the tumour and leaves surrounding tissues alone.

of treatment also shows promise as a treatment for early stage oesophageal cancer.

Colorectal Cancer

This type of cancer is highly curable if it is diagnosed early. Surgery is the front-line treatment for early stages of the disease. In more advanced cases of colorectal cancer, doctors use various combinations of surgery, radiation and chemotherapy.

• SURGERY Removal of the tumour and any surrounding cancerous tissue may be the only treatment necessary in some cases. More rarely, a colostomy may be required, in which an opening is created in the colon and abdomen through which wastes pass into a bag that is worn outside the body.

• RADIATION Radiation therapy uses targeted, high-energy X-rays to destroy tumours. External radiation employs a machine outside the body to direct radiation towards

cancerous tissues. Internal radiation uses a radioactive substance sealed in needles, seeds, wires, or catheters that are surgically placed into or near the tumour.

• CHEMOTHERAPY Cancer-fighting chemicals administered by mouth or injected into a vein are used to destroy malignant cells or stop them from dividing.

• BIOLOGICAL THERAPY Genetically engineered antibodies (proteins produced by the immune system to fight foreign substances) are now used to treat colorectal cancer that has metastasized, or spread to other tissues of the body.

Stomach Cancer

Radiation and chemotherapy, as described in the previous sections, may be used separately or in combination with the other treatments described here.

• SURGERY A subtotal gastrectomy is a surgical procedure in which the cancerous part of the stomach and any affected nearby tissues and lymph nodes is removed. The spleen, an organ in the upper abdomen that filters worn-out blood cells and other foreign materials from the body, may also be removed. In a total gastrectomy, the entire stomach, nearby lymph nodes and parts of the oesophagus, small intestine, other tissues, and sometimes the spleen, are removed. The oesophagus is then connected to the small intestine. Other procedures include placing a stent, or small tube, to keep the oesophagus open; a laser procedure that removes cancerous tissue with a laser beam; or electrocautery, which destroys cancerous lesions and controls bleeding with an electric current.

• BIOLOGICAL THERAPY For advanced stomach cancer that has not responded to standard treatment, some patients may be able to participate in clinical trials of biological therapy. In this treatment, genetically engineered antibodies are administered, which may help restore the body's natural defences against cancer.

Liver Cancer

This type of cancer is difficult to cure unless it is identified in the very early stages, when there may be few noticeable symptoms. Patient survival can be improved with some treatments. These treatments may be used in combination or by themselves, along with radiation and chemotherapy.

• SURGERY The removal of the cancerous part of the liver and any affected nearby tissues and lymph nodes is the only surgical

procedure that is effective in treating this type of cancer.

• CRYOSURGERY This is another method of destroying malignant tissues, cryosurgery is a procedure that involves freezing tumours with a metal probe.

• ETHANOL ABLATION Cancer cells are killed by injecting a type of alcohol directly into the malignant tumour in the liver.

• BIOLOGICAL THERAPY Also called biological response modifier (BRM) therapy, this approach uses medication or substances such as antibodies that are naturally made by the human body to strengthen the immune system's own defences against cancer.

Gallbladder Cancer

For tumours in the early stages, surgery will likely be the best option, possibly followed by radiation therapy. No other treatments are available for gallbladder cancer in the advanced stages.

• SURGERY When a very small tumour has not spread beyond the gallbladder, removal of the gallbladder alone may be performed. More commonly, a more extensive procedure may be necessary, in which a surgeon removes the gallbladder along with part of the liver and the nearby lymph nodes.

• RADIATION Cancer that has metastasized, or spread, beyond the walls of the gallbladder is considered inoperable. In this case, radiation therapy may be advised to slow its spread.

• PALLIATIVE CARE Pain control and comfort measures are the primary goal if gallbladder cancer is too advanced to treat.

Pancreatic Cancer

A malignancy of the pancreas is unpredictable, because most of the time it has metastasized before there are any identifiable symptoms. About 25 percent of people with pancreatic cancer can be treated in time to stop the spread of the tumour. More often, however, the tumour may grow for some time before the disease is discovered. Most treatments for pancreatic cancer are attempts to slow its progression.

• SURGERY Some patients have early stage pancreatic cancer that can be treated surgically. The cure rate for this cancer is very low.

• CHEMOTHERAPY Chemotherapy and radiation therapy may be administered after surgery in an attempt to extend survival time, although no cure is possible if the cancer has metastasized, or spread, beyond the pancreas into surrounding tissues.

• CLINICAL TRIALS Because the overall survival rate for pancreatic cancer is so low and the progression of the disease is normally very fast, some patients are advised to consider enrolling in a clinical trial – a medical research study that investigates experimental medication and treatments.

• SUPPORTIVE THERAPY Managing pain and addressing the dietary problems that result from pancreatic cancer, such as poor absorption of nutrients and difficulty digesting food, are important components of treating the disease.

See also: Gastric Ulcer, p.276 • Gastro-esophogeal Reflux Disease, pp.264–5 • Hepatitis, p.269

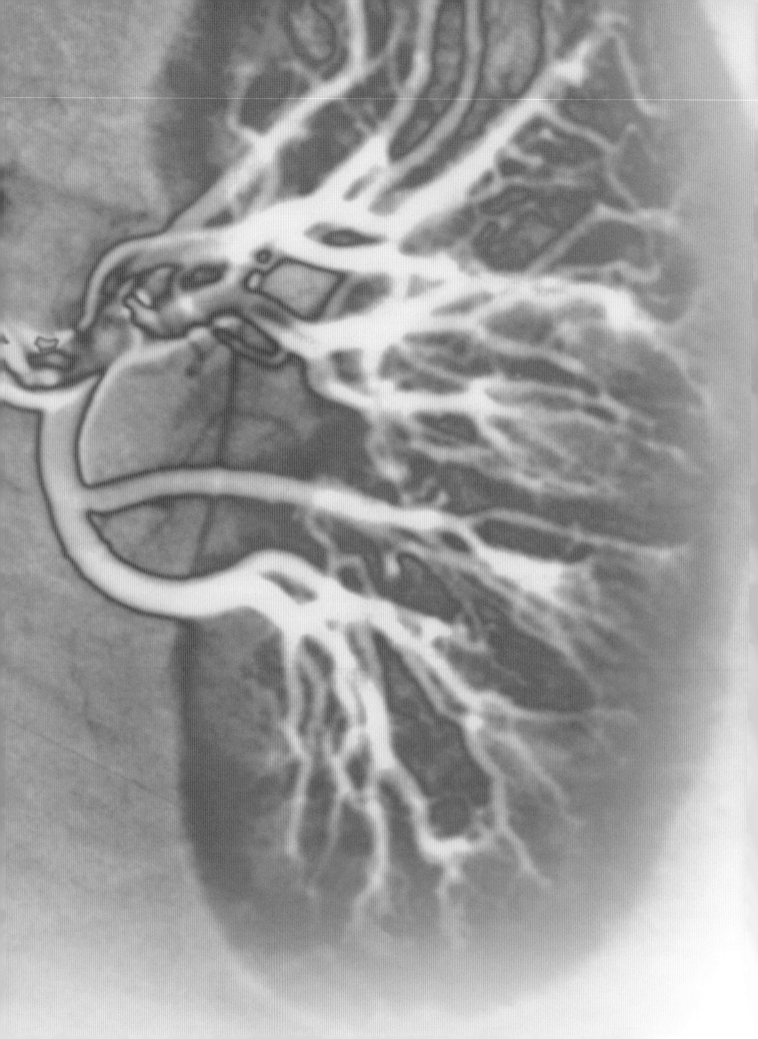

KIDNEYS & URINARY TRACT

10

The kidneys, located in the middle of the back on either side of the spine, filter excess water and waste products that accumulate in the blood as a normal result of metabolism. When the kidneys do not function properly, toxins build up in the body that can cause serious illness or death. The kidneys and urinary tract are vulnerable to bacterial infections. Kidney stones form when proteins and mineral crystals build up on the kidneys' inner surfaces, causing pain and irritation. More serious disorders, such as nephrosis, polycystic kidney disease and diabetes have different causes but can all result in kidney failure.

Drinking plenty of fluids and maintaining a healthy diet is the best way to prevent many common kidney disorders. Conditions such as diabetes type 1 and polycystic kidney disease may not be preventable, but managing risk factors can help minimize their severity.

Urinary Incontinence

Urinary incontinence is an involuntary loss of urine. It is not a disease but rather a symptom that can be caused by a wide range of conditions, including childbirth, diabetes (pp.338–41), stroke (pp.168–9), multiple sclerosis (pp.182–3), Parkinson's disease (p.181) and some surgeries. Especially common among women over 50, incontinence can affect men and younger women as well.

Unfortunately, many people fail to seek treatment because they are embarrassed or because they believe incontinence is a normal part of ageing. It is not; incontinence is treatable and often curable.

CAUSES

With age, several changes occur that affect a person's ability to control urination. Bladder capacity decreases, the rate of urine flow through the urethra and out of the bladder slows, and the ability to postpone urination declines. All of these changes increase the risk of incontinence.

However, the condition usually occurs only when there is an additional cause. In women, thinning and drying of the skin in the vagina or urethra after menopause are common factors; in men, prostate surgery or an enlarged prostate gland may be contributors. Weakened pelvic muscles, urinary tract infections (pp.302–3), diabetes, abnormally high calcium levels, constipation, and some prescription and nonprescription medications may also increase the risk of incontinence.

Pregnant women are also at risk, because of the pressure the foetus places on the bladder.

PREVENTION

Maintaining overall muscle tone and performing pelvic floor muscle (also called Kegel) exercises, which involve repeatedly tightening and releasing pelvic muscles, are helpful in many cases, particularly for women at high risk of incontinence following childbirth. Other ways to help prevent incontinence include keeping bowel movements regular, refraining from straining to empty the bladder and bowels, and drinking adequate but not excessive amounts of fluids (four to six 0.25 litre/8 fl.oz glasses a day is enough).

Discontinuing or cutting down on drugs and other substances that can irritate the bladder can also help. Some of the most common include alcohol, caffeine, some nasal decongestants, angiotensin-converting (ACE) inhibitors (a class of blood pressure medication), some antidepressant and antipsychotic drugs, calcium channel blockers, diuretics, pain-killers and sedatives.

WHO IS AT RISK?

The risk factors include:
- Bladder irritants
- Women over age 50
- Structural changes in the urinary tract
- Diabetes
- Anxiety
- Constipation
- Some medications
- Pregnancy
- Difficult/traumatic childbirth

DIAGNOSIS

Determining the cause of incontinence requires a medical history and a physical examination. In addition, patients may be asked to keep a 'bladder diary' in which they record how often and when they urinated, whether they lost control and approximately how much urine leaked each time.

A number of tests may be performed to pinpoint the cause of a patient's incontinence. These may include urinalysis to rule out infection; a post-void residual (PVR) examination to measure the amount of urine in the bladder after urination; and a urinary stress test, in which the patient is asked to stand with a full bladder and cough so doctors can determine how much leakage occurs. Other tests, such as pelvic or abdominal ultrasound, X-rays, cystoscopy (an examination of the bladder using an instrument inserted via the

On Call

There are several types of urinary incontinence:

Stress incontinence The uncontrollable loss of urine when coughing, sneezing, lifting heavy objects, jumping or doing anything that suddenly increases pressure within the abdomen. It is common among young and middle-aged women and can be caused by weakness of the urinary sphincter, which can result from childbirth or pelvic surgery.

Urge incontinence A sudden, intense urge to urinate quickly, followed by uncontrollable loss of urine. Also called overactive bladder, urge incontinence is most common in the elderly and may be a sign of an infection in the kidneys or bladder.

Overflow incontinence A constant dripping of urine caused by an overfilled bladder. This occurs more often in men and can be caused by something blocking the urinary flow, such as an enlarged prostate gland or tumour. Diabetes or certain medicines may also cause this.

Functional incontinence Urine loss resulting from an inability to get to a toilet. The most common reasons for this are conditions that cause immobility, such as stroke, severe arthritis, dementia and severe depression, or other emotional disturbances.

Mixed incontinence This involves more than one type of incontinence. The most common type of mixed incontinence occurs in older women, who often have both urge and stress incontinence.

MALE

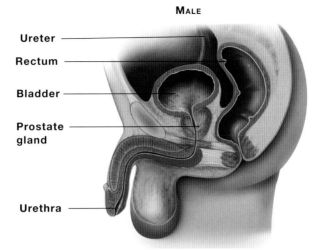

- Ureter
- Rectum
- Bladder
- Prostate gland
- Urethra

Illustration showing anatomy of the male urinary tract. In men, prostate surgery or an enlarged prostate gland may contribute to urinary incontinence. Diseases that affect the nervous system, such as Parkinson's, diabetes or multiple sclerosis, can also play a role.

urethra) and urodynamic evaluations to measure urine pressure and flow, may also be performed.

TREATMENTS

The treatment for urinary incontinence depends on the cause.

- **EXERCISE** Kegel exercises (see Prevention) may be helpful in treating incontinence. This may be done in conjunction with biofeedback (pp.504–7). Biofeedback-assisted Kegels use electronic or mechanical devices to relay visual or auditory evidence of pelvic floor muscle tone to assist patients in correctly performing the exercises.

- **MIND–BODY CONNECTION** Scheduled voiding involves deliberately urinating at regular intervals. The idea is to specifically set, and over time lengthen, the time between voids; in a sense, to set the bladder as one might set a clock.

- **ACUPUNCTURE** This Traditional Chinese Medicine (pp.464–5) technique can improve the symptoms of incontinence, including urgency and frequency of urination, in many patients.

- **MEDICATION** Drugs that increase the strength of the urinary sphincter, including oestrogen, alpha-adrenergic blockers, and beta-adrenergic blockers may be prescribed. Other potentially helpful medications include those that relax muscles and prevent bladder spasms, such as oxybutynin chloride and tolterodine tartrate. Imipramine hydrochloride, a tricyclic antidepressant that relaxes bladder muscles and tightens urethral muscles, may also be used. Oestrogen replacement therapy, which has been used in the past, has recently been shown to increase rather than decrease the risk of developing incontinence.

- **INJECTIONS** Collagen may be injected into tissues around the bladder neck and urethra to add bulk and close the bladder opening.

- **SURGERY** Severe cases of incontinence can sometimes be corrected using various surgical techniques to correct abnormalities.

See also: *Stroke, pp.168–9* • *Diabetes, pp.338–41* • *Urinary Tract Infections, pp.302–3*

Haematuria

Blood in the urine is called haematuria. Very small amounts of blood can make the urine look cloudy or smoky, and just slightly more of it can turn the urine pink, red or brown, like tea or cola. In some cases, haematuria may be accompanied by pain, a temperature, frequent urination, increased or decreased thirst, nausea, vomiting or diarrhoea. These symptoms may help in determining the likely cause.

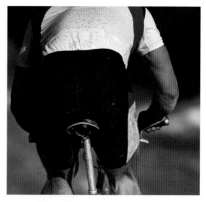

For cyclists, using an anatomically designed seat that relieves pressure on the groin may prevent haematuria.

CAUSES

Haematuria has many causes; some are serious, but many others are not. Common causes include urinary tract infection (pp.302–3), kidney stones (pp.304–5), injury, blood vessels broken by the strain of urinating with an enlarged prostate and strenuous exercise, as well as the use of certain medications, such as blood thinners, aspirin-type drugs and penicillin, among others.

All cases of blood in the urine should be investigated by a doctor, including cases in patients taking blood thinning medication. Additional causes of haematuria include tumours, glomerulonephritis – a family of illnesses characterized by inflammation of the filtering units of the kidneys – and bleeding disorders, such as haemophilia (p.320).

The urine may also look reddish after eating certain red foods, such as beetroot, rhubarb, items containing red food colouring, and soft drinks. This is called pseudo-haematuria, a condition in which urine looks pink or red but blood is not present.

PREVENTION

Runners may prevent injury-related haematuria by drinking plenty of fluid and running on soft ground. Cyclists can use padded seats and should rise from the seat when going over bumps. Diet and sometimes medication can help to minimize the risk of stone formation in people prone to kidney stones.

DIAGNOSIS

Usually a haematuria examination is not to definitively diagnose a specific cause, but to rule out a serious problem. In addition to a physical examination, a number of laboratory tests may be performed, including urinalysis and blood tests. Doctors may also take X-rays of the bladder, kidneys and abdomen, and perform a cystoscopy (visual inspection of the bladder and urethra through a tube inserted via the urethra). Sometimes a biopsy will be performed.

TREATMENTS

Treatment for haematuria depends on the cause, which often cannot be found, suggesting that nothing is seriously medically wrong.

• REST Exercise-induced haematu-
ria usually clears up with rest and adequate fluid intake.

• MEDICATION Infections can be eliminated with antibiotics.

• LITHOTRIPSY Stones that cause haematuria may pass out of the body on their own or may require treatment with sound waves (lithotripsy), which break up the stones so they can be passed.

• SURGERY Tumours or large stones may be surgically removed, depending on their size and location.

See also: *Fever, p.318* • *Kidney Stones, pp.304–5* • *Urinary Tract Infection, pp.302–3*

WHO IS AT RISK?

The risk factors include:

• Strenuous exercise
• Enlarged prostate
• Injury
• Underlying medical problems
• Certain medications

Nephritis & Nephrosis

An inflammation of one or both kidneys is called nephritis. It is more common in childhood and adolescence. Nephritis most often affects the glomeruli, tufts of microscopic vessels that filter blood. Less commonly, nephritis affects the tubules that surround the glomeruli or the blood vessels inside the kidneys. Nephritis may be acute or chronic. People with the acute form usually recover. Nephrosis is a non-inflammatory disease of the kidney also affecting the glomeruli.

WHO IS AT RISK?

The risk factors include:

- History of polycystic kidney disease
- Kidney disease or infection
- Drug allergies
- Hypertension
- Diabetes
- Sickle cell anaemia
- Long-term dialysis

Chronic nephritis can lead to severe hypertension (pp.236) which can, in extreme cases, result in death from kidney or heart failure.

Nephrosis occurs when the glomeruli are damaged; instead of filtering only wastes and water from the blood, the gomeruli also filter out protein. Without sufficient protein, a person may develop oedema (swelling) in the feet, ankles, abdomen and around the eyes. Nephrosis can occur in people of all ages, but is more common in children.

CAUSES

Acute nephritis can be caused by drug allergies, especially analgesics such as aspirin and paracetomol, immunosuppressant drugs such as cyclosporine, anti-cancer drugs such as cisplatin and carboplatin, and lithium, which is used to treat bipolar disorder. Other causes include bacterial and viral infections, metabolic and toxic disorders, and hypercalcemia, .

Chronic nephritis develops more slowly has many causes, including abnormal immune system reactions, bacterial kidney infection,

drug hypersensitivity or exposure to a toxin. It can also be caused by radiation exposure, obstruction of the urinary tract, hypertension, sickle cell anaemia and polycystic kidney disease (PKD, p.308), among other conditions.

Nephrosis can be caused by kidney disease or it may be a complication of another disorder, particularly diabetes (pp.338–41).

PREVENTION

Staying healthy and following a doctor's treatment plan are important in treating all kidney disorders. Also, be aware of the symptoms and to report them to a doctor promptly. Symptoms of nephritis may include appetite loss, fatigue, facial swelling, abdominal pain and dark urine. A key symptom of nephrosis is oedema.

DIAGNOSIS

Common diagnostic tests for nephritis and nephrosis include urinalysis to check kidney function and renal ultrasound to check size and shape of the kidneys and to determine whether there are any

blockages in the urinary tract. A renal scan may also be done to measure blood flow through the kidneys. A biopsy may also be performed.

TREATMENTS

The aim of all treatment is to reduce inflammation, limit damage to the kidneys, and support the body until kidney function is restored.

• MEDICATION Nephritis caused by infection is treated with antibiotics. Both nephritis and nephrosis may be treated with anti-inflammatory drugs. Diuretics or special diets may be prescribed. Nephrosis can sometimes be suppressed using corticosteroids, including prednisone and cortisone.

• DIALYSIS If either condition progresses to kidney failure, dialysis may be needed, which is a treatment that filters wastes from the blood.

• SURGERY For kidney failure, a kidney transplant may be needed.

See also: *Polycystic Kidney Disease, p.308 • Diabetes, pp.338–41 • Hypertension, pp.236–9*

KIDNEY & URINARY TRACT INFECTIONS

Kidney infections are one type of urinary tract infection (UTI). UTIs develop when bacteria enter the urethral opening and multiply in the urinary tract, which includes the urethra, bladder, ureters and kidneys. Usually, UTIs develop first in the lower urinary tract (the urethra and bladder). If they are not treated, they may progress to the upper urinary tract (the ureters and kidneys). An acute kidney infection starts suddenly with severe symptoms.

Urinary tract infections are more common in adult women than in men or children. Women who are sexually active tend to have more UTIs than women who are not, because intercourse can introduce bacteria and irritate the urethra, allowing germs to travel more easily up into the bladder. Uncircumcised boys and men are more likely to suffer from UTIs than those who have been circumcised.

CAUSES

Bacteria called *E. coli* cause about 80 percent of UTIs in adults. These bacteria are normally present in the colon and may enter the urethra from the skin around the anus and genitals. Girls and women are particularly susceptible to lower urinary tract infections because their urethral opening is closer to the anus than men's, and the anus is the source of the bacteria. In addition, women's urethras are shorter than men's, providing bacteria easier access to the bladder. Other organisms that cause UTIs

include *Staphylococcus saprophyticus*, *Chlamydia trachomatis* and *Mycoplasma hominis*.

There are many different factors that cause such infections, including sexual intercourse, especially when diaphragms or condoms are used with spermicide; long-term catheterization in the bladder; congenital urinary tract abnormalities; and bladder obstructions such as an enlarged prostate in men or kidney stones. UTIs occur also when the immune system is impaired in some way, by diabetes or some other chronic illness, or if someone is taking medication that lowers immunity, such as cortisone in high doses. People who have a history of urinary tract infections are more susceptible as are those who have conditions that cause incomplete emptying of the bladder, such as spinal cord injury.

PREVENTION

There are a number of ways sufferers from UTIs – especially women – can prevent them:

- Wipe from front to back following a bowel movement to minimize the chance that *E. coli* will enter the urethra.
- Avoid using potentially irritating feminine products such as deodorant sprays, douches and powders in the genital area, since these can irritate the urethra.
- Drink plenty of water to flush bacteria from the body.
- Drink cranberry juice or take vitamin C. Both increase acid in the urine and so inhibit bacterial growth; cranberry products also appear to prevent bacteria from sticking to bladder walls.
- Consuming fermented milk products containing probiotics – potentially beneficial bacteria and yeasts (pp.550–1) – can reduce incidence of UTIs. These foods include yogurt, kefir and acidophilus milk. Probiotics are also sold in capsules or powdered form as supplements.
- Urinate whenever you feel the urge. Bacteria can grow when urine remains in the bladder for too long.
- Always urinate after intercourse to flush away bacteria that may have entered the urethra during sex. Use lubricated condoms without spermicide.
- Wear cotton underwear and loose-fitting clothes to inhibit bacterial growth.

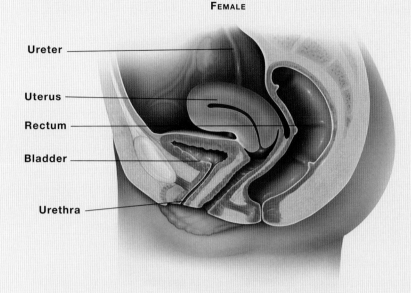

FEMALE

Ureter

Uterus

Rectum

Bladder

Urethra

Many doctors believe that urinary tract infections are more common in women because the urethra is relatively shorter. This difference allows bacteria easier access to the bladder, causing infection.

Clinical Query

I suffer from repeated urinary tract infections. Can anything be done to stop this unending cycle?

Currently, people with recurrent urinary tract infections can be placed on long-term suppressive doses of antibiotics. However, researchers are working to develop a vaccine for women who suffer repeated urinary tract infections. Researchers have found that women and children who tend to get recurrent UTIs are likely to lack proteins called immunoglobulin, which fight infection. Early tests indicate that a vaccine can help patients build up their own natural immunity. The dead bacteria in the vaccine prompt the body to produce antibodies that can later fight against live organisms. Researchers are testing injection and oral vaccines to see which works best. Application with vaginal suppositories is another method being considered.

DIAGNOSIS

Each type of UTI has a different name, and may cause specific signs and symptoms, depending on where the infection is.

• **URETHRITIS** An inflammation or infection of the urethra that causes burning urination and, sometimes, pus in the urine. In men, urethritis may cause penile discharge.

• **CYSTITIS** Inflammation or infection of the bladder that may result in pressure in the pelvis and lower abdomen and strong-smelling urine. Blood is often present with cystitis, but does not necessarily signify a more serious infection.

• **ACUTE PYELONEPHRITIS** This infection of the kidneys may spread from an infection in the bladder, or occasionally, from bacteria that make their way into the blood from other sources of infection. Kidney infection can cause pain in the sides, high temperatures, shaking, chills, and nausea or vomiting.

If symptoms of a urinary or kidney infection develop, it is important to contact a doctor promptly. A urinalysis, sometimes followed by a urine culture, can also reveal the presence of an infection. Although no simple test can differentiate between an upper and lower urinary tract infection, the presence of a temperature, pain in the sides, nausea and vomiting indicate that the infection probably involves the kidneys. A CT scan with dye to view the urinary tract may also be performed. Another test, cystoscopy, enables the doctor to get a good view of the bladder and urethra.

TREATMENT

Antibiotics will be prescribed for any bacterial infection. Typically, bladder infections can be treated and eliminated with as little as three days of antibiotics.

When an infection develops in the kidneys, the most important measures are to eliminate the bacteria with antibiotics given orally or intravenously, and to remove any obstruction such as kidney stones. Treatment may continue for one to two weeks after tests indicate that the kidneys are back to normal. When an obstruction cannot be eliminated and recurrent infections persist, long-term antibiotic therapy may be required.

See also: *Yeasts, pp.550–1* • *Kidney Stones, pp.304–5* • *Diabetes, pp.338–41*

Kidney Stones

These 'stones' are hard masses made of protein and mineral crystals that separate from urine and build up on the inner surfaces of the kidney. They may be as small as grains of sand or as large as golf balls. They may be jagged or smooth. The prevalence of kidney stones varies among ethnic groups and geographic locations. About 10 percent of all people will have a kidney stone at some point in their life.

CAUSES

Kidney stones are caused by the build-up of mineral salts in the urine. Repeated urinary tract infections (pp.302–3), kidney and metabolic disorders, such as hyperparathyroidism (p.350), and certain rare inherited conditions, such as polycystic kidney disease (p.308), have all been linked to kidney stone formation.

Certain diuretics, calcium-based antacids, and other medications can increase the risk of developing kidney stones. Although some foods, such as meat, fish and poultry, may promote stone formation in susceptible people, no specific food causes stones to form in people who are not susceptible.

PREVENTION

There is currently no known way to prevent stones from developing. Once a person has had a kidney stone, preventing additional stones depends on what kind of stone it is (see *On Call*) and whether there is an underlying disease that caused the stone to develop. Treating an underlying disease can reduce the likelihood of more stones. In almost all cases, increasing fluid intake – especially water – can help prevent additional stones from forming.

In the past, people who developed calcium phosphate stones were often told to avoid dairy products and other calcium-rich foods. Doctors now know that eating calcium-rich foods usually does not promote stone formation, and may even help prevent the formation of calcium phosphate stones. Taking large amounts of calcium supplements, however, may increase the risk of developing stones.

Patients with calcium oxalate stones may be advised to limit their consumption of animal protein such as meat, fish and chicken, as well as other foods and beverages that can increase the risk of these stones, including beer, black pepper, beetroot, berries, broccoli, chocolate, nuts, rhubarb, spinach, tea and wheat bran.

DIAGNOSIS

Blood in the urine or sudden pain are often the first signs. Other symptoms include excruciating pain, which is cramping and spasmodic, as well as painful urination, nausea, vomiting and fever. To confirm the presence of stones,

On Call

There are four common types of kidney stones:

Calcium stones About 80 percent of all kidney stones are composed of calcium and phosphate or calcium and oxalate. Calcium not used by bones and muscles goes to the kidneys and can form stones. About 60 percent of people who develop one stone will go on to develop additional stones.

Struvite stones Approximately 10 percent of kidney stones are struvite. These often form after repeated urinary tract infections caused by a type of bacteria that produces a substance called urease, which makes urine less acidic. Composed of magnesium and ammonia, they are especially dangerous because they can grow quite large.

Uric acid stones About 5 percent of kidney stones develop when uric levels in urine become so high that solid bits of uric acid form a solid mass.

Cystine stones Two percent of kidney stones are caused by the build-up of cystine, a type of amino acid. They form stones in people who cannot process amino acids in their diet. These stones tend to run in families.

doctors often take sonograms or X-rays. In a procedure called an intravenous pyleogram (IVP) or a CT, iodine dye is injected into a vein before an X-ray is taken. The dye is visible in the kidneys, ureters and bladder as it travels through them. When a stone is present, the dye will be halted or will only be able to pass the obstructing stone at a trickle.

When a kidney stone is suspected, the urine should be strained through a special sieve. The stone can then be collected and sent to a laboratory to determine what type it is. Collecting urine for 24 hours, followed by analysis of its chemical makeup, can often determine why a stone formed.

TREATMENTS

Initial treatment includes taking pain medication and large amounts of fluid to help the stone pass through the urinary tract. Often, a person can stay at home during this process. If a person

is vomiting or unable to drink because of the pain, doctors may provide fluids intravenously. If pain is intense, doctors may prescribe narcotic drugs such as morphine. If symptoms and urine tests indicate the presence of infection, treatment will also include antibiotics. When stones do not pass on their own, there are several ways to get rid of them.

• **EXTRACORPOREAL SHOCKWAVE LITHOTRIPSY (ESWL)** Shock waves are created that travel through the skin and tissue until they hit the stones and break them into sand-like particles that can pass easily through the urinary tract. The appropriateness of the procedure depends on the size and location of the stone.

• **SURGERY** A surgeon passes a fiberoptic wire called a ureteroscope through the urethra and bladder into the ureter, where the stone is located. The ureteroscope has a tiny camera attached to it that enables the doctor to see the stone. The surgeon then pulls the stone out with a cage-like device or shatters it with shock waves. Fragments then pass out of the body on their own or may be removed through a tiny incision. Percutaneous nephrolithotomy may be used if a stone is very large or is in a location that makes ESWL inappropriate. The surgeon makes a small incision in the patient's back and tunnels directly into the kidney. Using an instrument called a nephroscope, the surgeon locates and removes the stone.

• **MEDICATION** Patients with calcium and uric acid stones may benefit from taking medication

that control the amount of acid and alkali in urine, which are key factors in stone formation.

• **ACUPUNCTURE** This treatment (pp.464–5) is used to relieve the pain associated with kidney stones.

See also: *Urinary Tract Infections, pp.302–3 • Kidney Disease, p.308 • Acupuncture, pp.464–5*

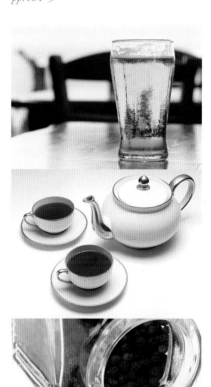

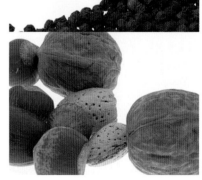

Limiting consumption of beer, black pepper, nuts and tea may help decrease the risk of developing kidney stones formed from calcium and oxalate.

Kidney Failure

Kidney failure occurs when the kidneys are unable to adequately filter metabolic waste products from the blood and control the amount and distribution of water, sodium, potassium, calcium, and phosphate in the bloodstream. Acute kidney failure is a rapid decline in kidney function; chronic kidney failure is when the decline is gradual. However, acute kidney failure can become chronic if kidney function does not recover after treatment.

Although kidney failure affects people of all ages, it is more common in older people. African Americans are four times more prone to kidney failure than Caucasians.

Many causes of kidney failure can be treated; the availability of dialysis has transformed kidney failure from a fatal disease into a chronic one.

CAUSES

Kidney failure may be caused by a primary disorder in the kidney or it may be secondary to other systemic diseases, such as diabetes, high blood pressure, and autoimmune diseases such as lupus (pp.324–5).

Acute kidney failure can result from any condition that suddenly decreases blood supply to the kidneys or obstructs urine flow anywhere along the urinary tact. It is likely to occur after surgery or severe injury, or when blood vessels leading to the kidneys become blocked.

Chronic kidney failure develops slowly. Many people with chronic kidney failure do not realize they have a problem until their kidney function has decreased to less than 25 percent of normal. The most common causes of chronic kidney failure are high blood pressure (pp.236–9) and diabetes (pp.338–41). Both of these conditions damage the kidneys' small blood vessels. Other causes of chronic kidney failure include urinary tract obstruction, kidney abnormalities such as polycystic kidney disease (p.308), and autoimmune disorders such as lupus, in which antibodies damage the tiny blood vessels and tubes of the kidneys.

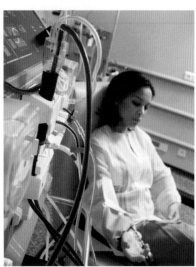

Haemodialysis machines use special filters to cleanse the blood of toxins and excess fluid after the kidneys have failed.

PREVENTION

Staying healthy is the best way to prevent acute kidney failure. When planning surgery, it is important to be aware of the risks and possible complications, and to report any changes in urine output to a medical professional. The most obvious symptom of acute kidney failure is a decrease in urine, which occurs in 70 percent of kidney patients.

Managing high blood pressure and diabetes is key to decreasing the chances of chronic kidney failure. It is also important not to use any prescription or over-the-counter medicines or herbal or nutritional supplements without first talking to a doctor, since some of these can affect the kidneys.

DIAGNOSIS

Urinalysis and blood tests can detect many abnormalities; ultrasound is often performed as well. Kidney biopsy may be the most accurate test for kidney failure, but

WHO IS AT RISK?

The risk factors include:

- Diabetes
- Hypertension
- Family history of kidney failure
- Autoimmune diseases such as lupus
- Over age 60
- African-American heritage

is not recommended if results of an ultrasound show that the kidneys are small and scarred. Many kidney biopsies will reveal scarring but will not help in determining what caused the kidneys to fail.

TREATMENTS

Treatment depends upon the cause and whether the problem can be reversed. Doctors will first treat any reversible illnesses that caused the kidney failure.

• MEDICATION Infections can be treated with antibiotics. Patients with high blood levels of potassium due to kidney failure can be prescribed medication to bring potassium levels under control. High blood pressure can be treated with antihypertensive drugs to prevent further impairment of heart and kidney function.

• NUTRITION Decline in kidney function can sometimes be slowed by restricting the amount of protein consumed. A recent analysis of published studies done jointly at L'Hôpital Edouard Herriot in Lyon, France, and the University of California–Irvine, concluded that low-protein diets delay end-stage renal disease in non-diabetic adults with chronic renal failure.

• LITHOTRIPSY Stones that cause kidney failure may pass out of the body on their own or may require removal or treatment with sound waves (lithotripsy), which breaks the stones up so they can be passed.

• SURGERY Tumours or very large stones may be surgically or medically removed, depending on their size and location.

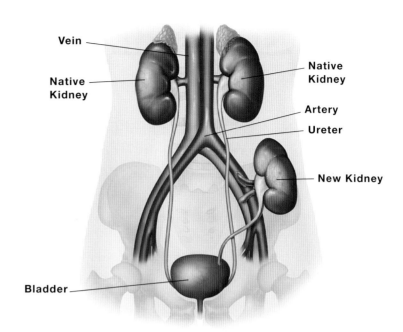

This shows the placement of a transplanted kidney. The new kidney is implanted through an incision in the lower abdomen near the groin. Native kidneys are not usually removed unless they are chronically infected or too enlarged to make room for the new kidney.

If the above measures prove to be inadequate, patients have two treatment options: dialysis and kidney transplant. There are two types of dialysis:

• HAEMODIALYSIS This is the most common method that is used to treat advanced and permanent kidney failure. The blood is allowed to flow gradually through a machine with a special filter that removes wastes and extra fluids. The clean blood is then returned to the body.

• PERITONEAL DIALYSIS A tube called a catheter is used to fill the abdomen with a cleansing liquid. The abdominal walls are lined with a membrane called the peritoneum, which allows waste products and extra fluid to pass from the blood into the dialysis solution. The solution contains a type of sugar that pulls wastes and extra fluid into the abdominal cavity. These wastes and fluid then leave the body when the dialysis solution is drained. The used, waste-filled solution is then discarded.

See also: *Kidney Disease, p.308* • *High Blood Pressure, pp.236–9* • *Diabetes, pp.338–41*

Clinical Query

I've heard that vitamin D may help people who are on kidney dialysis. Is this true?

Recent studies have found that vitamin D may significantly improve survival for many kidney failure patients on dialysis. Although vitamin D injections are currently recommended only for dialysis patients with elevated levels of parathyroid hormone, research suggests that vitamin D may extend the lives of most kidney failure patients. All categories of patients may benefit, including those with elevated phosphorous and calcium levels.

Polycystic Kidney Disease

In people with this genetic disorder, fluid-filled cysts grow out of nephrons, the tiny filtering units inside the kidneys. Over time, polycystic kidney disease (PKD) cysts can crowd out normal kidney tissue, reducing kidney function and eventually causing kidney failure.

CAUSES

Diseases with dominant inheritance occur when an abnormal gene received from only one parent is enough to produce illness. Recessive inheritance refers to a disease that requires genes from both parents.

Autosomal dominant PKD is the more common inherited form, accounting for about 90 percent of all PKD cases. (Autosomal means the gene involved is not one related to gender.) Symptoms of autosomal dominant PKD usually develop between the ages of 30 and 40. Autosomal recessive PKD is much more rare. Symptoms usually develop in early childhood.

Acquired cystic kidney disease (ACKD) is a non-inherited form of PKD. It develops in association with long-term kidney problems, especially in patients who have kidney failure (pp.306–7) and have been on long-term dialysis.

PREVENTION

Genetic tests can detect PKD mutations before cysts develop. Young people who know they have a PKD mutation may forestall the disease by controlling blood pressure.

DIAGNOSIS

Abdominal ultrasound imaging is used to detect multiple kidney cysts. The diagnosis is strengthened by a family history of PKD and the presence of cysts in other organs. Doctors can also detect cysts using computed tomography (CT) scans and magnetic resonance imaging (MRI). Urinalysis may also be performed.

TREATMENTS

Although PKD has no known cure, treatment can reduce symptoms, help prevent complications, and prolong survival. If patients with PKD develop kidney failure, they will require dialysis or a kidney transplant.

- **PAIN CONTROL** Pain, which typically occurs in the back and sides, may be controlled with over-the-counter analgesics. Surgical or radiologic drainage of PKD cysts can also relieve pain.
- **BLOOD PRESSURE CONTROL** Blood pressure can often be controlled with antihypertensive drugs or diuretics and a low-salt diet.
- **INFECTION CONTROL** People with PKD from a dominant gene tend to have frequent urinary tract infections (pp.302–3). These should be treated promptly with antibiotics to prevent them from spreading to the cysts in the kidneys, where such infections are difficult to treat.
- **DIET** Altering the diet may help retard the growth of cysts in PKD. Such alterations might include substituting soy protein for milk. While to date studies have only been conducted in mice, soy protein appears to retard the growth of kidney cysts. Other measures include reducing dietary protein to a low, yet growth-maintaining level, reducing dietary fat and adding flaxseed to the diet.

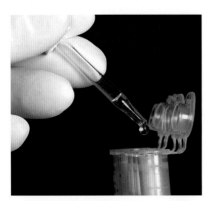

Genetic testing can detect polycystic kidney disease in patients before illness develops. Maintaining low blood pressure can help prevent the disease getting worse.

See also: *Kidney Failure, pp.306–7* • *Urinary Tract Infection, pp.302–3*

Kidney Cancer

Cancer in the kidneys accounts for just 2 to 3 percent of all adult cancers. It affects more men than women, is twice as likely to develop in smokers as in non-smokers, and is most often diagnosed in people between the ages of 50 and 70. When kidney cancer is found and treated early, the survival rate ranges from 79 to 100 percent.

There are several types of kidney cancer. The most common, renal cell carcinoma (RCC), accounts for approximately 90 percent of all cases. Transitional cell cancer (TCC), accounts for about 5 to 10 percent of all kidney cancers. TCC begins in the renal pelvis – the junction of the ureter and the kidney. There is also a type of kidney cancer called Wilms tumour that affects children.

CAUSES

Tumours that originate in the kidney are called primary tumours. Kidneys can also develop secondary tumours when cancer spreads from other parts of the body.

Although the exact causes of primary kidney cancer are not known, it is often associated with hereditary conditions like Hippel-Landau disease and tuberous sclerosis. Transitional cell cancer is linked to cigarette smoking and exposure to certain cancer-causing chemicals.

PREVENTION

Stop smoking and maintain a healthy weight. Get treatment for high blood pressure; eat adequate amounts of fruits and vegetables;

exercise; and avoid workplace exposure to harmful substances such as asbestos, cadmium and organic solvents. A study conducted at the Karolinska Institutet in Stockholm, Sweden, and published in 2005 in the International Journal of Cancer suggested that eating large amounts of fruits and vegetables might be associated with a reduced risk of RCC.

DIAGNOSIS

Today, the most common way to discover a kidney cancer is as an incidental finding on a CT scan performed for other reasons.

Specific symptoms may point to a kidney cancer diagnosis. Renal cell carcinoma occasionally presents as an abdominal mass, which may be accompanied by discomfort, pain or blood in the urine, which, if not visible to the naked eye, can be detected by urinalysis. Transitional cell carcinoma is signalled by similar symptoms, including blood in the urine and, sometimes, back pain.

If kidney cancer is suspected, the first test is usually an ultrasound, which may give enough information to confirm the presence and nature of a kidney tumour. CT or MRI scans may be done if ultrasound

WHO IS AT RISK?

The risk factors include:

- Being male
- Ages 50 to 70
- Smoking
- Obesity
- Hypertension
- Long-term kidney dialysis
- Exposure to asbestos and other toxic substances
- Von Hippel-Landau syndrome

results are uncertain. Finally, doctors will perform a biopsy.

TREATMENTS

When diagnosed at an early stage, kidney cancer is curable. Moreover, improved imaging techniques have increased the detection of small kidney tumours.

• SURGERY The standard treatment for kidney cancer is surgery to remove all or part of the kidney, called total or partial nephrectomy. Less invasive procedures include laparoscopic partial nephrectomy, cryoablation (freezing cancer cells), and radiofrequency ablation (using radio waves to kill tumours).

• IMMUNOTHERAPY In patients with advanced kidney cancer, immunotherapy with Interferon and interleukin 2 may be used to boost the immune system to fight tumours.

See also: *Obesity, pp.348–9 • Smoking Cessation, pp.216–17 • High Blood Pressure, pp.236–9*

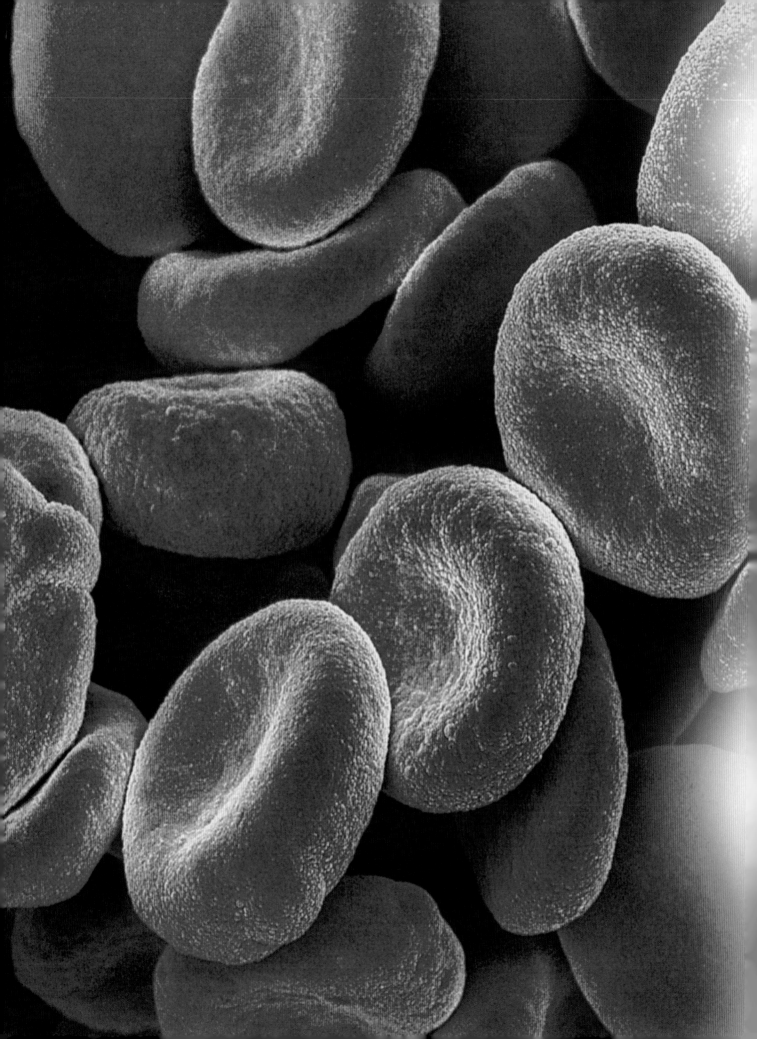

BLOOD & IMMUNE SYSTEM

11

The blood and immune systems transport oxygen and cells that fight foreign substances such as viruses and bacteria through the body. They do this with the help of several cellular components: red blood cells carry oxygen from the lungs to the organs and carbon dioxide from these organs back to the lungs. Platelets allow a clot to form if a person is injured. White blood cells – helper T-cells, killer T-cells, B-cells and phagocytes – attack and destroy any harmful substance within the body. Helper T-cells roam the body; if one finds a cell or microorganism that poses a danger, it sends a signal to the rest of the immune system to mount an attack. B-cells produce antibodies that can remember its characteristics and quickly surround a foreign substance if it returns. Killer T-cells destroy the substance or a phagocyte engulfs and neutralizes the invader.

Anaemia

With each breath, we inhale oxygen into our lungs. Oxygen is needed to nourish the organs and tissues that compose our bodies. Red blood cells work to carry oxygen molecules throughout the bloodstream with the help of a substance called haemoglobin. Anaemia occurs when there are too few healthy red blood cells to transport the oxygen throughout the body.

People with anaemia do not receive the optimal oxygen carrying capacity in their blood. They may feel tired, appear pale, have a shortness of breath and an elevated heartbeat.

CAUSES

Anaemia can occur as a result of several conditions: damage to existing red blood cells, blood loss, or inadequate production of red blood cells in the bone marrow. Below are the most common forms of anaemia.

• IRON–DEFICIENCY ANAEMIA This is the most common type of anaemia. It occurs when the body does not have enough iron to produce haemoglobin. The body recycles blood cells as a source of iron, and so blood loss, like that which can result from a heavy menstrual cycle or a bleeding ulcer can cause this iron–deficiency anaemia. Other causes include poor nutrition and pregnancy. During pregnancy, iron is taken from the woman's body to support the growing foetus.

• VITAMIN–DEFICIENCY ANAEMIA Vitamin B_{12} and folate are both necessary for the production of healthy red blood cells. A diet low in folic acid and vitamin B_{12} may cause this type of anaemia. If a person's body is unable to absorb vitamin B_{12}, a condition called pernicious anaemia may result, which affects the nervous system.

• APLASTIC ANAEMIA A serious condition called aplastic anaemia results when bone marrow is unable to produce blood cells. It is thought to be an autoimmune disease in which the body mistakenly attacks healthy cells. Aplastic anaemia has also been associated with exposure to toxic chemicals, radiation therapy, chemotherapy and certain medications.

• HAEMOLYTIC ANAEMIA This anaemia occurs when red blood cells are destroyed more quickly than the bone marrow can replace them. It can be caused by a malfunctioning immune system that destroys healthy red blood cells, or by medication such as antibiotics or blood pressure medication.

• SICKLE-CELL ANAEMIA This inherited condition frequently occurs in people of African and Arabic descent. It is often associated with painful crises and can sometimes be quite serious. In people affected with sickle-cell anaemia, abnormal haemoglobin causes the red blood cells to become crescent-shaped. These abnormal red blood cells are quickly destroyed by the body and are unable to pass through the bloodstream, which may cause severe episodes of pain.

• THALASSAEMIA In this condition, red blood cells are incapable of surviving for extended periods due to an abnormality. In severe forms of thalassaemia, iron is deposited in the skin and vital organs.

• GLUCOSE-6-PHOSPHATE DEHYDRO-GENASE (G6PD) DEFICIENCY The enzyme G6PD protects red blood cells from premature damage. Those born with insufficient levels of G6PD cannot sustain normal levels of red blood cells. Certain foods, such as fava beans, can precipitate an episode of haemolysis.

• ANAEMIA RESULTING FROM CHRONIC DISEASE Some chronic diseases inhibit the production of healthy

WHO IS AT RISK?

The risk factors include:

• Diet poor in iron and vitamin B_{12}
• Family history of anaemia
• Intestinal disorders
• Chronic diseases
• African-Americans are at increased risk of sickle cell anaemia
• Women are at increased risk of iron deficiency anaemia

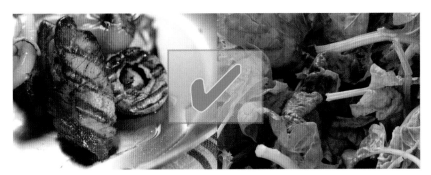
Iron-rich foods include red meat, green leafy vegetables, dried beans, dried apricots, prunes, raisins, almonds, seaweeds, parsley, whole grains and yams.

red blood cells. Examples include chronic infections and kidney disease. In kidney failure (pp.306–7), the body does not produce enough red blood cells due to a decrease in erythropoietin, a hormone produced in the kidney that stimulates production of red blood cells in the bone marrow.

PREVENTION

The best way to prevent iron and vitamin deficiency anaemia is to eat a well-balanced diet of foods rich in iron, vitamin B_{12} and folic acid. Examples of these types of foods include beef, leafy green vegetables, fortified breakfast cereals and nuts. Vitamin C increases the absorption of iron into the body; calcium decreases absorption. Certain other diseases such as Crohn's disease (p.266) may make it difficult to absorb enough of these nutrients even with adequate intake and anaemia may result. Many forms of anaemia cannot be prevented.

DIAGNOSIS

The common symptoms of anaemia include fatigue, shortness of breath, elevated heart rate, chest pains, dizziness, headaches, an inability to concentrate, and feelings of coldness in the arms and legs. If the anaemia is mild, there may be no symptoms at all. Blood tests are used to diagnosis anaemia. A complete blood count (CBC) indicates levels of red blood cells and haemoglobin circulating in the bloodstream. A blood smear analysis will also be performed. In this test, the blood is examined under a microscope to determine the colour, size and shape of the red blood cells, which offers clues to the type of anaemia present.

Additional testing may be required to pinpoint the cause of a patient's anaemia. Haemoglobin electrophoresis is used to determine if a patient's haemoglobin molecules are abnormal. A bone marrow biopsy indicates whether the bone marrow is producing sufficient quantities of healthy red blood cells.

TREATMENTS

Each kind of anaemia is treated differently. Depending on the type, doctors recommend the following.

• CHANGE IN DIET Eating foods rich in iron, folate and vitamin B_{12} can increase the production of healthy red blood cells.

• SUPPLEMENTS AND MULTIVITAMINS These are prescribed in patients with low levels of vitamin B_{12} and iron. They are taken for a period of time, until a patient is able to maintain sufficient levels of these substances in the bloodstream.

• DISCONTINUATION OF MEDICATION Certain medication can cause the development of anaemia. The doctor may change a prescription or lower its dosage.

• IMMUNE-SUPPRESSING MEDICATION If a patient's immune system is attacking healthy red blood cells, this medication is used to prevent their destruction by inhibiting the immune cells from functioning.

• BLOOD TRANSFUSION During a blood transfusion, red blood cells from a healthy donor are given by vein to increase the blood's oxygen-carrying capacity.

• BONE MARROW TRANSPLANT In severe cases, where the bone marrow is unable to produce healthy red blood cells, a patient may require this procedure. Many factors determine whether this is a potential treatment, including cause of the anaemia, patient's age and his or her underlying health.

• MEDICATION In some cases, medication can treat anaemia. Examples include hydroxyurea and erythropoeitin. Hydroxyurea increases the flexibility of abnormally shaped blood cells, allowing them to pass through the bloodstream of patients with sickle cell anaemia. A synthetic version of erythropoietin, a hormone that stimulates the production of red blood cells, is sometimes given to correct the condition.

See also: *Headaches, pp.166–7* • *Menstrual Bleeding Disorders, pp.384–5* • *Kidney Failure, pp.306–7*

IMMUNIZATIONS

In 1790, the English doctor Edward Jenner developed the first immunization after observing that milkmaids infected with cowpox rarely became ill with a similar and more deadly disease called smallpox. His discovery has revolutionized healthcare – it is now possible to prevent more than 20 infectious diseases with immunizations or vaccines. Today, scientists continue to develop vaccines through their newfound knowledge of genetics and molecular biology.

Immunizations protect humans from diseases by stimulating the body's immune system to respond to a less dangerous form of an illness. An immunization can consist of a less potent form of a microbe (a bacteria or virus), dead microbes, or inactivated toxins or proteins from microbes. The words immunization and vaccine are often used interchangeably.

Once the immune system is exposed to these substances, it can produce antibodies: proteins made by the body's immune system that fight infection. These antibodies can later recognize and eliminate the dangerous forms of the disease.

CAUTION

Most flu vaccines are very safe, but some groups should not be immunized. They include anyone with a severe allergy to chicken eggs, anyone who has had a severe reaction to a flu vaccination in the past, and anyone who has developed Guillain-Barré syndrome within six weeks of previously receiving an influenza vaccine.

CHILDHOOD IMMUNIZATIONS

Some parents wonder whether to vaccinate their children at all because they fear that immunizations are dangerous. The fact is that the benefits of immunizations far outweigh the risks. In many countries, persistent immunization campaigns have meant that the occurrence of most childhood illnesses is rare.

Vaccines are currently available for 12 childhood illnesses, each given according to a specific schedule. Below are descriptions of each immunization as well as information about when it is most commonly administered.

• **HEPATITIS B** This disease is life-threatening, especially in young children. Hepatitis B (p.269) can cause severe liver damage that can result in liver failure or cancer. This vaccine is usually the first given to an infant before leaving the hospital and again during follow-up visits to the paediatrician after two and six months.

• **DIPHTHERIA, TETANUS, PERTUSSIS** Diphtheria is a deadly disease that causes a thick grey membrane to develop in the throat. This membrane eventually affects an infected individual's airway and may cause difficulty with breathing. It also produces a toxic substance that is deposited through out the body during the illness.

Also known as lockjaw, tetanus is a disease that affects the nervous system and may cause permanent damage to the speech, memory and mental function of its victims. It can also result in the death of individuals with compromised immune systems.

Pertussis, or whooping cough, is an extremely dangerous disease to infants. It is highly contagious and can cause convulsions, coma and permanent brain damage.

Today diphtheria, tetanus and pertussis outbreaks are rare in many countries because of the vaccine, which is administered at regular intervals during childhood. Children are usually vaccinated against these three diseases in two injections, one when the child is between 2 and 4 months, and the second between 3 and 5 years old.

• **HAEMOPHILUS INFLUENZA TYPE B** Once the most common cause of bacterial meningitis in children, haemophilus influenza type b (Hib) meningitis can result in blindness, hearing impairment, joint damage or permanent brain damage in children. The Hib vaccine is administered by an injection given between 2 and 4 months old. It is also now possible to have a vaccination against meningitis C at this age.

• **PNEUMOCOCCAL DISEASE** This illness, also known as infantile paralysis, is prevented by the pneumococcal conjugate vaccine (PCV), which is recommended for at risk children aged 2 months to under 5 years of age. The bacteria that causes pneumococcal disease was the most frequent cause of ear infections in children before the introduction of this vaccine.

• **HEPATITIS A** The vaccine for hepatitis A (p. 269) is given only after a child's first birthday. Many children can be carriers of this virus and have no symptoms. If contracted, hepatitis A can later cause severe liver damage.

• **MEASLES, MUMPS, RUBELLA** The MMR vaccine protects children from the measles, mumps, and rubella. It is administered at around 13 months of age and between 3 and 5 years of age.

Measles was once a common childhood illness in the West. Those stricken sometimes suffered complications such as inflammation of the central nervous system, permanent brain damage or death.

Similarly, mumps was also once a common disease. It could cause infertility in boys, encephalitis (a viral infection of the brain), paralysis and seizures.

Rubella, or German measles, is known to cause serious birth defects if a pregnant woman becomes infected with the illness.

• **VARICELLA** Chicken pox, or varicella, causes tiny blisters to develop on the face, scalp and trunk of children. If contracted later in childhood, it can result in encephalitis and pneumonia. This vaccine is given to children in the United States between the first and second year of life.

ADULT IMMUNIZATIONS

Because most adults have healthy immune systems, the number of vaccines recommended for them is limited. Following are the most common adult immunizations. Note that, depending upon where one lives, travel to some parts of the world may require immunizations in addition to those listed below. For instance, yellow fever immunizations are required for people travelling to some parts of Africa and South America.

• **FLU VACCINE** Each year, the flu vaccine is recommended for adults, especially those who are over age 50, people whose immune systems are compromised (as is the case for those with HIV or AIDs), and people who suffer from chronic heart or lung conditions.

• **PNEUMOCOCCAL VACCINE** This vaccine can prevent the occurrence of pneumonia and is strongly recommended for those over age 65 and those with chronic disease.

• **TETANUS AND DIPHTHERIA** Adults should receive a booster shoot for tetanus and diphtheria every ten years for life.

• **OTHER CHILDHOOD ILLNESSES** Adults who were never ill with either the chickenpox, measles, mumps or rubella should receive these vaccinations.

• **HEPATITIS A AND B** Certain populations have an increased risk for contracting hepatitis A and B (p. 269) and should therefore receive vaccinations for both of these diseases. At-risk groups include people with chronic liver problems, healthcare workers, intravenous drug users, international travellers and those who participate in high-risk sexual behaviour.

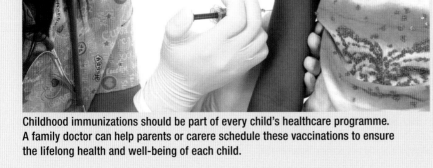

Childhood immunizations should be part of every child's healthcare programme. A family doctor can help parents or carere schedule these vaccinations to ensure the lifelong health and well-being of each child.

See also: *Hepatitis, pp.269* • *Pneumonia pp.202–3* • *Infertility, pp.420–1*

HIV/AIDS

The human immunodeficiency virus – more commonly known as HIV– is a life-threatening microorganism that has infected more than 40 million people worldwide. HIV can destroy the human immune system by attacking helper T cells, also known as CD4 lymphocytes. Helper T cells coordinate the entire immune response by signalling to other immune cells when to desbtroy an infected or abnormal cell.

Thus, HIV leads to a debilitating illness known as acquired immuno-deficiency syndrome, or AIDS. People with AIDS are unable to fight off infections and often contract certain cancers.

CAUSES

HIV is contracted once the virus enters the bloodstream; it is transmitted from contact with bodily fluids in the following ways:

• **SEXUAL CONTACT** Semen, vaginal secretions and blood of infected people contain HIV. During anal, vaginal or oral sex, the virus can be passed between sexual partners through small abrasions that routinely occur during sex. The covering of the anus is extremely susceptible to tearing, which makes it easy for HIV to spread between semen and blood. In addition, if a person has cuts in their mouth, HIV can enter at these sites during oral sex.

• **SHARING OF INFECTED NEEDLES** HIV can survive on the tip of a needle; therefore, intravenous drug users are at extreme risk of contracting the virus while sharing needles. Hospital workers and others can be exposed to HIV by an accidental prick from a needle that had been used by an infected individual.

• **BLOOD TRANSFUSIONS** Although in many countries blood is carefully screened for HIV, there are parts of the world where the screening process is not effective and so it is possible to contract HIV during a blood transfusion.

• **DURING PREGNANCY, CHILDBIRTH AND BREASTFEEDING** Mothers can pass HIV to their children. The

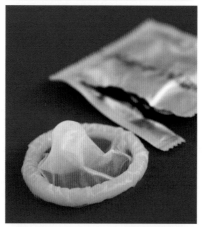

Latex condoms, when used correctly, can reduce the risk of transmitting HIV. Non-latext condoms, such as those made from sheepskins, do not protect against HIV.

risk of this occurring decreases dramatically if the mother immediately seeks treatment upon learning of the pregnancy.

Once the virus enters the bloodstream, it invades helper T cells and reproduces itself. The virus overtakes the ability of the helper T cells to function. Eventually, the number of helper T cells circulating within the body decreases to such an extent that the body can no longer protect itself, rendering the immune system defenceless.

PREVENTION

HIV and AIDS can be prevented by following these guidelines.

Before engaging in any form of sexual activity, both partners should be aware of their own – and each other's – HIV status.

Intravenous drug users should seek treatment for their addiction, and needles should not be shared.

Since infections with other sexually transmitted diseases (STDs, pp.392–3) increase the risk of HIV, people infected with any STD should be treated and tested for HIV immediately and abstain from any sexual contact until the illness is resolved.

Pregnant women should be pre-screened for HIV infection and treated immediately to prevent the transmission to their unborn baby.

In some countries, blood transfusions can be extremely risky. If a transfusion becomes necessary during an emergency situation, it is advisable to take an HIV test after the transfusion.

DIAGNOSIS

The symptoms of HIV and AIDS progress gradually over time. In fact, in the beginning stages of HIV infection, it is possible to experience no symptoms at all. It is common for newly infected people to complain of a flu-like illness that lasts for 2 to 6 weeks. Symptoms include a high temperature, vomiting, a sore throat and headaches. As the disease progresses, symptoms can include rashes, diarrhoea, weight loss, persistent fevers, shortness of breath, fatigue, night sweats, frequently reoccurring headaches, blurred vision and swollen lymph nodes.

HIV is diagnosed by blood tests that identify antibodies to the virus in the blood. Antibodies attach to microorganisms and abnormal cells within the body to destroy them. Once the antibodies have been identified, the HIV infection is confirmed with more specific tests.

The viral load test is important

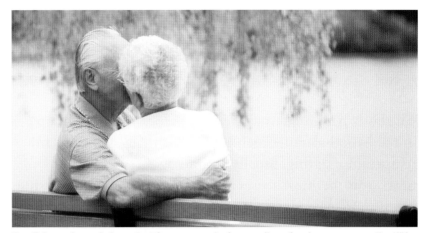

Practising safe sex is important for anyone who is sexually active. In some areas, the HIV infection rate of people over 50 is rising for many reasons, including not knowing the risk factors, lack of education and the mistaken belief that HIV affects only younger people.

for assessing the extent of the illness. The test measures the amount of HIV in the blood and helps to determine treatment options.

Diagnosis of AIDS is made if two conditions are met. First, the number of helper T cells must be below 200 per cu.ml. (A normal level is 600–1000 T cells per cu.ml.) Second, the individual must have developed an infection or cancer as a result of a weakened immune system. Examples include certain types of pneumonia, tuberculosis and Kaposi's sarcoma.

TREATMENTS

There is no cure for HIV or AIDS. Doctors strive to preserve the quality of life of an infected individual and prevent the virus from replicating. The approach used to achieve this is called Highly Active Antiretroviral Therapy (HAART).

• **MEDICATION** Treatment involves the use of antiretroviral drugs often in combinations of three or more medications. There are several classes of these drugs. They work to inhibit the replication of HIV, which is a retrovirus,

by suppressing the formation of certain proteins the virus needs to survive in the body. A new class of antiretroviral drugs, called fusion inhibitors, works by preventing HIV from attaching itself to the helper T cell.

• **MEDITATION AND MASSAGE** One treatment that has been shown to improve the overall quality of life for some individuals with HIV/AIDS is a combination of meditation (pp.514–19) and massage (pp.468–73). In addition, group therapy that focuses on mental health and stress management may also improve the quality of life of HIV/AIDS patients.

• **HERBAL TREATMENTS** Although there is insufficient evidence to suggest that the use of herbal medication are effective in treating HIV/AIDS, limited studies indicate that the Chinese herbal compounds such as IGM-1 and SH may provide some beneficial improvement in the quality of life of HIV/AIDS patients.

See also: *Fever, p.318* • *Diarrhoea, p.268* • *Pneumonia, pp.202–3*

Fever

The body has an internal thermostat located in the brain in the hypothalamus. Each person has their own standard temperature setting, usually around 37°C (98.6°F). At times, this thermostat rises to a higher temperature, causing a person to experience what is known as a fever. Medically, a fever is defined as a rectal temperature of 38°C (100.4°F).

In addition to a warm feeling, a fever can cause sweating, chills, headache, muscle pain, tiredness, thirst and a lack of appetite.

Children can suffer fever-induced seizures, which cause the limbs to shake from side to side. The condition occurs in approximately 4 percent of all children and generally does not cause permanent damage.

CAUSES

Although they can seem alarming, fevers are a normal response to viral and bacterial infections. A slight increase in body temperature makes the body an uncomfortable environment for microorganisms to thrive, which helps the body fight the infection.

Although less common, a fever can also occur as a result of heat exhaustion, sunburn or the presence of a malignant tumour. Medication to treat bacterial infections,

high blood pressure and seizures can also cause fever. Many children experience a fever after a routine immunization (pp.314–15).

PREVENTION

Good hygiene, such as frequent hand-washing, is the only way to prevent viral and bacterial infections that are the cause of most fevers. Hands should always be washed following toilet use, before meals and after touching animals. Contact with the mouth, nose and eye area should be avoided, because germs can easily enter the body through these openings.

DIAGNOSIS

Some fevers require a trip to the doctor: any temperature change in an infant; a fever higher than 38.3°C (101°F) that lasts more than three days in a child older than two; and a fever over 40°C (104°F) that lasts more than three days in an adult.

Fever is diagnosed with a thermometer. Temperature can be taken orally, in the inner ear or rectally. The doctor may also do additional tests to determine the cause. A physical examination,

medical history, blood and urine tests and chest X-ray may be done.

TREATMENTS

Fever in a newborn or young child can indicate a life-threatening infection such as meningitis, especially when accompanied by irritability, listlessness or increased crying. Consult a doctor immediately.

• **MEDICATION** Paracetomol, ibuprofen and aspirin are the most common treatments for fevers. Children should never be given aspirin as it can cause a serious condition, Reye's syndrome, to develop.

• **WATER TREATMENTS** A sponge bath in lukewarm water can help to lower temperature. It is also recommended to drink plenty of water, juices or sports drinks containing electrolytes to replenish fluids.

See also: *Headaches, pp.166–7 • Epilepsy and Seizures, pp.176–7 • Heat Injuries, pp.108–9*

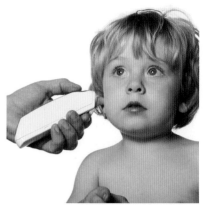

When taking a child's temperature from the ear or orally, a normal range is 36°C to 36.8°C (97.7°F to 99.1°F). An infant's temperature should be taken rectally.

WHO IS AT RISK?

The risk factors include:

• Infections
• Immunizations

Mononucleosis

Also known as mono and the kissing disease, this systemic illness affects mostly adolescents. The common symptoms include fatigue, high temperature, sore throat, enlarged tonsils, swollen lymph nodes, headache, skin rash and an inflamed spleen. Rarely, the liver can be involved and develop an associated mono-hepatitis. This condition can lead to abnormal blood-clotting and the risk of bleeding. Activity should be limited to prevent any risk of damage in patients with an enlarged spleen.

CAUSES

Mononucleosis is caused by the Epstein-Barr virus, a member of the herpes virus family and one of the most common human viruses. Approximately 95 percent of the population is affected with this virus before they reach adulthood. Most people contract it during childhood and suffer symptoms that resemble only a mild respiratory infection. Problems occur, however, when children are not exposed to the virus early in life but rather become infected during adolescence or later. Young adults are more susceptible to full-blown mononucleosis.

Mononucleosis is not highly contagious. The virus is found in saliva and mucus and is spread through close contact with an infected person, for example, by sharing a glass or food, coughing or sneezing near someone, or by kissing.

PREVENTION

The only method to prevent the spread of mononucleosis is to avoid contact with infected individuals. Those experiencing full-blown mononucleosis should not have close contact with another person; nor should they share food or eating utensils until the fever has been gone for several days. In addition, blood should not be donated for six months following the illness. Symptoms of mononucleosis commonly last approximately four weeks.

DIAGNOSIS

A doctor can usually diagnose mononucleosis based on a physical examination and the patient's symptoms. If necessary, the diagnosis can be confirmed with a blood test called the Mononucleosis spot test or Monospot. This test identifies the presence of antibodies to the Epstein–Barr virus in a patient's blood. In addition, the doctor many check for an elevated white blood cell count and an increased percentage of atypical white blood cells. A change in the number of white blood cells in the blood is an indication that the body is fighting off an infection.

TREATMENTS

The treatment for mononucleosis involves plenty of bed rest and the intake of fluids to relieve the discomfort associated with the fever.

- **MEDICATION** Pain medication such as paracetomol and ibuprofen can be used to ease the sore throat and headache.
- **GARGLING** Gargling with salt water can provide relief for the sore throat as well. A mixture of 225 ml (8 fl.oz) warm water and ½ teaspoon salt can be used as a gargle several times throughout the day.

See also: *Fever, p.318 • Headaches, pp.166–7 • Spleen, p.333*

CAUTION

Mononucleosis can cause an enlargement and rupture of the spleen (p.333). Because of this, contact sports and rigorous play activities should be avoided through out the duration of the illness and for an additional two months afterwards.

Bleeding Disorders

When a person receives a cut or injury, a complex array of events happens in the body that changes blood from liquid to solid, extensive blood loss. This process is called clotting. Platelets, tiny cells in the blood, cluster together at the site of the injury. Next, special substances called blood-clotting factors work with calcium and other components to form a clot over the wound. The clot serves as a protective covering over the injury. With time, the clot becomes stronger and eventually disappears into the wound once it is healed.

A bleeding disorder arises when this chain of events does not occur in an individual. People who suffer from bleeding disorders bleed for longer periods of time than healthy individuals and may loose significant amounts of blood spontaneously or even after minimal injury. In addition, they may experience excessive bruising and frequent nose bleeds.

CAUSES
Normally, the body contains many distinct clotting factors that aid in the process to control bleeding. Those with bleeding disorders may be missing a clotting factor or have clotting factors that do not work properly. Abnormalities of platelets can also lead to excessive bleeding.

Some bleeding disorders are inherited. Von Willebrand disease is a genetic condition in which individuals are missing a substance in the blood called van Willebrand factor or have an irregular version of this substance in their blood.

The van Willebrand factor helps the platelets bind together during clotting and carries clotting factor VIII through the blood.

Haemophilia is another genetic disorder that affects the body's ability to form a clot. Those with haemophilia do not have sufficient amounts of one of clotting factor VIII (this is the classic deficiency), IX or XI.

PREVENTION
Genetic bleeding disorders can not be prevented, because they are inherited from a parent. However, adequate vitamin K intake is important, as it is necessary for the formation of various clotting factors.

DIAGNOSIS
After completing a physical examination and medical history, the doctor may recommend special blood tests to measure the levels and functioning of blood clotting factors and platelets.

The first sign of a clotting

problem or bleeding disorder in young girls and women may be heavy bleeding during their menstrual cycles.

TREATMENTS
Depending on the cause of the bleeding disorder, the doctor may recommend one of the following treatment options:
- **REPLACEMENT THERAPY** Patients may be given infusions of the missing blood-clotting factor.
- **DESMOPRESSIN (DDAVP)** This synthetic hormone, which is administered as intravenous (IV) infusion, may decrease the risk of bleeding.
- **ANTIFIBRINOLYTIC DRUGS** These substances, which can be taken orally, by injection, or in IV form, prevent the destruction of clotting factors within the blood.
- **FIBRIN GLUE** This substance is applied directly to an injury, and can help produce an artificial clot.
- **PROGESTERONE** This hormone can be given to women who have heavy menstrual cycles. It works to increase certain clotting factors in the blood.

See also: *Menstrual Bleeding Disorders, pp.384–5 • Nosebleeds, p.70*

Candidiasis Fungal Infections

Candida is a common fungus found in the body and throughout the environment. These fungi can infect any part of the body; however, several types of candidiasis fungal infections are most commonly encountered.

- **ORAL THRUSH** This condition affects the mouth and surrounding area. Cancer and AIDS patients, diabetics, denture-wearers and infants frequently experience thrush. Symptoms include white patches in the mouth and around the lips.
- **OESOPHAGITIS** This mouth infection can also spread to the oesophagus. It is common after chemotherapy. Painful swallowing and chest pains are common symptoms.
- **CUTANEOUS** Candidiasis nappy rash is a common example of this infection. Patches of red moist areas with tiny bumps appear on the skin.
- **VAGINAL YEAST INFECTIONS** In this common infection, the vaginal area becomes itchy or sore. Other symptoms include a cottage cheese-like vaginal discharge, burning during urination and painful intercourse.
- **INVASIVE CANDIDIASIS** In this serious condition, candida invades the bloodstream. Those with a weakened immune system are more susceptible. Invasive candidiasis is also common at the site of catheters or surgical wounds and following intravenous drug use or severe burns.

CAUSES

The candida fungus, along with many bacteria, is normally found in the mouth, gastrointestinal tract and vagina. These bacteria, and the body's immune system, normally prevent it from causing an infection. If a change occurs in the level of bacteria or in the immune system, candida may be able to invade the body. These changes can occur due to sickness such as AIDS and diabetes; medication such as antibiotics, birth control pills and anticancer drugs; and malnutrition.

PREVENTION

Most candida infections can be prevented by maintaining clean and dry skin; eating a balanced diet, and limiting use of antibiotics.

DIAGNOSIS

A complete medical history is the first step in diagnosing any candida infection. Oral thrush, cutaneous candidiasis and vaginal yeast infections are diagnosed after an examination of a sample of cells from the infected area. Endoscopy, a procedure in which a tubular camera is inserted in the throat, can determine whether a patient has oesophagitis. Blood

WHO IS AT RISK?

The risk factors include:
- Weakened immune system
- Organ and bone marrow transplantation
- Feeding tubes and catheters
- Chemotherapy and radiation therapy
- Bacterial infections
- Corticosteriods
- Burns
- Antibiotics
- Prolonged hospital stays
- Severe trauma or surgery
- Premature birth

tests and, occasionally, biopsies are used for the diagnosis of invasive candidiasis.

TREATMENTS

- **MEDICATION** Antifungal medications, such as fluconazole, are used to treat most cases of candidiasis.
- **LIVE YOGHURT** Studies show that eating yogurt containing live lactobacillus can reduce the frequency of vaginal yeast infections and oral thrush in infants.
- **HERBAL TREATMENTS** In limited studies, oregano was shown to effectively treat vaginal yeast infections in rats and eliminate other candida species. Tea tree oil and garlic both show promise in treating vaginal yeast infections.

See also: *AIDS, pp.316–7* • *Diabetes, pp.338–41* • *Burns, p.110*

Chronic Fatigue Syndrome

Although little is known about the cause of chronic fatigue syndrome (CFS), the Centres for Disease Control's International Chronic Fatigue Syndrome Study Group defines it as unexplained fatigue that persists for at least six months, does not improve with rest or relaxation, and worsens following physical and mental activities.

CAUSES

The cause of chronic fatigue syndrome is unknown, although there is speculation that an infection due to a virus and/or a C pneumoniae, a common cause of human respiratory disease, may be the culprit.

PREVENTION

Because the cause of chronic fatigue syndrome is unknown, prevention methods cannot be specified. However, patients with CFS have discovered various ways to manage the condition, minimize the severity of the symptoms and prevent relapses.

• MINIMIZE STRESS Those with CFS should avoid stressful situations, limit their daily activity and practise relaxation techniques regularly such as deep breathing exercises or meditation (pp.514–19).

• GET SUFFICIENT SLEEP Healthful sleeping habits can minimize the symptoms of CFS. It is helpful to go to sleep and wake up at the same times each day.

• MAINTAIN AN EXERCISE ROUTINE Light exercise can improve the muscle and joint pain that are associated with CFS. Some

examples of helpful exercises include yoga, tai chi, water aerobics, swimming and cycling.

• MAKE HEALTHY CHOICES CFS patients should eat a balanced diet, drink adequate amounts of fluids, and avoid caffeine and alcohol consumption. Those suffering from CFS should also stop smoking immediately.

DIAGNOSIS

In order to receive a diagnosis of CFS, a person must be experiencing at least four of eight symptoms: difficulty sleeping; unexplained sore throat; memory loss or an inability to concentrate; tender and enlarged lymph nodes in the neck or armpits; muscle soreness; pain that moves from joint to joint without redness or swelling; headaches; extreme exhaustion after completing normal daily activities or exercises.

Those who have CFS may experience additional symptoms such as abdominal pain, earaches, intolerance to alcohol, chest pain, coughing, diarrhoea, dizziness, nausea, irregular heartbeats, shortness of breath, bloating, dry eyes

and mouth, jaw pain, joint stiffness in the morning, night sweats, depression and weight loss.

In order to diagnose chronic fatigue syndrome, a doctor must first rule out the presence of any other disorders or diseases. This can be a lengthy and difficult process that involves a complete medical history, a physical examination, and perhaps laboratory tests. The doctor may rule out other causes of a patient's fatigue by asking these questions:

• Do you have another medical condition that results in fatigue such as minimal levels of thyroid hormone or sleep apnoea?

• Are you using medication that causes fatigue?

• Do you have cancer or any other illnesses?

• Do you suffer from any psychological conditions such as depression, schizophrenia or an eating disorder?

• Are you severely overweight?

TREATMENTS

Current treatments for chronic fatigue syndrome are designed only to relieve the symptoms associated

WHO IS AT RISK?

The risk factors include:

• No proven risk factors exist for chronic fatigue syndrome. Women are diagnosed more often than men, but gender is not a proven risk factor.

healing hope

I made an appointment to see my doctor after I realized how many sick days I was taking from work each month. I felt as if I had reccurring bouts of the flu every couple of weeks and I just could not get back to my old energy level. It took several months for me to be diagnosed with chronic fatigue syndrome. Throughout the diagnosis process, I became depressed because no one knew what was going on with my body. Eventually, the emotional stress became overwhelming. Luckily, my doctor was able to refer me to a special support group for those with CFS. The counselling services offered through this group helped me cope with the limitations on the life I now experienced. They also helped me deal with my inability to lead an active lifestyle and to do the things I used to do in the past.   Mary K.

with this condition. Unfortunately, until a cause is identified, a specific treatment cannot exist. Nevertheless, the doctor may recommend the following to provide relief for symptoms associated with CFS:

• **LIFESTYLE CHANGES** The elimination of both physical and psychological stress can help patients with CFS maintain their energy levels throughout the day.

• **PHYSICAL THERAPY** An exercise regimen can help increase energy levels and reduce muscle aches. (See *Prevention,* left.)

• **DIETARY SUPPLEMENTS** Preparations that contain adenosine monophosphate, coenzyme Q 10, germanium, glutathione, iron, magnesium sulfate, melatonin, NADH, selenium, l-tryptophan, vitamin B_{12}, vitamin C, vitamin A and zinc (pp. 532–41) have been studied and may increase the energy levels of some patients who are suffering from CFS.

• **CARNITINE** This substance plays an important role in the body's energy production. As a dietary supplement, carnitine has been shown to improve the symptoms

associated with CFS. Meat, dairy products, beans and avocados are all naturally occurring sources.

• **ANTIDEPRESSANTS** Tricyclic antidepressants and selective serotonin reuptake inhibitors (SSRIs) have been used to relieve the depression associate with CFS as well as to improve sleep patterns and to minimize pain in patients who are not depressed.

• **PAIN–REDUCING MEDICATION** In order to reduce a high temperature and ease the muscle aches and joint discomfort associated

with CFS, medication such as paracetmol, aspirin and ibuprofen may be prescribed.

• **ANTIHISTAMINES** CFS Patients who suffer from allergy-like symptoms may benefit from taking decongestants.

• **MEDICATION TO INCREASE BLOOD PRESSURE** Fludrocortisone, atenolol and midodrine are used to raise the blood pressure of some CFS sufferers.

• **MEDICATION TO ALLEVIATE PROBLEMS OF THE NERVOUS SYSTEM** Dizziness and anxiety, which are sometimes associated with CFS, can be treated with medication that affects the nervous system such as clonazepam, lorazepam, and alprazolam.

• **KAMPO THERAPY** This system of Japanese herbal therapy, which uses herbal formulas, has been shown to effectively treat the mental fatigue, physical fatigue and sleep disorder associated with CFS.

See also: *Meditation, pp.514–9 • Chronic Fatigue Syndrome, pp.532–41 • Depression, pp.368–9*

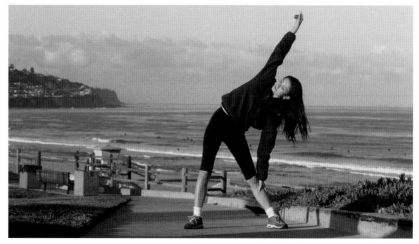

Exercise is an important component of any programme designed to cope with the symptoms of CFS. But care must be taken. Any exercise should be started slowly and increased gradually so as not to exacerbate the symptoms.

Lupus

The immune system consists of specialized cells that can recognize and attack foreign substances, such as viruses and bacteria, with the help of a variety of secreted chemicals and proteins, one class of which is called antibodies. Lupus is a condition in which the immune system becomes confused and begins to attack its own tissues. Auto-antibodies, or antibodies that work against one's own body, disseminate through the body, causing inflammation in various organs.

There are four forms of lupus. Systemic lupus erythematosus (SLE) is the most serious form of the disease. It often causes enlarged and tender joints, rash, fatigue, central nervous system symptoms and kidney damage.

Discoid lupus erythematosus is a chronic skin condition in which a raised red rash appears on the body, especially on the face and scalp. Rarely, discoid lupus erythematosus can develop into the more serious SLE.

Drug-induced lupus can occur after taking certain medications but quickly goes away once these drugs are discontinued.

Neonatal lupus erythematosus is the rarest form of the disease. It occurs in the newborns of women who have lupus. These babies receive their mother's auto-antibodies during birth.

CAUSES

The exact cause of this auto-immune condition remains unknown. One theory is that it occurs due to a combination of factors. Clearly genetics plays a role in this disorder because those with a family history of lupus are more likely to develop the condition themselves. Research also shows viral infections, such as Epstein–Barr, may cause the reoccurrence of SLE but are not felt to be the primary cause.

Prescription medication has been linked to lupus as well. It includes chlorpromazine, an anti-psychotic, hydralazine for lowering blood pressure, the tuberculosis treatment isoniazid, some antibiotics, and heart medications such as beta-blockers and procainamide.

Female hormones, such as oestrogen, appear to play a significant role in the development of the disease. This is evident by the fact that more women are diagnosed with lupus than men. In addition, birth-control pills and female hormone replacement may exacerbate the symptoms.

PREVENTION

Researchers continue to investigate ways to prevent lupus.

DIAGNOSIS

Lupus symptoms vary from person to person. One person may experience mild symptoms that come and go while another may be debilitated. This makes lupus a difficult disorder to diagnosis. The American College of Rheumatology recommends that all those diagnosed with lupus must have at least four of the most common symptoms associated with this disorder, which include the following.

- **RASH** The characteristic rash covers the bridge of the nose and checks. Rashes, though, may appear on any part of the body.
- **FATIGUE** Many patients with lupus are constantly tired, even after getting sufficient rest.
- **ARTHRITIS** Swollen and painful joints are common.
- **FEVER** A constant and unexplained temperature of 38°C (100°F) or higher.
- **PHOTOSENSITIVITY** An intolerance of natural sunlight or fluorescent lighting that exacerbates the occurrence of skin rashes.

- ULCERS Painful sores often develop in the mouth or nose.
- KIDNEY FAILURE Some patients suffer kidney damage and lose the ability to filter toxins through their kidneys. This can lead to the need for dialysis (pp.306–7).
- CENTRAL NERVOUS SYSTEM (CNS) PROBLEMS An autoimmune attack on the brain or CNS can result in many problems including dizziness, seizures, psychiatric problems and vision loss.
- HEART PROBLEMS The heart muscle, its lining and surrounding tissue can become inflamed, causing chest pain and the inability to breathe.
- LUNG PROBLEMS The most common lung problem involves the inflammation of the chest cavity known as pleurisy.
- IMPAIRED BLOOD CIRCULATION The blood vessels can become inflamed after an attack by the immune system.
- HAIR LOSS Scalp rashes sometimes cause hair loss in clumps.
- WEIGHT LOSS Abdominal pain, nausea and vomiting ultimately cause weight loss in lupus patients.
- RAYNAUD'S PHENOMENON Exposure to low temperatures causes the fingers, toes, nose and ears to become pale and numb (p.243).

Certain laboratory tests can give a doctor clues during the diagnosis process. Depending on the symptoms, the doctor may evaluate the circulatory system, kidneys, lungs, liver and heart function. The doctor may also order tests to identify auto-antibodies circulating in the blood. A skin and/or kidney biopsy may indicate whether lupus is causing the abnormalities. Lupus

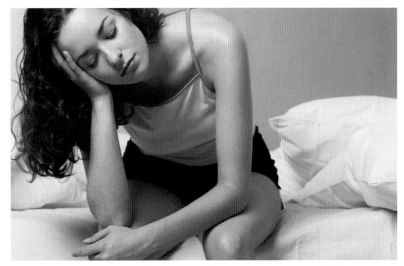

Diagnosing lupus is often difficult because the symptoms can vary widely from person to person. However, one of the most common symptoms is persistent fatigue that does not respond to adequate sleep or rest.

patients can experience low levels of complements – proteins that circulate in the blood and that aid antibody activation and control inflammation, and so these might also be measured.

TREATMENTS

An individualized treatment plan aims to prevent the reoccurrence of symptoms, relieve symptoms that do occur, and thwart complications of the disease. Examples of treatments include the following.

- NONSTEROIDAL ANTI-INFLAMMATORY DRUGS (NSAIDS) These medications help reduce joint pain and inflammation. Examples include ibuprofen, aspirin and naproxen sodium.
- ANTIMALARIALS These minimize fatigue, joint pain, ulcers, skin rashes and lung inflammation.
- CORTICOSTERIODS These are natural anti-inflammatory hormones.
- OMEGA-3 FISH OIL Fish oil supplements (pp.252–3) have been shown to improve lupus symptoms. Results of one study involving 52 lupus patients indicated that the

use of these supplements reduce the Systemic Lupus Activity Measure (SLAM-R) scores of participants.

- SUPPLEMENTS Calcium and vitamin D supplements are often used to reduce the degradation of bone structure in women with lupus.
- IMMUNOSUPPRESSIVES These medications are used in the hope that they may decrease the production of auto-antibodies and prevent the damage they cause. Because they are associated with dangerous side-effects, caution is necessary.
- RITUXIMAB Studies indicate that this drug may be effective in treating those with lupus by reducing the number of immune cells in the body.
- DEHYDROEPIANDROSTERONE (DHEA) Studies involving this steroid hormone illustrate that DHEA can be effective in reducing the number of flare-ups suffered by women with SLE.

See also: *Pregnancy, pp.398–400* • *Omega-3 Fatty Acids, pp.252–3* • *Kidney Failure, pp.306–7*

LYME & OTHER TICK-BORNE DISEASES

Ticks, insects that live in grassy and wooded areas, are responsible for a group of illnesses called tick-borne diseases. Ticks can harbour bacteria in their guts. Once they bite a human, they may transmit bacteria that cause illnesses such as Lyme disease, Rocky Mountain spotted fever, ehrlichiosis and tularaemia. Less common tick-borne diseases are tick paralysis, babesiosis, relapsing fever and Colorado tick fever.

Tick-Born Disease	Cause
Lyme disease	*Borrella burgdorferi*
Rocky Mountain spotted fever	*Rickettsia rickettsii*
Erlichiosis	*Ehrlichia chafeensis*
Tularaemia	*Francisella tularensis*
Babesiosis	*Babesia microti*
Relapsing fever	Borelia species
Colorado tick fever	Cotivirus
Tick paralysis	Neurotoxin produced in the mouth of a tick

The chart (right) identifies several tick-borne diseases along with the cause of each illness.

CAUSES

Tick-borne diseases are normally caused by microorganisms that live in the stomachs of ticks. These microorganisms are passed to the blood stream of a human by a bite. Usually, a tick must remain attached to the human for a period of time to transmit a disease.

PREVENTION

Tick-borne diseases can easily be prevented by following some precautionary measures.

Ticks often hide in overgrown grass and wooded areas. Wear light-coloured trousers, long sleeves and closed-toed shoes or boots when spending time outdoors in areas known to have a heavy tick populations. Light-coloured clothing allows ticks to be easily spotted. Also keep shirt tails tucked into trousers and trouser legs tucked into socks.

Avoid areas of heavy tick populations, especially during the summer months.

Apply products containing the insecticide N,N-diethyl-meta-toluamide (DEET) to any exposed skin and those that contain the insecticide permethrin to clothing.

Carefully check the entire body for any ticks. If found, gently and promptly remove the tick with tweezers, taking care not to squeeze the insect. Apply antiseptic ointment to the site of the bite.

Check pets for ticks as well; they can bring the insects into the home, where they can attach themselves to a person.

Research indicates that garlic works as a natural tick repellent. A study involving 100 Swedish

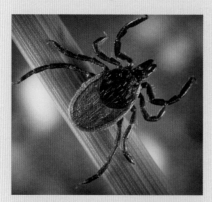

The blacklegged tick, *I. pacificus* (above) and *I. scapularis*, are known carriers of the pathogen that is responsible for causing Lyme disease.

soldiers found that daily digestion of garlic capsules reduced the frequency of tick bites by 30 percent.

DIAGNOSIS

Tick-borne illnesses are often difficult to diagnosis. The presence of a rash is often the most important step in diagnosing these diseases. Each tick-borne disease can cause a characteristic rash. For example, the Lyme disease rash resembles a bull's eye with a red outer ring, an unaffected clear patch, and a red centre. This is called an erythema migrans or EM rash.

Unfortunately, many patients never experience a rash. In these cases, the doctor relies on the other symptoms and a medical history. Other symptoms include high temperature, chills, body

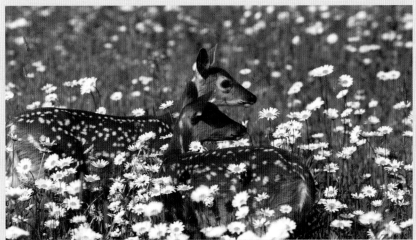

Some ticks are transported from place to place on wild animals such as deer, as well as domestic animals including dogs, sheep and cattle.

• **WESTERN IMMUNOBLOT TEST** If the ELISA test is positive, the laboratory confirms the results with this test, which identifies proteins or other substances produced by microorganism, such as the ones that cause tick-borne diseases,.

• **POLYMERASE CHAIN REACTION (PCR)** This test can detect microorganisms associated with tick-borne illnesses in spinal and joint fluid. This is especially important in cases where the patient is experiencing neurological symptoms.

aches, nausea, vomiting, diarrhoea and fatigue. Some of these illnesses cause joint pain, and neurological and heart problems.

During the medical history, the doctor may ask some or all of the following questions.

• Have you been in an area heavily populated by ticks?
• Did you take the necessary precautions to avoid bites?
• Have you seen ticks attached to your skin, and if so, for how long?

Because the symptoms of tick-borne diseases are similar to those of many other medical conditions, the information revealed during the medical examination is very important during the diagnosis process.

After the examination, laboratory tests are used to confirm a diagnosis of a tick-borne disease These tests look for antibodies to the organisms transmitted by ticks. Examples include:

• **SEROLOGY** These blood tests are designed to identify antibodies to the organisms associated with tick-borne disease.

• **MICROSCOPIC EXAM** The blood is examined under a microscope for the presence of microorganisms.

• **ENZYME-LINKED IMMUNOSORBENT ASSAY (ELISA) TEST** This procedure looks for specific antibodies in a sample of blood.

TREATMENTS

The chart below summarizes the available treatment options for tick-borne diseases.

See also: *Fever, p.318 • Nausea and Vomiting, pp.274–5 • Diarrhoea, p.268*

Tick-Borne Disease	Treatments
Lyme disease	Antibiotics such as amoxicillin and doxycycline are effective in treating lyme disease. In cases of neurological damage, ceftriaxone or penicillin G is administered to the bloodstream of patients through a tube called an IV.
Rocky Mountain spotted fever	The antibiotics tetracycline or chloramphenicol are used to treat Rocky Mountain spotted fever. Chloramphenicol is given in an IV to patients with neurological symptoms.
Erlichiosis	The antibiotics tetracycline and doxycycline work best to treat erlichiosis.
Tularaemia	The most effective antibiotics for tularaemia include streptomycin and gentamycin.
Babesiosis	Mild cases of babesiosis recover without treatment. A combination of quinine and clindamycin are used to treat more serious infections.
Relapsing fever	Tetracycline and erythromycin are most effective in treating relapsing fever. IV treatments with these antibiotics are used in severe cases.
Colorado tick fever	No treatment is available.
Tick paralysis	This condition is caused by an undiscovered embedded tick. Doctor remove the tick, often found in the scalp, and symptoms usually resolve shortly thereafter.

Lymphoma

The lymphatic system is an integral part of the body's network of protection against any foreign substances including viruses, bacteria and abnormal cells. Using the lymphatic vessels, a clear fluid called lymph is transported to the lymph nodes located in the neck, underarms, chest, abdomen and groin. The lymph nodes make and store special immune cells known as lymphocytes. The lymphocytes destroy foreign or harmful substances that may penetrate the body.

In lymphoma, some of the cells, or lymphocytes, in the lymphatic system multiply uncontrollably. The two main types of lymphocytes are B and T cells. Lymphomas are classified as either non-Hodgkin's lymphoma or Hodgkin's disease, depending on the kind of cells that are growing. Both types of lymphomas can spread to other lymph nodes and bodily organs.

CAUSES

The exact cause of lymphoma remains unclear, but it is known that the condition occurs following damage to the DNA within lymphocytes that causes them to grow abnormally, and produce a tumour.

PREVENTION

There is no known way to prevent lymphoma.

DIAGNOSIS

To diagnosis lymphoma, a doctor first takes a medical history and performs a physical examination. Lymph nodes in the neck, under-arms and groin are evaluated for swelling or enlargement, the most prominent symptom of lymphoma. Other symptoms can include night sweats, fatigue, weight loss and itchy skin.

Blood tests determine the number of blood cells in a patient's body and kidney and liver functioning. The doctor may look for compounds such as lactate dehydrogenase (LDH) in the blood; these levels are usually higher in patients with lymphomas. Later, a biopsy allows the study of lymphatic cells for abnormalities; imaging tests identify the organs affected by the cancer.

TREATMENTS

• CHEMOTHERAPY AND RADIATION These are frequently used to destroy cancerous lymphomas cell. In chemotherapy, potent drugs are administered that kills both abnormal and normal cells. In radiation therapy, high-energy rays target the tumour or radioactive materials are injected into the bloodstream.

• IMMUNOTHERAPY Antibodies that target cancer cells and destroy them are used here. Other substances can also be given to patients to strengthen their own system's ability to respond to the cancer. Polysaccharide K, a compound derived from mushrooms, has been shown to also improve immune function and have anticancer abilities.

• ACUPUNCTURE Some patients have success in relieving symptoms associated with treatment. Acupuncture (pp.464–5), a technique in which needles placed on certain areas on the skin, helps relieve pain and nausea associated with lymphoma and chemotherapy.

• ANTIOXIDANTS Coenzyme Q10 (pp.543) is an antioxidant that works to stimulate the immune system and protect against the side effects of chemotherapy and radiation.

See also: *Enzyme Replacement Therapy, p.543 -4 • Acupuncture, pp.464–5 • Fever, p.318*

Multiple Myeloma

The plasma cell is a special type of blood cell that creates antibodies. These antibodies are used by the immune system to attack harmful substances. Multiple myeloma is a type of cancer that affects plasma cells. Myeloma cells are abnormal plasma cells that reproduce themselves in abundance. As myeloma develops in the bone marrow, it may displace other healthy blood cells. Because the antibodies that myeloma plasma cells produce are not effective, patients are at an increased risk of infection.

Myeloma cells can also invade the solid part of bone. When this happens, large amounts of calcium are deposited into the blood. In addition, myeloma cells produce antibodies called the M protein. These factors cause the kidneys of those with multiple myeloma to work harder to filter out extra amounts of calcium and M protein. Thus, patients with myeloma are at risk for kidney failure.

CAUSES
No cause has been identified.

PREVENTION
Research indicates that limiting exposure to ionizing radiation and the pesticide dioxin may help prevent multiple myeloma.

DIAGNOSIS
Multiple myeloma is usually diagnosed after blood tests are performed because of symptoms such as fatigue and weight loss. (Other symptoms include painful bones, broken bones, exhaustion, weight loss, extreme thirst, high temperature, reccurring infections, nausea, vomiting, constipation, frequent urination and leg numbness.)

Blood tests identify elevated levels of plasma cells and calcium. The presence of M protein in the blood is also determined and a complete blood count is performed because most patients with this condition have anaemia (pp.312–13). The doctor may confirm the diagnosis with additional tests such as bone marrow aspirate and biopsy.

TREATMENTS
• **CHEMOTHERAPY** This is the primary treatment for myeloma. Stem cell transplantation is sometimes used to restore bone marrow after chemotherapy. Stem cells are removed from the patient before therapy, treated to remove the myeloma cells, and then returned to the patient. Or, a healthy person may donate stem cells to the patient.

• **LIFESTYLE** Patients can make lifestyle changes to limit the complications of myeloma. Regular exercise prevents bone damage and calcium loss. Staying hydrated helps the kidneys function. A well-balanced diet and avoiding large crowds or those with infectious diseases protects the immune system.

See also: *Anaemia, pp.312–3 • Obesity, pp.348–9 • Kidney Failure, pp.306–7*

The light spots at the base of the skull in this X-ray are excess plasma cells that have accumulated and formed plasmacytomas, which weaken the bone.

WHO IS AT RISK?
The risk factors include:
• Elderly
• African-American
• Exposure to radiation
• Family history
• Exposure to toxic chemicals
• Obesity

Parasitic Infections

Parasites are organisms that depend on another organism, such as a human or animal, to live. Parasitic infections occur once a parasite enters the body of a person. These infections are most common in warmer climates and in areas of poor personal hygiene and sanitation.

CAUSES

Parasitic infections are frequently contracted after eating contaminated food, walking barefoot in contaminated soil or placing soiled fingers in the mouth. Parasitic infections can be caused by many types of parasites.

• **PINWORM INFECTION** This parasite is spread mainly by children and is common in day-care centres, schools, and in the homes of small children. Pinworms usually live in the colon or rectum, but easily cling to the fingertips of children. Pinworm eggs can also remain in clothing or linen as well as attach to furniture, doorknobs and taps.

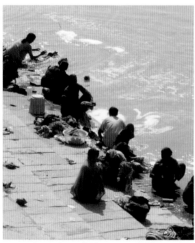

Parasitic infections are common in developing countries, where water supplies may be unsafe.

• **TRICHINOSIS** A trichinosis infection commonly occurs after eating undercooked pork. The parasite often infects meat-eating mammals such as pigs, rats and horses, and can be found in rubbish.

• **ROUNDWORM AND HOOKWORM INFECTION** These parasites are usually found in tropical areas where human faeces lies in heavily populated areas. Dogs and cats can become infected and spread it to people as well.

• **WHIPWORM DISEASE** Rectal prolapse, a serious condition involving bloody diarrhoea in young children, can occur as a result of this parasite. Children often ingest the whipworm eggs after eating or drinking something without first washing their hands.

• **TAPEWORM INFECTION** Eating contaminated pork or beef can cause a tapeworm infection.

PREVENTION

The best prevention is good personal hygiene. Hands should be washed after using the toilet and before eating or drinking. Children should be encouraged to wash their hands after playing outside or returning from school. Food items should be thoroughly

WHO IS AT RISK?

The risk factors include:

• Children

• Rural areas

• Warmer climates

cooked before consumption. And pets should be immediately treated for any infections.

DIAGNOSIS

The diagnosis of parasitic infections involves the following tests:

• **FAECAL EXAMINATION** Stool samples are examined for the presence of parasites or their eggs.

• **ENDOSCOPY** A thin tube is inserted into the mouth or rectum enabling the doctor to examine the upper or lower intestines.

• **BLOOD TESTS** These can be used to detect antibodies to the parasite.

• **IMAGING X-RAYS** MRIs, and CAT scans can determine if organs have been enlarged by a parasite or whether cysts have developed as a result of the parasitic infection.

TREATMENTS

Depending on the classification of the parasite, the doctor will choose from a number of anti-parasitic medications that can be given orally, injected into the bloodstream or applied as a cream.

See also: *Diarrhoea, p.268* • *Food Hygiene, pp.586–97*

Polycythaemia Vera

This is a rare condition in which the body makes too many red blood cells, causing the blood to thicken. The symptoms associated with polycythaemia include fatigue, headaches, shortness of breath, dizziness, itchiness, sweating, reddened or purplish skin, blind spots, double vision, burning sensation in the hands and feet, ulcers, excessive bleeding or bruising and blood clots.

CAUSES

Bone marrow, the spongy material found at the centre of the bones, is responsible for making blood cells. Polycythaemia occurs when the DNA notation of a blood cell becomes altered and begins to over-produce itself. Eventually, the altered cell is mass-produced, causing a thickening of the blood and inhibiting the production of healthy normal cells.

A secondary form of polycythaemia can be caused by low blood oxygen levels caused by living in high altitudes, heart and lung disease, and abnormal amounts of a hormone that stimulated blood cells production called erythropoietin.

PREVENTION

There is no known way to prevent polycythaemia, but those over age 60 and of Eastern European and Jewish descent are at higher risk.

DIAGNOSIS

Diagnosis is made following the completion of a medical history, an examination, blood tests and a bone marrow analysis.

Common complaints of the condition include fatigue, weight loss, itchy skin and the development of either bleeding or clotting disorders.

A complete blood cell count is taken to determine the number of red cells, white cells and platelets in the blood. Those with polycythaemia have an elevated haematocrit or number of red blood cells in their complete blood cell count. Sometimes there is also an elevated number of white blood cells and platelets.

In a bone marrow analysis, a doctor examines the cells in the marrow. People suffering from polycythaemia will have a higher than normal number of red blood cell precursors. Their blood may also contain lower levels of iron that is needed to manufacture additional red blood cells. Biomarkers (specific indicators of disease), such as c-Mpl and PRV-1, may also be searched for within the bone marrow. Scientists have learned that those with polycythemia have these unique combinations in their cells.

TREATMENTS

An individual treatment plan is designed for each patient with polycythaemia depending on their symptoms. The treatments chosen are designed to decrease the number of red blood cells in the body and minimize the risk of developing further complications as a result of polycythaemia.

• PHLEBOTOMY In this procedure a portion of the blood is removed from the body on a regular basis. This technique is used to lower the total number of red blood cells circulating in the bloodstream.

• MYELOSUPPRESSIVE AGENTS These are used to prevent the bone marrow from making too many read blood cells. Hydroxyurea is the most commonly prescribed myelosuppressive agent. Given in a pill form, it is able to reduce the number of red blood cells and platelets.

• OTHER MEDICATION Treatments involve using aspirin to reduce the occurrence of blood clots and antihistamines to relieve itching, a common complaint with the condition.

See also: *Vision Problems, pp.36–9* • *Bleeding Disorders, p.320* • *Headaches, pp.166–7*

WHO IS AT RISK?

The risk factors include:

• Elderly
• Jewish and Eastern European

Scleroderma

This relatively rare disease involves the gradual hardening of the skin and connective tissues. Scleroderma usually begins with the hardening of small patches of skin on the hands and feet. Over time, the hardened patches can spread to other parts of the body and involve the organs.

Scleroderma is loosely classified into two subsets; localized and systemic. Localized scleroderma involves only the skin and tissue below the skin. Systemic scleroderma is more dangerous, as it affects the blood vessels and major organs such as the lungs, heart, kidneys and gastrointestinal tract.

CAUSES
Scleroderma is caused by an increase in collagen production in the body's tissues. Research indicates that this may be as a result of genetic factors or exposure to certain toxic chemicals.

PREVENTION
There is no way to prevent scleroderma. The symptoms may be minimized by adhering to a regular exercise routine that keeps the joints flexible, quitting smoking, avoiding foods that cause heartburn and keeping warm while in colder climates.

DIAGNOSIS
Scleroderma is usually diagnosed based on the appearance of the hardened patches of skin. A medical history and physical examination may further

indicate symptoms characteristic of scleroderma. In addition, blood tests can identify certain antibodies within the body that attack connective tissues and a biopsy of the hardened skin is helpful in finding cellular abnormalities in these tissue samples. Biopsies are performed to confirm the diagnosis.

Raynaud's phenomenon is frequently seen in those with scleroderma. In this condition, cold climates and stress cause pain to occur in the fingers, toes, cheeks, nose and ears turning them numb and changing their colour. Additional symptoms of scleroderma include joint pain, ulcers on the elbows and knuckles, curling of the fingers, enlarged hands and feet, and digestive problems.

TREATMENTS
Treatments for scleroderma involve minimizing symptoms and complications. Skin problems that extend over limited parts of the body are treated with moisturizers or corticosteroid cream which helps to control inflammation.

• LIGHT THERAPY Skin treatments include a prescription of minocycline and phototherapy. Initial research shows that placing light

on the skin lesions – phototherapy – can help decrease the appearance of lesions.

• MEDICATION Circulatory problems caused by scleroderma are treated with medication that relaxes and opens the blood vessels, thus promoting circulation.

Joint stiffness is a common complaint among those who suffer from scleroderma. Anti-inflammatory medication, such as nonsteroidal anti-inflammatory drugs (NSAIDs), are used to alleviate joint pain and stiffness. In conjunction with NSAIDs, doctors sometimes prescribe disease-modifying anti-rheumatic drugs (DMARDs) or immuno-suppressants which help to control the immune responses causing the inflammation.

Digestive problems such as heartburn are treated with H-2 receptor blockers and proton pump inhibitors. These work to limit the amount of stomach acid produced in the body.

See also: *Smoking Cessation, pp.216–7* • *Yoga, pp.476–9*

WHO IS AT RISK?
The risk factors include:
- Women
- Adults between 30 and 50 years old
- Family history
- Exposure to certain toxic chemicals

Spleen Disorders

The spleen is a small organ the size of a fist that lies behind the rib cage on the left side of the body. It is composed of two types of tissues, white pulp and red pulp, which play a vital role in immune functioning. The spleen's blood vessels are surrounded by immune cells that remove abnormal cells and microorganisms from the blood. As the spleen receives blood from an artery, it serves as a gate keeper, preventing the passage of foreign substances and debris.

There are two types of spleen disorders: enlarged and ruptured spleen. Splenomegaly, or enlargement of the spleen, often occurs as a result of other medical conditions. A ruptured spleen is an extremely serious condition that requires emergency medical attention. Blood pours out of the spleen and into the abdomen.

CAUSES

Splenomegaly can be caused by conditions including viral infections, blood cancers, lymphomas, leukaemia, haemolytic anaemia, liver disease and lipid storage diseases. These conditions render cause the spleen to swell with the materials it can no longer filter and remove.

A ruptured spleen is common after road accidents, trauma during sports and assault. A blow to the abdomen can damage the spleen's covering and tissues.

PREVENTION

The only way to prevent an enlarged spleen is to prevent or cure the underlying medical condition. A ruptured spleen can be prevented by safe driving and wearing protective gear during sports.

DIAGNOSIS

Doctors can usually diagnosis an enlarged spleen during a physical exam. An ultrasound, CT scan or nuclear scan can confirm the diagnosis. Patients with splenomegaly may have low levels of blood cells and platelets. A ruptured spleen

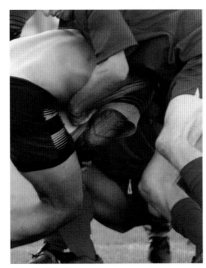

Spleen injuries occur in sports such as soccer and rugby in which participants often collide forcefully.

WHO IS AT RISK?

The risk factors include:

Ruptured spleen

- Athletics
- Car accidents
- Trauma to the abdomen
- Enlarged spleen
- Viral infections
- Blood cancers
- Lymphomas
- Leukaemia
- Certain anaemias
- Liver disease
- Gaucher's disease and Niemann-Pick disease

is diagnosed after testing in the appropriate clinical setting with procedures such as CT scans or procedures to look for blood in the abdominal cavity.

TREATMENTS

- SURGERY The surgical removal of the spleen, or splenectomy, is the usual treatment for spleen disorders. Attempts may be made to preserve the spleen after traumatic rupture. Although someone can live without a spleen, complications arise. The body's ability to fight infections and remove debris from the blood may be diminished, so patients are at higher risk of infections and are encouraged to receive regular vaccines.

See also: *Leukaemia, p.335* • *Liver Disease, pp.438–40* • *Lymphoma, p.328*

Anaphylaxis

Anaphylaxis is a sudden, severe and potentially fatal systemic allergic reaction. It can involve the gastrointestinal tract, the respiratory system, the skin and the cardiovascular system. Symptoms usually occur within minutes of contact with the allergy-causing substance but can occur up to four hours later.

CAUSES

Anaphylaxis is usually caused by allergies to food, insect bites (hymenoptera) and latex. After being exposed to the allergy-causing agent, basophils and mast cells in various body parts release a histamine, a substance that causes typical allergy reactions such as inflammation and itching.

In severe cases, it causes the airways of the throat to constrict because of swelling in the tissues; blood pressure drops, causing the body to go into shock. People who have asthma, eczema, hay fever and existing food allergies are at higher risk. Some patients have experienced anaphylaxis after routine vaccinations.

PREVENTION

People with allergies should avoid contact with allergy-causing substances. Antihistamines and corticosteroids can be taken regularly to prevent allergic reactions from occurring when exposure is unavoidable, such as when X-ray dye must be administered. Those who suffer from severe allergic reactions should always carry chewable antihistamine and injectable epinephrine to be used in emergency situations, if necessary.

Parents of teenagers who have allergies should take particular care in discussing the dangers of anaphylaxis. Teenager are most at risk for this condition because they often forget to carry their medication. They are also sometimes unable to recognize the early symptoms of anaphylaxis or ignore them, losing important time.

DIAGNOSIS

Because of its life-threatening nature, anaphylaxis must be diagnosed immediately. Hives and swelling of the eyes are most likely apparent during the initial moments of an attack. In addition, a patient's skin may appear blue or pale – this is caused by a lack of oxygen in the blood, which in turn is caused by the inability to breathe and also from shock.

During further examination, a doctor will use a stethoscope to listen for wheezing in the lungs. The heartbeat and blood pressure are also measured, because the pulse is usually elevated and blood pressure is lower than normal as anaphylaxis progresses. Blood

tests, which are, in most cases, postponed until after treatment, are used to detect the specific allergen that is causing the reaction.

TREATMENTS

• MEDICATION Epinephrine, which opens the airways and increases blood pressure, is injected in cases of full blown anaphylaxis.

• INTUBATION AND TRACHESTOMY The emergency medical personnel or the doctor place a tube in the mouth or nose of the patient. This procedure, called endotracheal intubation, assists the patient in breathing. Sometimes, a tracheostomy, in which the tube is placed directly into the trachea, is done.

Once these procedures are completed, the patient is given intravenous fluids and other medication such as antihistamines and corticosteroids.

See also: *Hay Fever, pp.50–1 • Asthma, pp.206–9 • Food Allergies, p.262 • Immunizations, pp.314–15*

> ## WHO IS AT RISK?
> **The risk factors include:**
> - Eczema
> - Asthma
> - Hay fever
> - Allergies to food especially nuts or fish
> - Allergies to latex
> - Previous history of anaphylaxis

Leukaemia

Cancer of the white blood cells, or leukaemia, is a serious illness that affects each person differently. White blood cells, also called leukocytes, travel throughout the body. Abnormal or cancerous leukocytes often accumulate in a particular area of the body, causing pain or other symptoms in the specific area. Examples include the testicles, brain, kidneys, lungs and the digestive tract.

Leukaemias are grouped by how quickly the disease develops and worsens. Chronic leukaemia gets worse slowly whereas acute leukaemia worsens quickly. They are also grouped by the type of white blood cell affected, lymphoid cells, or myeloid cells. Lymphotic leukaemia affects lymphoid cells; myeloid or myelogenous leukaemia affects myeloid cells.

CAUSES

The cause of leukaemia is unknown, but researchers have identified certain risk factors: exposure to high-energy radiation from an atomic bomb or nuclear power plant; exposure to chemicals such as benzene or formaldehyde; genetic abnormalities such as Down's syndrome; chemotherapy; blood disorders; and infection with the human T-Cell leukaemia virus (HTLV-1).

PREVENTION

There is no way to prevent the development of leukaemia other than to avoid exposure to known leukaemia-causing substances.

DIAGNOSIS

General symptoms of leukaemia include fever, night sweats, fatigue, recurrent infections, headaches, weight loss, joint pain, bleeding or bruising easily, swollen lymph nodes and an enlarged abdomen. Doctors use the following procedures to diagnosis leukaemia:
- **EXAMINATION** Lymph nodes, spleen and liver are checked for swelling.
- **BLOOD TESTS** A blood sample is analysed for the number of blood cells and platelets. A small amount of blood may be studied to identify any cellular abnormalities.
- **BIOPSY** A small amount of bone marrow is removed and examined for the presence of leukaemia cells.
- **CYTOGENETICS** This test analyses genetic material in blood cells, bone marrow and lymph nodes.
- **SPINAL TAP** Fluid around the brain and spinal cord may be tested for the presence of cancerous cells.

TREATMENTS

Leukaemia treatments depends on the type of leukaemia, parts of the body involved and if the patient has

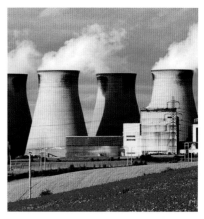

The cause of leukaemia is unknown, but risk factors include exposure to high-energy radiation.

been treated before. They include:
- **CHEMOTHERAPY** Administered between cycles of rest.
- **RADIATION THERAPY** Destroys cancerous cells and prevents them from regrowing.
- **BONE MARROW TRANSPLANTATION** Tissue damaged by chemotherapy and radiation is replaced.
- **IMMUNOTHERAPY** Immune enhancing drugs are given to help the body fight leukaemia.

See also: *Headaches, pp.166–7* • *Fever, p.318* • *Bleeding Disorders, p.320*

WHO IS AT RISK?

The risk factors include:
- Exposure to high energy radiation or certain chemicals
- Genetic abnormalities
- Blood disorders
- Chemotherapy
- HTLV-1 infection

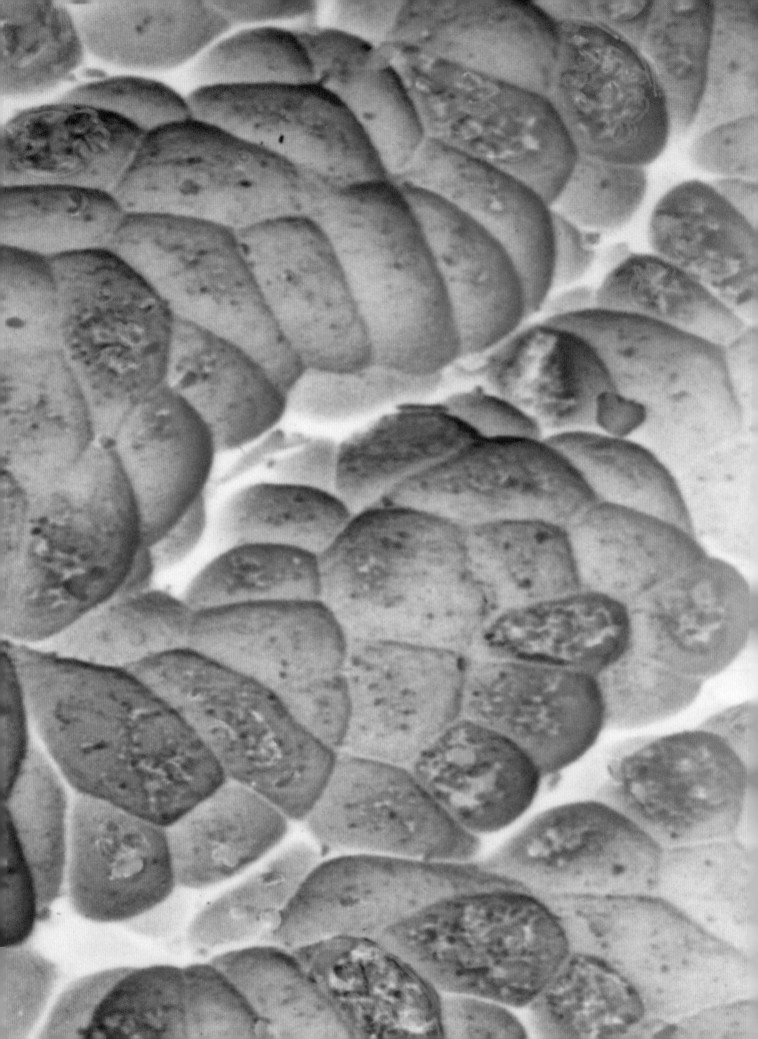

12 HORMONAL DISORDERS

The body's internal systems need chemical coordination in order to operate efficiently as a unit – work that is carried out by the endocrine system. This system is a collection of glands, located throughout the body, that regulate metabolism, growth, reproduction and body chemistry. Imbalances in the endocrine system can result in debilitating conditions, many of which can be difficult to diagnose because of the unusual nature of some of the symptoms. Graves' disease, for example, causes severe drying of the skin, muscle pain and in some cases bulging eyes, while an underactive thyroid can cause unexplained weight gain and extreme fatigue. Diet and exercise play an important role in maintaining healthy endocrine function. Eating the right foods and staying active can help avoid many of the more common hormonal disorders.

Diabetic Disorders

There are two primary types of diabetes, known as type 1 and type 2. In type 1 diabetes, the pancreas fails to make enough insulin – a hormone important for metabolism – because of damage by an autoimmune process. With type 2 diabetes, insulin resistance usually occurs first; the pancreas produces the insulin, but the body develops a resistance and requires higher and higher amounts for it to be effective. The pancreas makes more and more insulin, the cells become increasingly resistant, which results in high glucose and high insulin levels.

The pancreas, which is about the size of a hand, is located behind the liver and bowel, and is the organ responsible for producing insulin and other hormones that help the body turn food into energy.

When food is digested, it breaks down into glucose, which is the simple sugar that is the main source of energy for the cells in the body. The glucose then enters the bloodstream. When the pancreas does not make enough insulin or the body is unable to use the insulin that is present, the cells cannot use glucose and convert it to energy.

Excess glucose builds up in the bloodstream, and glucose intolerance results. Impaired glucose tolerance, sometimes called pre-diabetes, occurs in individuals with elevated blood glucose levels that are not high enough to be diagnosed as diabetes yet. Pre-diabetes generally has no symptoms, but in severe cases dark patches may appear on the skin around the neck, elbows or knees, a condition called acanthosis nigricans.

When blood glucose level fall too low, which can happen with either type of diabetes, hypogly-caemia occurs. It is usually the

result of too much insulin or other glucose-lowering medication, not enough food, too much activity or a combination of these. Hypo-glycaemia can result in a number of symptoms, such as weakness, double vision, shakiness, anxi-ety, convulsions and even loss of consciousness. If hypoglycaemia occurs, sugary sweets, a sweet drink such as orange juice, or glu-cose tablets (designed for such an emergency) can rapidly raise blood glucose to a safe level.

The two types of diabetes develop in different ways. Type 1

WHO IS AT RISK?

The risk factors include:

Type 1 Diabetes
- Family history

Type 2 Diabetes
- Family history, especially a parent or sibling
- Obesity, especially abdominal fat
- Age 45 or older
- Non-Caucasian
- Lack of exercise
- Gestational diabetes or delivering a baby who weighs more than 4 kg (9 lbs).
- High blood pressure
- Blood levels of triglycerides (a type of fat molecule) greater than 250 mg/dL
- High blood cholesterol level, with an HDL of less than 35 mg/dL
- Impaired glucose tolerance, identified by a doctor.

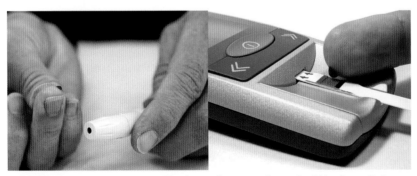

A portable glucose meter measures blood sugar from a small sample of blood, usually from a fingertip, that is collected onto a paper test strip coated with special chemicals. Some meters can use blood samples from alternate sites on the body, but these may be less accurate.

diabetes usually begins suddenly and may lead to hospitalization or a visit to casualty before a diagnosis is made. This type of diabetes – sometimes called insulin-dependent diabetes mellitus or juvenile-onset diabetes – usually occurs in children, teenagers and adults under age 30. But by far the most common type of glucose problem is type 2 diabetes, also sometimes called non-insulin-dependent diabetes mellitus. Historically, it typically occurred in adults, especially those over the age of 45, but recently there has been a surge in diabetes of this type in younger adults and children. Gestational diabetes is a temporary condition that occurs during pregnancy, although it increases the risk of a woman developing type 2 diabetes later in life.

Long-term complications from diabetes can include heart disease, stroke, kidney failure, blindness,

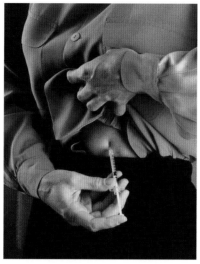

A person whose body is no longer making insulin, or does not make enough, must take insulin either by injecting it or by wearing an insulin pump.

high blood pressure, nervous system damage, amputations, dental disease and complications during pregnancy.

CAUSES

Why the pancreas fails to produce insulin or the cells become resistant is still unknown. Researchers believe genetic and environmental factors play a role in both types of diabetes, and autoimmune factors may play a major role in type 1.

When glucose cannot enter the cells, it cannot be used for energy. Excess amounts of glucose remain in the blood and must be removed by the kidneys, along with the water in which the glucose is dissolved. That causes the classic symptoms of increased urination and thirst, hunger and fatigue, which may occur with either type 1 or type 2 diabetes.

PREVENTION

There is no known way to prevent type 1 diabetes, but keeping weight normal, eating a balanced

diet and exercising regularly may prevent type 2 diabetes. Being overweight affects the way insulin works in the body. Extra fat tissue can make the body resistant to insulin, while exercise helps insulin work more efficiently.

In the Diabetes Prevention Program study, conducted between 1994 and 2004 by the National Institute of Diabetes and Digestive and Kidney Diseases in the United States, researchers found that people diagnosed with impaired glucose tolerance, or pre-diabetes, could cut their risk of developing type 2 diabetes by 58 percent if they lost 7 percent of their weight with moderate physical activity such as walking 150 minutes a week, or 30 minutes a day. The drug metformin, which is used to lower blood glucose levels, prevented the development of type 2 diabetes in 31 percent of patients in the same study, so lifestyle changes actually proved more effective.

Keeping blood glucose levels relatively stable throughout the day can also help prevent the development of type 2 diabetes. The glycaemic index ranks various carbohydrates according to their immediate effect on blood glucose levels. Learning how particular carbohydrates generally rate on the glycaemic index scale can help in making better diet choices. Ordinary sugar ranks at 100, for example, whereas foods such as whole grains and many vegetables that digest slowly rank much lower. Substituting high-fibre foods and complex carbohydrates for simple sugars and 'junk' foods helps stabilize blood glucose level.

Clinical Query

What is considered a normal blood sugar level?

Blood glucose level in a healthy person can range as high as 200 mg/dL throughout the day, but should be no higher than 99 mg/dL when measured after fasting. A measurement between 100 and 125 mg/dL after fasting is considered elevated and can mean you have pre-diabetes, which can lead to type 2 diabetes.

A blood glucose level above 126 mg/dL can mean you have diabetes. A doctor will perform a blood sugar test, such as the fasting plasma glucose test or the oral glucose tolerance test, at least twice to be sure.

DIAGNOSIS

Anyone with symptoms of diabetes or who has any of the risk factors should have their blood sugar level checked regularly. People over age 45 should get their blood glucose checked at least every three years.

People with type 1 diabetes may lose weight despite an increased appetite and may also experience nausea and vomiting. Those with type 2 diabetes may notice blurred vision, slow healing of infections or wounds; men may experience impotence. Or, in many cases, individuals may not experience any symptoms at all because of the slow onset of the disease. Many people with diabetes do not know they have it. Most people diagnosed with type 2 diabetes are overweight or obese; they may have high cholesterol as well.

Diabetes is diagnosed when a person has an abnormally high amount of glucose in the blood, which is determined using different types of blood tests. A fasting blood glucose test is done after not eating for at least eight hours; blood glucose should be lower than 126 mg/dL (milligrams of glucose per decilitre of blood) on two different occasions. A level between 100 and 125 mg/dL is considered impaired fasting glucose, or pre-diabetes, a condition that can lead to type 2 diabetes. A random blood glucose test may be done at any time, without fasting, and blood glucose should be 200 mg/dL or less. A result of 140 to 199 mg/dL indicates pre-diabetes.

The oral glucose tolerance test is used to diagnose type 2 diabetes when fasting glucose levels are normal, but the diagnosis is still in question. This test is more sensitive than the fasting glucose test, but it is less convenient to administer. It is also used to test for gestational diabetes during pregnancy. After fasting, blood glucose levels are checked and then the patient consumes a special drink with a high amount of glucose. Blood samples are drawn over the next two to three hours to measure glucose levels, which should never exceed 200 mg/dL. A result of 140 to 199 mg/dL indicates pre-diabetes.

People with uncontrolled type 1 diabetes are at risk of high levels of ketones, which are produced when fat and muscle break down and are discarded by the body in urine. High levels of ketones can be dangerous and even fatal by causing 'acidosis', or low blood pH. A simple urine test, using paper test strips, can detect the presence of ketones. Urinalysis can also reveal high level of glucose.

TREATMENTS

There is no cure for diabetes, but it is possible to manage the disease with a combination of exercise, diet, weight control and drugs. Although some supplements may help to stabilize blood glucose levels, they should not be substituted for diet and drug therapy, and should not be used without first consulting a doctor. Self-monitoring will help to ensure the disease is kept under control and that the risk of long-term complications is decreased.

• DIET What to eat, and just as important, when to eat it, are crucial in maintaining stable blood sugar levels. Consultation with a

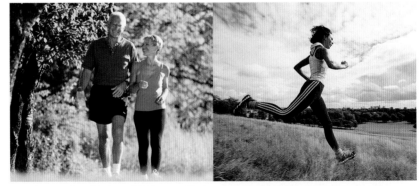

Regular exercise aids in weight loss and helps regulate blood pressure, both of which are critical to managing diabetes. However, it is important to check blood glucose levels before and after exercise, and to carry a snack to avoid a drastic drop in blood sugar.

registered dietitian is helpful in designing meal plans. It is important to avoid extreme highs or lows in blood glucose level, and that means adhering to regular meal times and snacks. A low-fat diet for people with type 2 diabetes is valuable in keeping cholesterol and triglyceride levels normal.

• WEIGHT MANAGEMENT Weight is generally more of an issue for those with type 2 diabetes. In fact, some people with type 2 who lose excess weight may be able to reduce or even stop their medications. Crash diets that recommend extremely low calorie intake should be avoided; instead, eat smaller portions, limit fats and increase exercise.

• EXERCISE At least 30 minutes a day of regular physical activity can help control blood glucose level, aid in controlling weight and reduce high blood pressure. It is important to check blood glucose level before and after exercise, and to carry a sugary snack in case blood glucose level fall too low. Be sure to drink extra fluids that do not contain sugar before, during and after exercise.

• INSULIN Daily insulin injections are required for people with type 1

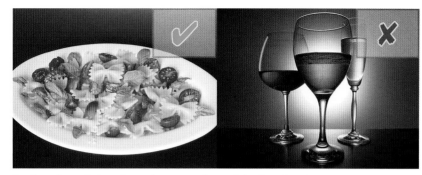

Foods such as whole grains and pasta are digested slowly and are better than sweets and sugary foods for regulating blood glucose. Avoid consuming alcohol; the body reacts to alcohol as if it were a toxin, and the liver will not put out glucose until the alcohol is metabolized.

diabetes and for some with type 2. Insulin is currently only available by injection, and one to four injections a day may be needed. An insulin pump with a needle under the skin near the abdomen can also be used; it is worn all the time and can provide a steady amount of insulin. Different types of insulin that are effective for different time periods are available.

• MEDICATION Oral hypoglycaemic agents can lower blood glucose levels for people with type 2 diabetes. These drugs work by increasing insulin production, increasing the body's sensitivity to insulin or delaying the absorption of glucose. Women who are pregnant should not take any of these medications, but instead should rely on diet and insulin to manage their diabetes.

• SUPPLEMENTS A chromium deficiency may impair the body's reaction to glucose and insulin. A daily supplement of 150 mcg of chromium picolinate may help treat hypoglycaemia and stabilize blood glucose levels. Chromium is also found in whole wheat and rye breads, beef liver, potatoes, green peppers, eggs, chicken, brewer's yeast, apples, butter, parsnips and cornmeal.

• SELF-MONITORING Infections, emotional stress, some medications, and even the time of day can affect blood glucose level. It is critical for individuals with diabetes to monitor their blood glucose levels with home monitors. Armed with that knowledge, they can modify their meals, activity levels and medications to help avoid emergencies caused by extreme levels of blood glucose.

• MEDICAL MONITORING The haemoglobin A1C blood test (also called glycolated or glycosylated haemoglobin), measures the percentage of the haemoglobin A1C protein in the blood. It can reveal the average blood glucose level over the previous three months. Most diabetics aim for an A1C under 7 percent; higher than 8 can increase the risk of complications. The test should be done at least twice a year, depending on the patient's general level of control. Studies show that tight control of blood sugar level (an A1C of 7 percent or less) can avoid many of the long-term complications from diabetes.

See also: *Obesity, pp.348–9* • *High Blood Pressure, pp.236–9* • *Heart Disease, pp.230–3*

On Call

People without diabetes can also experience hypoglycaemia, in which blood sugar levels become low and cause symptoms such as weakness, shakiness, fatigue, dizziness, sweating, anxiety, extreme hunger, poor vision and even irrational behaviour.

Adrenal Gland Disorders

The adrenal glands are two triangular organs that sit above the kidneys and secrete a variety of hormones. These hormones include cortisol and epinephrine, which help maintain metabolism and other functions, and aldosterone, which helps regulate sodium and potassium levels in the blood to help control water balance, blood volume and blood pressure. Levels of these hormones are either too high or too low in people with adrenal gland disorders.

Unless they are treated, these disorders can cause serious complications, including hypertension (p.236), diabetes (pp.338–41), osteoporosis (pp.146–7) and, in some cases, death.

CAUSES

Each of the adrenal gland disorders has a different cause. Addison's disease is a lack of adrenal hormones. The most common cause is an autoimmune reaction in which the immune system attacks the outer portion of the adrenal glands, which produce cortisol (a hormone that helps regulate blood pressure and blood glucose level). Other causes include tuberculosis, fungal infections, cancer and surgical removal of the adrenal glands. Addison's disease can also be a side-effect of anticoagulant medication, occurring when the drug bleeds into an adrenal gland.

Cushing's syndrome is an overabundance of cortisol. The most common cause is taking cortisone-like medicines, such as prednisone, every day for weeks to months. Another leading cause is an adenoma, a benign tumour of the pituitary gland. The tumour can make the pituitary gland produce too much adrenocorticotropic hormone (ACTH), which stimulates the adrenal gland to produce cortisol. (Cushing's disease is the term doctors use when the syndrome is caused by a pituitary tumour.) Other causes of Cushing's syndrome are tumours on the adrenal glands and elsewhere.

Pheochromocytoma is an adrenal gland tumour that causes the glands to secrete too much epinephrine and norepinephrine, which regulate heart rate and blood pressure. The cause of the tumour is unknown, but it is most likely to occur in young and middle-aged adults. More than 90 percent of pheochromocytomas are benign.

Hyperaldosteronism, also called aldosteronism or Conn's syndrome, is an excess of aldosterone, a hormone that regulates blood volume and levels of sodium and potassium. The main cause is an adrenal tumour, but it can also be a complication of heart failure (pp.234–5), cirrhosis (pp.282–3) or kidney failure (pp.306–7).

PREVENTION

Avoiding oral corticosteroid medications whenever possible can reduce the risk of adrenal gland disorders.

DIAGNOSIS

Adrenal gland disorders are diagnosed based on their symptoms, as well as laboratory tests and sometimes imaging tests. Weakness,

WHO IS AT RISK?

The risk factors include:

Addison's disease
- Type 1 diabetes
- Hypopituitarism
- Chronic thyroiditis
- Myasthenia gravis
- Pernicious anaemia
- Autoimmune disorders

Cushing's syndrome
- Adrenal gland tumour
- Pituitary gland tumour
- Ongoing corticosteroid medication
- Female

Pheochromocytoma
- Young adulthood to middle age

Hyperaldosteronism
- Adrenal gland tumour
- High blood pressure
- Cirrhosis
- Heart failure
- Kidney failure

fatigue, and unintentional weight loss or weight gain are signs of all adrenal gland disorders.

Addison's disease causes a loss of appetite but a craving for salt, as well as chronic diarrhoea and dark skin patches.

Cushing's disease causes physical changes – roundness and redness of the face and a hump between the shoulders – as well as increased thirst and urination, and high blood pressure. Men may experience impotence and women a cessation of menstruation. Common symptoms of pheochromocytoma are increased perspiration, headache and blood pressure fluctuations.

Signs of hyperaldosteronism include high blood pressure, headache, numbness and intermittent paralysis.

For a definitive diagnosis, blood tests are done to measure levels of adrenal hormones. Urine tests may be used to assess levels of the hormones and potassium, which is low in people with hyperaldosteronism. In an ACTH-stimulation test, a synthetic version of this pituitary gland hormone is given to stimulate the adrenal glands to produce cortisol. Other tests include imaging – such as MRI or CT scans – to detect tumours of the pituitary or adrenal glands.

TREATMENTS

Addison's disease
This illness is life-threatening.
• **MEDICATION** Corticosteroids must be taken for life to supplement the adrenal glands' low output of cortisol. Whenever an individual is under extra mental or physical stress, increased dosed of steroids may be required. Intravenous corticosteroids are needed during times of adrenal crisis, in which cortisol levels plunge dangerously low. Supplements of DHEA, a chemical produced by the adrenal glands that naturally declines with age, may improve mood and overall well-being. Some patients need aldosterone replacement therapy.
• **HERBAL MEDICINE** Various Chinese and Western herbs, known as adaptogens, are sometimes used in conjunction with steroid replacement, though research that definitively proves their effectiveness are lacking.

Cushing's syndrome
All treatment for Cushing's syndrome also involves regular medical visits to check for complications from the disorder, including diabetes, high blood pressure and osteoporosis.

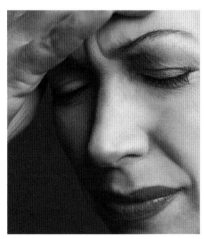

Headaches and intense anxiety are symptoms of pheochromocytoma. This condition, caused by non-cancerous tumours on the adrenal glands, results in an excess of adrenaline and can be fatal if left untreated.

• **SURGERY** Pituitary adenomas and tumours on the adrenal glands may be removed surgically.
• **RADIATION THERAPY** Following surgery, radiation may be needed for cancerous tumours.
• **MEDICATION** Corticosteroid medication is often needed either temporarily or permanently following surgery for pituitary tumours. When the syndrome is caused by corticosteroid medication given for another illness, treatment may involve gradually stopping the medication under a doctor's guidance.

Pheochromocytoma
• **SURGERY** This is often needed to remove adrenal tumours.
• **LIFESTYLE CHANGES** If hypertension persists following surgery, it may require treatment separately with careful attention to diet, exercise and medication. A diet low in saturated and trans fats, and rich in fruits, vegetables and whole grains, can reduce blood pressure.

Hyperaldosteronism
• **SURGERY** This may be performed to remove adrenal tumours, although sometimes medical treatment can control the problem.
• **MEDICATION** Aldosterone blockers may be prescribed in addition to, or instead of surgery to reduce the production of aldosterone.
• **DIET** A low-sodium diet is recommended to help maintain the proper balance of sodium and potassium in the blood.

See also: *Diabetes, pp.338–41* • *Heart Failure, pp.234–5* • *Kidney Failure, pp.306–7*

Thyroid Disorders

The thyroid gland, which wraps around the windpipe, secretes two hormones, thyroxine and triiodothyronine. These hormones regulate the rate of the metabolism (all the body's physiological processes). Thyroid disorders occur most often when the thyroid gland does not function properly and releases either too much or not enough of the thyroid hormones, but problems can also develop when the pituitary gland malfunctions.

Normally, the pituitary gland in the brain prompts the thyroid to produce hormones by releasing thyroid-stimulating hormone (TSH). Hyperthyroidism (overactive thyroid) is an excess of thyroid hormone production, causing such symptoms as protruding eyes, weight loss, restlessness, feeling hot and increased perspiration. Hypothyroidism (underactive thyroid) is a lack of adequate thyroid hormone production, with symptoms such as fatigue, weight gain, hair loss (pp.116–17), feeling cold, diminished sex drive, depression (pp.364–5) and brittle fingernails. Thyroid disorders can occur at any age, but they are especially common among middle-aged women.

CAUSES
Hyperthyroidism

Graves' disease, an autoimmune disorder in which the thyroid, skin and eyes are attacked, is the most common cause of hyperthyroidism worldwide. It most often affects women 20 to 60 years old, but it can also affect newborn babies. About 1 to 5 percent of babies whose mothers have Graves' disease are born with the condition. Graves' disease causes palpitations, rapid heartrate, fatigue and excess perspiration. A complication is Graves' ophthalmology, which is a bulging of the eyes.

Stress can trigger Graves' disease

by initially suppressing immune system activity and then causing too much activity. Pregnancy is sometimes enough to initiate this stress reaction, causing temporary hyperthyroidism. Smoking, though not a cause of Graves' disease, can aggravate the symptoms of Graves' ophthalmology. Left untreated, Graves' disease can be life-threatening.

Goitre is a swelling of the thyroid. Typically weighing less than 28 g (1 oz), the thyroid can swell to several times its normal size, creating a noticeable bulge in the neck. Symptoms also include hoarsness and difficulty swallowing. Goitre can be a side-effect of medications such as lithium and dopamine, or the result of a diet with too little iodine, a mineral that the thyroid uses to make thyroid hormones. In rare cases, goitre is caused by thyroid cancer.

Iodine deficiency has been eliminated in many countries through the use of iodized salt, but it is still a major health problem in much of the world, and a focus of both UNICEF and the WHO.

WHO IS AT RISK?

The risk factors include:

- Female
- Stress
- Adenoma of the thyroid
- Graves' disease
- Birth defect of the thyroid
- Pituitary gland disorders
- Viral infection of the thyroid
- Too much or too little iodine in the diet
- Pregnancy
- Thyroid cancer

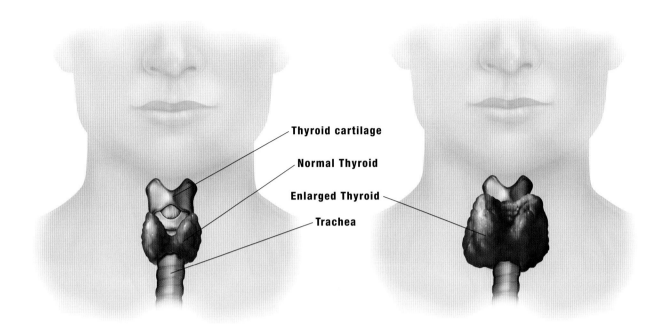

On the left is a normal thyroid and on the right an enlarged thyroid. The thyroid gland typically weighs less than 28 g (1 oz) but can become enlarged to many times its normal size and create a visible bulge in the throat, a condition called goitre. Goitre can arise as a side-effect of some medications, an iodine deficiency or as the result of cancer.

Thyroid cartilage
Normal Thyroid
Enlarged Thyroid
Trachea

Adenomas of the thyroid are benign growths that can also cause hyperthyroidism. Symptoms include small nodules on the thyroid that may cause pressure when swallowing.

Hypothyroidism

Autoimmune thyroiditis, which is an inflammation of the thyroid that occurs when the immune system attacks it, is a leading cause of hypothyroidism. In the most common form, called Hashimoto thyroiditis, the thyroid is increasingly unable to manufacture thyroxine because of the autoimmune process that has damaged it. Hashimoto thyroiditis progresses slowly over a number of years and leads to chronic thyroid damage.

Pituitary gland disorders (p.351) cause about 5 percent of cases of hypothyroidism. With these disorders, the pituitary does not signal the thyroid to secrete thyroid hormones.

Hyperthyroidism treatment causes permanent hypothyroidism in about 3 percent of patients each year. As many as 90 percent of hyperthyroidism patients develop temporary hypothyroidism in response to medical treatment with radioactive iodine, which absorbs into the thyroid and drastically slows output of thyroid hormones.

Other causes of thyroid disorders include birth defects of the thyroid, injury to the hypothalamus (the area of the brain that is connected to the pituitary gland), thyroid infections and pregnancy (pp.398–400). Hypothyroidism from infections and pregnancy are usually temporary. When a birth defect is the cause, it may be associated with cretinism, a form of mental and physical retardation.

PREVENTION

Taking either too much or too little iodine can lead to thyroid disorders. Iodine is absorbed by the thyroid where it is used to manufacture thyroid hormone. Ideally, humans should consume 150 mcg of iodine a day. Iodine is found in seafood, dairy products and iodized salt. In addition, eat plenty of foods that contain selenium, a trace mineral found in wheat germ, chicken, fish, red meat and sunflower seeds. Doctors recommend about 55 mcg of selenium a day. Selenium deficiency may increase the risk of thyroiditis.

DIAGNOSIS

Doctors diagnose thyroid disorders based on the symptoms, a medical history, a physical examination and various blood tests. The blood tests measure levels of thyroid hormones and TSH, and detect the presence of thyroid antibodies (which indicate Graves' disease or Hashimoto thyroiditis – the presence of thyroid antibodies means the body has developed an autoimmune reaction and is attacking the thyroid). If hyperthyroidism is suspected, the doctor may order a thyroid scan, which uses a radioactive chemical to produce an image of the thyroid, to see if it is inflamed, and if all or part of the gland is overactive. If hypothyroidism is suspected, the doctor may also test blood cholesterol because hyperthyroidism results in an elevation of cholesterol.

TREATMENTS

No treatment may be needed for temporary forms of the thyroid disorders. For chronic disorders, each type has different treatments that address the specific causes.

Selenium is a trace mineral found in eggs, seafood, sunflower seeds, chicken and turkey. Evidence suggests that eating foods that contain selenium may help control hyperthyroidism by decreasing the hormone output of the overactive gland.

Hyperthyroidism

• MEDICATION Propylthiouracil and methimazole block the production of thyroid hormones and the conversion to the more active form of the hormone, T3. They are used to lower overall hormone levels. Beta-blockers, which interfere with the activity of thyroid hormones, may be given to reduce symptoms associated with excess thyroid hormone levels, such as rapid heart rate, until the other medications take effect. Steroids are sometimes given in the short term to relieve severe hyperthyroid symptoms, including Graves' ophthalmology.

• RADIOACTIVE IODINE When medication is not sufficient, this therapy may be used to lower the production of thyroid hormones by destroying some of the thyroid cells. However, radioactive iodine will eventually lead to hypothyroidism in most patients. When this happens, thyroid replacement therapy is needed to increase levels of thyroid hormones. Radioactive iodine cannot be used during pregnancy, and in people with Graves' ophthalmology it can make the condition worse.

• SUPPLEMENTS Selenium, when given along with conventional treatments, may speed up the decrease in thyroid hormone levels.

• SURGERY A thyroid tumour may be removed surgically. Removal of all or part of the thyroid may be considered as an alternative to

Clinical Query

How do I know if I have a thyroid disorder?

Surprising changes in weight, hair loss, unusual sensitivity to hot or cold, and abnormal menstruation are all signs of thyroid disorders.

Symptoms of hyperthyroidism include swelling of the neck (a sign of an enlarged thyroid), protruding eyes, weight loss despite an increased appetite, restlessness, exceptional sensitivity to heat, sweating, insomnia (pp.170–2), hand tremors (p.173), hair loss (pp.116–17), high blood pressure (pp.236–9), and, for women, abnormal menstrual periods.

Symptoms of hypothyroidism include weakness, fatigue, memory loss or mental slowness, exceptional sensitivity to cold, weight gain, joint or muscle pain, brittle hair and nails, hair loss, pale dry skin, puffy face, hands, and feet, decreased taste and smell, hoarseness, depression, and, for women, abnormal menstrual periods.

medical treatment for pregnant women and others who cannot take thyroid medications or radioactive iodine.

In rare cases, a surgical procedure called orbital decompression is performed to enlarge the eye sockets enough to accommodate the swollen eyes that are symptomatic of Graves' ophthalmology. In this procedure, a bone that separates the eye sockets and the sinuses is removed, creating space behind the eyes and allowing them to slip back into the sockets.

• EYE TREATMENTS These include artificial tears to relieve dry eye associated with Graves' ophthalmology. Sunglasses can reduce discomfort by dimming the light and cool compresses can help by reducing swelling and adding moisture around the eyes. Radiation therapy to the eyes can also decrease swelling.

• MODIFIED ACTIVITY Avoiding strenuous physical activity can help minimize palpitations and rapid heart rate in people with Graves' disease.

Hypothyroidism

• THYROID REPLACEMENT THERAPY In this treatment, synthetic forms of thyroid hormones are used to raise and maintain hormone levels in the body. Levels then have to be checked periodically to make sure they are not too high, putting a person at risk for hyperthyroidism. Treatment often involves only thyroxine replacement, but using it in combination with triiodothyronine may have some benefit.

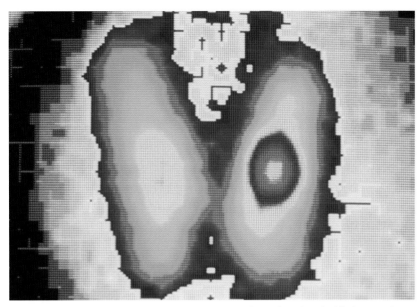

This coloured gamma scan has detected adenoma (shown in red and white), caused by a benign tumour, in the right lobe of the thyroid gland. This causes the production of excessive quantities of thyroid hormones, leading to a condition called hyperthyroidism.

• MEDICATION Anti-inflammatory medication may be given to reduce the inflammation of the thyroid gland if it is caused by a malfunction of the pituitary gland or autoimmune thyroiditis. The therapy often begins with nonsteroidal anti-inflammatory agents; if this medication is not effective, cortisone is prescribed.

Beta-blockers may also be prescribed to relieve symptoms.

• SUPPLEMENTS Selenium supplements appear to reduce levels of thyroid antibody, suggesting that they may also help treat Hashimoto thyroiditis.

See also: *Pregnancy, pp.398–400 • Depression, pp.364–5 • Hair Loss, pp.116–17*

healing hope I was successfully treated for an overactive thyroid but, unfortunately, I gained 9 kg (20 lbs). This came as a surprise, since I was always slim. My doctor explained that the thyroid treatment slowed my metabolism, so I didn't burn up as many calories as I used to. That meant I couldn't eat as much as before, or I had to find a way of burning those extra calories.

She advised me to try to boost my metabolism by increasing my physical activity level to about half an hour on most days. She didn't put me on a diet or recommend any weight loss supplements. But she did suggest that I pay closer attention to my body and eat only when I truly felt hungry and not for other reasons, like because I was feeling stressed out or because it was 'mealtime'.

Since I began following her advice, I've lost about 2.25 kg (5 lbs). I look better and I feel more energetic.
Zach S.

OBESITY

Obesity is reaching epidemic proportions worldwide, as one in six people around the globe is either overweight or obese. It increases the risk for diabetes (pp.338–41), heart disease (pp.230–3), stroke (pp.168–9), hypertension (p.236), gallbladder disease (pp.280–1), osteoarthritis (pp.136–9), sleep apnoea (pp.214–15) and other breathing problems, as well as many forms of cancer. Obese individuals have a 50 to 100 percent increased risk of death overall.

CAUSES

When more calories are consumed than expended, obesity is the result. However, how body weight is regulated is not yet well understood and the process may not be quite that simple. After looking at twin, adoption and family studies, researchers believe that genetic factors may account for 33 percent of the variation in body weight among individuals. Long-term studies show that factors, such as lower socioeconomic status, sedentary lifestyle and changes in diet due to the glut of processed foods and fast foods now available, account for the other two-thirds. Lower socio-economic status is particularly a risk factor for women.

PREVENTION

Consuming reasonable amounts of nutritious food and staying active are the best ways to prevent extra weight from accumulating. It takes 3,500 calories to add 0.45 kg (1 lb) of body weight. That means just an extra 250 calories a day (about 1 and a half cans of sugar-sweetened fizzy drinks) can add 9 kg (20 lbs) in a year; eliminating 250 calories a day can mean a 9 kg (20 lb) weight loss over the same period.

DIAGNOSIS

The relationship of weight to height in tables developed by life insurance companies was once the primary method of determining obesity, but now the Body-Mass Index (BMI) is considered a more accurate measurement. BMI is determined by dividing weight in kilograms by height in metres, squared. (To calculate BMI in pounds, multiply weight in pounds by 704.5, then divide the result by height in inches, then divide that number again by height in inches.) 'Overweight' is defined as a BMI of 25 to 29.9, while obesity is a BMI of 30 or higher. As the number increases, so do the health risks.

BMI is not foolproof. People who are very muscular may fall into the overweight category even though they are quite fit, and the elderly who have lost muscle mass may be classified as healthy when they are not.

Because abdominal fat may cause more health problems than fat distributed elsewhere such as the buttocks and thighs, especially increasing the risk for type 2 diabetes and cardiovascular disease, waist measurement is another way to determine obesity. Men whose waist measures 102 cm (40 in) or more and women with a waist measurement of 89 cm (35 in) or more are at higher risk. Measure the waist at the smallest circumference under the rib cage and above the navel.

TREATMENTS

Losing just 10 percent, or sometimes even 5 percent, of body weight will control or improve the complications of obesity. Anyone with a serious medical condition should check with a doctor before starting a weight-loss programme. Fortunately, extremely low-calorie diets of 400 to 800 calories a day have fallen out of favour. Many other diets work because they reduce the amount of calories consumed, but only for the short term. To keep the weight off, it is more important to change habits for life.

• DIET Choose more fruits and vegetables. Reduce fat with low-fat dairy products and substitute fish for fattier meats twice a week, and baked or grilled chicken for fried chicken. Increase fibre by replacing white bread, cereals, and pastas with whole-grain products. Reduce or eliminate simple carbohydrates found in biscuits and sweets. Replace sugar-sweetened fizzy drinks and fruit drinks with water and diet drinks. Limit alcohol to two drinks a day for men and one drink a day for women. When fast food is the only option, get a small hamburger instead of the giant cheeseburger, and skip the fries or get a small portion. Read labels when out shopping to find low-fat foods.

• EXERCISE Few weight-loss programmes will be successful in the long term without exercise or an increase in physical activity. Exercise, or any kind of physical activity, does not just burn calories, it

Clinical Query

I finally managed to lose 13.5 kg (30 lbs), but how do I make sure I keep it off – for good?

Few people keep off lost weight for five years or longer, despite the billions of pounds spent worldwide on weight loss products and services. Researchers at the National Weight Control Registry in the United States found that most of those who succeed do the following:
• Eat a low-fat diet high in complex carbohydrates
• Weigh themselves regularly (usually weekly)
• Have breakfast every day
• Spend at least 60 to 90 minutes a day in physical activity

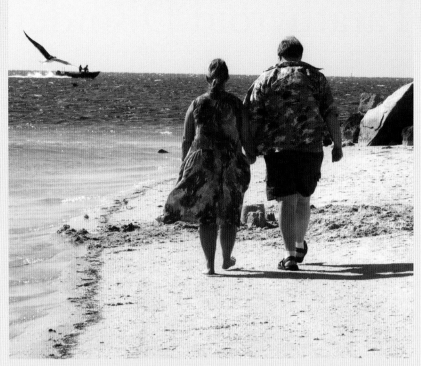
Dieting alone is not enough to reduce obesity. It is essential to exercise to burn calories and help control food intake. Simple ways to increase daily activity, include taking the stairs instead of the elevator and walking short distances instead of using transport.

also helps control food intake.

• BEHAVIOURAL THERAPY Many commercial weight-loss programmes, along with those offered by health professionals, include behaviour therapy designed to change eating habits and increase physical activity. Hypnotherapy (pp.508–13) and relaxation therapy (pp.474–5) help some people as well. Studies show people lose more weight with behavioural therapy with diet and exercise, than through diet and exercise alone.

• MEDICATION Researchers continue to work on developing medications that will suppress appetite safely and aid in weight loss. Sibutramine is sometimes used as an appetite suppressant, but it can sometimes increase blood pressure (pp.236–9) and pulse rate. Lipase inhibitors such as orlistat block the

absorption of fat but cause gastrointestinal side effects.

• SURGERY Surgical treatment may be considered for anyone with a BMI of 40 or higher, or with a lower BMI but serious or life-threatening complications. Resulting weight loss usually lasts five years or more. Two popular operations, vertical banded gastroplasty and gastric bypass, result in a smaller stomach, forcing patients to eat less and limiting their bodies' ability to absorb the food that is eaten. The surgery is fairly safe with a low mortality rate and few side-effects, but certain populations, including people over 65, have much higher mortality and complication rates.

See also: *Diabetes, pp.338–41* • *Stroke, pp.168–9* • *Hypertension, pp.236–9*

Parathyroid Disorders

The parathyroid glands are a cluster of four small glands in the neck on each side of the thyroid; they control the level of calcium in the body by secreting parathyroid hormone. Hyperparathyroidism is a disorder in which the glands are overactive and secrete too much hormone, leaving too much calcium in the blood and too little stored in the bones. Hypoparathyroidism is an underactive parathyroid that secretes too little hormone, causing blood calcium levels to drop too low.

Symptoms of hyperparathyroidism include fatigue, joint or muscle pain, increased thirst and sometimes fractures. Symptoms of hypoparathyroidism include tingling, muscle cramps (p.142), pain, dry hair and skin and cataracts (pp.34–5). It can be a complication of kidney disease.

CAUSES
The most common causes of hyperparathyroidism are adenomas (benign tumours on the parathyroid glands) or an enlargement of one of the glands. Less common causes are a malignant tumour of the parathyroid and serious calcium deficiency.

Hypoparathyroidism can develop as a result of other endocrine gland disorders that affect the thyroid, ovaries or adrenal glands. It can be a side-effect of treatment for an overactive thyroid (pp.344–7). It can also be caused by an injury to the parathyroid from trauma or by surgical removal of the parathyroid glands. Hypoparathyroidism may also be inherited.

PREVENTION
Getting enough calcium in the diet can help prevent hyperparathyroidism.

DIAGNOSIS
Doctors diagnose these disorders based on the symptoms, medical history, and various blood tests, including tests to measure calcium levels and levels of parathyroid hormone. Other tests may include bone X-rays, a bone density test, and an ultrasound of the kidneys.

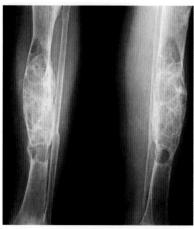

Over-activity of the parathyroid glands causes the formation of brown tumours, in this case along the shafts of the tibias in the legs. Brown tumours need surgery.

TREATMENTS
Hyperparathyroidism
If calcium levels are only slightly high, and the bones and kidneys appear normal, the doctor may recommend no treatment other than periodic evaluation of calcium levels and kidney function.

• LIFESTYLE CHANGES Drinking plenty of water throughout the day and exercising regularly can help protect the kidneys by stimulating them, keeping blood levels of calcium from getting too high.

• SURGERY Removing the parathyroid is often recommended if the condition causes complications such as kidney disease (p.308) or osteoporosis (pp.146–7).

Hypoparathyroidism
• SUPPLEMENTS Calcium and vitamin D are given to treat underactive parathyroid glands.

See also: *Thyroid Disorders, pp.344–7 • Muscle Cramps, p.142 • Cataracts, pp.34–5*

Pituitary Gland Disorders

The pituitary gland lies within the brain and functions as a master gland, secreting signalling hormones that trigger the release of other hormones, which help control a wide range of functions including blood pressure, growth, metabolism and reproduction. The gland produces several non-signalling hormones, including growth hormone, which stimulates the normal growth of tissues and bones, and prolactin, which prompts breast growth and milk production.

Disorders are characterized by abnormal levels of pituitary hormones and of the hormones that are either stimulated or lowered by pituitary hormones. Symptoms include weakness, abnormal growth, lack of menstrual periods in women and loss of sex drive in men. Without treatment, some pituitary disorders can lead to thyroid disorders (pp.344–7), adrenal gland disorders (pp.342–3), and other neurological and hormonal complications.

CAUSES

Tumours can damage the pituitary gland or hypothalamus. Other causes of damage include radiation, surgery, meningitis (p.180) and other infections. In some cases, the cause is unknown.

Acromegaly, an excess of growth hormone, is usually caused by an adenoma, a benign tumour on the pituitary gland. It occurs most often in middle age.

Galactorrhoea is the production of breast milk in women who are not pregnant or have not recently given birth and, in rare cases, men. Causes include a brain tumour that secretes prolactin and an intraductal papilloma, a benign growth in the breast. Galactorrhea can also be a side-effect of several medications, such as oral contraceptives, cimetadine for ulcers (p.276), methyldopa for high blood pressure (pp.236–9) and tricyclic antidepressants.

Hypopituitarism, a deficiency of one or more pituitary hormones, has many causes, including tumours of the pituitary gland or the brain (pp.196–7), head trauma, stroke (pp.168–9) and brain infections. In rare cases, it is a complication of pregnancy.

PREVENTION

Experts know of no way to prevent pituitary gland disorders.

DIAGNOSIS

A doctor can diagnose pituitary gland disorders based on the symptoms, medical history, blood tests for pituitary hormones and sometimes other blood tests. If the levels of any of the pituitary hormones is abnormal, the doctor will probably order a CT scan or an MRI to see if there is a tumour on the pituitary gland or abnormalities in the brain. Additional blood and urine tests may be needed. For galactorrhea, a biopsy may be taken if there is a lump in the breast.

TREATMENTS

• SURGERY Tumours from the pituitary gland and brain may have to be surgically removed.
• RADIATION THERAPY This may be used either as an alternative to surgery or in addition to surgery to shrink pituitary tumours.
• HORMONE THERAPY Hormones are used to compensate for deficiencies when a person has hypopituitarism. Hormone therapy may include cortisone and thyroid hormone.
• MEDICATION For acromegaly, medicines that suppress growth hormone secretion may be prescribed. For hypopituitarism, fertility medication may be needed.

See also: *Brain Tumours, pp.196–7* • *Stroke, pp.168–9* • *Thyroid Disorders, pp.344–7*

WHO IS AT RISK?

The risk factors include:
• Pituitary tumours
• Brain tumours
• Brain trauma
• Stroke
• Brain infection
• Intraductal papilloma
• Some medications, including oral contraceptives, cimetadine, methyldopa and tricyclic antidepressants

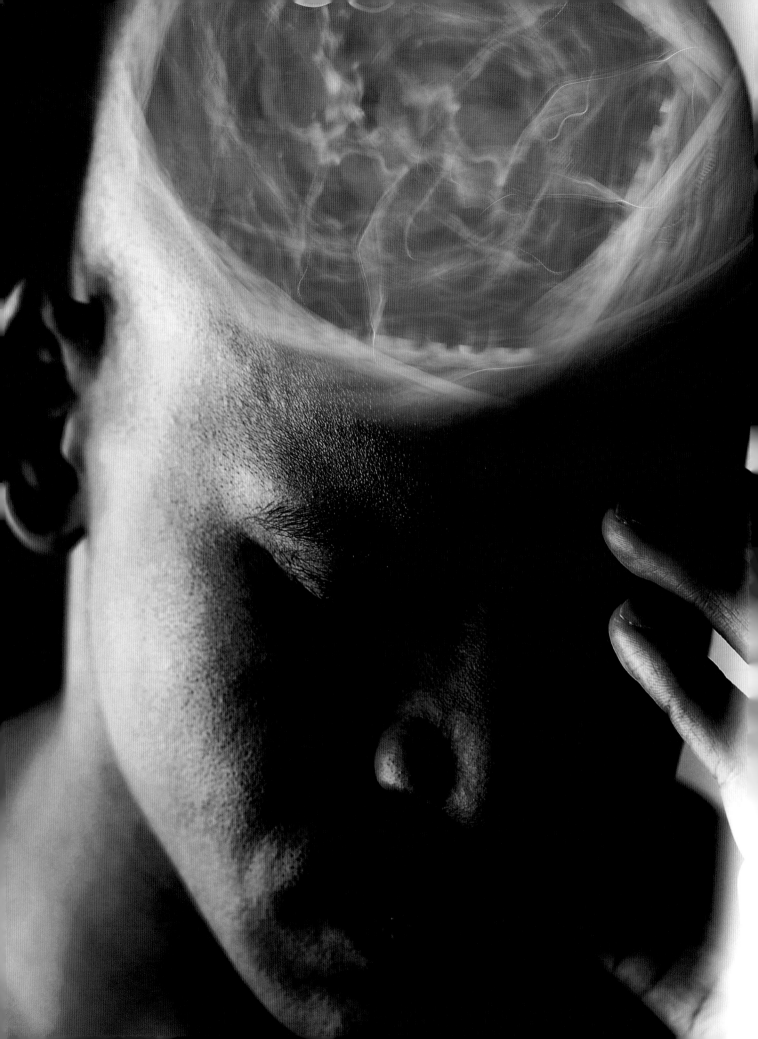

13 PSYCHIATRIC & EMOTIONAL DISORDERS

Psychiatric disorders disrupt thinking, behaviour and emotions, and range from mild depression that makes it hard to get up in the morning to schizophrenia so severe that all contact with reality is lost. Also referred to as mental illness, these disorders are often blamed on changes in brain chemistry or brain wiring, caused by genetics, injuries, infections or life events. They are not due to a lack of willpower or character.

Many of these disorders improve with a combination of approaches; some, such as medication, supplements, physical exercise or exposure to light work directly with the chemical balance of the brain. Others, such as psychotherapy, help rewire the brain by creating new connections and behaviour.

Anxiety Disorders

Stress and worry are a part of life, but when anxiety – a feeling of apprehension or fear – develops and becomes overwhelming to the point it is disabling, an anxiety disorder may be responsible. These anxiety disorders include panic disorder, obsessive-compulsive disorder, phobias (p.361) and post-traumatic stress disorder (pp.356–7). Anxiety disorders are the most common mental illnesses, affecting at least 10 percent of people in Western countries, including children and teenagers.

phobias (p.361) and post-traumatic stress disorder (pp.356–7).

WHO IS AT RISK?

The risk factors include:
- Family history
- Emotional neglect or abuse in childhood
- Traumatic events.

CAUSES

The causes of anxiety disorders are not completely known. They frequently develop after emotional neglect in childhood or stressful and traumatic events, and may continue for years after the initial event. They also do seem to run in families and some may be due to chemical imbalances in the brain; for example, some cases of OCD are blamed on an imbalance of a brain chemical called serotonin.

A physical disorder, such as an overactive thyroid gland, or the use of drugs like corticosteroids or cocaine, can produce the symptoms of an anxiety disorder.

PREVENTION

While it is not always possible to prevent anxiety disorders, teaching people to discern true risk from fears is central to prevention and treatment. In addition, some studies have shown the benefit of regular exercise and the use of relaxation methods such as meditation. Avoid caffeine, illegal drugs,

and stimulant-containing over-the-counter cold medication, which can all worsen the symptoms of an anxiety disorder.

DIAGNOSIS

Diagnosis is based on symptoms. A thorough physical examination can rule out any other possible causes. More than one mental illness can exist at a time; anxiety disorders may accompany depression, eating disorders, substance abuse, or another anxiety disorder.

- **GENERALIZED ANXIETY DISORDER** Twice as many women as men suffer from this constant, excessive worry and nervousness that lasts six months or longer. At least three of these symptoms must also be present for a diagnosis: restlessness, fatigue, difficulty concentrating, irritability, muscle tension and sleep problems.
- **OBSESSIVE-COMPULSIVE DISORDER** Disturbing, anxious thoughts or images are obsessions, while the rituals to get rid of them are called compulsions. These thoughts and

rituals feel out of control and may take up at least an hour a day, interfering with daily life. For example, a person with OCD may have an overwhelming fear of germs, and consequently wash their hands hundreds of times a day. OCD affects men and women equally and usually starts in childhood, adolescence or early adulthood.

- **PANIC DISORDER** This disorder is characterized by panic attacks that strike without warning, causing feelings of terror and physical symptoms of chest pain, heart palpitations, shortness of breath, dizziness, abdominal pain, feelings of unreality, and a fear of dying that may mimic a heart attack. Twice as common in women than in men, it often develops during late adolescence or early adulthood. Around one-third of people with panic disorder develop agoraphobia, a fear of being in situations where escape or help may be unavailable or embarrassing if a panic attack were to occur. Some people with panic disorder may become housebound, although this condition is one of the most treatable of the anxiety disorders.

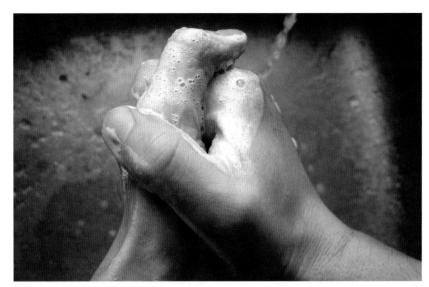

A person with obsessive-compulsive disorder who has obsessive fears about germs may wash their hands repeatedly – sometimes hundreds of times a day.

TREATMENTS

Many anxiety disorders can be treated with a combination of psychotherapy and medication. Other techniques may also help.

• MEDICATION Selective serotonin reuptake inhibitors (SSRIs), a class of antidepressants, are commonly prescribed for anxiety disorders, but they can take two to three weeks to be effective and sometimes may make symptoms worse at first. They are often used for generalized anxiety disorders and OCD. Other antidepressants such as the tricyclics or MAO inhibitors may be used in some cases. Antianxiety drugs such as the benzodiazepines are often used for anxiety, but can lead to drug dependence and must be tapered off. Buspirone, a non-habit-forming antianxiety drug, takes two weeks to be effective. Other drugs that may be prescribed include beta-blockers, antihistamines and certain sedatives.

• PSYCHOTHERAPY Cognitive-behavioural therapy is effective for many anxiety disorders. The cognitive therapy portion changes thinking patterns that in turn change reactions to feared situations. The behavioural therapy portion works to decrease avoidance of feared situations and allow patients to learn first-hand that such situations can be successfully handled.

People with OCD are often treated with 'exposure and response prevention' by exposing them to their fear while providing help in coping with the resulting anxiety. Exposure therapy carefully uses repeated imaginings in a safe environment to help the patient gain control of the fear. Desensitization uses a more gradual response and involves relaxation training.

• GROUP THERAPY This type of therapy may help individuals with generalized anxiety disorder realize others also experience the same excessive worry.

• MUSIC THERAPY Studies show that music therapy (p.565) can enhance mood and illicit the relaxation response, a physical state characterized by a reduction in heart rate, blood pressure and muscle tension. Listening to music that is a personal preference has a more beneficial effect on the outcome.

• MEDITATION Mindfulness meditation, a type of meditation (p.514–19) in which attention is focused on physical sensations in the present, may help reduce feelings of anxiety. Some studies show changes in brain wave patterns.

• KAVA Made from the dried roots of the shrub Peper methysticum, kava has been shown in human studies to be effective for anxiety, but more than 30 cases of liver damage have been reported and some countries no longer sell it. The U.S. Food and Drug Administration has issued a warning to consumers and doctors.

• HYPNOTHERAPY Hypnosis (pp.508–13) can reduce anxiety, especially that suffered before medical or dental procedures. It may be used as an adjunct therapy along with cognitive-behavioural therapy. While there is ample anecdotal evidence, no reliable research studies have compared hypnosis alone to antianxiety medication.

• YOGA Several studies have shown yoga (pp.476–9) effective in treating anxiety. Commonly used has been Kundalini meditation (p.478) and relaxation. However, more studies are needed.

• RELAXATION Regularly practised relaxation techniques reduce anxiety and are especially helpful when used with desensitization therapy for panic disorder or phobias.

See also: *Phobias, p.361* • *Post-Traumatic Stress Disorder, pp.356–7*

Post-Traumatic Stress Disorder

It was once called shell-shock or combat fatigue, but post-traumatic stress disorder affects many more people than war-weary veterans. Anyone who suffers a traumatic or disturbing event may fall prey to the disorder. PTSD is thought to affect about 10 percent of people in their life-time.

CAUSES

Once identified as the result of seeing heavy combat, post-traumatic stress disorder can happen to anyone after an over-whelmingly traumatic event such as a car accident, sexual assault, natural disaster, or even the diag-nosis of a life-threatening illness. Around 1 percent of women who experience a miscarriage may end up suffering from PTSD.

The body produces a hormone called adrenaline in response to stress. With PTSD, adrenaline levels may remain high, causing tenseness, irritability, an inability to relax and insomnia. That adrenaline may also prevent the hippocampus, the part of the brain that processes memories, from doing its job.

PREVENTION

Passive powerlessness during a traumatic event is related to a large risk of developing PTSD. Remain-ing active and focused on help-ing other people during combat exposure or natural disasters has been linked with a lower risk of symptoms. Opportunities to express distress after the event to other supportive people may also help prevent later symptoms.

DIAGNOSIS

Some of the most disturbing symptoms of PTSD include vivid memories and nightmares, which involve reliving the traumatic event over and over, often with the sounds, smells, pain and fear that were part of the original event. Because these traumatic memories are so painful, the person may be-come emotionally numb and avoid people and places that are remind-ers of the event. Finally, the PTSD patient may be 'on guard', always on the look out for danger, which is called hypervigilance. Irritability, depression, and physical symptoms such as headaches (pp.166–7), di-arrhoea (p.268), irregular heartbeat (pp.226–8), plus dependence on alcohol or drugs may be present. It affects more women than men.

Children can also suffer from PTSD. They may be prone to nightmares and lose interest in activities they once enjoyed. They may also recreate the traumatic event while playing, and suffer from headaches and stomachaches.

A mental health practitioner can diagnose PTSD based on the symptoms. A medical examination

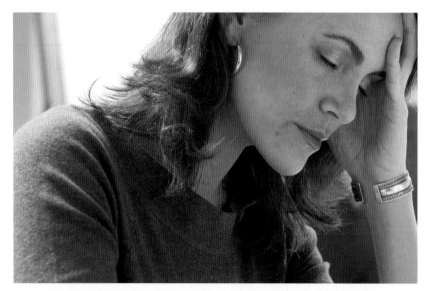

Post-traumatic stress disorder affects twice as many woman than men and can be triggered by life events that cause high levels of stress, including car accidents, natural disasters, or the diagnosis of a chronic or life-threatening illness.

should be done to rule out other possible causes of symptoms. PTSD generally co-exists with other disorders, such as depression (pp.364–5), alcohol or substance abuse (pp.358–60), panic disorder (pp.354–5) and other anxiety disorders.

The time-frame is important. Symptoms during the first four weeks after an event can actually be a positive sign that the mind is processing the event to recover. If symptoms persist for more than four weeks or longer and sometimes even worsen, then PTSD may be present.

TREATMENTS

Guidelines from the National Institute for Clinical Excellence in the United Kingdom recommend using cognitive-behavioural therapy or eye movement desensitization and reprocessing (EMDR) before medication for PTSD when possible.

• EMDR Although still controversial, eye movement desensitization and reprocessing (pp.372–3) has been shown effective in several studies for civilian and combat-related PTSD. The therapy combines elements of exposure therapy and cognitive-behavioural therapy along with rapid eye movements back and forth. During exposure to traumatic memories, the eye movements create an alternation of attention; researchers speculate this alternation somehow aids the mind in processing memories. The procedure usually requires fewer visits and costs less than conventional psychotherapy.

• EXPOSURE THERAPY This type of cognitive-behavioural therapy carefully uses repeated imaginings

of the traumatic event in a safe environment to help the patient gain control of the fear. Desensitization uses a gradual approach along with relaxation techniques. Flooding is an exposure technique in which the patient confronts all the memories at once.

• GROUP THERAPY Speaking with others who have shared similar experiences may be useful for those with PTSD, especially in helping deal with 'survivor's guilt'.

• FAMILY THERAPY Family members are often affected by PTSD as well and may benefit from therapy.

• COGNITIVE-BEHAVIOURAL THERAPY This therapy is effective when accompanied by repeated exposure of the self in imagination between sessions. This therapy changes thinking patterns so that reactions to certain situations also change. Behavioural therapy works to change specific behaviours with techniques including relaxation training and exposure.

• MEDICATION The most commonly prescribed drugs for PTSD are the antidepressants known as selective serotonin reuptake

inhibitors; they do not cure the disorder but instead relieve the symptoms, making treatment through psychotherapy more effective. Other antidepressants such as the tricyclics or MAO inhibitors may be used in some cases. Anti-anxiety drugs such as the benzodiazepines are often used to treat anxiety caused by PTSD, but are of limited benefit because they can lead to drug dependence and must be tapered off when discontinued.

• HYPNOTHERAPY Hypnosis can reduce anxiety, although no reliable research studies have compared hypnosis to proven effective methods. It may be used as an additional therapy along with cognitive-behavioural therapy or EMDR for PTSD.

• YOGA Relaxation techniques, including yoga (pp.476–9) and massage (pp.468–73), may reduce anxiety associated with PTSD. Promising results with yoga have been obtained in a preliminary study at Boston University.

See also: *EMDR, pp.372–3 • Depression, pp.364–5 • Substance Abuse, pp.358–60*

healing hope After the car accident, I told myself I was lucky to walk away unhurt. But it became harder and harder over the next few months to get behind the wheel and drive anywhere again – especially on the motorway. I would have to pull over because I kept seeing and hearing the crash that had happened months before. Dreams – nightmares, really – woke me. I had headaches. I yelled at the kids all the time, it seemed.

My husband did some research and told me about something called EMDR, or eye movement desensitization and reprocessing, which sounded pretty strange.

The therapist took me through the steps of reliving the accident while moving my eyes. Within weeks, I could drive again without symptoms. I'm not sure how it worked, but it gave me my life back.   *Cynthia R.*

Substance Addiction

An addiction is a dependence – either physical or psychological, or both – on a substance that creates an overwhelming craving for it, which can damage health, relationships and work. That substance may be legal, such as alcohol or prescription medications, or illegal, such as cocaine, heroin or methamphetamines.

Many substances may be 'abused'. That is, they are taken for a non-medical reason, such as an athlete using steroids or growth hormones, or a person with anorexia using laxatives or ipecac syrup to lose weight.

More than 76 million people worldwide have been diagnosed with an alcohol problem, and at least 15 million with drug use disorders. Intravenous drug use, which has been reported in 136 countries to the World Health Organization, is one of the major risk factors for the spread of HIV/AIDS (pp.316–7).

Alcoholism and substance abuse can cause premature death from overdoses, damage to the body or accidents caused by impaired judgment. Even something that may seem harmless such as sniffing model airplane glue or hairspray can cause sudden death.

Alcoholism

This is a disease that occurs when drinking alcohol affects physical or mental health as well as social, family, or work responsibilities. The disease is divided into dependence and abuse.

Dependence, the most severe form of alcoholism, is characterized by a physical dependency on alcohol, which results in withdrawal symptoms when intake is reduced or stopped, and tolerance, a need for greater amounts of alcohol to feel its effects.

Abuse has not reached the point of physical dependency but has developed into what might be called a problem drinker.

Alcohol can impair judgment and concentration, erode the lining of the oesophagus and stomach, interfere with the absorption of vitamins, result in liver disease (pp.282–3), affect the heart muscle and cause nerve damage, memory loss (pp.178–9), birth defects such as foetal alcohol syndrome and sexual problems such as erectile dysfunction (p.426) and cessation of menstruation (pp.384–5). It increases the risk of cancer of the larynx (p.74), oesophagus, liver and colon.

Illegal Drugs

A number of illegal drugs can cause addiction and serious health problems, even in young, otherwise healthy people.

The most common hallucinogens include LSD, mushrooms and peyote, as well as phencyclidine (PCP or angel dust), and ketamine (Special K). These drugs produce euphoria and decrease inhibitions, but in larger doses can cause numbness and changes in perception, paranoia, hallucinations, psychosis and even death.

Cocaine is highly addictive. Using the drug causes feelings of intense euphoria, increased confidence and energy, and decreased inhibitions.

Methamphetamine and ecstasy elevate mood, increase energy, stamina and alertness, and decrease inhibitions. These amphetamines also increase blood pressure (pp.236–9) and heart rate, and can cause heart attacks (pp.230–3) and strokes (pp.168–9) in healthy young people.

Heroin and other opioids, some of which are legal pain relief available by prescription, dull pain, produce euphoria and may enhance sexual pleasure. But tolerance can develop very quickly, and when it does, more of the drug is required for effectiveness, and numerous physical problems can develop as a result, including drug overdose. Withdrawal symptoms requires medical supervision.

CAUSES

Family history plays a role in substance addiction. Children of alcoholics and drug abusers have a higher chance of developing substance addiction themselves.

Depression (pp.364–5) and other mental disorders may make people more prone to alcohol and substance abuse. Low self-esteem, conflict with relationships and anxiety (pp.354–5) may also contribute, along with peer pressure and a stressful lifestyle.

PREVENTION

As the problem of drug abuse, especially among young people, has escalated over the years, more and more programmes have been designed to prevent substance addiction. Several research studies have shown that for each dollar spent on prevention, a savings of up to $10 in treatment for alcohol or other substance addiction is realized.

Families should be open about discussing substance abuse and its harmful effects. The goals of family-based prevention programmes are to improve family bonding with effective parent–child communication, parental involvement, education about drugs and moderate, consistent discipline.

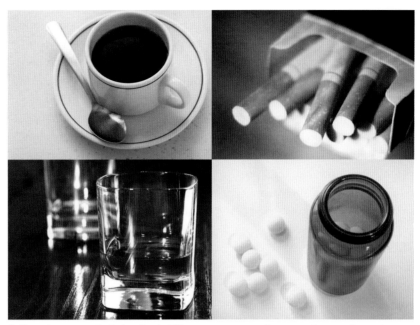

Coffee, cigarettes, alcohol and pain killers are common substances that people use in moderation, and at times, in excess. People with mental disorders such as depression and anxiety may be more susceptible to developing drug or alcohol abuse.

Prevention can, and should, begin as early as pre-school and continue through secondary school by focusing on such risk factors as aggressive behaviour, poor social skills and academic difficulties. Programmes are designed to improve skills such as self-control and to develop emotional awareness, communication skills and social problem-solving, and provide academic support, especially in reading. Prevention programmes can be presented in schools, clubs, faith-based organizations and through the media.

Peer pressure becomes a major factor by secondary school, and there are programmes that can reinforce anti-drug attitudes, teach drug-resistance skills, and strengthen personal commitment against drug abuse. Interactive techniques, such as peer discussion groups and parent role-playing, are effective in teaching children

about substance abuse and reinforcing drug-resistance skills.

DIAGNOSIS

When alcohol or another substance interferes with relationships and work, it is a problem.

A man who drinks five or more drinks a day, or 15 or more a week, or a woman who drinks four or more a day, or 12 or more a week, or anyone who drinks five or more drinks at one time at least once a week is at risk for alcoholism. One drink equals 4.5 cl (1½ oz) of liquor, a 15 cl (5 oz) glass of wine, or a 35.5 cl (12 oz) bottle of beer.

Alcohol is measured by units in the United Kingdom. Men are advised not to drink more than three to four units a day, women two to three. A unit equals 0.3 oz (10 ml) of pure alcohol – or one single pub measure of liquor, one small glass of wine, or a half-pint of regular-strength beer.

Different blood and laboratory tests can check for the presence of drugs or alcohol in the body, but cannot determine if the person is addicted. That diagnosis is based on symptoms of drug use. Other tests, such as liver function, complete blood count and serum magnesium, uric acid, total protein and folate can show damage from excessive drinking.

TREATMENTS

Treatment for alcoholism and drug addiction often requires a combination of behavioural therapies and medication. If physical withdrawal occurs, those symptoms must be treated first. The longer the treatment programme, the more chance of success; people who have spent three months or longer in a treatment programme have a higher success rate.

• **DETOXIFICATION** Suddenly quitting alcohol and some drugs, such as heroin, can cause physical withdrawal symptoms, so a process of detoxification, often in a hospital or other supervised setting, must be done. Delirium tremens (DTs) in alcohol withdrawal can be fatal without treatment.

• **MEDICATION** There are several medications that can help reduce the symptoms of withdrawal, suppress the craving for the drug and block the effects.

Disulfiram encourages abstinence by causing unpleasant side-effects if any alcohol is ingested. Naltrexone decreases the cravings for alcohol. It is sometimes also used to treat heroin addiction. Methadone, a narcotic itself, reduces the craving for other, more harmful narcotics such as heroin, and prevents withdrawal symptoms. The dose of methadone or other substitutes, such as LAAM, is gradually reduced, although some people may have to take a maintenance dose of methadone for months or even years.

Unfortunately, there is no medication available for treating addiction to many of the other popular street drugs, including cocaine and ecstasy. However, medication can be used to treat seizures and psychotic reactions that sometimes result from these drugs.

• **PSYCHOTHERAPY** There are several different types of behavioural therapies that are used to help patients abstain from alcohol or drug use. Cognitive behavioural relapse prevention teaches patients different ways to think and act in order to avoid drug use. Contingency management uses a system of rewards and punishments to make abstinence more attractive than drug use.

• **EDUCATION AND JOB REHABILITATION** Job skills are important so that the patient can find work and not return to old habits.

• **RESIDENTIAL TREATMENT PROGRAMMES** Some patients may find a programme in which they stay full-time for weeks or months to be most effective.

• **TWELVE-STEP PROGRAMMES** Alcoholics Anonymous (AA) is one of several support groups, and it has been very successful in treating recovering alcoholics by offering emotional support and encouraging abstinence. There are other groups available to provide support for family members.

• **THIAMIN** Also known as vitamin B1, thiamin is helpful in acute alcohol withdrawal. Thiamin supplements can be taken orally; but injections are more effective for the symptoms of alcohol withdrawal.

See also: *HIV/AIDS, pp.316–17 • High Blood Pressure, pp. 236–9 • Stroke, pp.168–9*

healing hope

My dad came home from work every day and had a few beers. He never seemed drunk, but now I wonder if he was ever really sober.

So having a few beers or a few shots of whisky didn't seem like a big deal to me. Except when I started drinking, I had trouble stopping.

Figuring out I was an alcoholic didn't happen overnight. My wife left me. My boss fired me for coming into work hung over. That's when my mum sat down and told me things about my dad I'd never realized. He was dead by then – from liver problems.

I went into a treatment centre. Going through detox was miserable. They gave me vitamin injections and made me eat right. I saw a counsellor every day. But I didn't believe I was an alcoholic. Sure, maybe I'd had a problem with alcohol, but I could drink in moderation. Well, no I couldn't. I can't have just one beer. AA helped me realize I had to stay off booze – and I haven't had a drink for over three years.

Jake G.

Phobias

Up to 10 percent of people suffer from phobias, the excessive or irrational fear of an object, situation, activity or animal that will not cause harm in most cases. Phobia is the most common of not only all anxiety disorders (pp.354–5), but of all psychiatric disorders as well.

Flying, bodies of water, dental visits – all of these can cause phobias. Women are twice as likely as men to suffer from these specific, or simple, phobias. Social anxiety disorder results in overwhelming anxiety and self-consciousness in social situations, such as public speaking, meeting new people or even using public toilets. Men and women are affected equally.

CAUSES

A parent's phobia may be passed on to children as learned behaviour. Sometimes a bad experience, such as a dog bite, may lead to a phobia. Phobias often appear during childhood or adolescence. Overprotective parents or limited opportunities for social interactions may contribute to the development of social phobia.

PREVENTION

Practising relaxation techniques such as deep breathing, muscle relaxation (pp.474–5) and yoga (pp.476–9) may help prevent symptoms from escalating. Do not rely on alcohol or illegal drugs for relief. Reduce the intake of caffeine and stimulants found in over-the-counter preparations.

DIAGNOSIS

Diagnosis is based on symptoms, their frequency and triggers. Phobias often cause physical symptoms such as difficulty breathing, elevated blood pressure, rapid heart rate and sweaty palms. A physical examination can rule out any physical causes. Phobias may accompany depression, eating disorders, substance abuse or another anxiety disorder.

TREATMENTS

Treatment is necessary only when phobias are disabling and disrupt work and relationships.

- MEDICATION Although medication does not treat phobias, it can lessen the symptoms for as long as it is used. Beta-blockers, which are used for heart disease, block the effects of epinephrine, or adrenaline, reducing the physical symptoms. Antidepressants can reduce anxiety; most commonly prescribed are the selective serotonin reuptake inhibitors. Benzodiazepines also reduce anxiety, but can lead to addiction and must be tapered off when discontinued. They should be avoided in patients with a history of alcohol or other drug abuse.

- PSYCHOTHERAPY Cognitive therapy changes thinking patterns that in turn change emotional reactions to feared situations. Behavioural therapy works to change specific behaviours with techniques such as relaxation training or exposure. Exposure therapy carefully uses repeated imaginings of the phobia in a safe environment to help the patient gain control of the fear. Preliminary studies of newer approaches to exposure therapy involving computer- generated virtual reality experiences show promise. Desensitization uses a gradual approach to facing the phobia.

- GROUP THERAPY Patients discuss their shared phobias and sometimes engage in role playing to help reduce the phobia.

- EMDR This technique (pp.372–3) reduces anxiety associated with fear of dental visits due to a past traumatic experience.

- HYPNOTHERAPY Hypnosis (pp.508–13) can reduce anxiety, especially that suffered before a medical or dental procedure. No reliable studies have compared hypnosis to other interventions.

See also: Anxiety Disorders, pp.354–5 • EMDR, pp.372–3 • Hypnosis, pp.508–13

Attention Deficit Disorder

Many children are active. They say and do impulsive things and have trouble concentrating. When those characteristics are severe and affect a child's schoolwork and social life, they are part of a group of chronic conditions known as attention-deficit hyperactivity disorder (ADHD), attention-deficit disorder (ADD), or hyperkinetic disorder.

ADHD has been a controversial diagnosis around the world. However, it is now recognized by such organizations as the World Health Organization, the Royal College of Psychiatrists and the American Psychiatric Association.

It is also recognized that ADHD persists into adulthood in somewhere between one-third and two-thirds of children with the disorder. Estimates vary widely as to how many people have ADHD – anywhere from 3 to 7 percent of school-age children and 2 to 4 percent of adults.

CAUSES

No one knows the cause, but a number of studies show that ADHD runs in families. Boys are more likely to have it than girls. It is not caused by bad parenting, although certain parenting styles may make it better or worse.

Low birth weight, prenatal maternal smoking or drug abuse, and other prenatal problems have been linked to ADHD.

Researchers have found that the neurotransmitters – the chemicals that carry signals within the brain – behave differently in children

with ADHD. Why this occurs is still a mystery.

The Royal College of Psychiatrists in the United Kingdom say that there is some evidence that diet affects children, while United States sources adamantly deny the role of sugar and food additives.

PREVENTION

Although ADHD may not be preventable, proper treatment of ADHD can help prevent problems with school and social relationships. Do not smoke or abuse alcohol or drugs during pregnancy, and get good prenatal care.

DIAGNOSIS

No test exists that can diagnose ADHD, so diagnosis can be difficult. It is based on symptoms and the exclusion of other conditions that could cause similar problems.

A physical evaluation, including hearing and vision assessments, is critical. Doctors may do blood tests, brain imaging studies such as CAT scans and MRIs, or an electro-encephalogram (EEG). However, these cannot diagnose ADHD;

> ### WHO IS AT RISK?
> **The risk factors include:**
> - Boys
> - Trauma during birth
> - Expectant mothers who use drugs
> - Family history

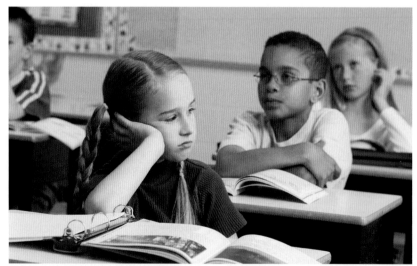
Children who have attention deficit hyperactivity disorder suffer from inattentiveness, are often easily distracted, and have difficulty paying attention to school work and completing homework on time.

they can, however, rule out other conditions, such as thyroid problems (pp.344–7). In as many as two-thirds of cases, other problems, such as depression (pp.368–9), anxiety (pp.354–5), sleep disorders (pp.170–2) and learning disabilities, may co-exist with ADHD.

Diagnosis is not usually made until after the age of six or seven, because many young children may show some of the symptoms. Information should be collected from parents, teachers and other carers. Symptoms must occur in more than one setting, be more severe than in other children, have started before the age of seven, last more than six months, and interfere with functioning at school, home or in social situations.

• INATTENTIVENESS A child who has ADHD with inattentiveness (ADD) will have six or more of the following symptoms: difficulty following instructions, difficulty paying attention, often loses things, looks like they are not listening, does not pay close attention to details, seems disorganized, has trouble planning ahead, forgets things and is easily distracted.

• HYPERACTIVITY/IMPULSIVITY A child with ADHD and hyperactivity/impulsivity will have six or more of the following symptoms: fidgety, runs or climbs inappropriately, cannot play quietly, blurts out answers, interrupts people, cannot stay in a seat, talks too much, is always on the go and has trouble waiting his or her turn. There are some children who have both inattentiveness and hyperactivity/impulsivity.

• ADULT ADHD Adults who have ADHD usually are not hyperactive but suffer from mood swings, a quick temper, an inability to complete tasks, and are easily distracted. They may have trouble organizing things, listening to instructions, remembering details and controlling their behaviour.

Symptoms of ADHD do not suddenly appear in adulthood; they must have been present since childhood. Otherwise, conditions such as depression, anxiety, thyroid or other hormonal problems, alcoholism, drug use, exposure to toxins or side-effects of prescription or herbal medicines may be to blame.

TREATMENTS

Treatment should take a multifaceted approach.

• MEDICATION Children and adults may benefit from treatment with psychostimulants such as methylphenidate, dextroamphetamine or pemolines. These drugs cannot cure ADHD, but may control many of the symptoms. Atomoxetine, a new nonstimulant medication, may also work. Some antidepressants and antihypertensives may also control symptoms.

• BEHAVIOURAL INTERVENTIONS Children with ADHD need consistent parenting strategies and positive reinforcement. Children, especially older ones and teenagers, should be involved in planning treatment. Children and adults need problem-solving, communication and self-advocacy skills to cope with the symptoms of ADHD. Individual and family counselling as well as support groups offer other coping strategies and build self-esteem.

On Call

Strategies for parenting a child with ADHD:

- Make a schedule for all daily activities
- Write down rules and their consequences
- Reward good behaviour
- Supervise children at all times
- Set a homework routine and reduce distractions like TV
- Focus on effort, not grades
- Communicate regularly with your child's teachers.

• SCHOOL SUPPORT Most children with ADHD can be taught with other students in the regular classroom. Some may need more positive reinforcement or special education services, especially if they have learning disabilities.

• OTHER STRATEGIES Sufferers of ADHD should have a structured environment and use organizational tools such as planners.

• HOMEOPATHY A study published in the *European Journal of Paediatrics* in 2005 found that a homeopathic remedy had positive effects in children with ADHD.

• OMEGA-3 FATTY ACIDS A Oxford University study published in *Paediatrics* in 2005 found that children with coordination disorders and problems with school performance had improved concentration and behaviour when given a mixture of omega-3 and omega-6 fatty acids.

See also: *Thyroid Problems, pp.344–7 • Pregnancy, pp.398–400 • Smoking Cessation, pp.216–17 • Omega-3 Fatty Acids, pp.252–3*

DEPRESSION

Depression goes beyond feelings of sadness or suffering from 'the blues'. It is among the leading causes of disability in the world and affects 121 million people globally. Some 850,000 people a year commit suicide, often due to depression. It can impact on physical health in other ways, and it can affect everyone from children to the elderly.

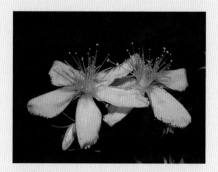

St John's Wort, a botanical therapy, has been used for centuries to calm nerves. Now, it is widely prescribed in Europe for mild to moderate depression.

CAUSES

Although the exact cause of depression is unknown, it is believed to be due to changes in brain function triggered by stressful events such as the death of a loved one, serious illness or job loss. A number of people may have a hereditary tendency to become depressed in the face of such events. Low self-esteem, a pessimistic attitude, difficulty dealing with stress and continuous exposure to violence, neglect or poverty may increase a person's risk for depression. Some medical conditions, such as a brain tumour (pp.196–7), hypothyroidism (pp.344–7), or a deficiency in vitamins (pp.532–41) such as folate can cause depression.

PREVENTION

No one should feel guilty for suffering from depression; sometimes it cannot be prevented. In general, the following healthy habits boost prevention: eating a balanced diet rich in fruit, vegetables and omega-3 fatty acids, getting enough sleep, exercising regularly, finding ways to relax, limiting alcohol consumption and not using drugs.

Counselling can also help prevent depression, teaching new ways to handle stressful events such as grief, stress or chronic disease. Social connection is particularly important when feeling isolated or lonely, especially for the elderly; volunteer or group activities can be quite helpful.

DIAGNOSIS

There is no medical test to diagnose depression. Major depression is indicated by at least two weeks of persistent sadness and/or loss of interest or pleasure in things that brought enjoyment. In addition, three to four of the symptoms below must be present:

- Feelings of hopelessness or helplessness
- Feelings of guilt or worthlessness
- Fatigue or lack of energy
- Difficulty concentrating, remembering, or making decisions
- Insomnia, early morning wakefulness
- Dramatic change in appetite, often with significant weight gain or loss
- Thoughts of death or the belief that one would be better off dead
- Restlessness, agitation
- Persistent physical symptoms, such as headaches, digestive upsets and chronic pain, that do not improve with treatment.

Dysthymia is considered a chronic but milder form of depression that lasts longer, usually as long as two years. Psychotic depression has unusual symptoms such as hallucinations or delusions.

Depression in children may be difficult to diagnose. Younger children may pretend to be sick or worry that a parent will die; older children may sulk or get into trouble at school. Symptoms in the elderly may mimic those of dementia (pp.178–9).

Depression may accompany serious illness, such as Parkinson's disease (p.181) or heart disease (pp.230–3), and slow down the amount of time it takes to recover. Men may mask their depression with alcohol or overwork. Women are more likely to suffer from depression and blame it on hormones. Post-natal depression lasting three weeks or longer occurs in about 10 percent of women after giving birth. Seasonal affective disorder, or SAD, is a type of depression that affects people during the winter months.

TREATMENTS

Antidepressants and psychotherapy can successfully treat 60 to 80 percent of those suffering from depression. Medication and psychotherapy are equally effective in the short term. Psychotherapy appears more effective in the long run.

• **PSYCHOTHERAPY** Cognitive-behavioural therapy teaches ways to fight negative thoughts and is considered the most effective non-medical treatment for depression.

• **EXERCISE** Regular exercise improves symptoms of depression. The positive effects of exercise also promote feelings of well-being and can help prevent subsequent depressive episodes from occurring.

• **MEDICATION** Several different types of antidepressants are available; it may be necessary to try different ones until finding what works best. They all require weeks to months produce a therapeutic effect. Some are safe for breast-feeding mothers with post-natal depression. Selective serotonin re-uptake inhibitors (SSRIs) have fewer side-effects than tricyclic antidepressants. Less frequently used are MAOIs, which require avoidance of foods with high levels of tyramine, such as many cheeses, wines and medications such as decongestants. Other medication, such as antianxiety drugs, sedatives, lithium, thyroid supplements and antipsychotics may also be needed.

• **SUPPLEMENTS** Make sure your diet includes omega-3 fatty acids (pp.252–3) from fish like tuna, salmon or mackerel, and take 400 to 800 mcg folate (vitamin B_9) in a multivitamin.

• **ST JOHN'S WORT** This herb (p.554) is widely prescribed for depression in Europe and has been shown in studies there to be useful for mild to moderate depression. It has few side-effects, though it can sometimes cause dry mouth and increased sensitivity to sunlight. It reduces the efficacy of birth-

CAUTION

Some antidepressants may increase the risk of suicidal tendencies in children. Get help immediately if you feel like harming yourself or others.

control pills and can also reduce the efficacy of HIV drugs, chemotherapy and anti-rejection medication. Talk to a doctor before using St John's wort. The usual starting dose is 300 mg of a product with 0.3 percent hypericin extract three times a day. Safety for children has not been proven.

• **LIGHT THERAPY** Thirty minutes of daily exposure to full spectrum lighting (p.564) may help reduce symptoms of seasonal affective disorder (SAD).

• **YOGA** Studies show promising results in both adults and children with using yoga (pp.476–9) to treat depression.

• **ELECTROCONVULSIVE THERAPY (ECT)** Electric shock therapy may work for the severely depressed or suicidal people who have not responded to other treatments.

• **TRANSCRANIAL MAGNETIC STIMULATION (TMS)** This treatment is similar to ECT, but with fewer side-effects, and is being evaluated by researchers for its effectiveness.

• **MUSIC THERAPY** This therapy (p.565) may increase the effectiveness of antidepressants and works especially well the elderly.

• **ART THERAPY** Creating art as a means of self-expression may be effective for suicidal teenagers.

Symptoms of depression can include a loss of energy and feeling tired despite lack of activity, and changes in sleeping patterns, such as difficulty sleeping, early morning awakening or sleeping too much.

See also: *Light Therapy, p.564* • *Yoga, pp.476–9* • *Art Therapy, pp.491–3*

Eating Disorders

Eating disorders have made headlines in recent years as celebrities have confessed to suffering from anorexia nervosa or bulimia, or sometimes even both. These conditions are medical illnesses that require treatment. Without, other health problems may develop, and consequences may be fatal.

WHO IS AT RISK?

The risk factors include:

- Family history
- Emotional insecurity
- High-performance athletes
- Models and dancers

CAUSES

The causes of eating disorders are not known, but society's attitudes toward appearance and family factors are thought to contribute, creating an obsession with thinness and an intense fear of being fat. Girls and women are ten times more likely than boys and men to suffer from an eating disorder, although the number of boys diagnosed is on the increase. It usually begins during the teenage or early adult years, but can occur later.

Body-building, wrestling, dancing, swimming, gymnastics and other athletics may demand a low body weight, encouraging the development of eating disorders.

Low self-esteem and depression may be contributing factors. Eating disorders may be triggered by traumatic events such as a death or relationship break-up.

Weight-control through anorexia may also give young girls a feeling of control that may be missing elsewhere in their lives.

PREVENTION

Unless society's positive view of thinness changes, preventing eating disorders remains a difficult task. However, by recognizing the symptoms and getting early treatment, possible complications of anorexia and bulimia can be prevented. Those complications include loss of enamel from teeth, serious heart conditions, kidney failure and suicide.

DIAGNOSIS

People with anorexia will lose weight to the point of becoming dangerously thin. Those with bulimia often maintain a normal weight. Binge-eaters may even be overweight. Some people suffer from a mixture of eating disorders, or develop bulimia after having anorexia for several years. Other conditions that may be present include substance abuse (pp.358–60), depression (pp.364–5) and anxiety disorders (pp.354–5).

A diagnosis is made after a clinical and behavioural assessment. Tests may be done to check for damage from weight loss or purging, including urine and blood tests, thyroid function and ECG.

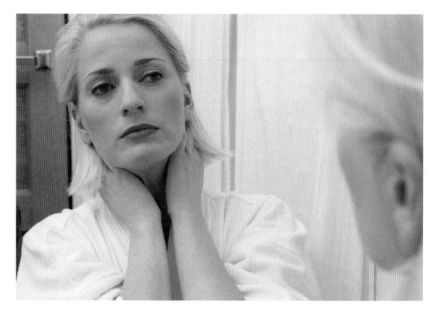

Girls and women with low self-esteem who have concerns over body image are at increased risk for developing eating disorders such as anorexia nervosa or bulimia that can impair the body's normal functioning and cause long-term health complications.

• **ANOREXIA NERVOSA** People with this disorder may literally starve themselves to thinness, as they fear they will get fat. About a third were overweight before dieting, but then cannot stop their efforts to lose weight. They mispercieve themselves as overweight, despite their extreme thinness. They eat less and less, while exercising more and more. Despite their dieting efforts, they are often preoccupied with food. Females often lose so much weight that their menstrual cycles are affected and they miss periods. The genitals of males may shrink back to pre-puberty size.

Patients will weigh less than 15 percent of the normal weight for their height. Symptoms include cessation of menstrual periods, thinning of the bones, brittle hair and nails, dry skin, anaemia, wasting of the muscles (including the heart muscle), severe constipation, low blood pressure, slowed breathing and pulse rates, feeling cold all the time, depression and lethargy.

• **BULIMIA** Rather than dieting to the point of starvation, people who suffer from bulimia get caught up in a cycle of 'binge and purge'. They eat huge amounts of food while feeling a loss of control, followed by intense guilt or self-disgust. In an effort to compensate, they then vomit, use laxatives, or excessive exercise – behaviours to rid the body of the excess calories.

CAUTION

Suicide is the most common cause of death in those with anorexia after complications of the disease itself.

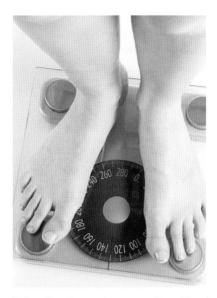

Eating disorders such as anorexia and bulimia are characterized by a preoccupation with weight that results in severe disturbances in eating and other behaviour.

Like those with anorexia, they have an obsessive fear of gaining weight and want to lose because of unhappiness with their appearance. It is most common in women who were overweight as children.

Symptoms include a constantly inflamed and sore throat, swollen salivary glands, puffy checks and face, erosion of tooth enamel from stomach acid, intestinal problems, GORD (pp.264–5), kidney problems, and severe dehydration. Laxative abuse may damage bowel muscles, making bowel movements impossible without laxatives.

• **BINGE-EATING** This disorder has not been approved as a formal diagnosis, although mounting evidence suggests it is a discrete diagnosis. It is basically what the name says: bingeing, or consuming huge quantities of food, while feeling unable to stop. A 'binge' is followed by feelings of shame and disgust. There is no purging, so sufferers usually gain weight. As

many as 30 percent of those who attend weight control programmes are thought to have this disorder.

TREATMENTS

Eating disorders often require a combination of treatments. In anorexia, it is critical to restore a healthy weight, and in severe cases, hospitalization may be needed to prevent death. The earlier treatment is started, the greater its chances for success.

• **HOSPITALIZATION** Intravenous feeding may be required to correct weight and malnutrition. The first step of treatment, especially for anorexics, involves getting weight back to a normal level.

• **NUTRITIONAL REHABILITATION** Counselling with a nutritionist can help establish new eating habits.

• **TALK THERAPY** Treatment for all eating disorders involves learning better ways to regulate emotion and tolerate distress. Cognitive-behavioural therapy, which examines thoughts and feelings in order to change distorted thought and behaviour patterns, is especially helpful for bulimics. If the eating disorder began after a trauma, treatment for the trauma may help resolve the eating disorder. Interpersonal therapy focuses on helping to rebuild supportive relationships. Sometimes it is helpful if family members participate in therapy.

• **MEDICATIONS** Certain SSRIs, a type of antidepressant, may relieve the mood and anxiety symptoms associated with anorexia.

See also: *Substance Abuse, pp.358–60 • Depression, pp.364–5 • Anxiety Disorders, pp.354–5 • GORD, pp.264–5*

Bipolar Disorder

Bipolar disorder is characterized by regular and abrupt mood swings from euphoric 'highs' or periods of intense irritability to severe 'lows'. Around one in 100 people suffer from the disorder, which affects men and women equally.

Bipolar disorder was previously called 'manic depression'. Two main types exist: people with bipolar I have experienced at least one fully manic episode with periods of major depression (pp.364–5). People with bipolar II also have periods of major depression, but without full-fledged mania. Instead, they have hypomania, a milder form of mania with increased energy and impulsiveness. Still milder is cyclothymic disorder, characterized by alternating periods of hypomania and mild, but not severe, depression.

CAUSES

Although the cause is unknown, there appears to be a genetic link: 80 to 90 percent of people with bipolar disorder have a family member with either depression or bipolar disorder.

Environmental factors like extreme stress, sleep disruption, and drug and alcohol abuse (pp.358–60) may trigger bipolar disorder in people who are vulnerable.

PREVENTION

There is no known way to prevent bipolar disorder, although it is likely that alcohol or drug abuse exacerbate symptoms.

DIAGNOSIS

Diagnosis is based on symptoms without other possible causes, both physical and mental. Bipolar II and cyclothymia are sometimes mistaken for depression and fail to receive adequate treatment.

The manic phase of bipolar disorder includes an elevated expansive or irritable mood, and can include racing thoughts, increased talkativeness, increased energy, inflated self-esteem, agitation, distractibility, decreased need for sleep or poor control of temper.

Reckless behaviour and impaired judgment may result in spending sprees, sexual promiscuity, binge eating (pp.366–7) and drinking, or drug use.

These manic phases can last for days, weeks or months. Sometimes mania co-exists simultaneously with depression in a type of bipolar episode called a 'mixed episode'.

Symptoms of depression include loss of interest or enjoyment in life, chronic unhappiness,

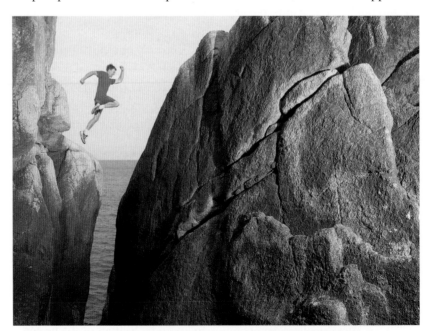

A manic phase of bipolar disorders may feel like a prolonged adrenaline rush that can last for days, weeks or months. In this state of increased energy, racing thoughts and euphoria, a person is more likely to engage in high-risk activities.

inability to concentrate, strong feelings of guilt or worthlessness and even thoughts of suicide. The most common physical symptoms include loss of appetite and weight change, trouble sleeping, fatigue or agitation and decreased libido.

Most individuals with bipolar I disorder return to full functioning between mood episodes.

Although unusual in children and teenagers, bipolar disorder can occur. However, the symptoms of mania are more likely to be irritability, aggressiveness and destructive tantrums, which may be confused with ADHD (pp.362–3), conduct disorder or oppositional defiant disorder.

To diagnose bipolar disorder, a mental healthcare provider will observe the person's behaviour and mood, take an individual and family medical history, ask about symptoms and talk to family members about the person's behaviour. Laboratory tests may be done to rule out other disorders. For example, thyroid disorders (pp.344–7) can cause changes in energy and mood, although it can also co-exist with bipolar disorder. Drug abuse may also cause some of the same symptoms as bipolar disorder, but it does not rule out the disorder because it can also be a symptom.

Other mental disorders can be present with bipolar disorder.

TREATMENTS

Bipolar disorder is a chronic illness that requires long-term medication treatment. Some patients stop taking their medication because their symptoms disappear or they miss

healing hope The symptoms of manic depression started when I was in my early 20s while I was working as a newspaper reporter. At first, I thought it was the adrenaline rush at meeting deadlines that was making me feel so euphoric.

Then the depression hit. I couldn't get out of bed. I thought of suicide but simply didn't have the energy to do it.

And then, without warning, I felt great again – the energy, the productivity, the creativity all came rushing back.

My mother got me to a doctor. She'd recognized the symptoms from her sister, who'd suffered from it and committed suicide years ago.

I'm on lithium for the rest of my life. But I'm calmer, and though I sometimes miss the highs, I don't miss those lows at all.   *Anne W.*

the euphoria of the manic phases. Because suicide occurs in 10 to 15 percent of those with bipolar disorder I, it is important to follow treatment plans.

• **MEDICATION** Mood-stabilizers such as lithium and anti-convulsants such as valproate and carbamazepine are often used to treat bipolar disorder. Blood tests are used to check the levels of lithium and, sometimes, that of the anti-convulsants. Newer anti-convulsant drugs such as lamotrigine, gabapentin, and topiramate are being prescribed. Although they require less monitoring, their effectiveness in bipolar disorders is still being studied. Antidepressants may be used for the depressive phase, but mood stabilizers are also given to prevent manic episodes once the depression is relieved. Antipsychotics may be prescribed for those with psychotic symptoms such as hallucinations and delusions. Anti-anxiety drugs such as the benzodiazepines may provide some relief.

• **HOSPITALIZATION** Hospitalization may be required for patients with severe symptoms until their moods are stabilized.

• **ELECTROCONVULSIVE THERAPY (ECT)** An electrical current is used to trigger a brief seizure while the patient is under anaesthesia in a hospital. It can relieve severe depression that does not respond to medication, but can cause temporary memory loss and confusion.

• **PSYCHOTHERAPY** Cognitive-behavioural therapy teaches the patient how to change negative or inappropriate thought patterns and behaviour. Psychoeducation teaches patients and family members about the illness, its signs and its treatments. Family therapy involves all family members so that stressful behaviour is reduced and coping strategies implemented. Interpersonal and social rhythm therapy aims to create regular daily routines and sleep schedules, improving interpersonal relationships and preventing manic episodes. Support groups can provide education and coping strategies.

• **SLEEP** Getting enough sleep can help patients keep stable.

See also: *Depression, pp.364–5 • Attention-Deficit Disorder, pp.362–3 • Substance Addiction, pp.358–60*

Autism

Autism refers to an entire spectrum of disorders that typically appear by the age of 3 and impact on social and communication skills. Symptoms can range from so severe that institutionalization is required to so mild that the child can be mainstreamed in school and live a near-normal life. Asperger's syndrome may be a mild form of autism; it is sometimes referred to as high-functioning autism.

WHO IS AT RISK?

The risk factors include:

- Family history
- Male

CAUSES

Scientists do not yet understand what, exactly, causes autism, but they suspect that genetics and environment are responsible. Irregularities in some areas of the brain have been discovered in people with autism. Some have abnormal levels of the neuro-transmitter serotonin.

Some cases of Asperger's syndrome have been reported after the mother was exposed to a viral infection during pregnancy. Bad

parenting does not cause autism.

PREVENTION

No known method of preventing autism exists, although good pre-natal care may prevent some cases of Asperger's.

DIAGNOSIS

Symptoms are mostly related to difficulty with social interactions and language, and typically fall into four categories: problems with verbal and non-verbal communi-cation, social interactions, pretend play and responses to sensory in-formation. Communication prob-lems include the inability to have a conversation, use of nonsense rhyming, a lack of language devel-opment, and referring to self with name instead of 'I'. In the realm of social interactions, children may be unable to make eye contact or to form friendships. Sensory infor-mation may be poorly processed, with a heightened or lowered sense of sight, hearing, touch, smell or taste. Children would rather play alone and do not engage in pretend play. Aggressive behaviour, towards others or self, may occur,

along with rhythmic movements. In some cases, development is normal until age 18 months or two years and then regressive behaviour occurs.

Three to four times as many boys as girls are diagnosed with autistic disorders, and an estimated one in 1,000 children suffer from an autistic disorder. The incidence is on the rise, but whether it is due to an actual increase in the num-ber of cases or to better diagnosis and the broadening of the defini-tion of the disorder is unknown.

Asperger's Syndrome

Children with Asperger's syn-drome have severe and sustained impairment in social interaction; they fail to understand nonverbal communication or to develop relationships. They have repetitive patterns of movement or behav-iours such as hand-flapping, or they have nonfunctional routines. However, many children with Asperger's have above-normal or even high intelligence and do not experience the language delays common to autism.

Several other disorders can produce behaviour that mim-ics that of autism. These include

On Call

An increase in the incidence of autism was reported since the MMR vaccine (pp.314–15) was introduced, but several major studies have found absolutely no link between the two. The Cochrane Library in Oxford, England, reviewed 31 studies and found no relationship be-tween MMR and autism. Both the United States Centers for Disease Control and the Ameri-can Academy of Pediatrics also say there is no connection.

mental retardation, metabolic degenerative central nervous system disorders and schizophrenia (pp.374–5). Almost one-third of children with autism will develop epilepsy by adulthood. About 6 percent will also have, in addition to autism, tuberous sclerosis, a little over 2 percent also have fragile X syndrome, and about 25 percent suffer from mental retardation.

No physical test exists to diagnose any of the autistic disorders. The decision is made based upon observation of the child in multiple settings, clinical interview of the parents and various questionnaires. The European company IntegraGen has announced it is developing a genetic test that could diagnose the risk of developing autism before symptoms appear. Research validating such a test has yet to be presented.

TREATMENTS

Although there is no cure for autism, treatment can reduce disruptive behaviour, improve sensory integration and other symptoms, and develop routines that are as functional as possible. A combination of treatments is usually needed, and may be required for life, although some children do grow up to lead normal or near-normal lives. More research is needed to identify better treatments.

CAUTION

Autism may lead parents to desperate measures: a five-year-old boy reportedly died after receiving chelation treatment (pp.576–7) for autism.

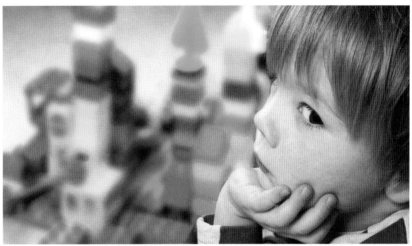

Children with Asperger's syndrome, a mild form of autism, do not understand nonverbal communication and have trouble developing relationships or engaging in social interactions. They prefer to play alone.

• **BEHAVIOUR MANAGEMENT THERAPY** Early intervention is extremely important. Two types of behaviour modification are commonly used: applied behaviour analysis (ABA) uses repetition of simple elements of behaviour followed by individualized rewards to increase functional behaviour. TEACCH, developed in North Carolina, uses picture schedules and other visual cues to compensate for deficits common to autism.

Whatever method is used, behaviour modification often relies on highly structured sessions done one-on-one with a therapist and requires involvement by parents, carers and teachers.

• **MEDICATION** There is no cure for autism, but medication can treat some of the symptoms. SSRI antidepressants may reduce the frequency and intensity of repetitive behaviour and decrease irritability and aggressive behaviour. In some cases, tricyclic antidepressants work better. Antipsychotics may decrease hyperactivity, withdrawal and aggression. Stimulants can

treat hyperactivity. Anti-anxiety medication is sometimes used to reduce anxiety and panic attacks.

• **OTHER THERAPIES** Small studies show that music therapy (p.565), provided by a trained professional, may help improve communication skills and expression of feelings, but may not impact behaviour. Occupational therapy can teach skills such as fastening buttons; physical therapy improves movement and coordination, and speech therapy helps with language skills. There are many other therapies that have not been tested scientifically.

• **DIET** Abnormal levels of peptides from gluten and casein have been found in the urine and cerebrospinal fluid of some people with autism. A study of 20 participants showed that a diet free of gluten and casein improved behaviour, and cognitive and social function. Gluten is found in foods with wheat, rye and barley; casein is in dairy products such as milk and cheese.

See also: Sound Therapy, p.565 • Schizophrenia, pp.374–5

EMDR

Eye movement desensitization and reprocessing, or EMDR, is a fairly new but controversial treatment for post-traumatic stress disorder (PTSD). It combines elements of cognitive, behavioural, psychodynamic and client-centred therapies, while adding a technique of eye movements, similar to the spontaneous eye movements of REM sleep, to alternate the patient's attention between statements associated with the trauma and these rhythmic eye movements.

Some researchers believe it is the alternation of attention that may somehow help the mind process the information from past traumatic events. Others argue that the effectiveness of EMDR results from its components found in other therapies, and that the eye movements offer nothing new. Regardless of the way it works, a number of randomized clinical trials suggest that it does work.

HISTORY

In 1987, Dr Francine Shapiro, then a PhD candidate in psychology at a California school, developed the technique of EMDR by chance. She discovered, while walking in a park, that rapidly moving her eyes back and forth reduced the intensity of negative thoughts. She then studied the effects of EMDR on treating the symptoms of post-traumatic stress disorder, basing her doctoral dissertation on that research. She is now a senior research fellow at the Mental Research Institute in California and executive director of the EMDR Institute in Pacific Grove, California. She has written three

books and more than 50 articles and book chapters on EMDR. In 2002, she received the Sigmund Freud award from the World Council for Psychotherapy.

PRACTICE

Some media reports have over-simplified EMDR to make it sound like nothing more than moving the eyes back and forth while recounting unpleasant memories. However, a standard EMDR treatment consists of eight phases that use specific

psychotherapeutic procedures. If those steps are not conducted by a trained professional, the process of recalling traumatic memories may cause additional harm.

EMDR should be performed by a psychiatrist, psychologist or licensed psychotherapist certified in EMDR. The EMDR Association in the United States and the European EMDR Association have established strict criteria for the certification process of a clinician. Training is offered by the EMDR associations and in several university-based programmes around the world.

EMDR is used to treat the consequences of psychologically or emotionally traumatic events. It has been studied most extensively for the treatment of non-combat-related post-traumatic stress disorder (PTSD) – for example, women who have suffered from sexual assault, which is not

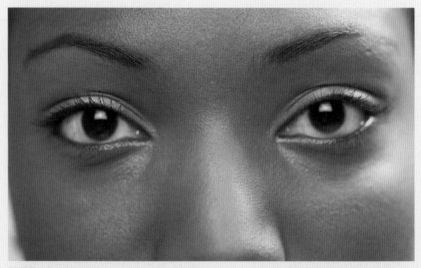

EMDR, a treatment approach used to treat the consequences of traumatic events, was developed by Dr Francine Shapiro, who by chance discovered that rapidly moving the eyes back and forth reduces the intensity of negative thoughts.

uncommon. In fact, some 8 to 15 percent of people will suffer from PTSD (pp.356–7) at some point in their lifetime and it is considered difficult to treat. Although some practitioners suggest EMDR may be useful for other psychological disorders as well, there is insufficient evidence at this time.

Since EMDR was first used, studies have shown that hand taps or sounds were as effective as the eye movements.

TREATMENTS

Each patient, and each EMDR session, will be unique, but eight steps should be followed.

• STEP 1: The therapist takes a thorough history of the patient to discover the problem and its negative behaviour and symptoms, leading to the development of a treatment plan. EMDR differs from other therapies in that specific details of the disturbing memory are not necessary to formulate treatment.

• STEP 2: The patient learns specific relaxation and self-calming techniques for dealing with any disturbing memories that will occur during therapy sessions.

• STEP 3: During the assessment phase, the patient chooses a picture or scene from the traumatic event identified earlier and then makes a statement expressing a negative self-belief associated with that event. Then the patient finds a positive self-statement to substitute. Emotions and physical sensations associated with the memory are brought out as well.

The next steps deal with reprocessing. It may only take three ses-

sions if a single event is responsible for the PTSD. Eye movements or other rhythmic taps or tones are used during these phases.

• STEP 4: Desensitization focuses on the emotions and sensations the patient associates with the traumatic memory. Additional events are frequently recalled during this time.

• STEP 5: Installation increases the strength of the positive belief that has come to replace the original negative belief.

• STEP 6: Body scan involves clearing any remaining physical responses, such as tension and headache, that are associated with the original disturbing memory.

• STEP 7: Closure ends each session with self-calming techniques and a briefing on what to expect between sessions. The use of a diary and other techniques are also discussed.

• STEP 8: Each new session begins with re-evaluation of results from the previous session, as well as identifying new areas to treat.

During each step, scales and other rating tools that are widely accepted in the counselling field are used to measure the patient's stress levels and feelings toward the traumatic event.

Does It Work?

EMDR has been studied more than any other treatment for civilian PTSD, but experts from several universities, including Harvard, still disagree on its efficacy. There have been numerous randomized clinical trials that have demonstrated some efficacy, with few trials finding negative

results. However, both sides have criticized the other for publishing research with flawed methodology – for setting up non-blind studies where the researchers actually know which subjects are receiving which treatments, for designing studies so that comparisons of EMDR with groups receiving no treatment take advantage of the placebo effect, and for failing to follow strict treatment protocols which results in the reduced efficacy of EMDR.

The American Psychiatric Association recognized in its 2004 practice guidelines for PTSD that EMDR may be as effective as other treatments, but called for more research. The United States Department of Veterans Affairs also issued clinical practice guidelines in 2004 that say EMDR is an effective treatment for PTSD. Frustrating some researchers is the mystery of the mechanism involved in EMDR, which may be the focus of the next round of research.

Next Steps

The challenge is to find a therapist trained in EMDR, as well as other techniques, who will be able to judge whether EMDR is appropriate and will be willing to recommend another treatment if EMDR does not work for a particular condition. EMDR usually takes fewer treatments to get results than cognitive-behavioural or exposure therapies, and most of the treatment can be done during the therapy visits.

See also: *Post-Traumatic Stress Disorder, pp.356–7*

Schizophrenia

Schizophrenia is a severe and chronic mental illness that affects one percent of the population – around 24 million people in the world. People with schizophrenia have psychotic episodes during which they lose contact with reality and suffer from delusions and hallucinations.

The behaviour responses of schizophrenics are difficult to understand, and they often cannot think logically. They do not suffer either from a 'split' personality or from multiple personalities.

CAUSES

The exact cause is unknown, but hereditary and environmental factors are involved. Anyone with a parent or sibling with schizophrenia has a 10 percent chance of developing the disease, and an identical twin of a schizophrenia patient has a 50 percent chance.

Contributing to the risk are problems during pregnancy, such as influenza or other viral infection in the second trimester, mother–baby blood type incompatibility, oxygen deprivation at birth or low birth weight.

The use of alcohol and street drugs, including ecstasy, LSD, amphetamines, crack and marijuana, may trigger schizophrenia. What is not fully understood is whether such drugs bring on schizophrenia in people already vulnerable to the disease, or whether these drugs cause the same risk of development in everyone. It is known that alcohol and other drugs can worsen psychotic symptoms in those with schizophrenia. Stress – as it does with many other ailments – can worsen symptoms. Childhood abuse may also increase the risk.

PREVENTION

There is no known way to prevent schizophrenia, although good prenatal care for pregnant women may help. To prevent psychotic episodes and other symptoms, it is important to get treatment and avoid alcohol and street drugs.

DIAGNOSIS

The symptoms of schizophrenia may appear suddenly or develop gradually over years, but they often begin between the ages of 15 and 35. The average age for onset is 18 for men and 25 for women. It is unusual for the disease to start in childhood or late in life.

CAUTION

Do not stop taking an antipsychotic drug without talking to your doctor first. It is important to taper off gradually under the supervision of a doctor. Stopping the medication suddenly can make symptoms worse and also have severe consequences.

WHO IS AT RISK?

The risk factors include:
- Family history
- Low birth weight
- Abuse of alcohol, marijuana and other street drugs

Symptoms must be present for at least six months and cause problems with work, school or social functioning. However, some people may suffer from just one or a few of the symptoms. Five different types of schizophrenia have been identified.

The symptoms of schizophrenia are often described as positive, negative and cognitive symptoms.

- **POSITIVE SYMPTOMS** These are the most common in schizophrenia, although they can occur in other mental illnesses. They include visual hallucinations, hearing voices, delusions, muddled thinking or thought disorder, feelings of being controlled and bizarre behaviour.
- **NEGATIVE SYMPTOMS** These are usually harder to recognize. They include emotional flatness, lack of pleasure or interest in life, difficulty communicating, and discomfort around others.
- **COGNITIVE SYMPTOMS** Schizophrenics have difficulty concentrating and remembering, organizing, planning and problem-solving.

Depression (pp.364–5) is apparent before treatment in around half of people suffering

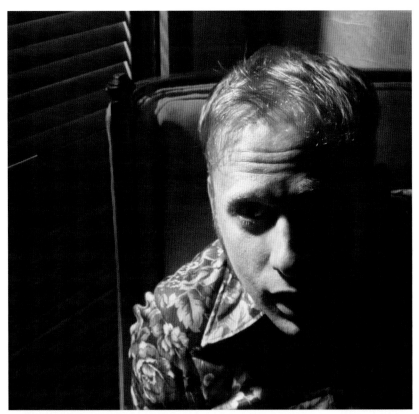

Negative symptoms of schizophrenia reflect a loss of normal function and can include social isolation, lack of emotion and inappropriate social skills.

from schizophrenia. In those with continuing symptoms, depression occurs in one out of every seven.

No test exists to diagnose schizophrenia, so other causes – both physical diseases and mental disorders – must be ruled out. Laboratory tests as well as CT or MRI scans may be done. Although schizophrenia does cause brain abnormalities which may show up on CT or MRI scans, they are not sufficient for a diagnosis.

TREATMENTS

Treatment for schizophrenia, which includes both medication and psychological interventions, is more effective the earlier it is started. One in five people with schizophrenia will resume functioning reasonably well, but 10 percent will commit suicide.

• HOSPITALIZATION In some cases, symptoms are severe enough to warrant hospitalization until the patient is stabilized on medication.

• MEDICATION Antipsychotics cannot cure schizophrenia, but they can keep symptoms like delusions and hallucinations under control. The 'typical' antipsychotics, developed in the mid-1950s, reduce the action of a neurotransmitter, dopamine, in the brain. Although effective, they may cause side-effects such as Parkinson's disease-like symptoms, uncomfortable restlessness, sex life disorders and tardive dyskinesia (TD), which are persistent involuntary movements, usually of the mouth and tongue.

Newer antipsychotics, developed in the 1990s and later, are referred to as 'atypical'. They affect other neurotransmitters, such as serotonin, and are less likely to cause the Parkinsonian side-effects although they may result in weight gain, problems with sexual function, type 2 diabetes (pp.338–41), and cardiovascular problems. They also have more effect on 'negative' symptoms than the typical antipsychotics.

It may take multiple trials to find the drug that provides the best symptom control and fewest side effects for each patient.

• TALK THERAPY Individual talk therapy can be used to help patients identify and work out problems in daily living. In addition, counselling can provide support in the process.

• FAMILY COUNSELLING These sessions help all family members understand better and cope with the patient who has schizophrenia and reduce emotional triggers that bring on symptoms.

• OCCUPATIONAL THERAPY Occupational therapists can help with identifying and improving skills and assist in the return to work.

• RELAXATION TECHNIQUES Learning ways to handle stress can help prevent symptoms.

• YOGA Good evidence suggests that yoga (pp.476–9), particularly Kundalini meditation (p.478) and relaxation can be useful in the management of schizophrenia.

• MUSIC THERAPY Music therapy (p.565), in addition to other treatments, may help improve the functioning of patients.

See also: *Substance Abuse, pp.358–60* • *Yoga, pp.476–9* • *Sound Therapy, p.565*

Personality Disorders

Each individual's personality is defined by certain traits and characteristics. But when these behaviour patterns become inflexible and long-lasting, interfering with relationships and work, they are known as personality disorders.

The severity varies, and some of the disorders increase the risk for substance addiction, depression and behaviour that is self-destructive, reckless or violent.

CAUSES

The causes of personality disorders are not well understood. A genetic predisposition is suspected; for example, schizotypal, schizoid and paranoid personality disorders are more common in families with a history of schizophrenia. Early childhood events, such as emotional neglect and physical abuse, are believed to cause personality disorders such as antisocial and borderline personality disorders.

Women are more likely than men to have avoidant, borderline, dependent, and paranoid personality disorders; men are more prone to develop antisocial and obsessive-compulsive personality disorders.

PREVENTION

It is not known if personality disorders can be prevented. However, some of the complications, such as substance abuse (pp.358–60), may be avoided with proper treatment.

WHO IS AT RISK?

The risk factors include:
- Family history
- Physical abuse
- Emotional neglect

DIAGNOSIS

The diagnosis of a personality disorder is based on a person's history of thought and behaviour patterns. Some symptoms, especially those of antisocial personality disorder, may appear in teenagers, and diagnosis is not made until adulthood. It is possible to have more than one personality disorder.

Many patients do not realize they suffer from a personality disorder and blame other people or circumstances for their problems.

Many personality disorders have been identified, most of which fall into three categories, or clusters. Following are the most common.

• **CLUSTER A** These are characterized by odd, eccentric behaviour. People with paranoid personality disorder suffer from extreme distrust and suspicion of others. Those with schizoid personality disorder are introverted and remain emotionally and socially distant, even from family members. The schizotypal personality is also withdrawn, like the schizoid personality, but thinks and communicates in ways similar to those with schizophrenia, although usually without hallucinations.

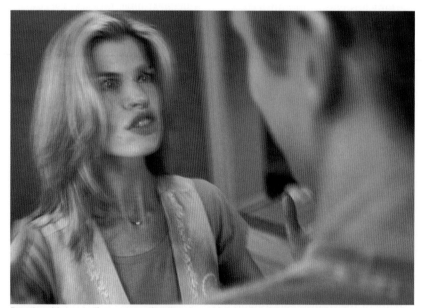

People with borderline personality disorder, which is characterized by mood swings, bouts of anger, and an inability to control emotions or impulses, tend to have conflict-ridden relationships and engage in reckless behaviour.

• **CLUSTER B** This group exhibits dramatic, emotional and erratic behaviour. One of the most common personality disorders is the borderline personality disorder, perhaps because they seek out help. They have trouble controlling emotions or impulses, resulting in reckless behaviour such as suicidal gestures and substance abuse, and may be involved in dramatic, stormy relationships. They fear being alone, yet push people away. People with antisocial personality disorder (formerly called psychopathic or sociopathic personality) act impulsively, may be belligerent and irresponsible, with no respect for others and no remorse for their behaviour. They are at high risk for substance abuse, especially alcoholism and criminal behaviour. The narcissistic personality disorder has an exaggerated sense of self-importance, feels oversensitive to failure, and lacks empathy for other people. Histrionic personality disorder is characterized by attention-seeking, concern with appearance and excessive need for approval.

• **CLUSTER C** Anxious, fearful behaviour characterizes this group. The most common personality disorder in the United States is obsessive-compulsive personality disorder, not to be confused with obsessive-compulsiveness (pp.354–5). Although conscientious and devoted to work, those with obsessive-compulsive personality disorder have a drive for perfectionism that makes it difficult to make decisions or finish tasks. They tend to be inflexible and often withdraw emotionally. People with avoidant personality disorder are extremely shy and overly sensitive to rejection; they avoid relationships yet deeply want them, and suffer from feelings of inadequacy. The dependent personality is dependent on others to make decisions and fulfil emotional and physical needs, and will suffer an abusive relationship to avoid being alone.

TREATMENTS

When the characteristics of these personality disorders interfere with functioning and relationships, treatment is needed. Often, psychotherapy combined with medication is more powerful than either treatment alone. Although there is no cure, some personality disorders improve with age.

• **PSYCHOTHERAPY** Therapy may be done with individuals, family or groups, and generally takes at least a year. Types of therapy include psychodynamic, which involves exploring the ways personal history contributes to the condition; cognitive behavioural therapy, which looks at how to change patterns of thinking and behaviour to more effective methods of dealing with situations and relationships; and dialectical behaviour therapy, a type of cognitive behavioural therapy that focuses on coping skills. Cognitive behavioural therapy is particularly useful for those with obsessive-compulsive personality disorder. It may help people with dependent personality disorder learn to make independent choices and people with narcissistic personality disorder to behave in a more positive and compassionate manner. Dialectical behaviour therapy may help those with borderline personality dis-

order. However, talk therapy may fail to work for those with schizoid personality disorder because they have trouble relating to others. It may be difficult to do talk therapy with people who have paranoid personality disorder because of they are suspicious of doctors.

• **GROUP THERAPY** People with borderline personality disorder may benefit greatly from one-on-one counselling.

• **PSYCHOANALYSIS** This type of talk therapy, developed by Sigmund Freud, involves several sessions a week delving into the patient's past relationships to understand their effects on current relationships so that new patterns of behaviour can be developed. This type of therapy may be useful for narcissistic and obsessive-compulsive personality disorders.

• **MEDICATION** Although no medication can cure personality disorders, it can relieve some of the symptoms. SSRI antidepressants may reduce the obsessions and compulsions in obsessive-compulsive personality disorder, reduce sensitivity to rejection in those with avoidant personality disorder, and help treat depression that occurs from failed romantic relationships in histrionic personality disorder. Mood stabilizers can level out the mood swings, and antidepressants can relieve depression in those with borderline personality disorder. Antipsychotic medication may help some patients with schizotypal personality disorder.

See also: *Substance Abuse, p. 358–60 • Schizophrenia, pp.374–5 • Anxiety Disorders, pp.354–5*

Adjustment Disorders

Adjustment disorders occur when the reaction to stress, such as a death, job loss or divorce causes symptoms more severe than would be expected – severe enough to impact on work or relationships.

This excessive reaction begins within three months of the stressful occurrence and usually does not last longer than six months after the stress subsides.

In some cases, adjustment disorders progress to depression (pp.364–5), generalized anxiety disorder (pp.354–5) or other mental health problems. They may result in a higher susceptibility to substance addiction (pp.358–60), suicide and violent behaviour.

CAUSES

Any severe, identifiable stressful event can cause an adjustment disorder. For teenagers, it may be school problems, family conflict or sexuality issues. For adults, it is often marital or financial problems. For people of any age, it may be the death of a loved one or unexpected catastrophes. It is not limited to negative events, either; marriage and pregnancy may result in adjustment disorder as well.

PREVENTION

Most stressful events cannot be prevented; how these affect people depends on their coping skills. Enough sleep, good nutrition, exercise and support from family and friends are all helpful. Stresses that disrupt the social network, such as the death of a loved one, may be very difficult to handle.

DIAGNOSIS

Symptoms vary from person to person and include agitation, trembling and palpitations. They may resemble symptoms of depression with feelings of hopelessness and sadness, or symptoms of anxiety with worry and nervousness. Other types of adjustment disorders can include violence, impulsive behaviour, or social withdrawal.

Adjustment disorders may be classified as acute, lasting less than six months, or chronic, lasting longer. When symptoms persist longer than six months after the termination of the trigger, the diagnosis may change to a more serious mental health problem. Other mental health disorders should be ruled out before a diagnosis of adjustment disorder is made.

TREATMENTS

Adjustment disorders often respond well to treatment.
• **PSYCHOTHERAPY** Talk therapy is the most effective method for dealing with adjustment disorders. Talking about the stressor that triggered symptoms helps the indi-

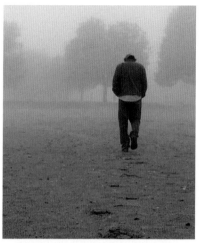

People with adjustment disorders often experience feelings of depression or anxiety, and may tend to withdraw socially.

vidual develop better coping skills.
• **SUPPORT GROUPS** Many groups are available for people who have suffered such stressors as bereavement, job loss and divorce.
• **MEDICATION** Anti-depressants or anti-anxiety medications may be prescribed for a short time to relieve certain symptoms.
• **STRESS MANAGEMENT** Biofeedback (pp.504–7) can be used to teach the mind to control body functions such as heart rate, blood pressure and muscle tension. Progressive muscle relaxation (pp.474–5) can aid in relaxation and relieving stress. Massage therapy (pp.468–73) relieves muscle tension and stress. Yoga (pp.476–9) may help individuals handle stress more effectively.

See also: *Substance Abuse, pp.358–60* • *Massage Therapy, pp.468–73* • *Biofeedback, pp.504–7*

Somatization Disorders

In somatization disorder, physical symptoms are present and are quite real, even severe, but no underlying medical illness or condition can be found to fully explain them. The condition is chronic, lasting for years, and often interferes with work and relationships.

CAUSES

No specific cause has been identified for somatization disorder, but symptoms may get worse after significant stressors, such as the loss of a loved one, a friend or even a job. Stress may also exacerberate existing symptoms.

It is important to remember that these symptoms are not 'faked'. The patient is not able to consciously turn these symptoms on and off and they should not be easily dismissed by the healthcare provider.

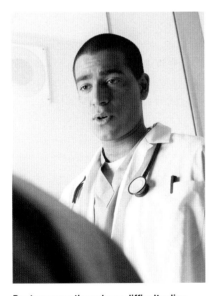

Doctors sometimes have difficulty diagnosing somatization disorder and may attribute chronic pain and problems with the nervous system to hypochondria.

PREVENTION

Somatization disorders cannot be prevented, but if correctly diagnosed, unnecessary and excessive medical tests may be avoided.

DIAGNOSIS

A physical examination and tests, based on symptoms, should be done to rule out any physical causes before a diagnosis of somatization disorder is made. Depression (pp.364–5) and anxiety disorders (pp.354–5) should be ruled out.

Symptoms usually include chronic pain and problems with the digestive system, the nervous system and the reproductive system: vomiting, abdominal pain, nausea, bloating, diarrhoea, pain in the legs or arms, back pain, joint pain, pain during urination, headaches, shortness of breath, palpitations, chest pain, dizziness, amnesia, difficulty swallowing, vision changes, paralysis or muscle weakness, sexual apathy, pain during intercourse, impotence, painful or irregular menstruation, and excessive menstrual bleeding.

TREATMENTS

The goal of treatment is to learn to control the symptoms of the

WHO IS AT RISK?

The risk factors include:
- Runs in families
- Personality disorders often present
- Dependence on others
- History of sexual abuse or emotional neglect

disorder. If a mood disorder exists, it should also be treated.

- **SUPPORTIVE DOCTOR** Establishing a supportive relationship with a sympathetic doctor is the most important aspect of treatment. Regular appointments give the patient an opportunity to review symptoms, enhance coping mechanisms and develop rapport. Test results should be explained. It is important – but difficult – to distinguish between somatic complaints that are due to a physical illness and those that are not.

- **MEDICATION** Antidepressants may help in some cases.

- **COUNSELLING** Cognitive-behavioural therapy may be beneficial. Improving methods of dealing with stress may reduce physical symptoms. Many people with somatization disorders refuse counselling.

- **SYMPTOM RELIEF** If possible, relief will be given for physical symptoms.

See also: *Depression, pp.364–5 • Anxiety Disorders, pp.354–5 • Nausea and Vomiting, pp.274–5*

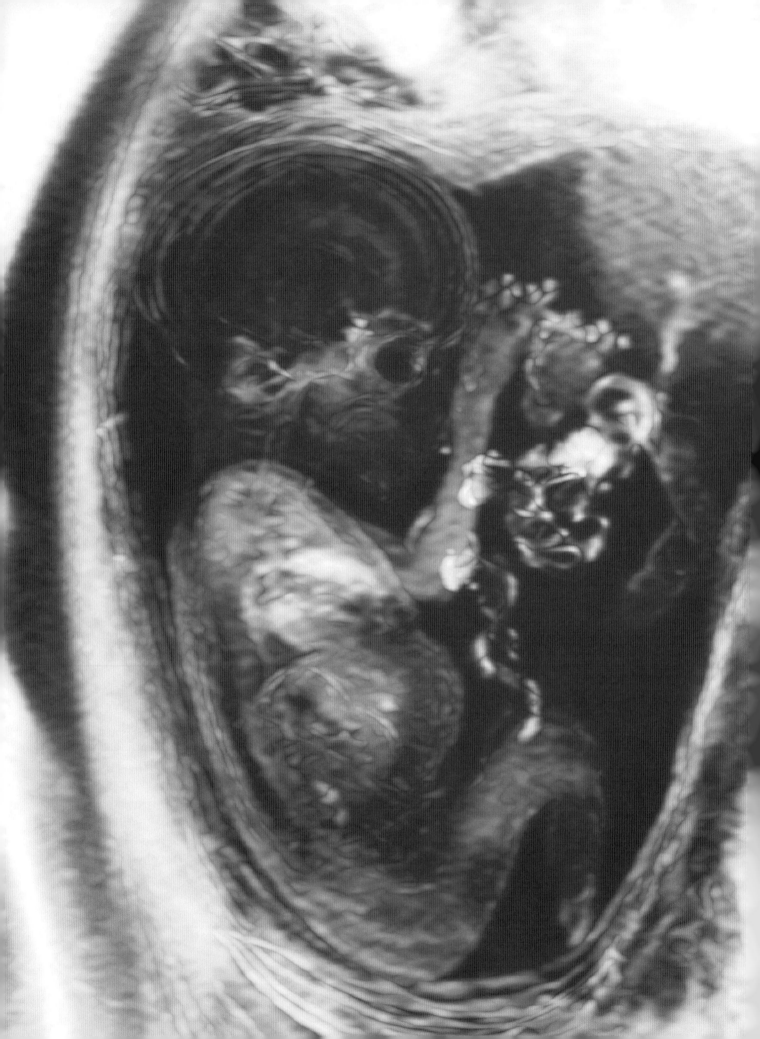

FEMALE
REPRODUCTIVE
SYSTEM

14

The female reproductive system includes the uterus, ovaries, fallopian tubes, cervix, vagina and vulva. The ovaries produce the egg, or ovum, and the female sex hormones oestrogen and progesterone. The uterus provides a nourishing environment for a developing foetus. The cervix expands and leads to the vagina, through which the baby is delivered. Each month, as oestrogen levels rise, the inner lining of the uterus thickens to prepare for a fertilized egg. Luteinizing hormone (LH) is released from the pituitary gland, signalling the ovaries to release an ovum. Progesterone levels increase to further prepare the uterus for possible pregnancy by inhibiting contractions and the release of another ovum. If pregnancy does not occur, progesterone levels drop and the menstrual cycle begins. If pregnancy occurs, the fertilized egg implants and grows in the uterus.

Benign Breast Disease

The breast consists of glandular and stromal tissues. The glandular tissues contain the lobules and ducts. In lactating women, the lobules produce milk that flows through the ducts and out of the nipples. Stromal tissues, which are made up of fatty and fibrous connective tissue, provide support for the breasts.

There are two common benign breast conditions: fibrocystic breast changes and fibroadenoma. Neither is life threatening, but both may cause worrying symptoms.

Fibrocystic breast changes are common; it is estimated that they affect over 60 percent of all women. The condition involves changes in the glandular tissue and stromal tissue of the breast.

Fibroadenomas are benign tumours that develop in the glandular or stromal tissues of the breast.

CAUSES

The cause of both conditions is unknown. However, it has been established that ovarian hormones play an important role in the development of both, because symptoms tend to vary during the menstrual cycle, and they subside during menopause.

PREVENTION

The American Cancer Society (ACS) recommends that women pay attention to any changes in their breasts, because early detection may allow for the best treatment outcome. The ACS has set the following guidelines.

- Yearly mammograms beginning at the age of 40.
- Regular clinical breast examinations during physical examinations, every three years for women under 30 and every year for women over 40.
- Breast self-examination may be done monthly beginning at the age of 20. Any changes should be immediately reported to a doctor. The best time to examine breasts is right after the menstrual period has ended – the breasts will be the least full and tender at this time in the cycle.
- Additional testing and mammography screening should be considered for women with a family history of breast cancer.

DIAGNOSIS

Symptoms of fibrocystic breast changes include a lumpy consistency in the breast tissue, development of cysts, breast discomfort, fullness or thickening in the breasts, pain and tenderness, and nipple sensations such as itching. These symptoms are usually more prominent before the menstrual period and tend to improve, or resolve, after the period is finished.

Symptoms of fibroadenoma include lumps in the breast that are usually moveable, painless, firm or rubbery and have well-defined outer edges. Fibroadenomas can increase in size, especially during pregnancy, and have been known to shrink and disappear following the development of menopause. These benign tumours frequently occur in young women under the age of 30. African-American women have an increased risk for the development of them.

During the diagnosis process, the doctor works to determine whether the symptoms indicate breast cancer or a benign breast disorder. The following diagnostic tools are used to identify and distinguish breast conditions:

- **MEDICAL HISTORY** Questions about the patient's personal and family medical history.
- **PHYSICAL EXAMINATION** A breast physical examination identifies any masses or lumps. If found, the texture, size and location are

noted. In addition, the doctor looks for changes in the nipples or skin of the breasts, and examines the lymph nodes under the armpits and above the collarbones.

• **MAMMOGRAPHY** This special X-ray of the breast tissue identifies masses and calcifications, small mineral deposits within the breast tissue.

• **BREAST ULTRASOUND** In this test, high-frequency sound waves produce images of the breast and differentiate between masses and fluid-filled cysts.

• **FINE-NEEDLE ASPIRATION** A thin needle is inserted into the breast lump and fluid is drawn out. The fluid is later analysed for cellular abnormalities.

• **SURGICAL BIOPSY** A portion or all of the mass is removed from the breast and later analysed for cellular abnormalities.

• **DISCHARGE EXAMINATION** Any nipple discharge is analysed for the presence of abnormal cells.

• **DUCTOGRAM** This test identifies any masses within the duct. A tiny tube is placed inside the opening of a duct within the nipple. A special dye is injected that allows a doctor to visualize the shape of the duct on a radiograph.

TREATMENTS

Various treatment options are available for benign breast conditions. Some women find that symptoms improve after making dietary changes, such as limiting their intake of dietary fat and eliminating caffeine and other stimulants found in soft drinks, coffee, tea and chocolate. Wearing a support bra may also provide relief from bothersome symptoms.

• **SURGERY** This is done to remove benign tumours or cysts is sometimes recommended. The benefits of this approach must be weighed carefully, because in many cases the tumors resolve on their own. In addition, the removal of a large

On Call

Mastitis is a breast infection that often affects women who are breastfeeding. An area within the breast becomes red, warm and tender. This occurs because bacteria from the surface of the skin enter the breast duct through a crack in the skin surrounding the nipple. Women with mastitis are encouraged to continue breastfeeding to drain the breasts and to apply warm compresses to open the ducts and to reduce discomfort. Over the counter non-steroidal anti-inflammatory pain medication can be helpful. If the mastitis is not completely resolved with these treatments, it will often respond to the use of antibiotics. In rare cases, an abscess develops and must be surgically drained.

number of masses can cause scar tissue to form, which changes the shape and texture of the breast. If a woman, with her doctor, chooses not to remove fibroadenomas, regular breast and monthly self-examinations are recommended to monitor the growth of the tumour.

• **CONTRACEPTIVES** A physician may prescribe oral contraceptives to treat benign breast conditions. These contraceptives change a woman's hormone levels and may provide some relief from some symptoms. Studies involving the use of vitamins E and B_6 and herbal preparations that contain evening primrose oil remain controversial.

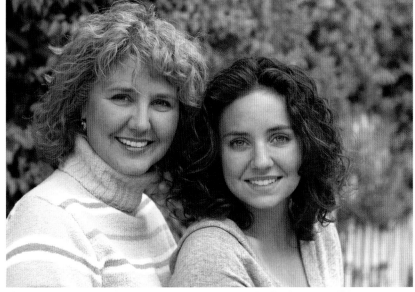

Fibrocystic breasts and fibroadenoma are two common benign breast conditions that have a genetic component and tend to run in families. Although symptoms may cause pain and tenderness in the breasts, neither condition is life-threatening.

See also: *Premenstrual Syndrome, pp.386–7* • *Menopause, pp.406–8* • *Supplements, Vitamins & Minerals, pp.532–41*

Menstrual Bleeding Disorders

Many women experience menstrual bleeding irregularities at some point in their lives. There are three primary types of menstrual bleeding disorders: menorrhagia, or heavy periods; amenorrhoea, or the lack of periods; and menometrorrhagia, or heavy bleeding during normal periods in addition to irregular bleeding throughout the rest of the month.

Symptoms of menorrhagia include a menstrual flow that soaks through one or more sanitary pads or tampons in one hour, having to change pads throughout the night, menstrual bleeding for more than a week, passing large blood clots, periods that interfere with daily activities, severe cramping, and anaemia (pp.312–13).

The two forms of amenorrhoea are primary and secondary. Primary occurs in young women who have not had their period before the age of 16. Secondary amenorrhoea occurs in a woman who previously cycled but has had no period for more than three months.

Excessive bleeding throughout the month, or menometrorrhagia, can indicate health concerns such as hormone imbalances, benign fibroid tumours, infections or cancer. Women with menometrarrhagia are also at increased risk for anaemia.

CAUSES

The two most common causes of menorrhagia and menometrorrhagia are hormone imbalances and uterine fibroids. To prepare for a fertilized egg, the uterus lining thickens in response to changes in the levels of the hormones oestrogen and progesterone. Normally, if pregnancy does not occur, the lining is shed during the menstrual period. In menorrhagia, the lining thickens in excess, causing a large amount of blood to be shed. Adolescent girls, women nearing menopause or with conditions that cause hormonal imbalances are at increased risk for menorrhagia.

Less common causes of the conditions include polyps or tiny benign uterine growths; adenomyosis, in which glands from the endometrium are embedded in the uterine muscles; ovarian cysts (p.389); ovaries that do not regularly release eggs; miscarriage or ectopic pregnancy (pp.398–400); female reproductive cancers (pp.412–15); endometriosis (pp.402–3); lupus (pp.324–5); and medications or conditions that prevent blood-clotting.

Primary amenorrhoea may be caused by several conditions, including a chromosomal abnormality that inhibits the ovaries from producing mature eggs; pituitary disease (p.351), a hypothalamus disorder; vaginal obstruction, or the lack of a component of the female reproductive system.

Among the many causes of secondary amenorrhoea are pregnancy; the use of birth-control pills or hormone injections (pp.410–11); breast-feeding; chronic illness; the use of medication such as antidepressants, antipsychotics, chemotherapy and oral corticosteroids; polycystic ovary syndrome (PCOS); thyroid problems (pp.344–7); pituitary tumours; low body weight caused by eating disorders such as anorexia or bulimia (pp.366–7); excessive exercise; uterine scarring; as well as the premature onset of menopause (pp.406–8).

WHO IS AT RISK?

The risk factors include:

Menorrhagia and Menometrorrhagia

- Young women who have just begun their periods
- Women approaching menopause
- Women with a family history of heavy vaginal bleeding
- Women with a history of fibroids

Amenorrhoea

- Pregnant or breast-feeding women
- Young women over 16 who have not begun menstruating
- Women who use oral contraceptives
- Women with eating disorders
- Women involved in intensive athletic training

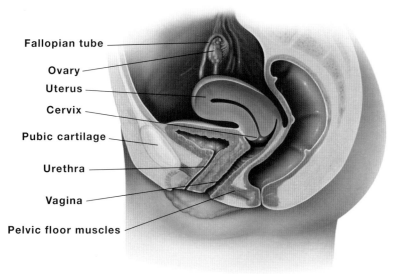

Fallopian tube
Ovary
Uterus
Cervix
Pubic cartilage
Urethra
Vagina
Pelvic floor muscles

Menstrual bleeding disorders may originate in the ovaries, fallopian tubes or the uterus. A thorough examination is required to determine the specific cause.

PREVENTION

To minimize the risk of developing a menstrual bleeding disorder, get plenty of rest, eat a well-balanced diet, minimize any mental stress and maintain an appropriate exercise routine.

DIAGNOSIS

To diagnose a menstrual bleeding disorder, the doctor may do the following:

• MEDICAL HISTORY The doctor may ask questions about the patient's menstrual cycle and family history. The patient may also be asked to keep a diary to record information about bleeding and non-bleeding days, the amount of flow, and the number of sanitary towels or tampons needed.

• PHYSICAL EXAMINATION A pelvic examination may reveal abnormalities of the reproductive organs and whether the patient is pregnant.

• BLOOD TESTS A sample of blood is used to test for pregnancy, hormonal deficiencies, and other abnormalities.

• PAP SMEAR This examination of cervical cells may indicate the presence of an infection or cancer.

• ENDOMETRIAL BIOPSY A tissue sample from the inside of the uterus is examined for cellular abnormalities.

• ULTRASOUND This test allows the doctor to view the uterus, ovaries and pelvis.

• SONOHYSTEROGRAM Fluid is injected into the uterus, which is then examined with an ultrasound.

• HYSTEROSCOPY OR LAPAROSCOPY A slender tube with a lighted end is inserted through the vagina and cervix into the uterine cavity (hysteroscopy) or a tiny incision in the abdomen allowing the doctor to see inside of the abdomen (laparoscopy) to see the outer uterus, fallopian tubes and ovaries. Laparoscopy is an outpatient surgery. Hysteroscopy may also be performed as an outpatient surgery.

• DILATION AND CURETTAGE (D AND C) After the cervix is opened, and then a spoon-shaped instrument is used to remove tissue from the lining of the uterus. The tissue is then examined for abnormalities.

• HYSTEROSALPINGOGRAPHY An X-ray is taken of the uterus and fallopian tubes after the injection of a dye to view the shape of the uterine cavity and determine whether the fallopian tubes are open.

TREATMENTS

Amenorrhoea can be treated with lifestyle changes including weight loss, exercise, and stress reduction.

• MEDICATION Menorrhagia and menometrorrhagia may be treated with oral contraceptives or progesterone pills. Iron supplements may be prescribed if anaemia has developed as a result of excessive bleeding. Nonsteroidal anti-inflammatory drugs (NSAIDs) such as ibuprofen may be used to soothe cramping and decrease flow.

• SURGERY The doctor may need to remove the lining of the uterus by performing a D and C, endometrial re-section, or endometrial ablation. Uterine polyps can be removed during an operative hysteroscopy. In this procedure a slender tube with a lighted end is inserted into the uterine cavity and used to locate and remove the polyps.

• HORMONE TREATMENT If uterine fibroids are found to be a cause of bleeding, the bleeding can be controlled with hormone medication, or the fibroids can be removed surgically with a myomectomy (removal of fibroids only) or hysterectomy (removal of the uterus).

See also: *Anaemia, pp.312–13 • Thyroid Disease, pp.344–7 • Birth Control, pp.410–11*

Premenstrual Syndrome (PMS) and PMDD

Premenstrual syndrome (PMS) is a collection of physical and psychological changes that occur before the menstrual cycle that are severe enough to interfere with a woman's normal function. As many as 75 percent of women report experiencing one or more of the many symptoms of PMS.

Premenstrual dysphoric disorder (PMDD) is characterized by severe physical and emotional symptoms that end after menstruation begins. Between 2 and 10 percent of women may suffer from PMDD.

CAUSES

The causes of PMS and PMDD are unknown, although several related factors have been identified. For instance, hormone fluctuations contribute to the changes experienced during PMS and PMDD. When these fluctuations cease, for example during pregnancy and menopause, the symptoms of PMS and PMDD end.

Research indicates that serotonin, a brain chemical that affects mood, may be involved in the disorders. Women who suffer from PMS and PMDD may have insufficient amounts of serotonin, which causes fatigue, food cravings and insomnia.

Other factors may include depression (pp.364–5), stress, vitamin or mineral deficiency, a high-salt diet, and excessive use of alcoholic and caffeinated beverages.

PREVENTION

Lifestyle changes may help women minimize the symptoms associated with PMS and PMDD. These changes include eating a balanced diet, establishing an exercise routine, managing daily stress, getting proper rest, and practicing relaxation techniques such as deep breathing exercises.

DIAGNOSIS

Symptoms of PMS may vary from month to month, but they end after the period begins. The symptoms include:

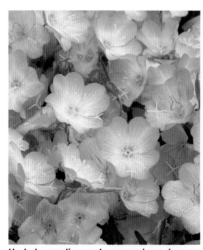

Herbal remedies such as evening primrose oil can help to relieve symptoms of PMS.

- weight gain as a result of fluid retention
- bloating
- constipation
- diarrhoea
- breast tenderness
- headaches
- joint and muscle pain
- anxiety
- tearfulness
- mood swings
- fatigue
- irritability and aggression
- food cravings
- sleep problems

Symptoms of PMDD include:
- depression
- despair
- anger
- low self-esteem
- difficulty concentrating

To be diagnosed with either PMS or PMDD, a woman must experience symptoms starting between five and ten days before the menstrual period begins; have symptoms for at least three consecutive menstrual cycles; the symptoms must resolve within four days after the beginning of the menstrual period; and the symptoms must interfere with a woman's daily activities.

During the diagnosis, the patient may be asked to keep a diary, recording any signs or symptoms they experience and the dates on which they occur. The dates of the menstrual period are also recorded. This diary-keeping is continued for two complete menstrual cycles.

Next, a physical examination that includes a gynaecological examination is performed. In severe cases, a psychiatric evaluation may be necessary to identify psychological symptoms such as depression.

Since many thyroid disorders (pp.344–7) have symptoms that mimic those of PMS and PMDD, the doctor may perform a thyroid test. This allows the doctor to determine whether a malfunctioning thyroid is the root of the problem.

TREATMENTS

Each woman with PMS and PMDD experiences the symptoms differently. Thus, the treatment approach must be specialized to meet the needs of each woman. The doctor may choose from one of the following options:

• **LIFESTYLE CHANGES** Avoiding caffeine, salt, sugar and alcohol and increasing consumption of whole grains, fruit and vegetables may alleviate some symptoms of PMS and PMDD. Exercise – at least 30 minutes of activity most days a week – can help women cope with symptoms and minimize stress.

Women who practise relaxation techniques experience fewer symptoms of PMS. Regular massage therapy (pp.468–73) and acupuncture (pp.464–5) has also been found to alleviate PMS symptoms for many women.

• **VITAMINS** Those that contain 1200–1600 mg calcium, 200–400 mg magnesium, and 50 mg vitamin B_6 can improve symptoms of PMS and PMDD, specifically breast soreness, bloating, and cramping.

• **HERBAL COMPLEXES** Black cohosh, chastetree berry (vitex), and evening primrose oil may provide relief for the symptoms of PMS.

• **NONSTEROIDAL ANTI-INFLAMMATORY DRUGS (NSAIDS)** Examples of these medications include ibuprofen and naproxen sodium. They reduce breast tenderness and abdominal cramping.

• **ORAL CONTRACEPTIVES** Doctors sometimes prescribe contraceptives, which can eliminate or reduce symptoms by inhibiting ovulation and stabilizing hormonal fluctuations.

• **ANTIDEPRESSANTS** Research indicates that some women with PMS and PMDD suffer from deficient levels of serotonin. The use of selective serotonin re-uptake inhibitors (SSRIs) such as flouxetine, paroxetine and sertraline can help minimize fatigue, food cravings and insomnia.

• **MEDROXYPROGESTERONE ACETATE** Injections of this medication temporarily stop ovulation and sometimes provide relief from the symptoms associated with PMS and PMDD. Unfortunately, medroxyprogesterone acetate is also associated with side-effects

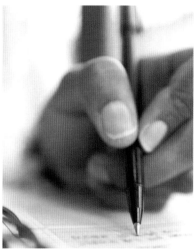

The first step in the diagnosis process may be the keeping of a diary. During this task patients record any signs or symptoms they experience.

that are similar to those of PMS and PMDD, including weight gain, increased appetite, headaches and mood swings.

• **PROGESTERONE CREAM** This cream contains derivatives of wild yams and soybeans. Although there are no studies that conclusively illustrate its benefits, some women report that it helps relieve their symptoms. Although many progesterone creams are formulated from derivatives of wild yam and soybeans, effective ones also actively contain the hormone progesterone. Other creams, such as those called wild yam creams contain no progesterone and are not recommended.

• **COUNSELLING** Whether in a group or individual setting, counselling helps women cope with stress, anger, anxiety and depression. Patient education helps many women deal with their symptoms and relate to their feelings.

See also: *Menopause, pp.406–8 • Depression, pp.364–5 • Breath Work, pp.526–7*

Bartholin's Cyst

Bartholin's glands are two small organs located on either side of the vaginal opening. They secrete fluid that helps to lubricate the vagina. If one of the ducts draining the glands becomes blocked, normal fluid builds up in the gland and forms a cyst. Under certain conditions, the cyst becomes infected, in which case it is called an abscess. An infection can occur as a result of bacteria normally found in the intestinal tract, such as E. coli or sexually transmitted diseases such as chlamydia and gonorrhoea.

Bartholin's cysts can be painless but are often tender. They can begin as a tiny mass and grow to be quite large. Some women with Bartholin cysts are unable to walk or sit comfortably due to the size of the enlarged gland. Bartholin's abscesses are extremely painful. The skin is often red and warm to the touch.

CAUSES
A Bartholin's cyst can be caused by fluid clogging the duct emptying the gland, or by the growth of skin over the opening of the gland.

PREVENTION
Poor personal hygiene and high-risk sexual behaviour, such as sex with multiple partners or without a condom, can increase the risk of infection of a Bartholin's cysts.

DIAGNOSIS
A pelvic examination can diagnose a Bartholin's cyst. The doctor will also ask about symptoms during the medical history.

If the cyst is infected, fluid from the abscess and the cervix will be analysed for the presence of bacteria. It is important to identify any sexual transmitted infections, as they can cause further problems.

An excision of the gland or a biopsy of the cyst may be recommended for women over the age of 40, who are at increased risk for developing a Bartholin gland tumour and other cancers of the reproductive system.

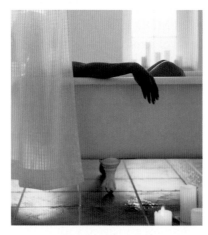
To treat a Bartholin's cyst, a doctor may recommend a sitz bath. Sitting in warm water several times a day can encourage the cyst to drain and heal.

WHO IS AT RISK?
The risk factors include:
- Women who are sexually active
- High risk sexual behaviour

TREATMENTS
Sometimes a Bartholin's cyst clears up on its own; sometimes the doctor may rely on one of the following treatments.
- SITZ BATHS Using a special basin or a bathtub, the vulva is soaked in some warm water for approximately 15 minutes. The sitz bath should be repeated three or four times per day. A sitz bath may cause the cyst to rupture and drain, which allows it to heal.
- ANTIBIOTICS Medications may be prescribed to resolve bacterial infections within the gland.
- SURGICAL DRAINAGE A small incision is made in the cyst, and then a tiny catheter is inserted that allows the gland to drain completely.
- MARSUPIALIZATION This procedure is used for recurring cysts. A permanent opening is made in the gland by creating a tiny incision with stitches on either side.
- SURGICAL REMOVAL The complete removal of one or both of the Bartholin glands is recommended in cases where it is important to avoid reccurring abscesses.

See also: *STDs, p. 392–3*

Ovarian Cyst

Fluid filled sacs, or cysts, on the ovaries develop monthly as a part of the female reproductive cycle. Two common types of ovarian cysts are follicular and corpus luteum. Both are classified as functional because they play a role in female reproduction. Follicular and corpus luteum cysts are usually painless and resolve on their own in two or three cycles.

Other common types of ovarian cysts include the following:

- **DERMOID CYSTS** An ovarian cyst that is filled with cells that can produce hair, teeth or other kinds of tissue.
- **ENDOMETRIOMAS** Cysts that develop in women suffering from endometriosis.
- **CYSTADENOMAS** A benign cyst containing watery or mucus-like fluid that forms on the ovary.
- **POLYCYSTIC OVARIES** This condition occurs when eggs are recruited to develop but do not mature are not released regularly at ovulation.

CAUSES

Each month, an egg bursts from the ovary out of a cyst-like structure, called a follicle. This process is mediated by luteinizing hormone (LH). An increase in the body's LH level signals for the release of the egg. Following the egg's release, the follicle turns into a structure called a corpus luteum, which produces progesterone to further prepare the uterus for conception. The corpus luteum normally resolves in 14 days if conception does not occur.

PREVENTION

Suppressing ovulation with hormone therapy can decrease the risk of forming ovarian cysts. Scheduling regular pelvic examinations can minimize the complications associated with the occurrence of cysts.

DIAGNOSIS

Ovarian cysts can cause a variety of symptoms, including pain in the pelvic area or abdomen, painful menstrual cycles, pain during sexual intercourse, a feeling of fullness in the abdomen, and pressure on the rectum or bladder. When ovarian cysts twist and cut off their own blood supply, it is called ovarian torsion. The condition usually causes a sudden onset of severe abdominal pain, nausea and vomiting. Other benign and less common cysts include fibroademonas and Brenner's tumours. Although cancerous cysts can occur, premenopausal woman rarely experience a cancerous cyst of the ovary. The lifetime risk of ovarian cancer is approximately 1 in 70.

Ovarian cysts are diagnosed during pelvic examinations. The doctor feels the area of the abdomen located near the ovaries to identify any unusual growths. A medical history helps the doctor and patient identify unusual symptoms or changes in the menstrual cycle. Other tests for ovarian cysts include the following.

- **PELVIC ULTRASOUND** An image of the uterus and ovaries is produced by high-frequency sound waves.
- **BLOOD TEST** Doctors analyse a blood sample for elevated amounts of CA 125, a substance often found in the body of some women with ovarian cancer (pp.412–15). This test is most helpful in menopausal women with an ovarian cyst.

TREATMENTS

Since most cysts resolve on their own, the doctor may choose to simply monitor the symptoms for a period up to three months.

- **BIRTH-CONTROL PILLS** These prevent ovulation, therefore lowering the probability of the formation of a new cyst so may be prescribed.
- **SURGERY** This may be performed in some cases to remove a large or persistent cyst, eliminate severe symptoms, or to ensure that a cyst is not cancerous.

See also: *Menstrual Bleeding Disorders, pp.384–5 • Ovarian Cancer, pp.412–15 • Birth Control, pp.410–11*

WHO IS AT RISK?

The risk factors include:
- All women

Polycystic Ovary Disease

Also known as Stein-Leventhal syndrome, polycystic ovary syndrome (PCOS) is a hormonal imbalance that causes irregular menstrual periods, weight gain, increased body hair, breast shrinkage, acne, infertility, diabetes, high blood pressure and cardiovascular disease. Some women with PCOS also have darkened skin on the nape of the neck, armpits, inner thighs, vagina and beneath the breasts.

CAUSES

Female reproductive cycles and ovulation are regulated by chemicals such as luteinizing hormone (LH) and follicle stimulating hormone (FSH), both of which are normally released by the pituitary gland. FSH and LH stimulate the ovaries to produce oestrogen, progesterone, and small amounts of male hormones called androgens.

Women with PCOS do not ovulate regularly; eggs mature, but are not released. The retained eggs die and are reabsorbed by the ovary, causing them to enlarge with a thick white outer layer.

PREVENTION

To prevent PCOS and its complications, maintain a healthy weight, eat a balanced diet and exercise regularly. This helps the body maintain hormone levels, reduces the risk of diabetes (pp.338–41), and limits cardiovascular risk.

DIAGNOSIS

A gynaecologist, a doctor who specializes in female reproductive issues, and endocrinologist, a doctor who specializes in hormone disorders, often work together to diagnosis PCOS. Both specialists use a detailed medical history to gather information about the symptoms a woman may be experiencing and any family history of the condition.

During a pelvic examination, the gynaecologist looks for an enlarged ovaries and clitoris. In addition, acne (pp.99–101), hair growth and darkened skin may be noted.

Several blood tests are used throughout the diagnosis process. Hormone levels, especially those of LH, FSH, testosterone, oestrogen and progesterone are measured. Fasting glucose level, cholesterol level and liver function tests are used to identify possible insulin resistance, and liver and cardiovascular complications associated with PCOS.

It is sometimes necessary to visualize the ovaries and the uterus with an ultrasound or laparoscopy. A laparoscope is a slender tube with a camera on the end. It is inserted through an incision in the abdomen, allowing the doctors to see the ovaries and surrounding organs as an outpatient surgery.

TREATMENTS

Several treatment approaches are available for PCOS.

- **WEIGHT LOSS** Healthy food choices along with regular exercise helps restore hormone balance.
- **HORMONES** Birth-control pills containing oestrogen and progesterone or progesterone alone work to regulate the menstrual cycle and prevent ovulation.
- **CLOMIPHENE CITRATE** This medication works to increase the likelihood of ovulation in the women who are ready for pregnancy.
- **ANTI-ANDROGENS** Spironolactone, a diuretic, is prescribed to block the effects of androgen and its production, to decrease unwanted hair.
- **METFORMIN** Research indicates that this medication enhances ovulation and lowers androgen levels in women with insulin resistance associated with PCOS.

See also: *Acne, pp.99–101 • Menstrual Bleeding Disorders, pp.384–5 • High Blood Pressure, pp.236–9*

Uterine Fibroids

Uterine fibroids are benign tumours that grow in the wall of the uterus. They can begin as small bumps and may grow to the size of a small watermelon. Some fibroids develop on the inside of the uterus (submucosal) and are mostly likely to cause painful periods of bleeding and problems. Others grow within the walls (intramural) or on the outside of the uterus (subserosal) causing pelvic pressure, lower abdominal bulging, frequent urination or back pain.

CAUSES

The exact cause of uterine fibroids remains unknown, but evidence indicates that fibroids begin after a single cell overly reproduces itself. This occurs because of changes in the genetic information of the cell. It is also believed that the female sex hormone oestrogen further stimulates tumour development.

PREVENTION

Uterine fibroids cannot be prevented, but eating a healthy, balanced diet and exercising regularly can limit complications.

DIAGNOSIS

Common symptoms of uterine fibroids include heavy menstrual periods, excessive menstrual cramps, bleeding between menstrual cycles, pelvic pain, frequent urination, backaches and discomfort during sexual intercourse. In addition, uterine fibroids can cause infertility if the tumour blocks the fallopian tubes, or distorts the uterine cavity and interferes with implantation of the embryo.

To diagnosis uterine fibroids, the doctor will ask several questions about symptoms a woman is experiencing and then perform a pelvic examination. To pinpoint the location and size of the fibroid, the doctor orders imaging tests such as an ultrasound.

Blood tests may be used to measure female hormone levels and to identify cases of anaemia that can occur due to excess menstrual bleeding. An endometrial biopsy may be helpful to distinguish bleeding due to uterine fibroids from other causes. The biopsy allows the doctor to examine a small sample of cells from the lining of the uterus for abnormalities.

TREATMENTS

Depending on the symptoms and severity of the tumours, there are many treatment options available.
- **MONITORING** If a woman is experiencing no symptoms, the doctor may simply monitor the development of a uterine fibroid during regular office visits.
- **MEDICATION** Certain medication, such as birth-control pills and gonadotropin-releasing hormone (Gn-RH) agonists, can work to decrease symptoms.
- **MYOMECTOMY** In this procedure, the fibroid is surgically removed while leaving the uterus in place. It is possible for a woman to have children after this surgery, but delivery must usually be by caesarean.
- **UTERINE ARTERY EMBOLIZATION** A surgeon blocks blood flow to the fibroid, causing it to shrink. This procedure is appropriate only for women who do not want to become pregnant in the future.
- **ENDOMETRIAL ABLATION** The lining of the uterus is permanently removed to minimize menstrual cramping and bleeding. This procedure is appropriate only for women who do not wish to become pregnant.
- **HYSTERECTOMY** For a complete cure, the doctor will remove the uterus completely. A woman who has had a hysterectomy will no longer be able to become pregnant.

See also: *Back Pain, pp.132–3 • Menstrual Bleeding Disorders, pp.384–5 • Obesity, pp.348–9*

WHO IS AT RISK?

The risk factors include:
- Family history of uterine fibroids
- African-American women
- Obese women

Sexually Transmitted Diseases

A sexually transmitted disease (STD) is an illness spread through sexual contact. These diseases can be transmitted by vaginal, anal or oral sex.

The most common STDs that affect women include chlamydia, gonorrhoea, herpes simplex virus (HSV), human papillomavirus (HPV), trichomoniasis, syphilis and human immunodeficiency virus (HIV).

• **CHLAMYDIA** This is a common STD. The greatest risk for infection occurs between the ages of 15 and 24. If left untreated, this bacterial infection can cause serious health problems such as infertility (pp.396–7), ectopic pregnancies (pp.398–400), and pelvic inflammatory disease (p.409). Many women with chlamydia are unaware that they are infected because the condition presents with very mild or no symptoms.

Symptoms of chlamydia may include vaginal itching, a vaginal discharge, painful urination, pain during sexual intercourse, lower abdominal pain, low back pain

CAUTION

Pregnant women suffering from an STD can pass these organisms onto their unborn children. In most cases, STDs in infants cause more serious consequences. Pregnant women should be screened for STDs during their prenatal visits and be treated immediately.

and bleeding between periods.

• **GONORRHOEA** Gonorrhoea is another common STD. Much like chlamydia, many women with gonorrhoea do not realize that they are infected because of the lack of symptoms or symptoms, that mimic those of a bladder infection or another vaginal infection. The symptoms of gonorrhoea include a vaginal discharge that can be yellowish, thick and cloudy, or bloody; a burning sensation during urination; frequent urination; pain during sexual intercourse; and bleeding between menstrual periods.

• **HERPES SIMPLEX VIRUS** There are two forms of the herpes simplex virus (HSV) that can cause genital herpes. HSV type 1 is normally associated with cold sores and fever blisters around the mouth. During oral sex, this virus can be spread by open sore or fever blister. HSV type 2 is more frequently associated with genital sores and is spread during intimate contact.

In addition to small bumps, blisters and bleeding ulcers, HSV can cause pain and itching in the genital area, buttocks or inner thighs; vaginal discharge; muscle aches; and pain during urinating. HSV is usually characterized by outbreaks of painful blisters and ulcers which come and go.

WHO IS AT RISK?

The risk factors include:

- Women with multiple sex partners
- Women who abuse intravenous drugs
- Women with impaired immune systems

• **HUMAN PAPILLOMAVIRUS** Human papillomavirus (HPV) is associated with genital warts and cervical dysplasia. Warts appear as small bumps or large cauliflower-like growths. These warts may be found on the vulva, within the walls of the vagina, on the outer lips of the vagina, on the anus, and on the cervix and neck of the uterus. Other symptoms of HPV are an itching or burning sensation in the vagina and pain or bleeding during sexual intercourse. Some HPV infections have been associated with cervical cancer as well as cancer of the vulva and anus.

• **TRICHOMONIASIS** Trichomoniasis can cause a yellow-green and sometimes frothy vaginal discharge. Other symptoms of trichomoniasis include vaginal irritation, lower abdominal pain, painful urination, and discomfort during sexual intercourse.

• **SYPHILIS** Syphilis can affect not only the genitals, but also the skin and mucous membranes. Late consequences of untreated syphilis can be debilitating, resulting in

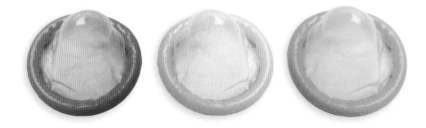

Other than abstinence from sexual activity, the only method of preventing sexually transmitted diseases is the use of condoms made of latex. Condoms are also available in other materials, such as animal skins. However, only latex condom provide protection from STDs.

mental illness and death. Syphilis has three stages – primary, secondary and tertiary. Primary syphilis is usually associated with a small painless sore (called a chancre) on the vagina, rectum, tongue or lips, as well as an enlargement of the lymph nodes in the groin.

The symptoms of secondary syphilis may include a reddish-brown rash, fever, fatigue and joint pain. Tertiary syphilis can involve neurological and cardio-vascular problems.

• HIV/AIDS Women and young girls maintain the fastest growing human immunodeficiency virus (HIV) rates all over the world. HIV (pp.316–7) causes a condition called the acquired immuno-deficiency syndrome (AIDS). The HIV virus destroys the immune system by destroying helper T cells or CD4 lymphocytes. Early in the illness there are few or no symptoms. Eventually, as the immune system is slowly destroyed, women may experience flu-like symptoms, swollen lymph nodes, diarrhoea and weight loss. When AIDS, a life-threatening condition, develops, recurring infections are common, as are night sweats, chills,

fever, lesions, fatigue, persistent headaches and impaired vision.

CAUSES
See chart, below.

PREVENTION
The best way to avoid contracting an STD is to avoid high-risk sexual behaviour. This includes avoiding anal sex without protection, oral sex, and sexual intercourse ouside that of a committed relationship. Latex condoms should always be used with any new sexual partner. In addition, regular pelvic examinations can help identify STDs early and prevent serious complications.

DIAGNOSIS
To diagnosis an STD, doctors may examine vaginal discharge, analyse a urine sample, perform a blood test that looks for antibodies to the causative agent of an STD, or remove a small sample of cells from any sores, warts or blisters.

TREATMENTS
See chart, below.

See also: *Pelvic Inflammatory Disease, p.409 • HIV/AIDS, pp.316–17 • Menstrual Bleeding Disorders, pp.384–5*

STD	Causative Agent	Treatments
Chlamydia	the bacterium *Chlamydia trochomatis*	Antibiotics such as azithromycin, erythromycin, tetracycline, or doxycycline
Gonorrhoea	the bacterium *Neisseria gonorrhoeae*	Antibiotics such as ceftriaxone, cefixime, ciprofloxacin, ofloxacin, cefuroxime axotal, cefpodoxime proxetil, enoxacin
Herpes simplex virus (HSV)	HSV-1 and HSV-2 viruses	There is no cure for HSV but outbreaks can be controlled with the use of antivirals such as acyclovir, famciclovir, and valacyclovir.
Human papillomavirus (HPV)	various strains of the HPV virus	HPV can never be cured but outbreaks can be minimized with the use of topical medications such as imiquimod, podofilox, and tricholoroacetic acid.
Trichomoniasis	the parasite *Trichomonas vaginalis*	Metronidazole pills
Syphilis	the bacterium *Treponema pallidum*	Penicillin
HIV	the HIV virus	Combinations of antiviral medications are used to control the virus.

Vaginitis

Inflammation of the vagina or vaginitis can occur as a result of bacterial or yeast infections, trichomoniasis, chlamydia, viral infections and low oestrogen levels. The symptoms of vaginitis may include a vaginal discharge with a foul odour, an itching or burning sensation in the vagina, abdominal discomfort, pain during urination or intercourse, and light vaginal bleeding.

WHO IS AT RISK?

The risk factors include:
- Menopause
- Diabetes
- Use of antibiotics
- Use of synthetic underwear
- Douching
- Unsafe sex practices

CAUSES

A number of bacteria normally grow in the vagina. These bacteria, which are also called the normal flora, help maintain a healthy environment in the vagina and fight off other more harmful organisms. Bacterial vaginosis occurs when one organism from the normal flora outgrows the others, disrupting the natural balance within the vaginal environment. Often, women who have bacterial vaginosis experience a greyish–white discharge that has a 'fishy' smelling odour. This odour may be more prominent after sexual intercourse.

Yeast infections are caused by fungi, the most common of which is *Candida albicans*. When the flora of the vaginal environment changes, fungi that are normally present become overgrown.

Although yeast infections are generally not serious, they can be uncomfortable. They often cause vaginal itching and a thick white curdled discharge that resembles cottage cheese. The discharge may also be watery, and it is odourless. Wearing underwear made of synthetic material and tight-fitting clothing may increase the risk of developing a yeast infection. Yeast infections can be caused by taking some antibiotics, which kill the 'friendly' flora in the vagina. Woman with diabetes also have an increased risk of developing yeast infections.

Several different sexually transmitted diseases (STDs, pp.392–3) can cause vaginitis. Trichomoniasis is caused by a parasite and spreads through sexual contact. Women who have trichomoniasis sometimes experience a greenish-yellow, frothy, foul-smelling discharge.

Other sexually transmitted diseases, such as chlamydia, herpes simplex viruses and the human papillomavirus (HPV) can cause irritation of the vagina.

Herpes simplex viruses may cause the growth of painful ulcers or blisters within the vagina. The development of warts inside the

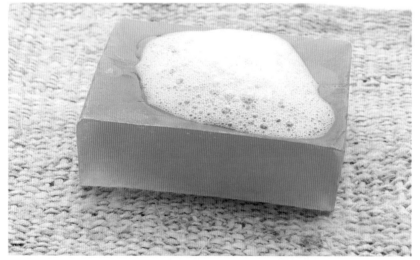

Some types of vaginitis can be prevented by practising good personal hygiene. Clean the genital area daily with a mild, fragrant-free, non-irritating soap, and always rinse soap from the genital area and dry it well.

vagina is also a symptom of some strains of human papillomavirus. HPV is also associated with cervical cancer (pp.412–15).

Menopausal women or those whose ovaries have been removed may also experience vaginitis because of changes in their hormone levels. A drop in oestrogen can cause the vaginal lining to become dry and irritated. In addition, some women develop vaginitis following the use of vaginal sprays, perfumed soap, scented detergents and spermicides that contain nonoxynol-9.

PREVENTION

Some types of vaginitis can be prevented by the following practices:
- **PRACTISE GOOD HYGIENE** Clean the genital area daily with a mild, fragrance-free, non-irritating soap. Always rinse soap from the genital area and dry well.
- **LIMIT BATHS** Also avoid hot tubs and whirlpool spas.
- **WEAR COTTON UNDERWEAR** Wearing pants that are made of synthetic material and tights with synthetic crotches allows yeast to thrive in the moist environment of the vagina. Underwear should not be worn to bed.
- **AVOID SCENTED SANITARY TOWELS AND TAMPONS** The chemicals used to add fragrance to these products may irritate the vagina.
- **WIPE FROM FRONT TO BACK** After using the toilet and especially after bowel movements, the vaginal area should be wiped from front to back to avoid the spread of bacteria to the vagina.
- **NEVER DOUCHE** Douching disrupts the normal flora of the

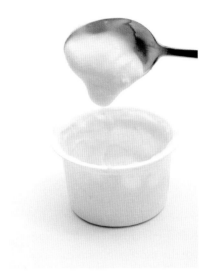

Eating yoghurt containing active lactobacillus cultures may prevent the development of recurrent vaginal yeast infections.

vagina and allows organisms to overgrow, which in turns causes infections to develop.
- **CONSUME YOGHURT CONTAINING ACTIVE LACTOBACILLUS CULTURES** These organisms inhabit the normal flora of the vagina and may discourage or prevent the development of recurrent vaginal yeast infections.
- **PRACTICE SAFER SEX** Condoms should be used to protect against STDs unless the relationship is a monogamous one in which both partners have tested negative for infection.

DIAGNOSIS

Vaginitis can be diagnosed using one or more of the following:
- **MEDICAL HISTORY** The doctor may as questions concerning symptoms and past vaginal infections or STDs.
- **PELVIC EXAMINATION** During this procedure, the physician examines the genital area for any discharge or lesions.
- **LABORATORY ANALYSIS** A doctor may collect samples of vaginal discharges and have them analysed in order to identify the cause of the vaginitis.

TREATMENTS

The treatment process for vaginitis depends on the cause of the inflammation. Bacterial vaginosis can be treated with metronidazole or clindamycin, drugs commonly prescribed to treat infections. These medications are available in the form of pills or vaginal gels and creams.
- **MEDICATION** Antifungal medications are also widely used to treat yeast infections. Creams and suppositories containing miconazole and clotrimazole are sometimes given to women suffering from a vaginal yeast infection. These are available by prescription or as over-the-counter preparations. Another option includes oral antifungal medications such as fluconazole.

Trichomoniasis can be treated with metronidazole pills. Antibiotics such as azithromycin, erythromycin, tetracycline or doxycycline are used to treat chlamydia.

There is no cure for herpes simplex virus and human papillomavirus. Doctors can prescribe antiviral medication such as acyclovir, famciclovir and valacyclovir to minimize discomfort and outbreaks. Topical medications or surgery can be used to remove genital warts.

See also: *STDs, pp.392–3* • *Menopause, pp.406–8* • *Diabetes, pp.338–41*

Infertility

A woman may be evaluated for infertility if after a year of unprotected intercourse she does not become pregnant. Many women do not experience any symptoms. Other women may have irregular menstrual periods as well as pain during menstruation or sexual intercourse.

CAUSES

Conception is a natural, yet complex, process. The timing of ovulation and fertilization must be exact. The process begins with a signal from the pituitary gland in a woman's brain. The pituitary gland produces follicle-stimulating hormone (FSH) and luteinizing hormone (LH), which stimulate the ovaries to release an egg, or ovum. Once it is released, the egg enters the fallopian tube and waits for a sperm with which to unite. If this occurs, the fertilized egg moves to the uterus, where it implants and develops into a baby over the next 40 weeks.

Approximately 40 percent of infertility is due to a male factor. If a woman is ovulating regularly and has a normal uterus and fallopian tubes, it is advisable that her partner have a semen analysis to check the number, appearance and movement of the sperm. Other factors can inhibit conception for women:

• AGE Fertility naturally decreases as women age. Peak fertility for women is in their twenties.

• DAMAGE TO THE FALLOPIAN TUBE Inflammation of the fallopian tube can lead to scarring that blocks

movement of the egg or sperm. Recurrent chlamydia infections are the most common cause of fallopian tube damage.

• ENDOMETRIOSIS This condition decreases the body's ability to transport, fertilize and implant a developing embryo (pp.402–3).

• POLYCYSTIC OVARY SYNDROME (PCOS) This disorder causes irregular periods and ovulation and sometimes hair growth and obesity (p.390).

• OVULATION DISORDERS Deficiencies in FSH and LH can cause female infertility.

• ELEVATED PROLACTIN High levels of prolactin – a hormone that stimulates breast milk production – are normal in pregnant and breast-feeding women. Excess amounts can affect a woman's ability to ovulate and may indicate the presence of a pituitary gland tumour.

• PREMATURE MENOPAUSE In rare cases, a woman's eggs may be depleted before the age of 35. This condition may be associated with smoking, chemotherapy, radiation therapy and autoimmune diseases that attack ovarian tissue.

• UTERINE FIBROIDS Benign tumours that grow in the walls of the uterus can alter the shape of the uterus

WHO IS AT RISK?

The risk factors include:

• Women in their 30s and 40s
• Smokers
• Women who consume large quantities of alcohol
• Over- or underweight
• Women who do not ovulate regularly

and block the fallopian tubes.

• PELVIC ADHESIONS Scar tissue can form in the pelvis. This prevents passage of eggs and sperm through the fallopian tubes and implantation in the uterus, and may occur as a result of endometriosis, or previous pelvic or intra-abdominal infections.

PREVENTION

Maintaining a healthy lifestyle is the best way to prevent infertility. This includes maintaining a healthy weight, following a moderate exercise routine, and limiting the use of medication and alcohol. Smoking and illicit drug use is known to impair a woman's ability to become pregnant. Practising safer sex will protect against complications of sexually transmitted diseases (pp.392–3). Fertility naturally declines as women age, so planning pregnancy is important.

DIAGNOSIS

A number of fertility tests are available. After performing a medical history and physical examination, the doctor may use one of the following to diagnose infertility:

• BASAL BODY TEMPERATURE A women may be asked to chart her waking body temperature to identify the days when she is ovulating.

• BLOOD TESTS These can confirm whether a woman is able to ovulate by monitoring hormone levels in the body, or whether one or more medical conditions are prohibiting ovulation.

• URINARY LUTEINIZING HORMONE DETECTOR KITs These tests may help a woman determine whether she is ovulating.

• HYSTEROSALPINGOGRAPHY This test is used to determine whether an egg is able to pass through the fallopian tubes to uterus. A special fluid is injected into the uterus. Using an X-ray to visualize the reproductive system, the doctor can identify any blockages.

• LAPAROSCOPY In this outpatient procedure, a slender tube with a lighted end is inserted into the abdomen. The doctor uses this test to examine the fallopian tubes, ovaries and uterus.

TREATMENTS

There are several treatments from which to choose.

• FERTILITY MEDICATION The most common treatment for female infertility is the use of fertility medication that regulates or induces ovulation. Clomiphene citrate helps the pituitary gland release FSH and LH, inducing ovulation. Human menopausal gonadotropin (hMG) contains both FSH and LH. This drug is used to stimulate the ovaries to produce more mature eggs. FSH

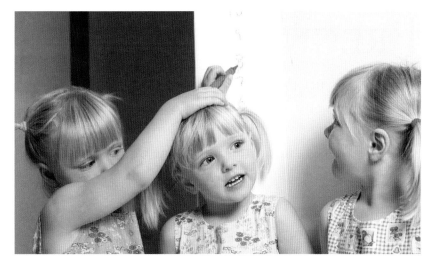
The use of fertility drugs can increase the chance of a woman having multiple births.

is sometimes given alone to stimulate the ovaries to produce mature egg follicles. Clomiphen, hMG and FSH are sometimes used in conjunction with human chorionic gonadotropin (hCG) to induce ovulation. Gonadotropin-releasing hormone (Gn-RH) analogues may be given along with hMG to prevent premature ovulation. Metformin can be used to boost ovulation in women with insulin resistance or bromocriptine to treat the overproduction of prolactin.

• SURGERY Blockages in the fallopian tubes may need to be removed.

• ASSISTED REPRODUCTIVE TECHNOLOGY (ART) This treatment consists of artificial insemination, in which the sperm is injected into the cervix or uterus, or in vitro fertilization, in which a fertilized egg is implanted within the uterus.

• VITAMINS AND SUPPLEMENTS Some nutritional supplements (pp.532–41) have been shown to aid fertility: vitamins C and E have been shown to increase fertility in women deficient in those vitamins. The amino acid L-arginine, when taken during in vitro fertilization,

may increase the success rate of conception. Vitex, also known as chastetree, is a herb that grows in Mediterranean countries and central Asia. Trials indicate that it can help correct deficiencies in the menstrual cycle and correct elevated levels of prolactin. Women with anaemia may also experience infertility; iron supplements may improve their chances conceiving.

• ACUPUNCTURE Treatment (pp.464–5) involves the placement of fine needles in specific sensory locations on the body. In studies using this technique, infertile women had increased success conceiving and suffered none of the side-effects associated with hormonal treatments.

• COUNSELLING Working on fertility is often very stressful for couples. Having a relaxation practice or going to counselling together to deal with stress in a healthy way also improves a couple's chances of becoming pregnant.

See also: *Pregnancy, pp.398–400* • *Menstrual Bleeding Disorders, pp.384–5* • *Polycystic Ovarian Disease, p.390*

PREGNANCY

Pregnancy occurs after a fertilized egg moves to the uterus, implants in the uterine lining, and then grows and develops into a baby. The process usually takes from 37 to 42 weeks. For a couple it is a normal, healthy time of significant physical, emotional, hormonal and life changes.

HEALTHY PREGNANCY

New demands are placed on a women's body during pregnancy. She should increase her daily calorie intake by 300 kcal during the first trimester, 400 kcal during the second trimester, and 500 kcal in the third trimester. Focus should be on fruit and vegetables (organic if possible), whole grains, and high-quality proteins such as lean meats, eggs and fish oils.

Omega-3 fatty acids (pp.252–3) are particularly important during the third trimester both for the developing baby's spinal cord, and for the mother. Decreased dietary levels of omega-3 fatty acids is associated with post-natal depression.

Pregnant and lactating women should limit the amount of cold water fish to one to two servings per week to avoid high mercury intake. There is no danger of mercury contamination in fish oil supplements.

Pregnant women should not eat soft unpasterized cheeses to avoid listeria infection. They should also limit the following to one or fewer serving per day: peanuts, peanut products, processed meats and artificial sweeteners. Tobacco and alcohol are unsafe during pregnancy.

Caffeine is associated with miscarriage, particularly in the first trimester. Large amounts of isoflavones are associated with infantile leukaemia. Normal dietary intake of isoflavones is generally safe in pregnancy, but concentrated forms, such as those in pills and powders should be avoided.

Pregnant women who have no problems with preterm labour or hypertension should maintain a moderate level of physical activity, such as prenatal yoga or walking 20 to 30 minutes daily. Women who were already atheletic before pregnancy may continue a more strenuous program with advice from their physician. While exercising, a pregnant woman's heart rate should not exceed 80 percent of her maximum heart rate. Women who maintain fitness while pregnant may lower their risk of gestational diabetes, restrict weight gain to the recommended 11–16 kg (25–35 lb), experience less back pain and improve postpartum recovery.

Regular massage (pp.468–73) by a certified pregnancy massage therapist can ease discomfort. Acupuncture has a long history of use during pregnancy to ease nausea and pain, to induce labour, and to turn babies from a breech position.

COMPLICATIONS

Some of the possible complications of pregnancy include:

• GESTATIONAL DIABETES MELLITUS This form of diabetes affects only pregnant women and develops when hormones produced by a pregnant woman to support the baby prevent the body from using insulin effectively. Eventually, the build-up of sugar in the mother's blood causes the condition.

In some women, gestational diabetes mellitus cannot be prevented. Others can decrease their risk by eating a balanced diet, exercising regularly and managing their weight gain. Those most at risk for the condition include women who are: obese; over the age of 30; African-American, American Indian, Hispanic, Asian-American or Pacific Islander.

Doctors check most pregnant women for gestational diabetes. To treat the condition, a doctor will design a healthy meal plan for the woman and recommend exercise. If diet and exercise do not return blood sugars to normal, medication will be prescribed to limit the body's blood glucose levels. Mind–body approaches for stress reduction may also be helpful in treating gestational diabetes mellitus.

• PRE-ECLAMPSIA AND ECLAMPSIA In pre-eclampsia, which occurs after 20 weeks of gestation, blood pressure increases, protein is excreted into the urine, and hands and feet swell. It can cause serious complications for the baby, including

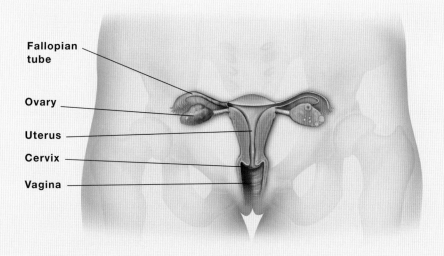

Fallopian tube

Ovary

Uterus

Cervix

Vagina

In pregnancy, the foetus develops in the uterus, which enlarges as the baby grows. During labour and delivery, the cervix dilates to around 10 cm, which allows the baby to pass through the vaginal canal, which also expands for delivery.

premature delivery, low birth weight, early separation of the placenta (abruption), low amniotic fluid levels (oligohydramnios), and rarely, stillbirth.

If pre-eclampsia is accompanied by seizures it is called eclampsia. Complications of severe pre-elampsia or eclampsia for the mother can include the risk of bleeding, liver and kidney damage, and rarely, brain damage or death.

Pre-eclampsia and eclampsia cannot be prevented; but proper prenatal care can prevent complications. During each prenatal visit, a doctor monitors the woman's blood pressure, weight and urine, and checks for the presence of pre-eclampsia. If found, blood tests may be ordered for a blood platelet count (cells that help the blood to clot) and liver and kidney functioning, which may be affected in severe pre-eclampsia.

Those at risk for pre-eclampsia and eclampsia include women who have a family history of the disorders, are younger than 20 or older than 35, are obese, are pregnant with more than one child or for the first time, or suffer from chronic high blood pressure (pp.236–9), diabetes (pp.338–41), kidney disease (p.308) or lupus (pp.324–5).

The best treatment for pre-eclampsia and eclampsia is the delivery of the baby. If it is too early in the pregnancy, bed rest, medication to lower blood pressure and steroids to help prepare the baby's lungs for birth may all be prescribed. During delivery, the mother may receive IV magnesium to decrease risk of seizure. Mind–body approaches to stress reduction may be particularly helpful.

• ECTOPIC PREGNANCY Normally, a fertilized egg implants itself in the lining of the uterus. If the implantation occurs outside the uterus, the condition is called an ectopic pregnancy. Ectopic pregnancies can cause life-threatening blood loss, because an embryo outside of the uterus cannot survive and can destroy the tissue in which it is implanted.

The causes of ectopic pregnancy are not always known, nor can one be prevented. However, those at increased risk include women who have had endometriosis; had surgery to any reproductive organ; had infection in the fallopian tube; have taken fertility drugs that stimulate ovulation (pp.396–7); or have experienced a previous ectopic pregnancy. Sexually transmitted diseases (pp.392–3) and pelvic inflammatory disease (p.409) can damage the reproductive organs and lead to ectopic pregnancies.

An ectopic pregnancy must be removed. In its early stages, an injection of methotrexate stops cell growth and dissolves the existing cells. During the later stages of an ectopic pregnancy, the embryo is surgically removed. If the fallopian tube ruptures from the pressure of the growing embryo, immediate surgery is required as this is a life-threatening situation.

• PLACENTA PRAEVIA This condition occurs if the placenta (an organ that provides nutrients for the growing foetus) implants in the lower region of the uterus, covering part or all of the cervix.

The symptoms of placenta praevia may include spotting during the first and second trimesters of pregnancy, and heavy vaginal bleeding during the third trimester. Causes of placenta praevia can include multiple gestations, prior uterine surgery and multiple prior pregancies. There is no way to prevent placenta praevia.

An ultrasound is used to diagnosis placenta praevia. During the procedure, the doctor can determine whether the placenta is covering the cervix as well as the position of the foetus.

The doctor may recommend bed rest and that a woman avoid having intercourse to prevent bleeding. In addition, the doctor may replace blood with a transfusion, and prescribe medication to prevent labour.

Mind–body approaches such as visualization and guided imagery may be particularly helpful during this time to reduce stress. After 36 to 37 weeks of gestation, or if heavy vaginal bleeding is endangering the mother or baby, the baby is delivered via caesarean section.

Among those at increased risk of developing placenta praevia are women who have already had children; had uterine fibroids removed, had a caesarean section or are over the age of 35.

LABOUR AND DELIVERY

The signs of labour include persistent lower back pain, rupture of the membranes or passage of the mucous plug that blocks the cervix, and the opening or dilation of the cervix by strong, consistent uterine contractions.

Depending on the condition and health of the mother, birthing options include the following.

• VAGINAL BIRTH The muscles of uterus contract to push the baby through the cervix and vaginal canal, which widens to allow room for the baby to pass.

• VACUUM ASSISTED VAGINAL BIRTH A suction device is placed on the baby's head and helps it pass through the vaginal canal.

• FORCEPS ASSISTED VAGINAL BIRTH The obstetrician gently guides the baby through the vaginal canal using forceps.

• CAESAREAN SECTION This is a surgical procedure in which an incision is made in the abdominal wall and the uterus through which the baby is delivered. After delivery, the uterus is repaired, and the rest of the layers of the abdominal wall are closed.

• OTHER MEASURES During labour and delivery, some women request pain relief medication and/or use techniques such as breathing exercises to manage pain. Supportive relationships are particularly important. Many women want a partner or family member with them as they go through the process of labour and delivery.

It is normal for the phase known as early labour to last for up to 24 hours in a first pregnancy. Once a woman is in active labour, the cervix normally dilates 1 cm (0.5 in) per hour. It is normal for the 'pushing' phase to last two to three hours. During this time, active emotional and physical support are needed.

Women who are in healthy early labour may eat and drink lightly, but should avoid heavy and spicy foods. Nausea and vomiting are common in active labour. Clear liquids and ice cubes are usually recommended during this time.

Women who are able to have acupuncture during labour may have shorter labours and less pain. Back massage and support can also be helpful. Although no large studies support this, some women report increased pain control with the use of hypnosis during labour.

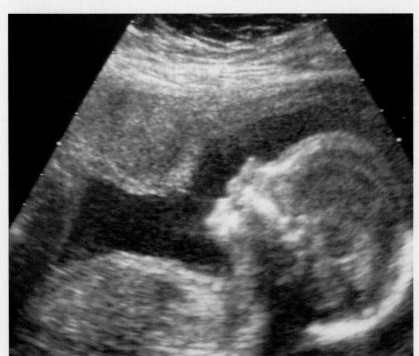

An ultrasound is a test performed during pregnancy to produce a picture of the foetus, the placenta (a temporary organ that nourishes the baby) and the amniotic sac, a fluid-filled membrane that surrounds and protects the baby during pregnancy.

See also: *Substance Abuse, pp.358–60 • High Blood Pressure, pp.236–9 • Yoga, pp.476–9*

Chronic Pelvic Pain

Steady or recurring pain in the lower abdomen area that lasts more than six months and interferes with a woman's daily life is termed chronic pelvic pain. Women with this condition may experience pain during sexual intercourse and with bowel movements.

CAUSES

Among the causes of chronic pelvic pain are intense levels of life stress, a history of abuse, anxiety or depression. Endometriosis (pp.402–3), fibroids (p.391), chronic pelvic inflammatory disease (p.409), irritable bowel syndrome (pp.270–1) and interstitial cystitis can also cause the condition.

PREVENTION

The best way to prevent chronic pelvic pain is to learn and use self-relaxation, stress relief and safe sex practices. Caring for one's body with good nutrition (pp.586–97), exercise and body work such as massage (pp.468–73) is important. In addition, medical conditions should be treated immediately to avoid further complications.

DIAGNOSIS

The diagnosis of chronic pelvic pain involves a process of elimination as doctors try to pinpoint the responsible condition. During a detailed medical history, the doctor asks questions about the severity of the pain, when it usually occurs, and what helps the pain to subside.

A pelvic examination allows the doctor to identify abnormal areas. The cervix and vagina are also cultured to check for infections such as chlamydia, herpes and gonorrhoea (STDs, pp.392–3). Imaging techniques allow the doctor to see abnormal tissues. A laparoscopy allows the doctor to inspect the abdomen and pelvis area. A long, thin instrument with a light and video camera on the end is inserted into the pelvic region in outpatient surgery. Other useful imaging tools include ultrasound, computerized tomography (CT) scans and magnetic resonance imaging (MRI).

TREATMENTS

The treatment regimen is designed around the cause of the pain and may include the following.
 • PAIN MEDICATION Including aspirin, ibuprofen, and paracetamol.
 • HORMONE OR GNRH (GONODOTRO-PIN-RELEASING HORMONE) AGONISTS THERAPY Birth-control pills can prevents chronic pelvic pain by halting ovulation.
 • ANTIBIOTICS Infections, such as STDs, are treated with antibiotics.
 • NERVE SEPARATION Nerve tissue can be removed surgically, destroyed with heat or lasers, or

desensitized using injections of certain medications to numb pain.
 • SURGERY Hysterectomy or less invasive surgeries to remove endometriosis lesions, remove fibroids or fallopian tubes damaged by infection might eliminate underlying causes of chronic pelvic pain.
 • PHYSICAL THERAPY Exercises to strengthen the pelvic muscles, massage, stretching and applications of heat and cold packs can help reduce chronic pelvic pain.
 • COUNSELLING Regular therapy can help a woman identify and deal with stress or depression.
 • ANTIDEPRESSANTS Tricyclic antidepressants, such as amitriptyline and nortriptyline, can treat clinical depression and chronic pain.
 • ACUPUNCTURE has been shown in several studies to improve pain symptoms in women suffering from chronic pelvic pain.

See also: Depression, pp.364–5 • Massage, pp.468–73 • Health and Healing Guidelines, pp.586–97

Endometriosis

The ovaries release eggs and produce the female hormones oestrogen and progesterone. These hormones help prepare the uterus for the implantation of a fertilized egg. At the beginning of the menstrual cycle, hormone levels increase; that signals the uterus to thicken its inner lining, making it easier for a fertilized egg to adhere inside the womb.

If pregnancy does not occur, hormone levels drop, and the thickened lining is shed from the body during menstrual bleeding.

Endometriosis occurs when the tissues that make up the inner lining of the uterus, the endometrium, begin to grow outside of the uterus in areas such as the fallopian tubes, ovaries, the outer layer of the uterus or the lining of the pelvis. The endometrial tissue outside of the uterus still responds to oestrogen and progesterone, causing it to grow and thicken each month. It also results in bleeding; however, there is no mechanism for the blood from displaced endometrial tissue to be released from the body. Often the trapped blood forms cysts that later develop into scar tissue and adhesions. The trapped blood also irritates surrounding tissue, which may cause severe pain.

It is estimated that 40 percent of women with endometriosis are infertile. Some women discover that they have endometriosis when seeking treatment for infertility. Infertility may occur because scar tissue and adhesions produced from endometriosis prevent the egg from leaving the ovary moving through the fallopian tubes. Inflammation caused by the displaced uterine lining may result in a less ideal environment for fertilization. If pregnancy is achieved, it often helps alleviate some of the symptoms of endometriosis.

CAUSES

The cause of endometriosis is unclear, but there are four theories: first, that endometrial cells travel backward in the fallopian tubes, adhere there and begin to grow; second, that the bloodstream transports endometrial cells to locations outside of the inner lining of the uterus; third, that some cells in the abdomen are able to develop into endometrial cells; and finally, that endometriosis is genetic and runs in families.

PREVENTION

Endometriosis is prevented when the menstrual cycle is inhibited, for instance during pregnancy and the use of oral contraceptives.

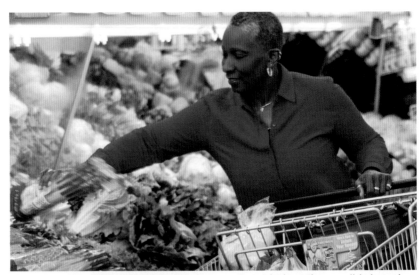

Although making dietary changes will not cure endometriosis, eating a well-balanced and healthy diet of fruit, vegetables, whole grains and high-quality protein will improve overall health, helping the body cope with the condition.

WHO IS AT RISK?

The risk factors include:
- All women, especially those who have not had children

Women who have given birth are at a decreased risk of developing endometriosis.

DIAGNOSIS

The symptoms of endometriosis can range from mild to severe. In fact, some women with endometriosis have no symptoms. Other women experience pelvic pain and cramping before their period begins. This pain sometimes radiates to the lower back and abdominal area. Women with endometriosis have also reported that they experience pain during ovulation, sexual intercourse, urination and bowel movements.

Endometriosis is diagnosed using the following techniques:

• MEDICAL HISTORY The doctor may ask questions about the location and severity of the pain, as well as the time of month it is usually experienced. In addition, questions about menstrual bleeding provide valuable information during the diagnosis process.

• PHYSICAL EXAMINATION During a pelvic examination, the doctor will look for cysts and scar tissue that may be located on the reproductive organs.

• TRANS-VAGINAL ULTRASOUND Images of the reproductive organs are produced that may indicate the presence of cysts, adhesions and scar tissue. During this procedure, a thin cylindrical device is inserted into the vagina. The device produces sound waves that are analysed by a computer to provide images.

• GNRH (GONODOTROPIN-RELEASING HORMONE AGONIST THERAPY) This is an injection that puts the ovaries at rest, simulating menopause.

It lasts for one to three months. If a women's pain improves with this treatment, it is considered diagnostic of endometriosis. Side-effects of the medication include hot flushes like those experienced with menopause; these can be controlled with progesterone and/or oestrogen.

• LAPAROSCOPY A laparoscope, a slender tube with a camera on one end, is inserted into the pelvic area through a small incision. The surgeon uses this device to look for damage to the reproductive organs that may have been caused by endometriosis.

TREATMENTS

A woman, working with her doctor, can choose the best treatment option depending on the severity of her signs and symptoms. These may include the following:

• APPLICATION OF HEAT Hot baths, warm compresses, and heating pads can help relax the muscles, thereby minimizing pelvic pain and cramping.

• PAIN MEDICATION Non-steroidal anti-inflammatory pain medication can help relieve cramping and pelvic pain. Depending on the severity of the pain, prescription-strength doses may be needed.

• LIFESTYLE INTERVENTION Studies have shown that women who maintain a regular exercise regimen, participate in a relaxation practice such as meditation, and/ or have acupuncture treatments (pp.464–5) experience less pain and possibly improved fertility.

• HORMONE THERAPY Oral contraceptives, progesterone, gonadotropin-releasing hormone (GN-RH) agonists and danazol may be

used to help alleviate the symptoms associated with endometriosis by inhibiting ovulation and the menstrual cycle.

• LAPAROSCOPIC SURGERY After finding the location of the affected tissues with the use of a laparoscope, a surgeon uses heat or a laser to treat any cysts, adhesions or scar tissue within the reproductive system.

• HYSTERECTOMY During this surgical procedure, the uterus, fallopian tubes and ovaries are removed. This option is used only for women who are no longer of childbearing age, wish to have no future pregnancies, or if there are no other options available to treat severe cases of endometriosis.

See also: *Menstrual Bleeding Disorders, pp.384–5* • *Acupuncture, pp.464–5* • *Infertility, pp.396–7*

Clinical Query

My teenage daughter often complains of painful periods. She sometimes misses school because of the severity of the pain. Is it possible for a young girl to have endometriosis?

Yes. Any female of childbearing age can develop endometriosis. In fact, many teenage girls experience endometriosis. It is important to have your daughter examined by a gynaecologist or family doctor as soon as possible to prevent the occurrence of further complications such as infertility. Your doctor will know the best way to treat this condition in young women.

Hirsutism

In the condition called hirsutism, dark, thick hair grows on the face, chest, stomach and back. Generally, hirsutism first appears during puberty and tends to run in families.

CAUSES

Hirsutism can result from elevated levels of male hormones in a woman's body, which can be caused by certain conditions, including polycystic ovary syndrome (p.390), Cushing's syndrome (p.342), congenital adrenal hyperplasia, and tumours in the ovaries or adrenal gland. Some women with hirsutism have hair follicles that are simply sensitive to the normal amounts of testosterone and other male hormones in their bodies. Medication such as birth-control pills, hormones and anabolic steroids can also cause the development of hirsutism in women.

PREVENTION

Maintaining a healthy weight may help prevent hirsutism. Obesity (pp.348–9) is associated with an elevation in levels of male hormones in the body. Medication that cause hirsutism, such as body-building steroids should be avoided to minimize unwanted hair growth.

DIAGNOSIS

A woman's menstrual cycle gives important clues during the diagnosis of hirsutism. For example, excessive hair growth in women with regular periods is usually due to genetic factors. Excessive hair growth in conjunction with irregular menstrual cycles may be an indication of a more serious complication such as polycystic ovary syndrome or a tumour of the ovaries or adrenal glands.

Blood tests are used to diagnosis the underlying cause of hirsutism. Hormone levels of testosterone and dehydroepiandrosterone (DHEA) and 17 alpha-hydroxy progesterone (17-OHP) are measured to determine whether a woman has polycystic ovary syndrome, ovarian tumours, adrenal gland tumours or adrenal gland hyperplasia. Prolactin levels are also evaluated. The test provides the doctor with information that may point to a tumour in the pituitary gland. A steroid suppression test may be performed to evaluate for Cushing's syndrome. In addition, glucose and cholesterol levels are checked because hirsutism has been associated with both diabetes and elevated levels of cholesterol.

TREATMENTS

Depending on the cause, a woman's doctor may recommend one of the following treatment options:

• WEIGHT LOSS Losing weight and maintaining a healthy diet can decrease male hormone levels in women and reduce hair growth.

• BIRTH-CONTROL PILLS Combination pills of oestrogen and progesterone can minimize the effects and decrease the production of male hormones by the ovaries.

• ANTI-ANDROGEN MEDICATION This medication counteracts male hormones and reduces excessive hair growth.

• HAIR REMOVAL Many hair removal techniques are available – plucking, shaving, waxing, bleaching and using hair removal creams. These techniques must be repeated for continued success and in some instances can cause skin irritation. More effective hair removal treatments include laser hair removal and electrolysis. During laser hair removal, light is used to generate heat within the hair follicles, destroying the ability of hair to grow within the follicle. Electrolysis also prevents hair growth in the follicles. It involves the use of electricity to destroy the ability of the follicle to function.

See also: *Polycystic Ovary Syndrome, p.390* • *Obesity, pp.348–9*

WHO IS AT RISK?

The risk factors include:

- Women with a family history of hirsutism
- Women with polycystic ovary syndrome
- Women with tumours in the ovaries or adrenal glands

Female Sexual Dysfunction

Female sexuality involves a complex array of factors encompassing the emotional, the psychosocial and the physical – which in turn involves the neurologic, vascular and endocrine systems. A disruption in any of these can result in female sexual dysfunction (FSD), a common condition.

Woman with FSD are divided into four categories: those with a lack of sex drive; those with an adequate sex drive who experience difficulty in becoming aroused or remaining aroused during sexual activity; those who have difficulty in achieving orgasm; and those who experience pain during sexual stimulation or vaginal contact.

CAUSES

FSD can be caused by physical or psychological problems, social issues or hormonal imbalances. Arthritis (pp.136–9), fatigue, headaches (pp.166–7), multiple sclerosis (pp.182–3), urinary problems (pp.302–3), bowel conditions (pp.266–7, 270–1) and recovery from pelvic surgery or trauma can cause FSD. Medication including antidepressants, blood pressure medications (pp.236–9), antihistamines and chemotherapy drugs can exacerbate it. Psychosocial issues include poor body image, relationship problems, stress, depression (pp.364–5), cultural and religious norms, and past or ongoing abuse.

Oestrogen and testosterone deficiency, which may occur after menopause or hysterectomy, can cause changes to the genitals that reduce sensitivity and cause pain. In these cases, the vaginal lining may become thin and have difficulty in becoming lubricated. Low levels of these hormones may also diminish sexual desire.

PREVENTION

FSD cannot always be prevented. But maintaining a healthy weight and regular exercise can contribute to a positive body image and enhanced sexual desire. Recognizing that the sexual response is a mind–body connection may help a woman and her partner deal openly with relationship issues. Allowing adequate time for sexual arousal helps prevent sexual dysfunction.

DIAGNOSIS

The initial steps of diagnosis involve a medical history and physical examination. The medical history helps the doctor pinpoint the dysfunction and its cause. A physical examination of the genital area may identify any diseases or abnormalities. Cultures and vaginal samples are obtained if the doctor suspects vaginitis, cervical infection, or inflammation.

Pelvic floor tenderness may indicate either involuntary contraction of the vaginal muscles (vaginismus) or a chronic inflammation of the vestibular glands (vestibulitis).

TREATMENTS

Treatment depends on the condition's cause, and may include:

• HORMONE REPLACEMENT THERAPY Oestrogen or testosterone levels may be restored.

• PHYSICAL THERAPY Kegel exercises (p.507) strengthen the vaginal muscles. Exercise and vaginal dilators can be used to treat vaginismus.

• PSYCHOTHERAPY Social or psychological issues contributing to the dysfunction are addressed. The doctor may also recommend sex education and relaxation techniques.

• OTHER MEDICATION Women with vestibulitis may respond to high dose steroid creams, treatment for yeast infections or low doses of antidepressant medication.

See also: Depression, pp.364–5 • Obesity, pp.348–9 • Vaginitis, pp.394–5

WHO IS AT RISK?

The risk factors include:

- Women who have been abused
- Women with a history of depression
- Women undergoing chemotherapy or on medication causing sexual side-effects

---

MENOPAUSE

Menopause is a transitional period marked by hormonal, physical and psychosocial changes in a woman. It occurs naturally, usually between the ages of 45 and 55. This is a powerful time of reflection for many women, frequently corresponding with life changes involving career and personal goals. It is a time to consider all dimensions of a woman's health and well-being.

There are two phases to the physical process—peri-menopause and menopause. Peri-menopause is the time in which symptoms begin and hormone levels fluctuate. It is normal for this phase to last for several years. A woman is still ovulating during peri-menopause, although her menstrual cycles may become increasingly irregular. Menopause is defined by a woman's periods stopping for twelve consecutive months. A menopausal woman's ovaries do not release eggs so produce a decreased amount of oestrogen and progesterone.

A TIME OF CHANGE

Many women experience few, if any, uncomfortable symptoms during peri-menopause and menopause. Others may experience some or all of the following.

• IRREGULAR PERIODS Women in peri-menopause may experience heavy bleeding at some times, periods that are closer together or many months apart, prolonged periods of more than ten days, shorter periods of fewer days with lighter bleeding, and spotting between periods.

• HOT FLUSHES Due to sudden drops in oestrogen levels, some women experience a feeling of warmth that radiates upwards from the chest to the head. This may cause perspiration followed by chills that are caused by the evaporation of the perspiration. Hot flushes can also cause the face to flush and blotchy red areas to appear on the chest, neck and arms.

• DECREASED FERTILITY Peri-menopausal fluctuations in hormone levels cause ovulation to occur less frequently. A woman can still become pregnant during peri-menopause, but it is less likely.

• VAGINAL DRYNESS A decline in oestrogen levels causes the vaginal lining to become dry and thin, losing its elasticity. This can cause burning and itching. Some women may experience pain and discomfort during sexual intercourse.

• INCONTINENCE The urge to urinate frequently and having trouble holding one's urine are symptoms sometimes associated with menopause.

• DIFFICULTY SLEEPING Hot flushes and night sweats make sleeping very difficult.

• BREAST CHANGES Some women's breasts become more tender during menopause.

• WEIGHT GAIN Sometimes women can experience a 2.25–5.5 kg (5–10lb) weight gain during the perimenopause phase. Other women experience a change in the distribution of their weight from the hips and thighs to the abdominal area.

• HAIR LOSS AND SKIN WRINKLES These may develop at an accelerated pace.

• FACIAL HAIR Although the body's oestrogen levels decline, it continues to produce trace amounts of the male sex hormone testosterone, which can cause course hair to grow on the chin, upper lip, chest and stomach.

• EMOTIONAL ISSUES Stress, fatigue, anxiety, irritability and the inability to concentrate and remember some things can occur.

Clinical Query

I began to experience the symptoms of menopause a few months ago. It is true that I no longer need to be concerned about getting pregnant?

No, it is important to emphasize that peri-menopausal women can still become pregnant. Women experiencing the symptoms of menopause should continue to practise birth control if they do not wish to become pregnant. In addition, although postmenopausal women cannot become pregnant, they are still susceptible to sexually transmitted diseases and should practise safer sex techniques.

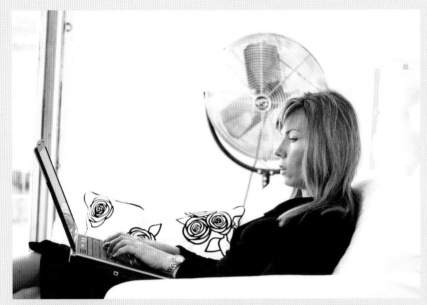

Hot flushes are one of the most discussed symptoms associated with menopause. As warmth spreads through the body, perspiration begins. As the perspiration evaporates, the woman begins to feel chilled. Fortunately, therapies exist to ease this symptom.

These symptoms are frequently associated with or exacerbated by disturbed sleep.

WHY IT HAPPENS

Menopause is a natural process experienced by all women. It occurs because the ovaries deplete their eggs and decrease production of the female hormones oestrogen and progesterone, which regulate the menstrual cycle.

Women in their late thirties usually begin to experience a decline in progesterone production. These women may also find it difficult to become pregnant, because their eggs are less likely to become fertilized.

HEALTH DURING MENOPAUSE

Menopause is a natural, powerful time in a woman's life. Choices of care regarding menopausal symptoms, bone, heart and breast protection should be individualized and reevaluated as personal goals and symptoms change, and as new research data becomes available. An integrative approach that prioritizes effective lifestyle choices – including nutrition, exercise, as well as mind–body approaches – is essential, whether the treatment approach is hormone replacement therapy (HRT) or herbal preparations.

Becoming an active partner with one's healthcare provider, making well-informed decisions, and being mindful that much is still unknown about this area of healthcare, will help a woman make choices that support her optimal vitality and well-being.

Until recently, hormone therapy has been a common therapy for easing menopausal symptoms. A study conducted by the Women's Health Initiative (WHI) of more than 16,000 women that was funded by the National Institutes of Health (NIH), found that women taking a certain combination of oestrogen and progesterone had increased risk for suffering heart attack, stroke and breast cancer. Although these findings are quite alarming, it is important to understand that fewer than 0.01 percent of the participants of the study experienced adverse affects each year. It is also unknown whether and how risks differ with different hormone preparations.

Hormone therapy may still be a viable option for many women, but they should discuss the risks and the benefits with their doctor before beginning treatment.

Oestrogen therapy can help some women control hot flushes and vaginal dryness and other discomfort. The lowest possible dose is usually provided to patients, and treatment may be weaned after the first three to five years of menopause, the period of greatest symptoms and bone loss.

Many types of hormone replacement therapies are available today. Popular formulations include bio-identical hormones, which are often called natural hormones, of estradiol, estrone, estriol, and progesterone. In addition, some women find that their symptoms are alleviated with the addition of small amounts of testosterone. Some of these formulations are available through conventional pharmacies; others are made available through compounding pharmacies – pharmacies that prepare customized medication for clients. These formulations are available in many different forms including pills, patches, creams, vaginal rings and suppositories.

Other treatments that may be used to minimize the discomfort experienced during menopause include the following.

• **MIND–BODY THERAPY** Stress can increase the intensity, frequency and discomfort of hot flushes. Inducing the relaxation response can be very effective in decreasing these symptoms and increasing a sense of self-control. Mind–body interventions to consider include breathing exercises (pp.526–7), progressive muscle relaxation (pp.474–5), meditation (pp.514–19), yoga (pp.476–9), diary-writing and music and art (pp.491–3).

• **EXERCISE** Doing 30 minutes of aerobic, weight-bearing exercise (such as walking or jogging) 5 to 6 days per week, has been shown to decrease the risk of heart disease (pp.230–3), osteoporosis (pp.146–7), and obesity (pp.348–9), and to improve positive mood and effective sleep.

• **NUTRITION** Food is a potent and frequently underused component of well-being, particularly during menopause. Reducing consumption of alcohol, hot and spicy foods, caffeine, and tobacco can manage symptoms (pp.586–97).

• **PHYTOESTROGENS** Isoflavones and lignans are naturally occurring

CAUTION

The following women should not undergo hormone therapy during menopause:
• Women with breast or uterine cancer
• Women who have had a stroke or heart attack
• Women who tend to develop blood clots

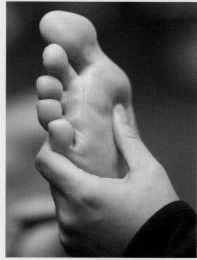
Some women find that reflexology can help ease some of the symptoms associated with menopause.

oestrogens found in foods such as soybeans, chickpeas, flaxseed, whole grains, and some fruit and vegetables. Although studies remain inconclusive, some women report that eating these foods eases symptoms, especially those of hot flashes. The mixed results of these studies are likely due to the difference among women's bodies in their ability to digest the isoflavones to their active components. Taking 30–60 g/day affects symptoms and 90 g/day affects bone loss.

Keep in mind that the role of increased use of phytoestrogens in post-menopausal women is controversial. Excessive use of phytoestrogens may increase the risk of hormonally sensitive cancers (breast and uterine) and blood-clotting.

• **VAGINAL OESTROGEN** Combinations of oestrogen in suppository, cream or ring form can be inserted into the vagina to relieve dryness, incontinence and discomfort that occurs during sexual intercourse.

• **VITAMINS** Calcium, magnesium and vitamin D will reduce perimenopause or menopause symptoms as well as slow bone loss.

• **HERBAL COMBINATIONS** Many women report that the use of herbs including black cohosh, dong quai, chastetree berry, evening primrose oil and red clover helps to reduce discomfort experienced with menopause. The use of black cohosh has the most support from scientific studies which show best results with the herb at a dose of 20–80 mg/day. Studies of the other preparations have been mixed.

• **ANTIDEPRESSANTS** Low doses of antidepressants may help decrease hot flushes in menopausal women.

• **CLONIDINE** Distributed in patch or pill form, this medication can reduce the number of hot flushes that occur during menopause.

• **LUBRICANTS** Use water-based personal lubricants to alleviate vaginal dryness.

POSSIBLE COMPLICATIONS

Menopause is associated with a number of health complications. As oestrogen levels decrease, cholesterol levels may increase, putting a woman at risk for developing cardiovascular disease (pp.234–5), high blood pressure (pp.236–9), and stroke (pp.168–9). Bone density begins to decline, increasing risk of osteoporosis (pp.146–7), a disorder in which bones may become brittle and break. Hip, wrist, and spine fractures are more common among post-menopausal women.

See also: *Menstrual Bleeding Disorders, pp.384–5 • Anxiety, pp.354–5 • Cardiovascular Disease, pp.234–5*

Pelvic Inflammatory Disease

An infection of the female reproductive organs such as the uterus, fallopian tubes, or ovaries can cause serious life-long complications. The condition is called pelvic inflammatory disease (PID). Left untreated, this condition can result in the formation of extensive scar tissue, that partially or completely blocks the fallopian tubes.

The blocking of the fallopian tubes in turn prevents the passage of the ovum (egg) and sperm. As a result, a woman may become infertile or experience ectopic pregnancies (pp.398–400). In addition, the damage to tissues from the infection can lead to chronic pelvic pain (p.401).

CAUSES

PID occurs when bacteria travels up through the vagina and through the cervix to the uterus and fallopian tubes. Sexually transmitted diseases (STDs, pp.392–3) such as chlamydia and gonorrhoea account for the majority of PID cases. PIDs also develop without exposure to an STD, because bacteria that normally inhabit the vaginal area can cause the infection. Why this occurs is unclear; but douching changes the environment of the vagina, allowing harmful bacteria to grow. Douching can also force bacteria to flow up the reproductive tract.

Less common causes of PID include infections after childbirth, miscarriage, abortion or the use of IUDs (pp.410–11).

PREVENTION

The best ways to prevent PID are to practise sexual abstinence, limit the number of sexual partners, and practise safer sex with the consistent use of male latex condoms.

DIAGNOSIS

Symptoms of PID include abdominal pain, an unusual vaginal discharge that is often green or yellow with an unpleasant odour, irregular menstrual cycles, pain during sexual intercourse or a pelvic examination, a temperature, chills, nausea and vomiting. Unfortunately, PID is often unrecognized due to the

WHO IS AT RISK?

The risk factors include:
- Sexually active women, especially under age 25
- Women with sexually transmitted diseases (STDs)
- Women with multiple sex partners
- Women whose sex partner has multiple sex partners
- Women who douche

mild symptoms or no symptoms at all, even though it severely damages the female reproductive system.

During a pelvic examination, the doctor will look for pain, fever and abnormal cervical or vaginal discharge. Gonorrhoea or chlamydia tests may be ordered. The doctor may need to visualize the reproductive organs by using a pelvic ultrasound or laparoscopy, which allows a view of the internal organs and take tissue samples as well.

TREATMENTS

Antibiotics are used to treat PID. Usually more than one antibiotic is prescribed to cover a range of infectious organisms. When PID is caused by an STD, a woman and her partner should be treated to prevent reinfection during sexual relations. Occasionally, surgery is required to drain a pelvic abscess or remove scar tissue.

See also: *Pregnancy, pp.398–400 • Fever, p.318 • Nausea and Vomiting, pp.274–5*

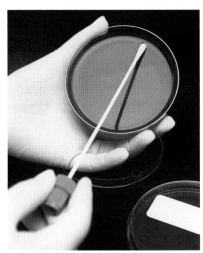

In a vaginal culture, vaginal fluids are transferred to a slide or petri dish and examined under a microscope.

BIRTH CONTROL

Birth control is used to prevent unintended pregnancy. Conception is a complex process that involves both the female and male reproductive systems. Each month an egg or ovum is released from the woman's ovaries and begins to travel through the fallopian tubes.

During sexual intercourse, the ejaculate from the penis contains sperm. The sperm enters the vagina and can travel to the ovum and fertilize it in the fallopian tube. The fertilized egg then travels to the uterus and implants in the uterine lining. Each birth-control method seeks to inhibit one or more of the steps needed for contraception to occur.

Many birth-control methods are available (some are explained below). Each option has advantages and disadvantages that may impact a woman's and her partner's life. Choices about birth control are personal decisions that many women make with input from their partners and gynaecologists.

Condoms and Spermicide
Usually made of latex, plastic or animal skin, the condom covers an erect penis before sexual intercourse. It holds the ejaculate of the male and prevents the sperm from reaching an ovum.

The condom is about 85 percent effective in preventing pregnancy. Improper use, breakage and slippage are the primary reasons that condoms fail.

The chief advantage of the latex condom is that is reduces the risk of the spread of sexually transmitted diseases (STDs, pp.392–3) such as HIV (pp.316–17). Condoms made from animal skin do not protect against STDs because tiny pores allow the passage of viruses and bacteria.

Spermicides can be used alone or with a condom. They are available in the form of foams, creams, gels, suppositories and vaginal films. Most spermicides containing nonoxynol-9 prevent conception by killing sperm before it can reach the uterus. Spermicides are about 70 percent effective in preventing pregnancy if used alone.

Spermicides do not protect against STDs. In fact, they may increase the likelihood of contracting a STD because they can

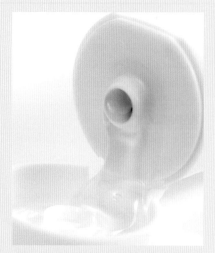

When choosing lubricants for condoms, make sure to select one that is water-based; others can damage a condom.

irritate the skin of the vagina. In addition, the use of spermicides can lead to increased risk of vaginal infections, because chemicals in the spermicides disrupt the bacterial environment usually found within the vagina.

Diaphragm, Cervical Cap, Sponge
These devices prevent pregnancy by providing a shield over the cervix, the opening to the uterus, and inhibiting the entrance of the sperm. The diaphragm is a dome-shaped rubber cup. Its flexible outer rim allows the diaphragm to be squeezed and inserted in the vagina, where it is placed on top of the cervix. The cervical cap is also rubber, but it is smaller and shaped like a thimble. Both the diaphragm and the cervical cap must be properly sized and fitted by a medical practitioner. The cervix can change shape after childbirth or if a woman loses or gains more than 4.5 kg (10 lb). In these cases, a new size may be needed.

The sponge is a soft, disk-shaped device that is manufactured from polyurethane foam. In addition to blocking the cervix, it can absorb semen and releases small amounts of spermicide.

Each of these devices is approximately 85 percent effective in preventing pregnancy but none provides protection from STDs. Furthermore, with extended use the risk of urinary tract infections, vaginal infections, and toxic shock syndrome is slightly higher with the use of these devices. Some women experience allergic reactions to the materials used to make these devices and may experience vaginal dryness as well.

Hormonal Methods

The birth-control pill, skin patches, vaginal rings, and hormone injections all work through the use of hormones, such as oestrogen and progesterone, which regulate the menstrual cycle. They work to prevent pregnancy by inhibiting ovulation, decreasing uterine lining build-up, and thickening cervical mucus. These hormones can be ingested in pill form, absorbed transdermally through a skin patch or vaginal ring, or injected intramuscularly.

The birth control pill is available in a combination formula of both oestrogen and progesterone and in a progesterone-only version. A woman must take it daily for it to be effective.

The skin patch contains both oestrogen and progesterone. It must be changed weekly. The vaginal ring also releases oestrogen and progesterone through the vagina and is left in place for three weeks each month. Injection of progesterone provides protection from pregnancy for up to three months.

These birth-control methods are popular and are approximately 99 percent effective in preventing pregnancy. They do not protect against STDs.

Natural Family Planning

This is also called the rhythm method. Women who use this technique check their temperature before getting up every morning

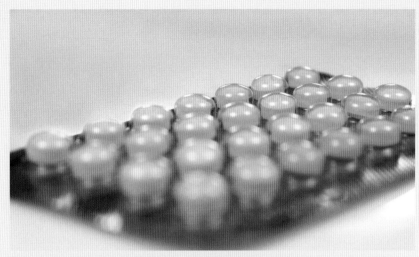

To work effectively, birth-control pills must be taken regularly. Some newer forms of the pill limit a woman's period to only four times each year.

and also the consistency of their cervical mucus to predict ovulation. Couples who choose this method have sex only on less-fertile days. The method is 80–87 percent effective. It does not provide protection from STDs. Natural family planning takes time and dedication on the part of both the woman and her partner.

IUD

The IUD, or intrauterine device, is a T-shaped apparatus placed inside the uterus. Some IUDs contain hormones that prevent ovulation. The nonhormonal IUD can be associated with heavier, crampier periods. The progesterone-containing IUD is effective for five years and results in less uterine lining build-up and light to absent periods. It is more than 99 percent effective, but does not protect against STDs.

Tubal Ligation

This birth-control choice is permanent and difficult to reverse. During tubal ligation, the fallopian tubes are cut and tied or cauterized to prevent the passage of an ovum or sperm. This is done at an outpatient surgery or in the hospital after delivery of a baby.

This method is 98 percent effective, but does not provide protection against STDs. If it fails and a woman becomes pregnant, she needs to be evaluated for an ectopic pregnancy (a pregnancy outside the uterus).

VASECTOMY

This permanent method of birth-control for men is a minor surgical procedure that prevents sperm from exiting the testes. During the procedure, a small incision is made in the upper part of the scrotum, and then the vasa deferentia, the tubes through which sperm travels from the testicles to the semen, are sealed. Vasectomy is 99 percent effective in preventing pregnancy, but does not protect against STDs. In some cases, vasectomy is reversible.

See also: Vaginitis, pp.394–5 • STDs, pp.392–3 • Urinary Tract Infections, pp.302–3

Cancer

A number of cancers affect the female reproductive system. Among them are breast, cervical, endometrial, ovarian, and vulvar cancers. Cancer occurs when cells start replicating in an out-of-control way and invading normal tissue. Cancerous changes can begin in any tissue and later move to surrounding tissues and other organs. A cancer's name always refers to the primary site (the tissue in which it originated).

BREAST CANCER

One in eight women in western countries will develop breast cancer during her lifetime. The most common symptom of breast cancer is a painless lump or thickened area in the breast. Many women discover the lump during self-examination. Other symptoms of breast cancer include a clear or bloody discharge from the nipple, indentation of the nipple or skin over the breast, changes in the shape or size of a breast, and redness or pitting of the skin over the breast.

CERVICAL CANCER

This cancer is one of the most common female reproductive system cancers. In its early stages it can grow unnoticed, because it produces no signs or symptoms. However, symptoms may develop as the cancer progresses. These can include irregular menstrual cycles with bleeding between periods, bleeding after menopause, bleeding after sexual intercourse, a vaginal discharge that can be heavy and have a pungent odour, and persistent pelvic pain.

ENDOMETRIAL CANCER

Each year, approximately 40,000 women in the United States are diagnosed with endometrial cancer. It involves the lining of the uterus (also called the endometrium) and usually occurs after menopause in women in their 60s and 70s. The most prominent sign of endometrial cancer is bleeding between periods or after menopause. In addition, some women may experience weight loss, longer than normal periods, a vaginal discharge that can be pink and watery, or pelvic pain.

OVARIAN CANCER

Typically, the symptoms of ovarian cancer are vague and non-specific, making early diagnosis difficult. These symptoms include abdominal pressure or bloating, the frequent need to urinate, changes in bowel movements from diarrhoea to constipation, pelvic and lower back pain, persistent indigestion and nausea, loss of appetite, unexplained weight fluctuations, painful intercourse and fatigue. Ovarian cancer often spreads to surrounding tissues and organs

WHO IS AT RISK?

The risk factors include:

Endometrial and ovarian cancer
- Over age 40
- Caucasian
- Extended years of menstruation
- Women who have never been pregnant
- Women with irregular ovulation
- Obese women
- Diabetics
- Women who have received hormone replacement therapy with oestrogen alone
- Women with hormone producing ovarian tumours
- Family history of endometrial or ovarian cancer
- Tamoxifen treatment (endometrial cancer only)

Breast cancer
- Over age 30
- Caucasian
- Family or personal history
- Obesity
- High exposure to oestrogen
- Smoking
- Alcoholics

Cervical and vulvar cancer
- Women with multiple sex partners

before being noticed. Seventy-five percent of ovarian cancers are diagnosed as Stage III (extensive local and regional spread of the cancer, usually to draining lymph nodes) and Stage IV (the cancer

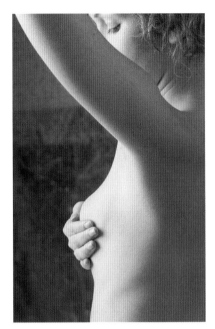

The optimum time to perform a breast self-examination is about seven days after the start of the period. Breasts are unlikely to be sore or tender at that time.

cancer has spread beyond the regional lymph nodes to distant parts of the body) of the disease.

VULVAR CANCER

This rare cancer involves the outer part of the female genitalia called the vulva. Vulvar cancer is most frequently diagnosed in elderly women and appears to be a type of skin cancer. Symptoms may include an itching or burning feeling in the vagina, unexplained bleeding, a change in the colour or texture of the vagina, and the presence of an ulcer.

CAUSES

Each kind of cancer has its own unique cause.

Breast Cancer

The primary function of the breast is lactation for a nursing baby. Therefore the breast consists of glandular tissue that is made up of small lobules that can produce milk. Ducts provide a passageway for the milk to exit the nipple. Between the lobe and the ducts are areas of fat and lymph vessels that collect immune cells. In breast cancer, malignant cells usually originate in the ducts or lobules. Scientists have identified a number of inherited genetic abnormalities that may contribute to abnormal cell growth in breast tissue. These include breast cancer gene 1 (BRCA1), breast cancer gene 2 (BRCA 2), and mutations in the cell-cycle checkpoint kinase 2 (CHEK 2) gene and in the p53 tumour suppressor gene. Environmental factors can also contribute to the development of breast cancer such as radiation exposure.

Certain risk factors may increase one's chances of developing breast cancer. Many relate to an increased lifetime exposure to oestrogen. Those who may have an increased risk include women over 50, women with no children, those who have a first birth after the age of 30, early onset of periods, late menopause, Caucasian women, alcoholic women, women with a family history of breast cancer, women with a genetic predisposition, overweight women, and women who have received hormone replacement therapy after menopause.

Cervical Cancer

The human papillomavirus (HPV) had been linked to the development of cervical cancer. In most cases, the virus lays dormant in the body as it is suppressed by the immune system. In certain women, though, the virus is able to infect the cells on the surface of the cervix, causing them to become cancerous, usually many years after the initial infection with HPV.

HPV is a sexually transmitted disease (pp.392–3). Having sex at an early age, many sexual partners and unprotected sex increase one's chances of developing cervical cancer. Other risk factors include infection with more than one STD, a compromised immune system and smoking.

Endometrial Cancer

The cause of endometrial cancer remains unknown. However, it is thought that oestrogen contributes to its development. Certain factors have been identified that put a woman at risk. If the balance between oestrogen and progesterone in the body shifts to such as degree that more oestrogen is released by the ovaries, a woman is at increased risk. In addition to elevated levels of oestrogen, extended exposure to this hormone increases the risk for endometrial cancer as well. Women who began menstruating before the age of 12 and continue until their late 50s or those who received oestrogen-only hormone replacement therapy have an endometrium that has been exposed to more oestrogen and are at increased risk for the cancer. Obese women, women who ovulate irregularly and diabetics are at increased risk for endometrial cancer as well. Other risk factors include oestrogen-producing ovarian tumours, tamoxifen treatment and genetic predisposition.

Ovarian Cancer

The cause of this cancer is unknown; however, it is theorizes that it is due to genetic errors that occur during tissue repair that follows the release of an ovum each month. It is believed that the rupture site is susceptible to damage in the cellular genetic machinery. Over time, changes to the DNA are reproduced and a tumour develops. In addition, elevated hormone levels may further stimulate the growth of abnormal cells.

The risk factors for ovarian cancer include genetic mutations in the BRCA1 and BRAC2 genes, hereditary nonpolyposis colorectal cancer (HNPCC) syndrome, age over 50, and a family history of ovarian cancer.

Vulvar Cancer

Like cervical cancer, most cases of vulvar cancer develop as a result of exposure to the human papillomavirus (HPV).

PREVENTION

The best way to prevent the development of these cancers is by making healthy lifestyle choices. This includes maintaining a healthy weight, eating fruit, vegetables, lean meats and foods high in fibre. Cooking with olive oil is beneficial, because it contains healthy monounsaturated fats. Regular physical activity, managing stress, and limiting exposure to smoking and pesticides are beneficial in preventing cancer.

All women should adhere to safe sex practices to limit the possibility of contracting a sexually transmitted disease such as HPV.

The use of birth-control pills and tubal ligation can decrease the likelihood of some female reproductive cancers. The use of oral contraceptives lowers the woman's risk of developing ovarian or uterine cancer by 50 percent. Avoidance or limiting hormone replacement therapy after menopause to less than five years decreases the risk of breast cancer. Avoiding unopposed oestrogen use decreases the risk of endometrial cancers. Routine breast self-examinations, gynaecological visits, and pap smears increase the chances of a successful treatment outcome by diagnosing cancer early.

DIAGNOSIS

A number of diagnostic tools are available to doctors when diagnosing cancers of the female reproductive system.

- **CLINICAL EXAMINATION** Breasts are examined for irregularities such as lumps or enlarged lymph nodes.
- **MAMMOGRAM** X-rays produce an image of the breast tissue, allowing for the detection of tumours. The American Cancer Society recommends beginning yearly screening mammograms at age 40.
- **DUCTAL LAVAGE** A small sample of cells are removed from a duct in the breast and tested for cellular abnormalities.
- **IMAGING TESTS** Ultrasound, magnetic resonance imaging (MRI) and CAT scans allow doctors to identify and pinpoint the location of a tumour.
- **BIOPSY** A tissue sample is removed from a suspicious area and tested for the presence of malignant tumour cells.

- **OESTROGEN AND PROGESTERONE RECEPTOR TESTS** Certain cancer cells respond and grow as a result of exposure to hormones. These tests are commonly used in breast cancer to look for the presence of hormone receptors on cancerous cells to determine if treatments that prevent the binding of hormones to tumour cells are beneficial.
- **GENETIC TESTING** The discovery of genes that increase one's risk of a female reproductive cancer may give the doctors clues as to the best treatment approach.
- **PAP SMEAR** Cells from the cervix are examined for the presence of abnormalities that suggest precancerous dysplasia or cancerous changes.
- **HPV DNA TEST** This test identifies the presence of the genetic material of HPV in cervical cells.
- **CA-125 BLOOD TEST** Cancer antigen (CA-125) is a protein-levels are sometimes elevated in the blood of women with ovarian cancer. Although results are not definitive, doctors may look for this compound when diagnosing ovarian cancer. This blood test is most helpful in menopausal women with an ovarian mass.

TREATMENTS

Many integrative medicine strategies can support the body, mind and spirit's ability to fight cancer in combination with conventional medical approaches such as chemotherapy, radiation and surgery. First and foremost, relationships play a pivotal role in health. Facing physical struggles and questions of mortality, finding peace, strong relationships with family and friends, and a supportive spiritual foundation can strengthen immune functioning and well-being.

• DIET AND SUPPLEMENTS These are powerful tools. Focusing on organic foods, fruit and vegetables rich in antioxidants, whole grains, and high-quality proteins and fats help the body to function optimally.

Melatonin supplements have been shown in multiple research studies to improve outcome on some solid tumours. High-quality medicinal mushrooms may help in some cancers. Antioxidant vitamins such as C and E are not recommended during radiation and chemotherapy. Herbal therapies may have interactions with chemotherapeutic regimens and should always be discussed with a doctor.

• ENERGY AND BODY WORK These therapies may also improve outcome and quality of life in people facing cancer. Acupuncture (pp.464–5) can ease pain and nausea. Energy medicine therapies

such as Reiki (p.573) and healing touch (p.562), may lessen side-effects associated with therapy and speed healing. Massage therapy (pp.468–73) improves immune functioning and may ease pain and stress.

• MEDICAL TREATMENTS The five main cancer treatments in conventional medicine are chemotherapy, radiation therapy, surgery, hormone therapy and immunotherapy. Doctors may use one or a combination of a few to treat cancers of the female reproductive system.

In chemotherapy, toxic drugs are administered to destroy cancer cells. Often, a combination of two or more chemicals are given either intravenously or in pill form. Chemotherapy can be used for all cancers, either before or after surgery or in combination with radiation to improve survival and cure rates.

During radiation therapy, cancer cells are targeted with high-energy X-rays that work to

shrink the tumour. It may be used before surgery to make the tumour more manageable to remove, after surgery to improve outcomes, or as complete therapy in some cases of advanced cervical cancer.

Surgical removal of a tumour or an affected organ may sometimes be necessary. For example, in cases of breast cancer the doctor may choose to remove the lump or the entire breast, depending on the progressive nature of the cancer. A hysterectomy, during which the cervix and the uterus are removed, may be necessary to treat cervical or endometrial cancers.

Certain cancers grow in response to the presence of hormone such as oestrogen. Hormone therapy is designed to prevent the adherence of oestrogen to tumour cells. Receptor sites that would normally bind oestrogen are blocked by drugs such as tamoxifen. Another class of hormone therapy drugs prevents the conversion of hormone precursors into oestrogen within the body. The hormone progesterone inhibits growth of endometrial cancer cells. Thus, a synthetic form of progesterone is sometimes administered to treat endometrial cancer.

The cutting edge of cancer treatment is the use of immunotherapy. These treatments boost the body's own defences to destroy cancer cells. An example is herceptin, a chemical that tells the immune cells to destroy tumour cells. This treatment is very effective in some women who have breast cancer.

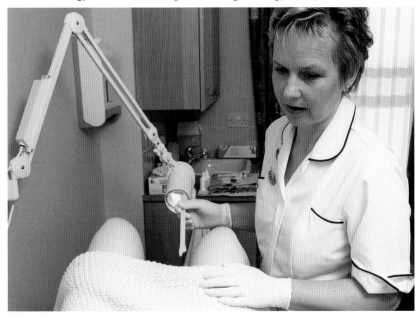

An annual pelvic examination is one way to find some cancers of the female reproductive system at an early stage, thereby increasing the chances for successful treatment.

See also: *Menstrual Bleeding Disorders, pp.384–5 • Diarrhoea, p.268 • Obesity, pp.348–9*

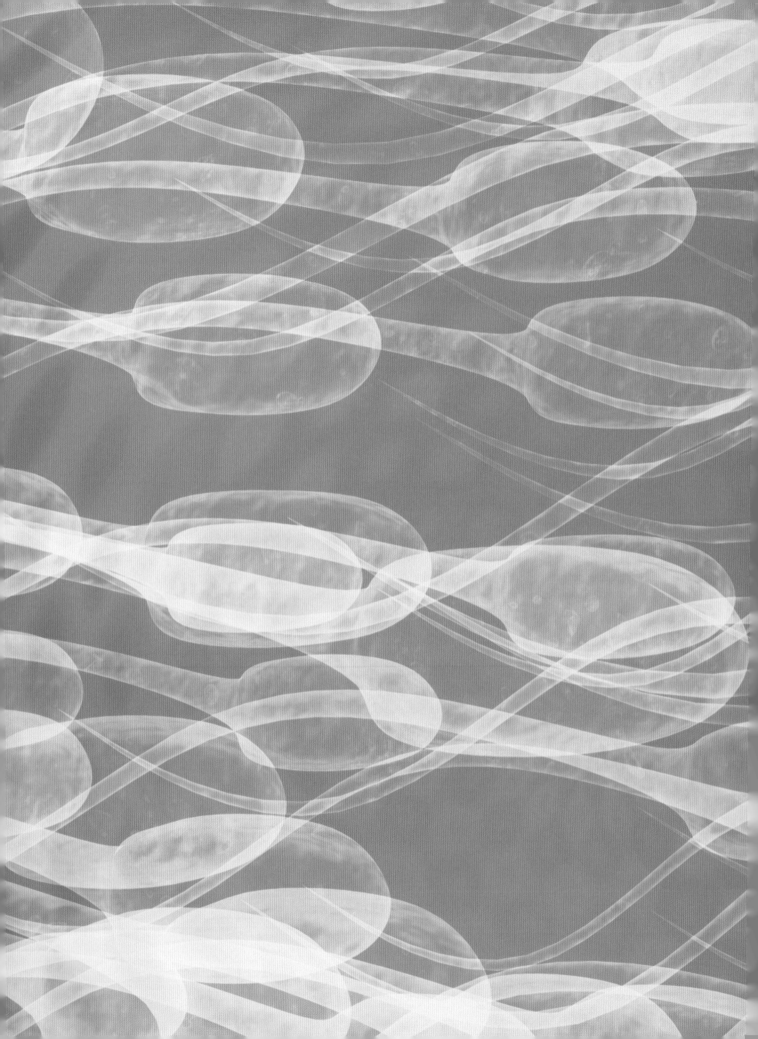

MALE
REPRODUCTIVE
SYSTEM

15

The male reproductive system consists of several organs that function together to produce and transport sperm. The penis contains a tube, the urethra, through which both urine and sperm travel. A small gland called the prostate encircles the urethra; it produces semen, a milky fluid that helps carry sperm (through a tube called the vas deferens) to the penis during ejaculation. The testicles are housed in a pouch of skin called the scrotum; they produce the male hormone testosterone, and sperm, which is released into the urethra during orgasm. Behind each testicle is a coiled tube, the epididymis. Sperm remain in the epididymis until they can fertilize a female's egg. During sexual arousal, blood flow increases in the penis, causing it to become erect. After climax, the muscles surrounding the testicles and prostate work simultaneously to ejaculate the semen from the penis.

Prostate Problems

Prostatitis and benign prostatic hyperplasia (BPH) are common prostate conditions. Prostatitis, or inflammation of the prostate – the gland located between the bladder and uretha – may be characterized by a swollen, red and warm prostate gland. Men suffering from prostatitis experience a burning feeling during urination, the urge to urinate frequently, pain in the lower back or between the legs, temperatures, chills and fatigue.

Benign prostatic hyperplasia (BPH), enlargement of the prostate, is associated with a frequent and urgent need to urinate, the inability to start a stream of urine, leaking from the penis and difficulty in stopping urine flow. It may also lead to small amounts of blood in the urine. Some men with BPH hardly notice these symptoms, while others suffer from one or more of them. Left untreated, BPH can lead to further complications, such as urinary tract infections and kidney damage.

CAUSES

Prostatitis is often caused by a bacterial infection. The presence of bacteria triggers the body's defences and may lead to significant inflammation. Recurrent bacterial prostatitis may indicate an abnormality in the prostate that allows the bacteria to repeatedly cause infections.

BPH is the result of the natural aging process. As men age, their prostate continues to grow in response to the male hormone testosterone. Eventually, the prostate becomes so large that it squeezes the urethra and inhibits urination. Pressure from the enlarged prostate can also affect bladder control.

PREVENTION

A healthy lifestyle is the best way to strengthen the body's defences and delay the ageing process. Maintaining a healthy and balanced diet of fruit, vegetables and whole grains, yet low in saturated fats may decrease the risk of prostatitis and BPH.

DIAGNOSIS

Doctors may use one of several methods to diagnose prostate problems, several of which are highlighted below.

• **DIGITAL RECTAL EXAMINATION (DRE)** A doctor inserts a gloved finger into the rectum to determine the size and condition of the prostate.

• **URINALYSIS** A doctor tests a urine sample for the presence of bacteria. A dipstick, which changes colour in the presence of bacteria, is inserted into the sample. If bacteria is present a microscope is used to classify the bacteria.

• **INTRAVENOUS PYELOGRAM (IVP)** A doctor injects dye into a vein. The dye passes through the blood and into the urine, allowing the urinary tract to be viewed on an X-ray machine.

• **CYSTOSCOPY** A thin tube with a microscopic lens, or a cystoscope, is inserted through the urethra and into the bladder, allowing the doctor to see the location and amount of urethral blockage.

• **RESIDUAL URINE TEST** A small tube, or catheter, is inserted into the bladder to determine the amount of urine remaining in the bladder after urination and the bladder pressure.

TREATMENTS

Several treatment options are available for prostate problems depending upon the cause.

WHO IS AT RISK?

The risk factors include:

- BPH
- Men over 50 years of age
- Prostatitis
- Men under 50 years of age
- Multiple sex partners and high risk sexual behavior
- Excessive alcohol consumption
- Physically inactive
- Poor diet

• **ANTIBIOTIC MEDICINE** Oral antibiotics are used to treat bacterial prostatitis.

• **PROSTATE MASSAGING** A doctor massages the prostate to reduce the fluid and relieve the symptoms in cases of chronic prostatitis.

• **WARM BATHS** Those suffering from recurrent prostatitis can take warm baths to relax the muscles and reduce the burning sensation that occurs during urination.

• **MONITORING** A patient, in conjunction with his doctor, monitors the symptoms and reports any changes. This tactic is employed only when the symptoms of BPH are not a nuisance.

• **MEDICATIONS** A doctor may prescribe medication, such as finasteride and alpha adrenergic blockers, which are used to to block the hormone that causes the prostate to enlarge.

• **SAW PALMETTO** (*Serenoa repens*) A natural extract of this herb has been shown to reduce the symptoms of BPH. In addition to improving urine flow, saw pal-memetto has been found to

decrease the burning sensation during urination, and the frequency of urination.

• **BETA-SITOSTEROLS** A preparation containing B-sitosteryl-B-D-glucoside has been shown to improve urinary symptoms and urine flow in a clinical trial of patients suffering from BPH.

• **STINGING NETTLE** (*Urtica dioica*) This herb is often used in conjunction with saw palmetto to treat BPH. Studies indicate that it inhibits the growth of certain prostate cells thus improving urinary flow and bladder control.

• **SURGERY** The removal of a portion or the entire prostate can reduce the constriction of the urethra and relieve bladder pressure. Depending on the size of the prostate, surgeons choose from a number of methods.

During a procedure called transurethral resection of the prostate (TURP), a surgeon removes a section of the prostate using a tool called a resectoscope, or wire loop. The procedure involves making a series of small incisions

Clinical Query

Does having BPH put me at risk for developing prostate cancer?

No. Although some men with BPH also have prostate cancer, the two conditions are not associated with each other. In fact, most men with BPH will never develop prostate cancer. It is important to realize, however, that both BPH and prostate cancer cause similar symptoms so your doctor should evaluate you for each condition.

in the prostate and bladder neck that loosen the muscles surrounding the bladder and improve urine flow.

Sometimes, when the prostate is extremely enlarged, a surgeon performs open surgery to remove prostate tissue. The skin above the pubic bone is cut in order to reach the prostate, which is then removed, layer by layer, using a scalpel, cauterization or laser.

• **NON-SURGICAL PROCEDURES** During transurethral microwave thermotherapy (TUMT) and transurethral needle ablation (TUNA), a catheter is inserted through the urethra and controlled heat is applied to the prostate. In both of these treatments, a doctor removes a portion of the prostate without the patient needing to stay overnight in the hospital or undergo general anaesthesia. Most patients are able to return to work and normal activities after three days.

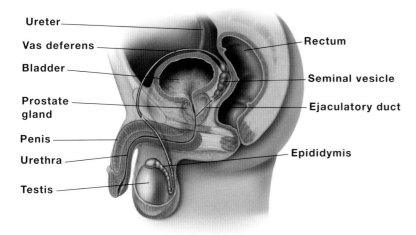

Benign prostatic hyperplasia (BPH), the enlargement of the prostate, causes a frequent and urgent need to urinate, the inability to start a stream of urine, leaking from the penis, difficulty in stopping urine flow and small amounts of blood in the urine.

See also: *Alcoholism, pp.358–60* • *Obesity, pp.348–9* • *Back Pain, pp.132–3*

Infertility

The inability of a couple to conceive a baby after one year of unprotected sexual relations is labelled infertility. An estimated 10 to 15 percent of couples are considered to be infertile. Male infertility involves the inability to produce healthy sperm which are able to reach the woman's fallopian tube and fertilize her ovum.

CAUSES

Under normal conditions, the male reproductive system is able to produce, store and transport sperm. The testicles produce both sperm and the male hormone testosterone. During orgasm, the sperm travels through the penis in a fluid called semen and is released from the body. This process is regulated by hormones and relies upon the ability of the entire reproductive system to function. So a number of factors can cause infertility in men.

Some men release too few sperm from their testicles as a result of genetic factors or life-style choices such as alcoholism, smoking and drug abuse. Some prescription medications, sexually transmitted diseases (pp.392–3), long-term illnesses, childhood infections and hormone deficiencies also diminish sperm production. Exposure to radiation, steroids, chemotherapy and toxic chemicals may affect sperm formation.

Structural abnormalities, such as varicoceles (p.428), can reduce the amount of sperm transported from the penis. Azoospermia is a condition in which a male is completely unable to produce sperm. It can occur as a result of damage to the reproductive system or a hormonal imbalance.

Erectile dysfunction (p.426) and retrograde ejaculation are also causes of male infertility. During retrograde ejaculation, the semen does not exit the penis, but travels backward toward the bladder.

PREVENTION

Some cases of male infertility cannot be prevented, such as those caused by structural abnormalities and genetic factors. Healthy lifestyle choices such as eating a balanced diet and participating in regular physical exercise can help men maintain a strong reproductive system. Men should also minimize their consumption of alcohol and avoid illicit drug use or high risk sexual behaviour.

DIAGNOSIS

Doctors may diagnosis and evaluate infertility with a variety of tests.

- **PHYSICAL EXAMINATION** A complete examination may give clues about a hormonal deficiency, a structural abnormality in the reproductive system, or an illness that is causing infertility.
- **MEDICAL HISTORY** The patient is asked questions concerning his childhood, his sexual history,

healing hope My wife, Jenny, and I had been trying to have a baby for nearly two years. I always assumed that it was her fault that she was not getting pregnant and I was apprehensive about seeing the doctor. When I finally met with an urologist that specializes in male fertility issues, he found a lump on the back of my left testicle. The doctor called it a varicocele and said that it is quite common in men who are having problems trying to conceive a baby. The condition was quickly fixed at a vein centre the next week. Best of all, I only missed a day of work and was able to return home the same night of the procedure. Today, I am proud to say that our son will soon be two years old and we are expecting his baby sister next month. John E.

current medication being taken, previous illness or infections, past surgeries, exposure to toxins and lifestyle habits.

• **SEMEN ANALYSIS** After a short period of abstinence, the ejaculate of a patient is analysed. This test, also called a sperm count, reveals how much semen is produced during ejaculation and whether it contains a sufficient number of healthy sperm.

• **BLOOD TESTS** These tests are used to measure the levels of hormones circulating in the patient's body.

• **GENETIC TESTS** A blood sample is used to check for missing or abnormal chromosomes, genetic information read by body cells.

• **ULTRASOUND** High-frequency sound waves are used to produce an image of the reproductive tract and to identify any blockages.

• **POST-EJACULATION URINE SAMPLE** A patient's urine sample is analysed for the presence of semen. This test is used to diagnosis retrograde ejaculation.

• **TESTICULAR BIOPSY** A tissue sample from the testicles is examined for cellular abnormalities that may inhibit healthy sperm production.

TREATMENTS

Treatment depends on the underlying cause of the infertility.

• **HORMONE DEFICIENCY** Hormone injections are given on a regular basis for six months or more.

• **GENITAL INFECTION** Antibiotics are prescribed to treat infections.

• **RETROGRADE EJACULATION** Because this condition is usually permanent, sperm retrieved from a urine sample is used in assisted fertilization techniques.

• **VARICOCELE** A surgeon blocks the enlarged vein and redirects blood flow into other healthy veins.

• **OBSTRUCTION** A surgeon removes the obstruction or creates a bypass in the reproductive tract.

> ## CAUTION
>
> With both in vitro fertilization (IVF) and intracytoplasmic sperm injections (ICSI), there have been conflicting reports of a higher risk of birth defects. Couples should discuss this information with their doctor.

• **ACUPUNCTURE AND MOXA** Studies of these therapies (pp.464–5) – in which a cone or stick of the herb moxa (mugwort or *Artemisia vulgaris*) is burned on or near an acupuncture point – indicate that they can be used to improve sperm quality. For example, 19 infertile men were treated with acupuncture and moxa for a period of ten weeks. At the conclusion of the study, the participants experienced an increase in the percentage of normal formed sperm.

• **IVF AND ICSI** Sometimes these techniques fail and a couple chooses to seek assistance in order to conceive. Many couples try in vitro fertilization (IVF) and intracytoplasmic sperm injections (ICSI). During IVF, eggs are removed from the woman's ovaries and placed in a laboratory dish along with the man's sperm. If the sperm fertilizes the egg, the doctor uses a tube to gently release the embryos into the woman's uterus, where it can fully develop into a baby. ICSI is a procedure in which sperm is injected directly into the egg in a laboratory dish. Sometimes, the sperm is removed directly from the male's testicle rather than from ejaculate.

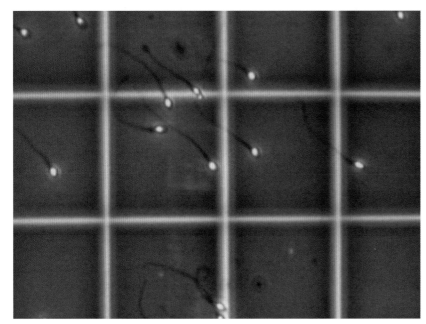

A graticular screen shows a field of human sperm occurring in abnormally low numbers. Screen lines assist in the counting of sperm. Here, 60 to 70 million sperm per ml of ejaculate are seen; a normal count is about 113 million sperm per ml.

See also: *STDs, pp.424–5* • *Erectile Dysfunction, p.426* • *Pregnancy, pp.398–400*

Epididymitis

The inflammation of the epididymis, the tiny spiralled tube behind the testicle that serves as a passageway for sperm, is often caused by a bacterial infection that may or may not be a sexually transmitted disease (STDs, pp.424–5). Common symptoms include swelling and tenderness of the testicles, scrotum or groin, pain during urination or sexual intercourse, fever, and a discharge from the penis that is only rarely bloody.

WHO IS AT RISK?

The risk factors include:

- High risk sexual behaviors
- Chronic urinary tract infections (pp.302–3) or prostate infections (pp.418–19)

CAUSES

Sexually transmitted diseases (pp.424–5), especially chlamydia and gonorrhoea, cause the majority of epididymitis cases in younger men. High-risk sexual behaviour, such as unprotected sex, greatly increases a man's chances of contracting epididymitis.

Bacterial organisms growing in the urinary tract or prostate can travel up the vas deferens, the tube within the penis that carries sperm to the epididymis, causing this site to become inflamed. Other less common causes of epididymitis are anatomical abnormalities of the urinary tract that allow bacteria to grow easily, an enlarged prostate, as well as a catheter or surgical instrument that has been inserted into the penis. Tuberculosis can

also bring about epididymitis if the bacteria move from the bloodstream into the epididymis.

Chemical epididymitis may occur after episodes of heavy lifting or straining. In this condition, urine flows backward from the urethra and irritates the epididymis. The drug amiodarone has also been shown to cause soreness of the epididymis.

PREVENTION

Epididymitis can be prevented by avoiding of high-risk sexual activity. Abstinence or a monogamous relationship are recommended. In addition, medical treatment should be sought for bacterial infections that may spread to the epididymis such as urinary tract infections (pp.302–3) and prostatitis (pp.418–9) to prevent episodes of epididymitis.

DIAGNOSIS

A doctor will first conduct a physical exam to diagnose epididymitis. The doctor may check for the enlargement or tenderness of the

testicles, prostate and lymph nodes in the groin. Blood and urine tests can identify any bacteria. Any discharge at the tip of the penis will be examined for the presence of infectious organisms.

The symptoms of epididymitis are similar to those of a condition called testicular torsion (p.427); however, each is treated quite differently. Epididymitis can be distinguished from testicular torsion by an increase of blood flow to the testicles. An ultrasound or nuclear scan of the testicles is occasionally used to produce images of blood flow allowing the doctor to distinguish between the two conditions.

TREATMENTS

Antibiotics are prescribed to treat epididymitis that occurs as a result of bacterial infections. Patients are encouraged to get plenty of rest, elevate their scrotum, wear undergarments that support the scrotum, and apply ice packs to help relieve the symptoms.

See also: *Urinary Tract Infection, pp.302–3 • Prostate Problems, pp.418–19 • Fever, p.318*

CAUTION

In some cases of epididymitis, both sex partners must be treated or the infection will be passed back and forth during sexual relations.

Peyronie's Disease

In 1743, François Gigot de la Peyronie, King Louis XV of France's personal physician, reported the first case of this sexually debilitating disease, in which a hard lump or plaque forms on the penis.

Peyronie's disease usually occurs in middle-aged and elderly men but can occasionally be seen in young men. The lump, typically found at the top of the shaft, causes the penis to bend upwards. Sometimes, though, the lump develops on both the top and bottom of the penis, causing a bottleneck to form that shortens the penis. These deformities often lead to painful erections and low self-esteem because of the inability to have sexual relations.

CAUSES

It is believed that Peyronie's disease develops after an injury to the penis. The elastic covering surrounding the corpora cavernosa, a two-chamber cavity that runs the length of the penis, and the septum become inflamed. The damaged tissue hardens or becomes fibrous. Evidence also indicates that some genetic factors may be involved in the development of Peyronie's disease, because men who have a family member with this disease are more likely to be diagnosed themselves.

The chances of developing Peyronie's disease from medication are very low, but some blood pressure and heart medications called beta blockers list this condition as a side effect. Other drugs that may cause Peyronie's disease include interferon, which is used to treat multiple sclerosis, and phenytoin, an anti-seizure medicine.

PREVENTION

The only way to prevent Peyronie's disease is to safeguard the penis from any type of injury or trauma.

DIAGNOSIS

Peyronie's disease is diagnosed by a physical examination of the penis in both a flaccid and erect state. Sometimes an ultrasound is used to identify the location of the lump.

TREATMENTS

The goal of treatment is to reduce the deformity of the penis and restore a patient's ability to have sexual relations and pain-free erections. In approximately 10 percent of cases, the penis will heal on its own and return to normal. Doctors usually wait a year before performing any corrective surgery.

• **NON-SURGICAL OPTIONS** The majority of the non-surgical options are still in the experimental phase and data on their effectiveness is not fully conclusive. Examples include oral medications such as vitamin E supplements, tamoxifen, and colchicine. Potassium para amino benzoate (POTABA) can be effective. However, large doses of POTABA are required which may cause intestinal discomfort. Chemical injections into the penis and radiation therapy have also been used as treatment options. Collangenase is an investigational drug that enzymatically digests scar tissue.

• **SURGERY** This becomes necessary if the lump does not heal on its own, the pain increases, or the deformity worsens. Three surgical options are available:

Grafting The surgeon removes the lump and replaces it with a graft. The graft can be tissue taken from another part of the patient's body, tissue harvested from another human or animal, or tissue made from a synthetic material.

Nesbit Procedure Tissue is removed from the penis on the side opposite of the lump which eliminates the bending effect.

Penile Prosthesis A surgeon implants a device in the penis which straightens it.

See also: *Erectile Dysfunction, p.426 • Supplements, Minerals & Vitamins pp.532–41*

WHO IS AT RISK?
The risk factors include:
• Men between the ages of 40 and 70 years

SEXUALLY TRANSMITTED DISEASES

The number of cases of sexually transmitted diseases (STDs) is on the rise, especially among men and women under the age of 25 years and in minority populations. Health professionals at the National Institute of Allergy and Infectious Diseases (NIAID) attribute this change to the fact that people today become sexually active at younger ages and have more sexual partners throughout their lives.

SYMPTOMS

Sometimes men and women with STDs experience no symptoms or only very mild discomfort. Anyone who is sexually active should be screened for STDs on a regular basis, especially if they participate in any high-risk sexual behaviour, such as having multiple sex partners, anal sex and unprotected sex. If any of the following symptoms are experienced, contact a doctor immediately.

- Burning or itching in the penis
- Pain during sex or urination
- A discharge from the urethra
- Sores, warts or lumps in the genital or anal area.

CAUSES

Sexually transmitted diseases can be caused by bacteria, a virus or a parasite. The most common STDs are highlighted below.

Chlamydia

The most commonly diagnosed STD is chlamydia. It is frequently associated with urethritis (inflammation of the urethra), epididymitis (p.422) and orchitis (irritation of the testicles). Chlamydia is treated using antibiotics such as azithromycin.

Gonorrhoea

Another common STD, gonorrhoea is caused by a bacteria. Gonorrhoea may cause an infection of the urethra, epididymis, testicles, throat or rectum. A culture can confirm the presence of the bacteria and treatment usually involves antibiotics such as ceftriazone.

Genital Warts

This condition is characterized by small, hard, and painless bumps on the penis or anus. These bumps can develop into a large mass that resembles a cauliflower. Genital warts are caused by the human papilloma virus (HPV), which is associated with the occurrence of genital cancers in both men and women. They are treated with the application of topical drugs such as podophylin resin to the skin, cryotherapy during which the warts are frozen off with liquid nitrogen, laser surgery or interferon injections, which boost the body's immune system to destroy the HPV virus. Preliminary studies suggest that lentinan, a natural substance derived from the Shiitake mushroom, may reduce the reoccurrence of genital warts.

Genital Herpes

Painful blisters or open sores on the penis and anal area are characteristic of a herpes infection. Similar outbreaks can also occur in the mouth of an infected individual or any area of the body that comes in contact with the herpes simplex virus (HSV). Once infected, the virus periodically recurs, causing outbreaks of the sores and blisters. There is no cure for herpes; however, the condition can be controlled with antiviral medications, such as acyclovir, famciclovir or valacyclovir. These can be applied directly to the skin, taken orally or injected. In addition, in initial studies a substance created by bees called propolis has been shown to destroy the herpes virus.

Syphilis

A chancre, or large open sore, is the first symptom associated with syphilis. The sore can appear on the penis, mouth, anus or hands. This infection can progress, causing a recurring rash as well as damage to the heart and central

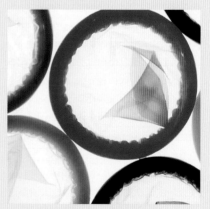

To prevent STDs, use a condom for sexual intercourse of any kind.

nervous system. Syphilis is diagnosed by examining secretions produced by the chancre with a specialized microscope (called a dark field) as well as blood and other screening tests. Since the dark field is not readily available, screening tests are also used in the diagnosis. Syphilis is treated with penicillin or other antibiotics.

Chancroid

This relatively rare STD is usually characterized by swollen lymph nodes and a painful open sore on the genitals, anus or mouth. Oral antibiotics such as azithromycin are used to treat this STD.

Pubic Lice and Scabies

Both pubic lice and scabies are caused by tiny parasites that can be seen by the naked eye. They live in the pubic hair and suck blood from the skin. Men with pubic lice or scabies find themselves constantly scratching their genital area. Scabies may cause itching on the hands, arms, legs and buttocks as well. A doctor may prescribe a cream containing permethrin or lindane to treat both pubic lice and scabies. Men diagnosed with either of these parasites must wash their clothes and bedding with hot water, because pubic lice and scabies can live in the fibres of the thread.

Trichomoniasis

This common STD is often repeatedly passed between sexual partners, as many men experience no symptoms. Some patients with trichomoniasis complain of pain within the penis, a discharge from the urethra, and a burning

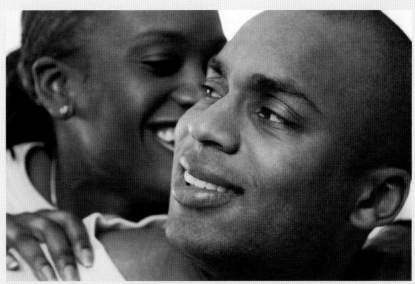

When one partner is infected with an STD, both partners need to be treated to prevent the infection from being passed back and forth between the partners.

sensation during urination and ejaculation. Trichomoniasis is caused by a parasite called trichomonas vaginalis. It is easily treated with the antibiotic metronidazole.

Human Immunodeficiency Virus

The human immunodeficiency virus (HIV) causes a disruption in a man's immune defences and destroys his body's ability to fight off infections. Eventually, men with HIV become diagnosed with a condition called AIDS–acquired immune deficiency syndrome. (pp.316–17). Infection with another STD, especially the presence of an open sore as a result of genital herpes, syphilis or chancroid, increases a man's risk of contracting HIV. Men who have contracted HIV often first complain of fatigue and fever. A blood test is used to confirm the presence of HIV.

There is no cure for HIV or AIDS. Many treatments are available that slow the progression of the disease, including antiviral

medication and prescription drugs that are administered to boost the immune response.

PREVENTION

The most effective way to prevent STDs is to practise abstinence outside any monogamous relationship. Statistics prove that the chances of contracting a STD are minimal if sex is practised only between two sexual partners who have no other sexual partners outside their relationship. In addition, the risk of contracting a STD can be minimized by using a male condom for all sexual relations, including oral sex, since the mouth can also become infected with an STD. An oral STD may be indicated by an irritated throat, or sores on the tongue or throat. Consult a doctor immediately. Because the anus and rectum are home to organisms that cause STDs, unprotected anal sex increases the risk of these diseases.

See also: *HIV/AIDS, pp.316–17 • Epididymitis, p.422*

Male Sexual Dysfunction

The inability to achieve or maintain an erection, premature ejaculation or the inability to orgasm are examples of male sexual dysfunction. A survey of men between the ages of 40 and 70 indicates the approximately half of the participants experience some degree of sexual dysfunction.

CAUSES

Male sexual arousal occurs when the brain sends a message to the nerves in the penis that causes muscles surrounding it to relax. Blood then flows in and fills the penis, causing an erection. Any event that disrupts this process results in male sexual dysfunction.

Men with diseases such as diabetes (pp.338–41) and high blood pressure (pp.236–9) are at higher risk of developing sexual dysfunction. Vascular diseases such as atherosclerosis (pp.230–3), peripheral vascular disease (pp.254–5), myocardial infarction (pp.230–3) and arterial hypertension (pp.236–9), cause almost half of the cases in men over age 50. Decreased testosterone levels, smoking, alcohol and drug abuse, prescription medication, depression, and relationship issues or stress are also causes.

PREVENTION

Maintaining one's physical and psychological health is the best way to prevent sexual dysfunction.

DIAGNOSIS

Physical and psychological factors are considered when diagnosing male sexual dysfunction.

- **PATIENT HISTORY** A doctor asks questions that may reveal diseases, medication or lifestyle choices that impair sexual function.
- **PHYSICAL EXAMINATION** The penis, testes and overall physical health of the patient are checked for abnormalities.
- **LABORATORY TESTS** The patient's blood counts, including his testosterone levels, are measured to identify hormonal deficiencies.
- **NOCTURNAL PENILE TUMESCENCE** A patient's erections are monitored during sleep.
- **PSYCHOSOCIAL EXAMINATION** Interviews with the patient and his sexual partner can help to reveal psychological issues inhibiting sexual function.

TREATMENTS

If psychological factors are found to be a cause of male sexual dysfunction, doctors suggest psychotherapy or counseling. In the case of dysfunction due to medications, the doctor may change or discontinue the medication. Other treatment options include the following.

- **PHOSPHODIESTERASE (PDE) INHIBITORS** This drug relaxes the muscles of and increases blood flow in the penis during sexual stimulation.
- **TESTOSTERONE REPLACEMENT THERAPY** Hormone imbalances are treated with pills, injections, skin patches or gels that contain testosterone.
- **INJECTIONS** Medications, such as alprostadil, are injected into the penis or inserted into the urethra to increase blood flow.
- **VACUUM DEVICES** These pumps are placed on the penis. They create a partial vacuum, which draws blood into the penis, which causes an erection.
- **IMPLANTS** Surgeons insert devices into the penis that allow men to manually control erections.
- **SURGERY** Blocked or torn arteries are repaired to restore blood flow to the penis.
- **ACUPUNCTURE** In patients with psychogenic sexual dysfunction, acupuncture has been shown effective in helping some regain their sexual functioning.
- **SUPPLEMENTS** Clinical trials indicate that yohimbe hydrochloride, pine bark extract (pycnogenol), *Butea superba* and L-arginine can be used to treat sexual dysfunction.

See also: *Acupuncture, pp.464–5 • Diabetes, pp.338–41 • High Blood Pressure, pp.236–9*

Testicular Torsion

This is a relatively rare – but extremely painful – condition in which the spermatic cord that supplies blood to the testicle becomes twisted, preventing the flow of blood. It is considered a medical emergency. Symptoms of testicular torsion include severe testicle pain, swelling of the scrotum, light-headedness, fainting, nausea and vomiting.

CAUSES

Most cases of testicular torsion are caused by one of the following:
- Birth defects
- Testicles that have not yet descended
- Sexual arousal or activity
- Injury
- Inadequate connective tissue within the scrotal sac
- Active cremasteric reflex (retraction of the testicles caused by stimulation of the upper or inner thigh)
- Cold weather.

PREVENTION

There is no way to prevent testicular torsion. However, young men and boys should always take particular care of their genital area.

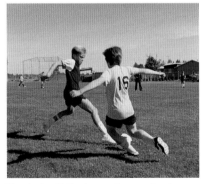

Physical activity does not cause torsion, but it may occur during sports or exercise.

Any severe pain or discomfort should be immediately reported to medical personnel.

DIAGNOSIS

Testicular torsion is most commonly diagnosed in boys and non-sexually active adolescents. The majority of the cases involve males under the age of 30 years. The condition must be diagnosed and treated rapidly in order to prevent permanent damage to the testicle. A physical examination may reveal that one of the testicles is raised high within the scrotum.

Since the symptoms of testicular torsion are similar to other conditions, such as epididymitis (p.422), the physician must first identify the cause of the pain. An ultrasound test or a testicular scan will be used to visualize the blood flow within the testicle if the physical examination is not definitive. During a testicular scan, small amounts of a radioactive material are injected into the bloodstream. The radioactive substance travels through the bloodstream to the testicle and accumulates, highlighting the testicle. A camera is then used to view the testicle.

If the patient has testicular torsion, the tests will show a lack of blood flow to one of the testicles.

Occasionally, the only way to diagnosis testicular torsion is surgery. The surgeon makes a small incision in the scrotum to see whether the cord is twisted.

TREATMENTS

Testicular torsion must be treated within a few hours – a lack of blood flow to the tissues will result in shrinkage of the testicle, infertility, or the need for amputation. Patients who receive treatment within six hours have a salvage rate of 80 to 100 percent. A urologist may first try to untwist the testicle by hand. Rarely, the testicle may untwist on its own. Surgery is needed immediately if the testicle cannot be manually untwisted.

See also: *Epididymitis, p.422, Nausea & Vomiting, pp.274–5 • Infertility, pp.420–1*

CAUTION

Seek medical attention immediately at the nearest casualty unit for any pain that occurs in the testicles, scrotum, penis or groin area and lasts more than several minutes.

Varicocele

When one of the veins within the scrotum becomes enlarged, it is called a varicocele. Normally, blood is supplied to the testicle through an artery that runs in the spermatic cord and drained from the testicles by the pampiniform venous plexus, a group of veins within the scrotum and above the testicles. Dilation of one of these pathways can occur, which prevents normal blood flow from the genital area.

Estimates say that up to 20 percent of males have a varicocele. This condition is a major contributing factors to male infertility (p.420) because it may cause problems in the regulation of optimal scrotum temperature. The presence of a varicocele may cause a decrease in sperm production, poor sperm mobility and the reoccurrence of abnormal sperm formation.

The formation of a varicocele usually begins during puberty; it can grow quite large over a long period of time. Varicoceles generally form in the left testicle due to the angle at which the veins enters this side. Most men experience no symptoms associated with a varicocele; the condition often develops undiscovered until a man seeks a fertility evaluation or has a physical examination. In rare instances, pain in the scrotum may follow physical activity that subsides following a period of relaxation.

CAUSES

Varicoceles are thought to be caused by abnormal valves within the veins. Like doorways that can open and shut, valves regulate the flow of blood within a vein. When the valve is in the open position, blood can flow upwards. A closed valve, on the other hand, prevents blood from flowing backwards. If a valve does not close properly, a back-up of blood occurs, restricting blood flow. Ultimately, the vein will widen due to the extra blood.

Infertility in men with varicoceles is believed to be caused as a result of the increase of temperature in the scrotum. Sperm requires a specific temperature for production, and normally blood is cooled to this temperature in the testicular veins. However, when the back-up of blood flow occurs, the veins are not able to cool the increased amount of blood.

PREVENTION

There is no known way to prevent the development of a varicocele.

DIAGNOSIS

A varicocele can be diagnosed during a physical examination. It appears as a mass above the testicles and feels like a bag of worms.

A large varicocele can be felt while a patient is standing. In the case of a small varicocele, the doctor may ask the patient to perform the valsalva manoeuvre, during which a deep breath is held while a man bears down on his groin area.

An ultrasound of the scrotum can also pinpoint the location of the enlarged vein.

TREATMENTS

- **MEDICATION** The treatment of a varicocele is usually performed only in cases of infertility or if the patient complains of pain. If a varicocele is causing only minor discomfort, a doctor may recommend painkillers, such as paracetomol or ibuprofen, and the daily use of supportive athletic undergarments to relieve pressure.
- **SURGERY** Some urologists suggest surgery in cases that the size difference between the two testicles is more than 20 percent. During the procedure, the enlarged vein is sealed off and the flow of blood is redirected to a healthy vein.

See also: *Infertility, pp. 420–1* • *Pregnancy, pp.398–400*

Priapism

A priapism is a painful condition in which a man has a persistent erection for four or more hours. This condition can occur in males of any age, including newborn babies. Without immediate treatment, priapism can lead to disfigurement and permanent erectile dysfunction.

CAUSES

Priapism develops when blood becomes trapped in the penis. There are two forms of priapisms: low-flow and high-flow. A low-flow priapism occurs after blood is trapped in the inner chambers of the penis. It can occur in healthy men for no apparent reason or in those diagnosed with sickle-cell disease (pp.312–13), leukaemia (p.335), or malaria. A high-flow priapism usually happens as a result of an injury to the penis or the perineum, the area between the scrotum and the anus. During the trauma, arteries become ruptured, disabling the normal circulation of blood.

Additional causes of a priapism include medication for depression, mental illness and erectile dysfunction, a spinal cord injury, trauma to the genitals, black widow spider bites, carbon monoxide poisoning, drug abuse and cancer.

PREVENTION

While low-flow priapisms cannot be prevented, the best way to protect oneself from a high-flow priapism is to safeguard the genital area from injury.

DIAGNOSIS

A physical examination and medical history are used to diagnosis a priapism. The doctor checks the genitals, rectum and abdomen for clues to the cause. A patient's medical history can identify when the priapism began, the usual amount of time a patient's erection last, any medication or illegal drugs being taken that cause priapisms, and whether the patient has experienced a recent injury to the genitals or spinal cord.

TREATMENT

A varity of treatment options are available for both low-flow and high-flow priapism.

• **DECONGESTANT MEDICATION** Pseudoephedrine and terbutaline, ingredients in many decongestants, are used in cases of an erection that has lasted fewer than four hours. They work by decreasing blood flow to the penis.

• **ICE PACKS** Applying an ice pack to the genitals can ease the discomfort of priapism by reducing swelling in the penis and the perineum.

• **SURGICAL LIGATION** A ruptured artery is repaired in order to restore blood flow to the penis.

• **ALPHA-AGONISTS** This drug is used in the case of a low-flow priapism. It is injected into a penis, and works by constricting veins, which in turn limits blood flow to the penis and causes the erection to stop.

• **SURGICAL SHUNT** In this procedure, a surgeon inserts an artificial passageway into the penis that serves as a bypass for the flow of blood. This enables circulation to return to normal.

• **SELECTIVE EMBOLIZATION** This relatively new technique involves the use of an object such as a tiny coil, a polyvinyl chloride or vinyl pellet, or a metal sponge introduced in the bloodstream to block the flow of blood to the penis.

• **ASPIRATION** The doctor uses a needle to remove blood from the penis to eliminate the erection.

See also: *Leukaemia, p.335 • Sickle-Cell Disease, pp.312–13 • Substance Abuse, pp.358–60*

WHO IS AT RISK?

The risk factors include:

• Drug abuse
• Sickle-cell disease
• Leukaemia
• Malaria
• Spinal cord injury
• Trauma to the genitals
• Bites of a black widow spider
• Carbon monoxide poisoning
• Cancer

Cancer

Malignant or tumour cells can originate in any part of the body and are characterized by their ability to reproduce uncontrollably and to invade surrounding tissue through the circulatory and lymphatic systems. Common cancers of the male reproductive system are prostate cancer and testicular cancer.

CAUSES

Tumour cells result from disruptions or mutations to cellular DNA. Exposure to radiation, drugs, smoking, infections and characteristics inherited from one's parents, can all cause DNA mutations.

PREVENTION

The best way to prevent cancer is by maintaining a balanced diet. At present, nothing can prevent testicular cancer, and regular testicular examinations are recommended for men between the ages of 15 and 40. This screening may help identify the disease in

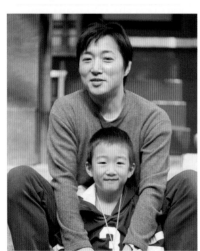

The risk of cancer is higher if you have a relative who has experienced prostate cancer or testicular cancer.

the early stages and increase the chances of successful treatment.

Drinking 0.25 litre (8 fl.oz) a day of pomegranate juice may reduce the risk of the developing prostate cancer. Pomegranate prevents the rise of prostate specific antigen (PSA) levels in the body and controls cellular regeneration. Research on supplements of vitamin E and selenium has suggested they may also decrease the risk of developing prostate cancer.

DIAGNOSIS

Most cancers of the male reproductive system can be diagnosed during a physical examination or by tests performed by a doctor.

Prostate Cancer

The prostate is a walnut-sized gland that surrounds the urethra. It produces semen, the fluid that makes up the largest component of the ejaculate and is important for sperm function. The symptoms of prostate cancer include problems starting or stopping the flow of urine, painful urination or ejaculations, and persistent pain in the hips or back. It is important to remember that these symptoms

can be caused by a number of conditions. The following tests may diagnose their cause.

• **DIGITAL RECTAL EXAMINATION** The doctor examines the prostate by inserting a gloved finger into the rectum.

• **PROSTATE SPECIFIC ANTIGEN (PSA) TEST** This test measures the amount of PSA, a substance produced by cells in the prostate, in the bloodstream. Although an elevated level of PSA may be an indication of prostate cancer, many men with a high score do not have cancer.

• **TRANSRECTAL ULTRASOUND** A small probe is placed in the rectum that produces sound waves, allowing the prostate to be visualized by a computer monitor.

• **BIOPSY** A small amount of tissue is removed. A pathologist examines the cellular structure within the tissue sample. Other tests include the following.

- **BONE SCAN** Radioactive material is injected into the blood and travels to damaged areas, where it can be seen with a special camera. The doctor determines whether the damage is due to prostate cancer.
- **COMPUTED TOMOGRAPHY (CT)** X-rays are used to take pictures of sections within the body.
- **MAGNETIC RESONANCE IMAGING (MRI)** With the use of special magnets, radio waves can be absorbed into the body and produce images at various angles.

Testicular Cancer

This type of cancer is usually discovered during self-examination or a physical examination. A doctor may perform an ultrasound to evaluate the mass or do a biopsy (see above) of the testicles. Blood tests are also used to measure tumour markers. A tumour marker is a substance frequently produced in abundance if cancer is present.

On Call

Many people erroneously believe that breast cancer affects only women. The truth is that both men and women have breast tissue within which breast cancer cells can multiply.

There are a number of factors that put men at risk for developing breast cancer.
- Over the age of 60
- Radiation exposure
- The presence of certain genes
- Having an extra X chromosome
- Exposure to oestrogen
- Liver disease
- Obesity
- Alcoholism

TREATMENTS

Potential treatments are based on the stage of the cancer.

Prostate Cancer

- **MONITORING** A patient, in conjunction with his doctor, monitors the symptoms. This tactic is used when the extent of prostate cancer and the associated symptoms are at a minimum. The doctor may recommend watchful waiting in elderly patients or those with other medical conditions.
- **SURGERY** A surgeon removes the prostate and surrounding tissues, such as the seminal vesicles, if the cancer is localized to the prostate. This option may be most effective during the early stages of the cancer for healthy men under age 70.
- **RADIATION THERAPY** This treatment destroys cancerous cells and reduces the size of the tumour. Small doses of radiation are given over a period of time. Unfortunately, radiation therapy also damages healthy cells. Spacing out the dosages appropriately allows the healthy cells time to recover. Radiation may be given externally or internally with special beads.
- **HORMONAL THERAPY** Testosterone causes prostate cancer cells to multiply. Medication is given to decrease the amount of testosterone in a patient's body. Examples include luteinizing hormone-releasing hormone (LHRH), antagonist therapy, and anti-androgen therapy. Sometimes the testicles are removed as they are responsible for the production of testosterone. These treatments are usually reserved for the later stages of prostate cancer.

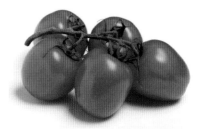

Lycopene, a substance found in tomatoes, pink grapefruit and watermelon, prevents damage to the genetic material found in cells and may help prevent both prostate and testicular cancer.

- **CHEMOTHERAPY** Toxic chemicals are used to destroy any rapidly multiplying cells in the body. As with radiaion, both healthy cells and cancer cells can be destroyed. Chemotherapy is an option only in the later stages of the disease.

Testicular Cancer

The two varieties of testicular cancer are seminomas and nonseminomas. Nonseminomas are more aggressive. In contrast, seminomas are slow-growing and remain in the testicles for long periods of time. Treatment options are:
- **ORCHIECTOMY** A surgeon makes an incision through the groin and removes the testicle containing the tumor and affected lymph nodes.
- **RADIATION THERAPY** This option is used only in cases of seminomas, as they are sensitive to radiation. After removing the tumour, the doctor may treat the affected area with radiation to ensure all the cancer cells have been eliminated.
- **CHEMOTHERAPY** A doctor may choose to administer chemotherapy after surgery to remove the tumour and any affected lymph nodes.

See also: *Supplements, Vitamins & Minerals, pp.532–41*

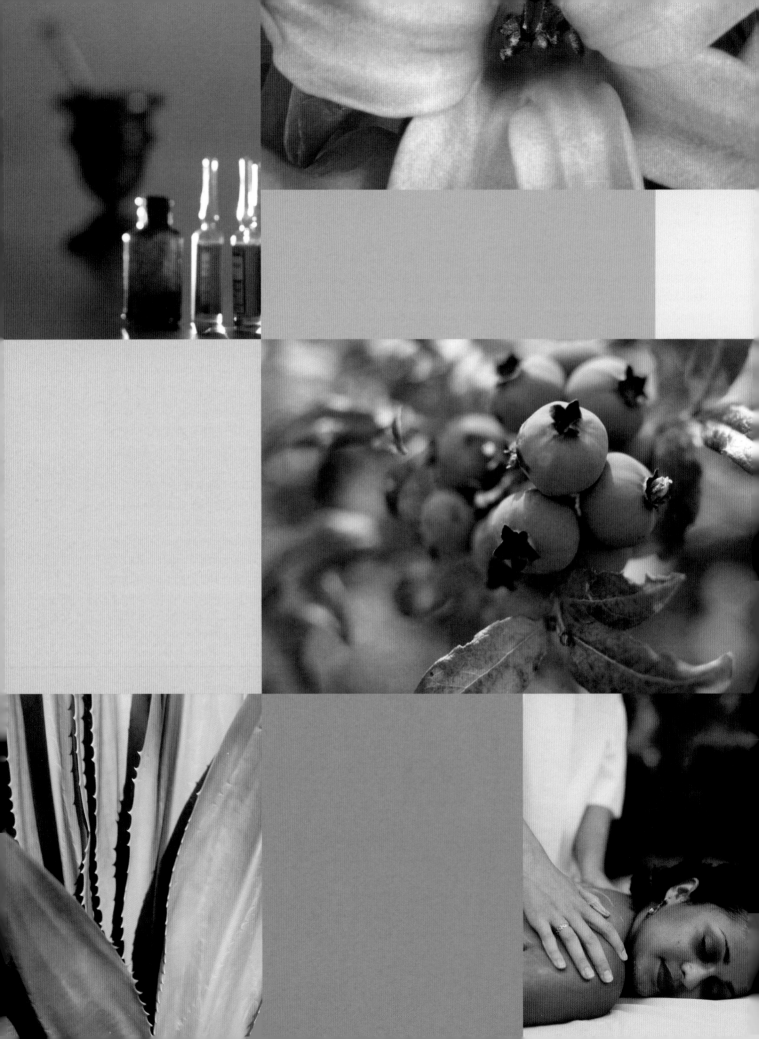

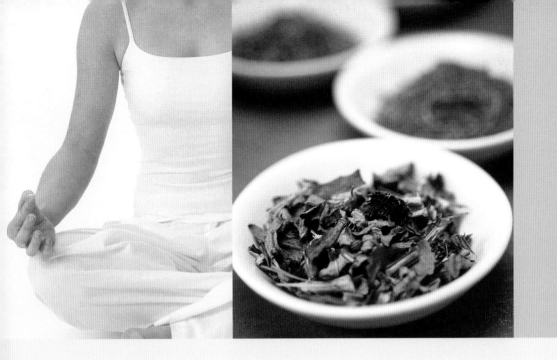

PART II

Complementary & Alternative Therapies

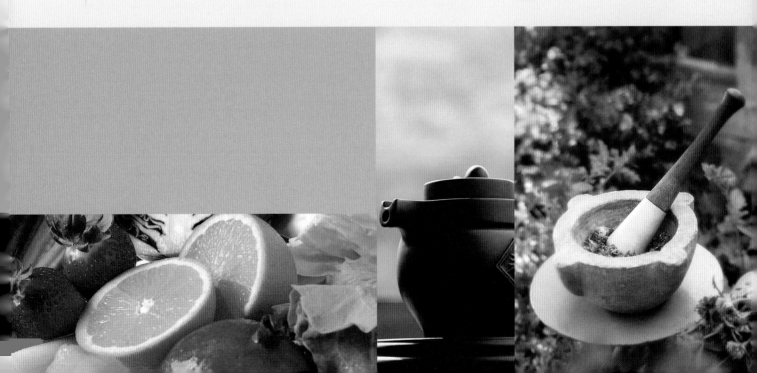

About CAM Therapies

Most patients contemplating complementary/alternative medicine (CAM) therapy want to know two things: Does it work? and Is it safe? This book provides answers by presenting the best evidence there is, based on the most up-to-date research.

More and more people are turning to CAM therapies. They may be seeking a 'whole person' approach to healthcare consistent with their values. They may be looking for the most effective treatment available after orthodox medicine has failed, or they may want to avoid side-effects of conventional pharmaceuticals.

CAM has much to offer modern healthcare. There is evidence that suggests that particular treatments achieve similar or even better results than their orthodox counterparts, some with fewer adverse effects. Glucosamine to treat knee osteoarthritis is a good example of an effective treatment with reduced side-effects when compared to over-the-counter remedies.

The Research Paradox

Although there is now an increasing body of quality evidence to support many uses of CAM, there is still a relative dearth of formally designed research studies. Such research is vital to ensure that valuable therapies are made available while ineffective or harmful ones are avoided, and in the process safeguard users. Unfortunately, research into CAM is fraught with difficulties. As well as inadequate funding, the approach of many CAM systems is so different from that of conventional medicine that it is difficult to conduct studies within similar frameworks.

Scientific Trials

Before being approved for public use, conventional drugs must pass an elaborate series of tests and be licensed. Clinical trials usually involve a single agent or procedure intended to act against either an isolated symptom or characteristic – such as a cough, nausea or high blood pressure – or a set of features distinguishing a particular condition, for example influenza, joint inflammation or vascular disease. These are defined with measurable outcomes: the coughing improves, the blood pressure comes down or inflammation is reduced. Typically, the active agent is compared either with another, or with a placebo (an inert substance made to appear identical to the active treatment).

Most trials are randomized – patients are selected for active or control groups purely by chance. They are also conducted 'blind'. In a single-blind trial, patients do not know which treatment they are receiving. In a double-blind trial, the researcher does not know either. Such precautions are attempts to reduce the influence of factors that might otherwise bias the outcome, such as sicker patients being preferentially selected for active treatment. In most trials, a significant proportion of patients taking placebos also experience improvement as well as side-effects.

The double-blind, placebo-controlled randomized clinical trial has long been regarded as the gold standard in medical research. The problem is that this model often does not fit the approach of CAM therapies.

Trials of Complementary Medicine

It is difficult to find valid control treatments for some CAM therapies – patients can readily recognize acupuncture or chiropractic manipulation, for example.

CAM therapies generally address multiple factors such as personality, lifestyle, nutrition and relationships. Treatments are tailored to the individual rather than the condition, and often involve several components targeted at improving overall well-being. It is hard to assess individual elements, and difficult to provide a control comparison. In addition, the approach to patients with similar symptoms or diagnoses may differ.

Since many CAM practitioners have a philosophical bias towards promoting self-healing, their aims – and how they assess outcomes – can be quite different from those of conventional doctors. Inevitably there is also more variation in training and practice between practitioners. Even when the benefits of a CAM treatment for a given condition are demonstrated, its mechanism of action often remains unknown within existing concepts of Western science.

Integrating CAM

Research is beginning to provide some explanations. Researchers have devised sham treatments for both chiropractic manipulation and acupuncture, enabling better comparative trials. CAM therapies are also increasingly recognized as playing a valuable role as an adjunct to conventional medicine, for example to improve sense of well-being among cancer patients. Chinese researchers have shown that adding moxibustion to the treatment improves the effectiveness of orthodox treatment for rheumatoid arthritis, and reduces the need for conventional drugs. Similarly, hypnosis may reduce the use of drugs in chronic pain.

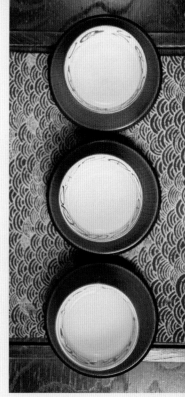

Other studies have demonstrated that CAM treatments may mitigate the side-effects of pharmaceutical drugs. Conventional medicine is also beginning to take note of ideas of health that CAM practitioners have been espousing for centuries, for example a greater focus on nutritional approaches to disease.

Improving the research into CAM therapies will enhance the prospects for evidence-based, patient-centred healthcare that will incorporate any therapy demonstrated to be safe and effective – and this is the future of integrative medicine.

SCALE OF EVIDENCE

For each of the complementary/alternative treatments discussed in Part II, we have provided our estimate of how well benefits of the treatment have been established. The green scale ranges from 1 – minimal to no evidence of benefit, to 3 – strong evidence of benefit. In the red scale, we have also provided our estimate of how much risk or danger may be involved in using the treatment. For example: meditation involves minimal risk, whereas ozone therapy can lead to serious side-effects such as anaemia, while some natural supplements such as kava-kava have been associated with liver failure and death and cannot be recommended in most circumstances.

We have not given a rating to any of the total systems of complementary/alternative medicine. These systems (pp.436–61) use many different treatment methods, most of which have been individually rated. The methods chosen to treat each patient depend on the patient's individual condition.

BENEFIT SCALE

 Treatments for which there is little or no evidence of benefit.

 Treatments for which there is some supportive data (anecdotal evidence, case reports, practitioners' consensus) that are possibly/probably helpful.

 Treatments for which there is strong supportive data that are probably/definitely helpful, including well designed clinical trials.

RISK SCALE

 Treatments for which there are *minimal risks* when used appropriately to treat specific conditions (as described in each section).

 Treatments for which there are *known risks* but that may be recommended to treat some conditions in circumstances when benefits outweigh risks.

 Treatments for which there are *definite risks* and are *not* recommended.

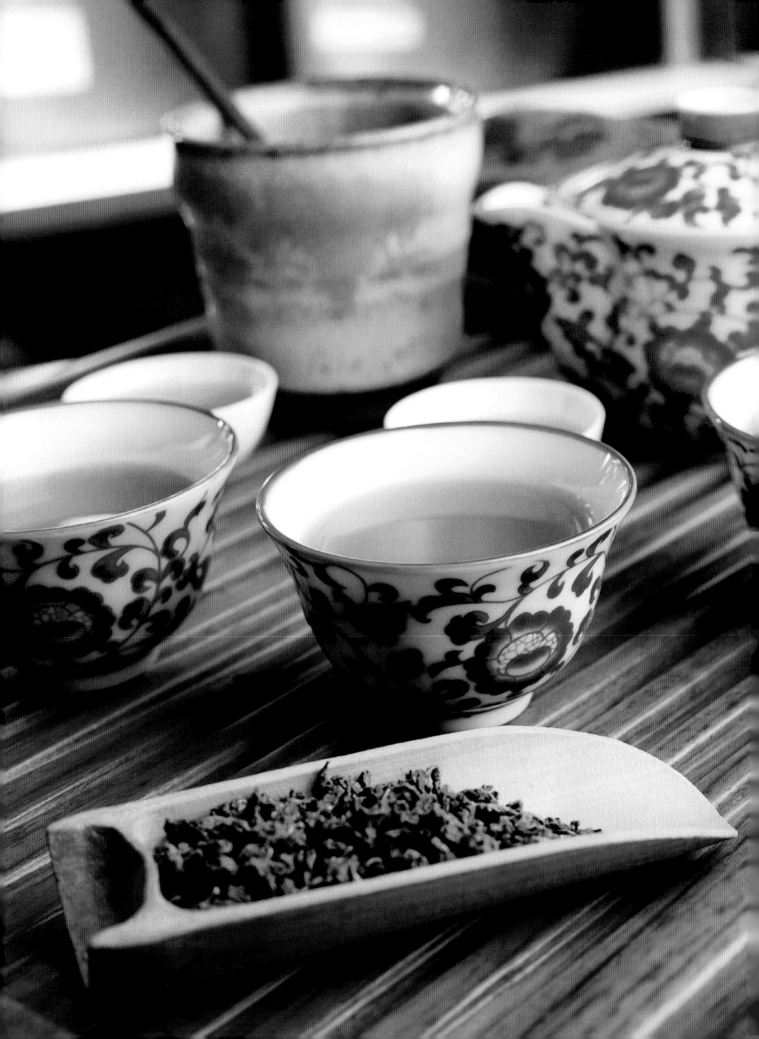

16 | SYSTEMS

The medicine of ancient cultures, such as Indian Ayurveda, Traditional Chinese Medicine or Tibetan Medicine, was refined by many people over millennia, usually as the only form of medicine available at the time. More recent systems of medicine were often fashioned by just a few people – for example, naturopathy and anthroposophic medicine – or even single individuals, as with homeopathy, osteopathy, and functional medicine. What they all have in common, other than offering an overall 'healthcare package' based on a particular philosophy, is their ability to pay attention to everything about a person. This attention is generally directed as much to the preservation of health as to the treatment of disease, and coupled with an awareness of the importance of the person's constitution, circumstances, personality, preferences and lifestyle, and of the mind–body connection and self-healing capabilities. All are truly holistic therapies – concerned with the whole person.

Osteopathy

This system of preventative medicine and treatment focuses on the relationship between the musculoskeletal system and the internal organs. Misalignment in any part of the musculoskeletal system (due to a variety of causes, including muscle injuries, tension and poor posture) is believed to impair health by blocking the free flow of blood and lymphatic fluids. Doctors of osteopathy use various manipulative techniques to correct these misalignments and improve overall health. Stress-reduction techniques and nutrition advice are other important aspects of treatment. Many osteopaths also practise conventional medicine: they prescribe medication, provide obstetrical care and perform surgery.

HISTORY

Osteopathy was developed in the United States by a doctor, Andrew Taylor Still. Following the death of three of his children from spinal meningitis in 1864, Still concluded that the orthodox medical practices of his day were frequently ineffective and sometimes harmful. Based on research and personal observation, he decided that the musculoskeletal system was central to the health and well-being of the rest of the body. In his view, by correcting problems in the body's structure using manual manipulation techniques, the body's ability to function and to heal itself could be greatly improved.

Still also promoted the idea of preventative medicine and endorsed the philosophy that doctors should focus on treating the whole patient, rather than just the disease. Today, osteopathy is practised throughout the world.

PRACTICE

Osteopaths, also called doctors of osteopathy, are trained at osteopathic medical schools. Their education is similar to that of medical doctors, but also includes training in osteopathic manipulation and holistic health. Osteopaths are licensed medical professionals in many countries. In the United States their licence conveys the same privileges as that of a medical doctor, allowing them to order laboratory tests, prescribe medicine and perform surgery. Osteopaths also have full hospital privileges in the United States.

The practice of osteopathy varies from country to country. In the United States, osteopaths use conventional medical diagnostic and treatment practices along with osteopathic manipulation, physical therapy and patient education about good posture. In many other countries, osteopaths primarily use holistic approaches to diagnosis and treatment.

During a visit, an osteopath will evaluate a patient's medical history and ask questions about symptoms, illnesses and lifestyle

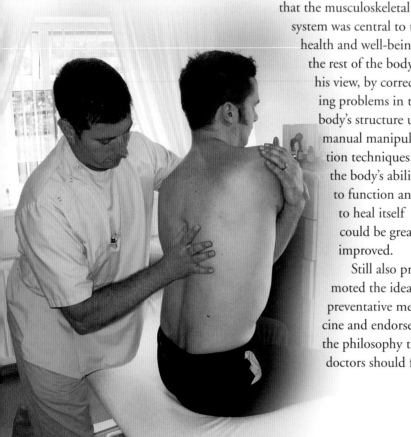

Osteopathic manipulation helps the body heal itself by properly aligning the body's organs, skeleton and muscles. Correct alignment ensures the free flow of blood and lymphatic fluids.

Clinical Query

What is the difference between osteopathic manipulation and chiropractic manipulation?

Osteopaths and chiropractors have different philosophies of health and illness. Osteopaths focus broadly on imbalances and misalignments throughout the musculoskeletal system, while chiropractors tend to focus on subluxations, or misalignments of the spine and the neck. For the most part, osteopathic manipulation is gentler than that carried out by chiropractors (pp.466–7), which is characterized by quick thrusts. An osteopath will gently move a joint to increase its range of motion or place a patient in a certain position to enable the body to release muscle spasms caused by an injury. When range of motion is severely restricted, however, osteopaths may use a quick thrusting manipulation, similar to chiropractic manipulation.

issues such as exercise and nutrition. Osteopaths use the following methods to evaluate health problems:

- Observation of posture and gait.
- Testing the range of motion of different parts of the body.
- Attention to symmetry – whether a person favours one side of the body or has a curvature of the spine.
- Palpation and inspection of the skin to test reflexes and detect such symptoms as excess fluid, tenderness and tight muscles.
- Conventional diagnostic tests such as blood and urine tests, and X-rays.

TREATMENTS

The aim of osteopathy is to treat health problems and educate patients about ways to prevent illnesses. The same prescription and over-the-counter drugs and surgical procedures used by traditional medical doctors are also used by many osteopaths to treat a wide range of health conditions, including upper respiratory infections, high blood pressure and gastrointestinal illnesses. The following treatments are also used.

- **MOVEMENT AND EXERCISE** Osteopathic manipulation includes several techniques to increase mobility and release muscular tension, including soft tissue massage, gentle mobilization, strain–counterstrain, myofascial release, articulation and craniosacral therapy (pp.480–1). Gentle mobilization involves slowly moving a joint to increase its range of motion. Strain–counterstrain is the movement of joints away from their restrictions to improve their functioning. Myofascial release (p.469) is a soft tissue massage used to release tension and improve muscle functioning. Articulation is a sudden, thrusting manipulation intended to mobilize a joint when its range of motion is very limited. Craniosacral therapy is a rhythmic manipulation of the head and base of the spine to relieve headache, neck pain and other conditions.

Many osteopaths also use techniques to improve posture, such as the Feldenkrais (pp.494–5) and Alexander techniques (pp.488–9).

- **NUTRITION** Osteopathic treatment draws on research into the connection between nutrition and the risk of certain illnesses. Advice on particular foods to eat or nutritional supplements to take is tailored to individual patients based on their conditions.

- **MIND–BODY CONNECTION** Osteopathic doctors educate patients on ways to prevent health problems by reducing stress. Methods include relaxation techniques, exercises and diaphragmatic breathing.

Myofascial release massage is a technique used to ease pressure within the fibrous bands of connective tissue that surround and support the muscles.

CAN OSTEOPATHY HELP ME?

Using conventional medicine, doctors of osteopathy can treat the same health conditions as primary care physicians. They can also provide prenatal care, deliver babies and provide paediatric care. In addition, osteopathic manipulation has been found beneficial for treating low back pain and there is evidence that it can help a wide range of other conditions. Most of the trials that have tested osteopathic manipulation therapy were small pilot studies, and therefore, the evidence is preliminary.

- **Low back pain** Several clinical trials have found osteopathic manipulation therapy beneficial for low back pain when administered within the first month after symptoms begin. Its effectiveness is comparable to that of conventional medical treatment. But a key difference is that patients treated with osteopathic manipulation therapy use fewer pain relievers, anti-inflammatory agents and other drugs, and need less physical therapy than do patients receiving conventional medical care.

- **Arthritis** People with arthritis who have osteopathic manipulation therapy and conventional medical care have less pain and greater mobility than similar people who have only conventional medical care.

- **Sprains and strains** A session of osteopathic manipulation therapy for a sprained ankle can significantly reduce swelling and pain. It is also effective in treating tennis elbow.

- **Fibromyalgia** Osteopathic manipulation therapy has been shown to reduce pain and improve daily functioning in women with fibromyalgia (pp.144–5).

- **Postoperative pain** A combination of osteopathic manipulation therapy and pain medicine appears to be better than pain medicine alone for relieving pain following various kinds of surgical procedures.

Patients given osteopathic manipulation therapy have less pain, need less pain medication, and are able to get out of bed sooner than patients given only pain-relieving drugs.

- **Depression** Osteopathic manipulation therapy, combined with antidepressant medication, is more effective than antidepressants alone in relieving symptoms of depression.

- **Recurrent middle ear infections** The children who had osteopathic manipulation therapy in addition to conventional medical treatment have fewer recurrences of ear infection and need fewer surgical procedures to drain ear fluid than do children who receive only conventional medical care.

- **Cerebral palsy** In infants with cerebral palsy, osteopathic manipulation therapy can lead to a host of benefits, including better sleep, improved mood, and better coordination of arms and legs.

- **Other conditions** Some people with asthma, chronic obstructive pulmonary disease, menstrual pain, neck pain and pneumonia will also benefit from osteopathic manipulation therapy.

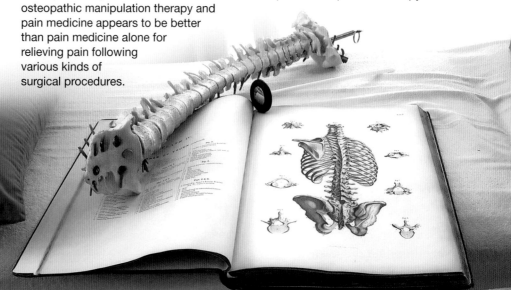

The philosophy that all of the body's systems are interrelated and dependent on one another for optimal health is the founding principle of osteopathy. Wellness is achieved by treating the whole body, not just the individual symptoms.

Functional Medicine

This relatively new holistic approach uses information about an individual's predisposition for certain illnesses to devise strategies to prevent those illnesses and enhance overall health. Each person is prone to certain health problems based on their genetic makeup, as well as external factors such as where they live and work, their diet, their level of physical activity level and the quality of their social relationships. Functional medicine takes all of these factors into account to help each individual devise a plan to prevent or control the health problems they are likely to develop.

HISTORY

The term 'functional medicine' was coined in 1993 by Dr Jeffrey S. Bland, an American biochemist specializing in nutrition. Since then, a broad range of healthcare providers have embraced the functional medicine approach, including medical doctors, osteopaths, nurses and acupuncturists. This approach to healthcare provides a way of helping individuals prevent and manage health problems that are caused by risk factors a person can control, such as diabetes and heart disease.

PRACTICE

Functional medicine does not treat acute medical conditions or medical emergencies. It is preventative medicine – intended to help individuals reduce their risk of developing chronic diseases by identifying and eliminating risk factors that are within their control, such as smoking, poor diet and a sedentary lifestyle. Although genetics influences each person's risk of disease, modifiable risk factors can increase or decrease that risk by affecting the expression of those genes. For example, modifiable risk factors cause 70 percent or more cases of stroke, colon cancer (pp.288–95) and type-2 diabetes (pp.338–41).

A healthcare practitioner who uses a functional medicine approach will assess an individual's personal risk factors by asking them about their family medical history (which will reveal any genetic predispositions); 'environmental inputs' that influence health, including the quality of the air and water in the area in which they live and work, as well as toxic chemicals to which they may have been exposed; their diet, exercise habits and psychosocial factors. The practitioner will also do a physical examination and may perform certain laboratory tests, such as blood tests. The results, along with an individual's genetic and environmental profile, help determine whether they suffer from any functional imbalances (physical or mental disturbances that can be precursors to disease). These sorts of imbalances include nutritional insufficiencies, weakness in immune function, inflammation, and psychosocial and emotional stress.

TREATMENTS

A variety of proven therapies are used in functional medicine, such as stress-reduction techniques and nutrition counselling. Supplements are sometimes prescribed.
- **MIND-BODY CONNECTION** Stress-reduction techniques are recommended for reducing psychosocial stress.
- **MOVEMENT AND EXERCISE** If the patient does

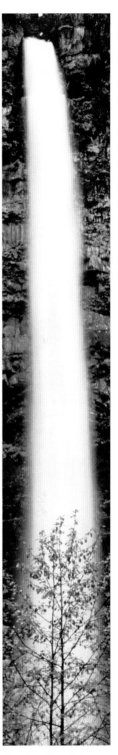

Functional medicine is tailored to the individual, helping patients avoid illness by managing environmental and lifestyle factors that can cause disease.

not get enough exercise, the practitioner may suggest a regular exercise regimen.

• NUTRITION Practitioners may advise dietary changes to reduce the risk of certain illnesses. For example, reducing the amount of saturated fats and trans fatty acids in a diet and increasing the consumption of fish lowers the risk of heart disease. Proper diet also promotes weight loss – obesity increases the risk of developing a number of illnesses, including diabetes.

• PHYSICAL ENVIRONMENT If a patient is exposed to dangerous substances at home or at work, the practitioner may be able to advise them on how to reduce their exposure. For instance, if there is lead in the local drinking water, installing a carbon filter can remove much of it. If a patient smokes, or if someone in the household smokes, the practitioner can counsel them on ways to quit (pp.216–17).

• PHARMACEUTICALS AND SUPPLEMENTS Nutritional supplements (pp.532–41) may be used in functional medicine for a range of purposes, including detoxification, boosting the immune system and weight loss.

Regular exercise promotes well-being by increasing energy and reducing stress, and can play a key role in correcting functional imbalances.

CAN FUNCTIONAL MEDICINE HELP ME?

Although there are few scientific studies of functional medicine as a system, it has the potential to help virtually anyone reduce their risk of chronic illnesses such as cardiovascular disease, diabetes and cancer by identifying and changing modifiable risk factors. Beneficial therapies used in functional medicine include getting regular exercise, eating a healthy diet and reducing stress. Making positive lifestyle changes can also help improve everyday functioning by making people feel more energetic and alert and improving their mood. The judicious use of nutritional supplements with strong scientific merit, such as omega-3 fatty acids (pp.252–3), can be beneficial in reducing the risk of certain health problems, such as hypertension, inflammatory bowel disease and rheumatoid arthritis.

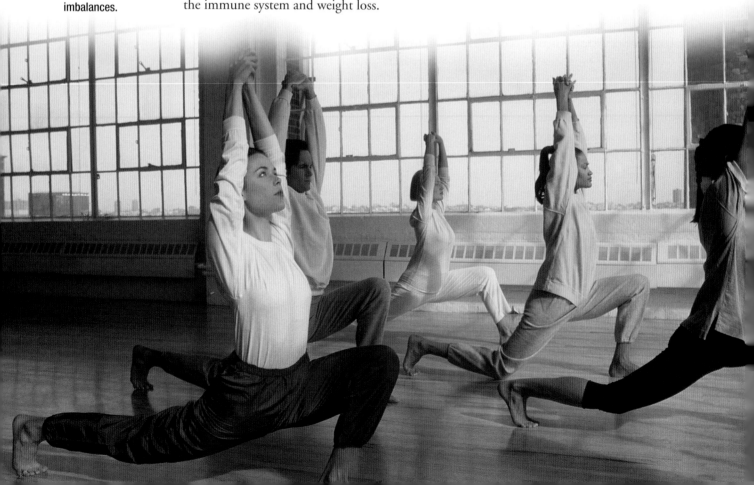

Naturopathy

The aim of naturopathy is to educate patients on how to prevent illness and, if they are sick, to support the body's capacity to heal itself. Practitioners use a wide range of natural healing tools, including nutritional supplements (pp.532–41), botanical medicine (pp.552–9), spinal manipulation, hydrotherapy (pp.482–3), exercises, counselling, Traditional Chinese Medicine (pp.446–50) and Ayurveda (pp.451–4) – all of which emphasize addressing the cause of a health problem. These tools may be prescribed individually or in combination. Naturopathy is used mainly to treat chronic and degenerative diseases, such as asthma and osteoarthritis. It is not intended to treat medical emergencies.

HISTORY

Naturopathy as a discipline began in Europe in the 19th century as part of a growing interest in natural medicine. Known simply as 'the nature cure', it spread to North America in the early 1900s. Today, naturopathic doctors are trained in graduate-level schools throughout Europe and North America. Some degrees are granted by web-based programmes, which are less rigorous than conventional naturopathy schools. Naturopathy is increasingly being integrated into conventional medicine to manage a wide range of health issues, including pregnancy and childbirth, arthritis and migraines.

PRACTICE

In contrast to conventional physicians, whose main focus is diagnosing illness, naturopathic doctors aim primarily to teach their patients how to maintain good health and prevent illness. A consultation with a naturopath involves taking a medical history, and a detailed interview about the patient's diet and other aspects of their lifestyle. If they have symptoms of an illness, the naturopathic doctor will use conventional diagnostic procedures, such as blood and urine tests, to help identify the cause.

A plan of preventive medicine, treatment, or both is then tailored to each individual patient's needs.

TREATMENTS

Naturopathic treatments include dietary changes, exercise, counselling, therapeutic manipulation, acupuncture (pp.464–5) and natural remedies, including both herbal remedies (pp.552–9) and homeopathy (pp.455–7).

• **COUNSELLING** Doctors of naturopathy use cognitive–behavioural therapy and other counselling techniques to treat depression and other psychological illnesses. Cognitive–behavioural therapy combines traditional 'talking' therapy with behavioural modification that helps naturopathy patients weaken the connections between difficult situations and their reactions to them.

• **ELECTRICAL STIMULATION** Transcutaneous electrical nerve stimulation (TENS) involves stimulating tissue with electrical currents. TENS sends a painless, mild electrical current to specific nerves through patches placed on the skin. The current generates heat, which helps relieve muscle pain and promote circulation, and is also believed to stimulate the body's production of natural pain-killers. Pulsed electromagnetic field stimulation sends

Naturopathic doctors use hydrotheraphy to improve circulation to the organs that detoxify the blood, such as the liver and kidneys, thereby stimulating the body's ability to heal itself.

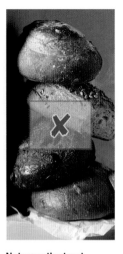

Naturopaths treat food as medicine and stress the importance of a diet high in whole grains, fruit and vegetables and low in processed foods.

CAN NATUROPATHY HELP ME?

Naturopathic doctors often work with conventional doctors to help care for patients with a variety of chronic conditions. Systematic reviews of naturopathy have not found evidence of its overall effectiveness. However, studies of individual treatments have shown some benefit for the following conditions.

- **Osteoarthritis** Glucosamine sulphate (a building-block of the fluid that cushions the joints) and SAMe (S-adenosyl-methionine, a compound that supports the production of joint cartilage), two natural supplements that are widely prescribed for relieving joint pain, are as effective as the drug ibuprofen in relieving symptoms of osteoarthritis, but with fewer side-effects. Other effective naturopathic therapies include a topical cream made from the herb capsaicin, pulsed electromagnetic field stimulation and acupuncture.

- **Asthma** To reduce the incidence and severity of asthma attacks, naturopaths recommend an elimination diet (a diet designed to identify food allergies), vitamin C supplements, and stress-reduction techniques such as deep breathing from the diaphragm.

- **Heart disease** A Mediterranean diet (rich in omega-3 fatty acids, vegetables, fruit, whole grains and fish, and low in meat and dairy products) can reduce the risk of heart attacks and death from heart disease. Naturopaths recommend niacin supplements for people who have had heart attacks, because niacin can help reduce mortality.

- **Back pain** Exercise, relaxation techniques and cognitive–behavioural therapy are used to control chronic back pain.

- **Benign prostatic hypertrophy** Naturopaths recommend herbs and supplements to relieve symptoms of enlarged prostate. For example, saw palmetto can improve urination problems and flow rate, and *Pygeum africanum* and a pollen extract can decrease prostate size.

- **Depression** The herb St John's wort is effective for relieving mild to moderate depression. For seasonal affective disorder (depression that recurs during the winter), naturopaths recommend light therapy.

- **Eczema** Naturopaths use nutrition therapies to treat and prevent eczema – for children and adults, eliminating eggs and cow's milk from the diet; for infants, delaying the

pulses of electromagnetic energy into the body, through coils and other devices placed on the body, and is believed to aid in wound healing and fusion of bone fractures.

• ACUPUNCTURE Naturopaths recommend acupuncture (pp.464–5) and acupressure (p.472) for acute and chronic pain relief.

• HYDROTHERAPY Techniques, such as soaking baths, whirlpools, ice packs and colonic irrigations (p.482), are used to treat health conditions such as migraine headaches.

• NUTRITION Diet modification is one of the primary forms of therapy used in naturopathy. Practitioners often recommend eliminating foods from the diet that may cause allergies or intolerances to see if a condition improves. Fasting or diets designed to cleanse the body by eliminating toxins may be prescribed. In addition, drawing on the

growing research on the connection between diet and health, naturopaths stress consumption of whole grains, fruit and vegetables as a means of preventing illness.

Naturopathy also uses probiotics (foods with beneficial bacteria, see pp.550–1), such as yogurt containing active cultures of *Lactobacillus acidophilus*, the bacteria that normally live in the intestines help regulate digestion and stool patterns. Their populations can become depleted due to competition with other bacteria, such as yeast, or when antibiotics are ingested. Replenishing the beneficial bacteria helps maintain overall health.

• PHARMACEUTICALS AND SUPPLEMENTS Naturopaths are trained in herbal medicine traditions and may prescribe herbs to prevent and treat various conditions (see Botanicals Therapy, pp.552–9). They also recommend nutritional

introduction of solid foods until they are over four months old. In addition, naturopaths may recommend a salve made of extracts of *Lupinus termis* seeds, used in Traditional Chinese Medicine. Cognitive-behavioural therapy and relaxation techniques may also be recommended to relieve the rash and reduce reliance on topical steroids.

- **Irritable bowel syndrome** A naturopathic approach to controlling this disorder includes a diet that eliminates allergy-provoking foods and stress-management techniques.

- **Migraine headache** Naturopaths use TENS to help prevent migraine headaches. They also recommend magnesium supplements to prevent migraines. To relieve migraine symptoms, naturopaths may suggest cold compresses (a form of hydrotherapy).

- **Middle ear infections and pain** To prevent these conditions, naturopaths advise new mothers to breast-feed infants exclusively for at least four months. When older children have recurrent ear infections, naturopaths advise an elimination diet to identify allergy-provoking foods. Avoiding these foods may reduce the incidence of middle ear infections. Eardrops that contain specific herbs and vitamin E in olive oil can reduce pain in children with middle ear infections.

- **Upper respiratory infections** Naturopaths often recommend taking zinc lozenges at the first sign of a cold, because zinc is believed to shorten the duration of the cold. For influenza, naturopaths use oscillococcinum, a homeopathic preparation, and elderberry, both of which may hasten recovery. For sinusitis, the herb goldenseal mixed with a nasal wash of salt water is used to help clear nasal passages.

- **Vaginitis** For women who are prone to vaginitis, naturopaths recommend regular consumption of yogurt containing active cultures of *Lactobacillus acidophilus*, which helps inhibit the growth infection-causing bacteria such as yeast.

- **Premenstrual syndrome** Practitioners recommend regular exercise as well as various herbal and nutritional supplements to help reduce mood swings, breast pain and pelvic cramps. These include calcium, magnesium, vitamin B_6 and chasteberry.

- **Pregnancy and childbirth** Naturopathic doctors work alone or with midwives to counsel women on nutrition during pregnancy and after delivery, as well as to assist with natural childbirth.

- **Menopause** Black cohosh is used to relieve night sweats and hot flushes, as is eating foods that contain soy.

supplements with therapeutic potential, such as zinc and omega-3 fatty acids (pp.252–3).

• MIND-BODY CONNECTION Naturopaths receive training in psychology to recognize and treat psychosocial difficulties, such as stress, addictions, developmental disorders and sexual dysfunction. They use mind–body therapies to control pain and aid in wound healing. They also use stress-reduction approaches, such as guided imagery (pp.520–2), when stress is contributing to a patient's health problems.

• EXERCISE Exercise recommended to reduce stress, relieve certain types of pain (such as back pain), and as a way of reducing the risk of certain illnesses, such as cardiovascular disease.

• PHYSICAL ENVIRONMENT Light therapy (pp.564), which involves exposure to bright, specially designed lights, is used to alleviate seasonal depression as well as to aid the body's healing process by increasing physiological functions such as blood circulation and metabolism.

Naturopathic healing relies on a combination of therapies that includes herbal remedies from a variety of cultures, such as Traditional Chinese Medicine, homeopathy and Ayurveda.

Traditional Chinese Medicine

One of the most ancient and complex systems of preventing and treating illnesses, Traditional Chinese Medicine (TCM) includes acupuncture, herbal medicine, massage and other hands-on techniques, nutrition and exercise. In its approach to diagnosis and treatment, it takes into account the correlations between body, mind and spirit, as well as the effects of the natural and social environments on an individual.

TCM incorporates elements of the religious and folk healing practices developed in China thousands of years ago. TCM is routinely taught in medical schools in China and other parts of Asia, and is often used along with Western medicine to treat conditions such as chronic pain, chemotherapy-related nausea and arthritis.

Like all herbal products, Chinese herbs carry some potential risks. There have been examples in recent years of Chinese herbal preparations being mis-identified, adulterated, mixed with pharmaceuticals not identified on the label, contaminated with heavy metals, and in other ways improperly processed or prepared. Herbs can cause adverse effects for a variety of reasons, such as the toxicity of the herbs themselves, overdose, interactions with conventional medication and allergic reactions. Still, some components of TCM have shown promise under scientific scrutiny.

HISTORY

TCM derives from folk healing practices that were used in China for thousands of years. *The Yellow Emperor's Classic of Internal Medicine*, the text that lays down the basic principles of Chinese medicine, was completed in 4 B.C.E. and describes the use of medicinal herbs and acupuncture. During the 17th through 19th centuries, missionaries, traders and Chinese immigrants helped introduce TCM throughout the world.

Use of TCM declined during the first half of the 20th century in favour of Western medical practice. But TCM was revived in China when the Communist Party came to power in 1949. Communist rulers sent researchers into the countryside to learn from peasant healers about traditional medicine practices. These researchers tested the treatments to see what worked, and Chinese medical schools incorporated the traditional treatments that seemed effective into their curriculums.

Acupuncture was introduced to the West by Georges Soulié de Mourant in the 1920s. Today, acupuncture and other elements of TCM are used along with Western medicine in many parts of the Eastern and Western world. Acupuncturists are generally licensed by state or national boards.

PRACTICE

Unlike Western medicine, which diagnoses disease based on physical or psychological symptoms, Traditional Chinese Medicine views symptoms in the context of the whole body, mind and spirit. Because TCM does not separate the symptoms from the whole person, people with similar symptoms – nasal congestion or a stomach ache, for instance – may actually be diagnosed with different problems that require different treatments.

Practitioners of TCM view wellness in terms of the balance, or harmony, of different qualities. The fundamental force that enlivens a person and is reflected through these qualities is qi (pronounced 'chee'). Qi is the life-giving energy that flows through all living things as well as the universe. Qi courses through the body in a system with 12 major pathways,

Herbalism is a key component in the practice of Traditional Chinese Medicine which, in addition to herbs, uses substances derived from animal and minerals in the treatment of illness.

or meridians, which reach the surface of the body at various points as well as all of the internal organs. When qi is in balance, which means it is flowing smoothly throughout the body, a person will be in good health. But an excess, a deficiency, a blockage or an imbalance of qi in a person's system will cause poor health or illness.

Other qualities that need to be in balance for good health are yin and yang. Yin and yang are two opposites that characterize everything in the universe, including the organs of the body. Yin represents feminine, passive, dark and inner qualities (see the chart on p.448 for the yin and yang organs) and yang represents masculine, active, light, and outer qualities.

Yin and yang are subdivided into the five elements: fire, earth, metal, water and wood. Each element corresponds to a yin organ and a yang organ. The five elements and their associated organs affect one another. For example, the metal element organs (lungs and large intestine) control the liver and gall bladder (wood organs).

It is important to note that the TCM concept of 'organ' is different from and broader than the anatomical body parts of the same name. A classic example of this is the triple heater or triple burner, an organ that even Chinese physicians say has a name but no shape. The triple heater is considered to integrate and harmonize the functions of the other organ systems.

Illnesses may arise from within the body because of various undesirable influences, such as negative emotions, hunger and overuse. They may also arise from undesirable influences experienced in the natural world, including those of wind, dampness and cold. These undesirable influences can lead to a deficiency of qi in an organ system, which in turn can cause disharmony among the five elements leading to further imbalances in the flow of qi through the body.

PART 2: COMPLEMENTARY AND ALTERNATIVE THERAPIES **447**

	Fire	Earth	Metal	Water	Wood
Yin organs	Heart, pericardium	Spleen	Lungs	Kidneys	Liver
Yang organs	Small intestine, triple heater	Stomach	Large intestine	Urinary bladder	Gall bladder
Sense organs	Tongue	Mouth	Nose	Ears	Eyes
Environment	Heat	Dampness	Dryness	Cold	Wind
Taste	Bitter	Sweet	Pungent	Salty	Sour

Diagnosing Illness

As with Western medicine, TCM relies on a physical examination as well as description of symptoms, a personal medical history and a family medical history. TCM practitioners use the checkup to assess qi and identify imbalances.

During the examination, TCM practitioners pay especially close attention to the pulse and the tongue. They look for 28 qualities of the pulse by feeling it at six places and at three depths on each wrist. (In TCM, the various pulses convey information about several organs and organ systems, not just blood flow.) They note the tongue's colour, texture, thickness, indentations and coating. The results of this examination and a description of symptoms lead a TCM practitioner to make a diagnosis.

TCM diagnoses are not labelled according to a single illness, such as the flu, but are identified as syndromes or patterns of disharmony. These syndromes can be described in terms of eight parameters: hot versus cold, external versus internal, excessive versus deficient and yin versus yang. Herbs, particular foods and other remedies may be prescribed to correct these imbalances.

TREATMENTS

Because every illness is a result of complex imbalances unique to each individual, TCM therapies vary from person to person – even when two people have what seems in Western terms to be the same illness. The following therapies may be used alone or in combination.

• ACUPUNCTURE This therapy has evolved over thousands of years. Fine needles are inserted into acupuncture points, which are points along the meridian system that, when stimulated, are believed to influence the circulation of qi. Several sterile disposable needles are usually inserted for an acupuncture treatment, and the acupuncture points used depend on the syndrome that is diagnosed. Moxibustion or cupping (see below) is sometimes used to augment the effects of needle acupuncture.

Today, various styles of acupuncture are practiced, some of which vary considerably from the TCM approach. Some styles are used with limited or no other TCM-based therapies. This kind of acupuncture, used alone, is often prescribed to control problems such as chronic pain and nausea, while the more holistic styles used in TCM also aim to restore overall health by correcting imbalances of qi.

Electro-acupuncture, a variation on the traditional needle method, involves sending an electric current pulse through the acupuncture needles to stimulate specific acupuncture points. In some cases, an acupuncturist uses methods other than needles to stimulate acupuncture points, including ultrasound, laser beams and heat.

Some doctors dismiss the notion of meridians and, instead, say that acupuncture works by triggering biochemicals, including painkilling endorphins and mood-altering neurotransmitters. There is some evidence

CAN TRADITIONAL CHINESE MEDICINE HELP ME ?

Of all the therapies used in TCM, acupuncture has been studied most extensively and established most firmly as an effective treatment for a number of conditions. Research has also looked at many Chinese herbal treatments and found some of them promising.

- **Pain** Acupuncture can ease chronic and acute pain, such as neck pain, myofascial pain, carpal tunnel syndrome, menstrual cramps, low-back pain and tension headaches.

- **Nausea** Acupuncture can relieve nausea associated with pregnancy, and acupuncture and electro-acupuncture may help reduce nausea from some types of chemotherapy.

- **Postoperative dental pain** Acupuncture reduces pain following dental procedures.

- **Depression** One Chinese study found that acupuncture was comparable to anti-depressants in relieving depression. After five weeks of treatment, 70 percent of those who had acupuncture were significantly improved, compared with 65 percent of those who had taken medication.

- **Stroke rehabilitation** Acupuncture can help people who have had strokes increase mobility, balance and quality of life.

- **Skin conditions** Acupuncture may help clear up acne, atopic dermatitis and psoriasis.

- **Tension headaches** In a randomised controlled trial of 270 patients, researchers at the Centre for Complementary Medicine Research in Munich, Germany, found patients receiving traditional acupuncture reported their headache rates dropped by almost half over the eight-week treatment period. Improvements continued for months after the acupuncture treatment, though they began to rise slightly as time went on. Those in the 'no treatment' group were subsequently given acupuncture for eight weeks after the main study period. These patients also improved significantly after the treatment, though not to the same level as those given acupuncture initially.

- **Fibromyalgia** Research on the use of acupuncture for fibromyalgia is inconclusive. A consensus panel of the National Institute of Health (NIH) included fibromyalgia among conditions for which acupuncture "may be useful as an adjunct treatment or an acceptable alternative or included in a comprehensive management programme." A review of alternative therapies for fibromyalgia, published in the *Annals of Behavioral Medicine* in 1999, concluded that evidence for acupuncture's effectiveness is relatively strong compared to other alternative therapies. So, while there is uncertainty about its use as a first-line treatment for relieving pain and other symptoms, acupuncture may be beneficial in combination with other therapies or when other therapies fail.

- **Arthritis** Anti-inflammatory and acupuncture medication provide greater relief and improvement in function in patients with osteoarthritis of the knee than medication alone. Patients with rheumatoid arthritis have been helped with hook F (*Tripterygium wilfordii*), a TCM herb.

- **Alzheimer's disease** Extracts prepared from the nuts and leaves of the *Ginkgo biloba* tree lead to temporary improvement in memory in people with Alzheimer's disease. The extracts may be as effective as standard medications for the early stages of this disorder.

- **High blood pressure** People with high blood pressure who practise qigong have been shown to have lower mortality rates than people who do not practise qigong. Qigong may also help reduce high blood pressure in pregnant women.

- **Asthma** TCM herbal formulas and acupuncture can help control asthma symptoms.

- **Terminal illness** TCM can help patients be more comfortable and reduce the need for painkilling drugs, especially in people with AIDS and cancer. Several anticancer drugs have been derived from TCM, including indirubin and irisquinone.

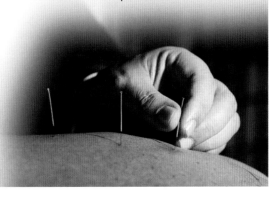

Acupuncture has repeatedly proven to be an effective treatment for a number of ailments, including pain and nausea.

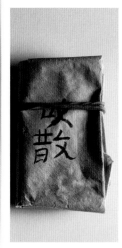

TCM uses a unique system for addressing illness, which is considered to be the result of syndromes, or imbalances, that are unique to each individual. Two people with the same disease will receive different treatments that address the cause, location, mechanism and nature of their specific condition.

that electrical currents do flow along the meridian pathways, but unequivocal scientific verification is lacking.

Despite uncertainty about how acupuncture works, it is effective for many conditions. Some practitioners use it along with or in place of anaesthesia for surgery. In addition, the World Health Organization has identified numerous conditions that acupuncture can help alleviate, including colds, sinusitis, migraines, asthma, ulcers, arthritis and depression.

• MOXIBUSTION This technique of burning a herb over an acupuncture point is used either with acupuncture or separately. Research in China shows that the herb, called moxa (also known as mugwort, or *Artemisia vulgaris*) has the unique ability to stimulate acupuncture points and, therefore, to support the body's capacity to heal itself. Moxibustion may be direct, with moxa applied and burned on the skin over an acupuncture point, or indirect, with a lighted moxa stick used to heat an acupuncture needle that is already placed in an acupuncture point.

• CUPPING This treatment uses suction to stimulate an acupuncture point or increase circulation around a sore muscle. Suction is created by placing a heated glass or a jar on the skin over an area to be treated.

• MASSAGE Acupressure, which uses finger or hand pressure to stimulate acupuncture points, and Chinese massage, which combines massage with herbal medicine, have beneficial effects. As it is practised today, TCM also uses osteopathy (pp.438–40) and chiropractic manipulation (pp.446–7). Massage is used to promote relaxation and treat pain, for example headaches, backache and sciatica.

• PHARMACEUTICALS AND SUPPLEMENTS TCM uses a unique Chinese system of herbal medicine. Among the more commonly used herbs are ginseng, ginger root, cinnamon and peony root. Dried insects, minerals, and

animal horns and bones may also be incorporated into Chinese medicines. They are selected according to a complex system that considers their relationship to the five elements. Herbs can be boiled to make decoctions or strong teas, or dried and ground into powder, then combined to make pills. Several TCM herbs show promise in providing symptomatic relief of asthma, arthritis, Alzheimer's disease, cancer and AIDS.

• NUTRITION Each of the five elements has an associated taste quality (see the chart on p.440), and certain foods that have these taste qualities are believed to nourish their associated element. For example, cherries nourish fire, pumpkins nourish earth, rice nourishes metal, kidney beans nourish water and lettuce nourishes wood. When a diagnosis of imbalance is made, the patient is advised to eat specific foods that strengthen the elements that are weak and avoid foods that further weaken those elements.

• QIGONG. This an ancient system of exercise integrates movement, breath and meditation to help stimulate the flow of qi. Qigong means 'working with energy'. Tai chi, perhaps the best-known and most popular form of qigong, combines martial arts and meditation. Tai chi exercise routines, called forms, are done very slowly with all attention focused on the movement. Tai chi and other forms of qigong are done for stress reduction, preventative therapy and personal development.

CAUTION

The safest way to use Chinese herbs is to get them from a reputable practitioner of Traditional Chinese Medicine. If you are taking any conventional medication, make sure to tell all your health practitioners if you also use herbal treatments. That way, they can be alert in case there are any potentially adverse interactions.

Ayurveda

This ancient system of holistic healing originated in India. The name is derived from the Sanskrit words *ayur* (life) and *veda* (knowledge). The aim of Ayurveda is to balance the physical, spiritual and psychological aspects of each individual because when a person is out of balance, illness and emotional and spiritual negativity can result. Specific treatments are prescribed to achieve detoxification, release of negative thoughts and emotions, palliation and rejuvenation. Therapies are individualized to each person's constitution, or profile of health strengths and weaknesses, and include dietary changes, yoga (pp.476–9), meditation (pp.514–19), massage (pp.468–73) and herbal medicines (pp.552–9).

HISTORY

Ayurveda is India's traditional system of medicine. It originated more than 3,000 years ago, and it was the medicine used by Buddha. As a system, Ayurveda puts equal emphasis on physical, spiritual and emotional well-being. In recent years, Ayurveda has become integrated into some Western medical practices around the world. Ayurvedic institutes in India, Europe and the United States provide training to medical doctors, naturopaths, homeopathic practitioners and others, although Ayurvedic practitioners are not licensed in most countries. Deepak Chopra, an endocrinologist in the United States, has helped increase awareness of Ayurveda through several popular books, including *The Book of Secrets: Unlocking the Hidden Dimensions of Your Life*, and *Perfect Health: The Complete Mind/Body Guide*.

PRACTICE

According to Ayurveda, all aspects of nature, including every living thing, can be characterized in terms of five basic elements: space (akash), air (vayu), fire (agni), water (jala) and earth (prithvi). In the human body, health is achieved when these five elements are held in balance. Such imbalances result in disharmony, which in turn ultimately leads to disease.

The five basic elements combine differently in each human being. These combinations fall into three general groups, known as doshas or biological forces. Each person is born with a unique combination of these three doshas, and this combination is known as their prakriti, or constitution.

Although all three doshas are present in each individual, one dosha usually predominates. The dominant dosha indicates which conditions an individual is most susceptible to and guides the recommendations for preventive and therapeutic treatment. Keeping the doshas in balance – that is, keeping the dominant dosha from expressing itself in excess – is key to maintaining good physical and mental health. (The physical and emotional characteristics of the doshas are explained in the chart on p.453.)

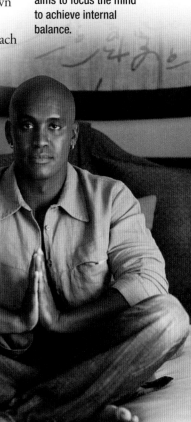

Ayurveda is an ancient system of traditional Indian wisdom that teaches wellness by balancing an individual's specific overall constitution, or prakriti. Chief among Ayurvedic techniques is meditation, which aims to focus the mind to achieve internal balance.

While a person's dominant dosha is an intrinsic quality that influences their health, outside factors also play a role, including viruses and bacteria, as well as the seasons and even the time of day. Dietary changes are often recommended based on the seasons. When the doshas are out of balance, a person may become vulnerable to ailments caused by infections and environmental stressors. When the doshas are in balance, people are able to fight off infections and withstand stress.

During an examination, practitioners use several strategies to establish a person's dominant dosha and determine if it is in balance. They look at the nails and tongue, for example, because particular physical traits give information about the doshas. Practitioners also ask about medical history and take a person's pulse, paying attention to qualities that are typical of the different doshas. They take a urine sample, noting the colour and odour for important clues about the doshas. Integrative practitioners also use conventional medical tests to help diagnose illnesses.

TREATMENTS

Ayurvedic treatments are tailored by the practitioner to the individual. They aim to rid the body of harmful substances and negative emotions, rebalance the doshas, and fortify body, mind and spirit. There are four main approaches to treating and preventing illness.

Ayurvedic medicine employs herbal formulations and mineral supplements that are taken orally or applied topically as a means to detoxify the body.

- **CLEANSING AND DETOXIFICATION (SHODAN)** This rids the body of toxins, which are considered the root of disease. A major source of toxins is food that has not been properly digested. The techniques used, which include enemas and emetics, are called pancha karma.

CAUTION

Although many Ayurvedic medicine formulations are effective, ingest them with caution. A study published in the *Journal of the American Medicine Association* in 2004 found that 20 percent of Ayurvedic herbal products contained high levels of lead, mercury and arsenic. Taking these products daily could be toxic, the scientists found.

- **PALLIATION (SHAMAN)** Palliation aims to spiritually balance the doshas. In contrast to Shodan, the approaches used tend to be gentler and more spiritually oriented, and may include fasting, yoga and herbs.
- **REJUVENATION (RASAYANA)** After the body is purged of toxins, it is energized with exercises and supplements. The goals are to improve overall function and balance, including sexual performance and fertility, and extend longevity.
- **MENTAL HYGIENE AND SPIRITUAL HEALING (SATVAJAYA)** The aim here is to release psychological stress and negative thoughts – toxins of the mind that are predisposing factors for physical illness. Just as Shodan cleanses the body to help improve functioning, Satvajaya cleanses the mind with the goal of achieving personal development and spirituality. The following therapies are part of the process for supporting mental hygiene and spiritual healing: mantra (chanting a sacred or mystical word or verse to awaken internal awareness), yantra (concentrating on geometric figures to promote fresh and creative thinking), and tantra (mentally channelling energy through the body).
- **SUPPLEMENTS** Herbs, taken orally and used topically, as well as mineral supplements, are part of the regimen of cleansing and detoxification, palliation and rejuvenation. Scientific studies have found several Ayurvedic herbal medicines to be beneficial for a number of ailments (see the box on p.454).

Dosha Constitutions

Vata	Responsible for	All movement-related functions in the body, such as respiration, circulation and thought
Elements: air, space	Physical characteristics	Thin body type, cool, dry skin, prominent features, joints and veins
	Personal characteristics	Quick thinking and acting, vivacious, creative, imaginative, flexible, moody
	Possible problems	Irregular eating and sleeping habits, constipation, anxiety and other nervous disorders, insomnia, digestive problems, fear, memory loss, worry
Pitta	Responsible for	Metabolism, including hunger and thirst, digestion of food and assimilating life's experiences
Elements: fire, water	Physical characteristics	Medium build, muscular, light hair, ruddy complexion
	Personal characteristics	Smart, determined, regular habits, passionate, well-organized, good leadership skills, warm, courageous, ambitious, proud, short-tempered
	Possible problems	Irritability, aggressiveness, ulcers, acne, haemorrhoids, excessive emotional intensity, addictions, workaholism, rage
Kapha	Responsible for	Cohesion, providing the body's structure
Elements: water, earth	Physical characteristics	Heavy, strong, oily skin
	Personal characteristics	Calm, kind, loyal, relaxed, eats slowly, sleeps soundly, tolerant, forgiving, greedy, jealous
	Possible problems	Weight gain, congestion, obstinacy, procrastination, obesity, allergies, sinus problems, high cholesterol, lethargy, sluggishness, trouble accepting change, attachment to material things, depression

• MIND–BODY CONNECTION Meditation, which is a technique used to focus the mind on the present moment and quiet mental chatter, is used for palliation as well as mental hygiene and spiritual healing. Herbal massage is an approach that is used for cleansing and detoxification.

• EXERCISE Stretching exercises are done for palliation and rejuvenation. Yoga (pp.476–9), a system of exercises developed for spiritual and physical well-being, is used for palliation and rejuvenation.

• NUTRITION Ayurvedic medicine (pp.451–4) emphasizes a diet high in fruit, vegetables, whole grains, legumes, and unsaturated fats such as fish oils, olive oil and nuts. Food should be organic and fresh to ensure optimum nutrition. However, there is no single 'Ayurvedic diet' – only a way of structuring diets according to each individual's dosha, as well as the season.

Food, drinks and spices are categorized according to their taste (sweet, salty, sour, bitter, pungent or astringent), the energetic

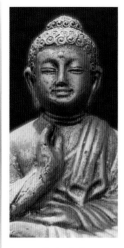

Ayurvedic techniques have been used for thousands of years, although much of it remains scientifically unproven. Still, certain facets of Ayurveda, such as herbalism, have shown some promise treating illness in clinical trials.

effect they have on the doshas, and their post-digestive effect on the body's tissues. Other qualites such as the food's form (solid or liquid), whether it makes a person feel hot or cold, whether it is heavy or light, and whether it is oily or dry are also important in determining the right food combinations. Not all foods are compatible, and certain foods, when eaten or cooked together, can disturb the normal digestive functions and promote the accumulation of toxins. For example, heavy foods such whole grains, dairy, meats and starches do not combine well with light foods such as fruit, which is digested more quickly.

Fasting may be part of the palliation process, to help the body detoxify itself. Fasting gives all the digestive organs a rest and reduces the influx of new toxins.

• OTHER THERAPIES Enemas, nasal douching, emetics, herbal steam saunas and even bloodletting are used for cleansing and detoxification. Lying in the sun for limited periods is done for palliation. Crystals, gems and metals are worn to promote mental hygiene and spiritual healing.

CAN AYURVEDA HELP ME?

Many clinical trials of Ayurvedic treatments are scientifically flawed or of poor quality. But several of the better ones show some preliminary benefit from various formulations of Ayurvedic medicines in treating the following conditions.

- **Acne** Sunder vati tablets (an Ayurvedic formulation) taken three times a day may reduce acne lesions. A mixture of seven herbs taken orally and applied topically in a cream have also been found useful. The herbs are aloe vera (*Aloe barbadensis*), neem (*Azardirachta indica*), turmeric (*Curcuma longa*), hemidesmus (*Hemidesmus indicus*), chebulic myrobalan (*Terminalia chebula*), arjuna (*Terminalia arjuna*) and winter cherry (*Withania somnifera*).

- **Rheumatoid arthritis** RA-1, a standardized formulation of winter cherry, boswellia (*Boswellia serrata*) and ginger (*Zingiberis officinale*), may help reduce joint swelling.

- **Obesity** Ayurvedic herbal preparations that include Indian bedellium (*Commiphora mukul*), chebulic myrobalan, belliric myrobalan (*Terminalia belerica*) and Indian gooseberry (*Emblica officinalis*) may help lower body weight, skin fold thickness, cholesterol and triglycerides in overweight patients.

- **Atherosclerosis** An integrated Ayurvedic medicine approach may slow the advancement of atherosclerosis.

- **High cholesterol** An Ayurvedic medicine derived from arjuna tree bark may help lower cholesterol.

- **Insomnia** Ayurvedic herbal treatments for insomnia may help reduce the time it takes to fall asleep.

- **Cognitive function** The herb thyme-leaved gratiola (*Bacopa monniera*) may help people learn faster and remember more new information.

- **Colitis** Boswellia may be helpful in the remission of chronic colitis.

- **Asthma** Boswellia may also reduce the symptoms of asthma.

- **Parkinson's disease** Ayurvedic herbal preparations (which include cow's milk), combined with cleansing therapy, may help patients improve motor function and general daily functioning.

- **Morphine-induced constipation** An Ayurvedic purgative may relieve constipation induced by morphine given to patients with advanced cancer. The Ayurvedic treatment, called misrakasneham, is a liquid made from 21 herbs, castor oil, ghee and milk.

- **Diabetes** A mixture of Ayurvedic herbs known as pancreas tonic may improve glucose tolerance in people with type 2 diabetes. Other Ayurvedic herbs and supplements that also either lower blood glucose or improve glucose tolerance include fenugreek (*Trigonella foenum-graecum*), holy basil (*Ocimum tenuiflorum*), Indian fruit gourd (*Coccina indica*), gurmar (*Gymnema sylvestre*) and chyawanprash, an Ayurvedic herbal jam made from a base of amalaki fruit, a rich source of antioxidants.

Homeopathy

This 200-year-old system of medicine uses dilutions of substances from plants, minerals and animals to treat illness. The word homeopathy comes from the Greek words *homo*, meaning similar, and *pathos*, meaning suffering. It rests on the belief that 'like cures like' – in other words, the very substances that induce the symptoms of an illness can, when highly diluted, treat it. Homeopathy is one of the most widespread modes of treatment in the world. It is practised by homeopathic physicians and is used as a form of self-care. It is also incorporated into many practices in dentistry and veterinary medicine.

It has been repeatedly studied in rigorous clinical trials, and in 1997, the British medical journal *The Lancet* published an analysis of all previously published studies which showed that of 89 clinical trials comparing the effectiveness of homeopathic remedies to a placebo, 44 reported homeopathy to be significantly more effective than the placebo. None of the 89 trials found the placebo to be more effective than homeopathy.

HISTORY

Homeopathy was developed in the late 18th century by Dr. Samuel Hahnemann, a German medical doctor who sought an alternative to bloodletting, arsenic and other harsh medical therapies that were standard at the time. In the course of his investigations into other medical therapies, he came across the bark of the cinchona tree, which is the source of quinine. Quinine was known to cure malaria, but Hahnemann found he developed symptoms of malaria after ingesting it. This experience lead him to theorize that the same substance can be helpful or harmful, depending on whether it is taken by someone who is ill or healthy and in minute or large amounts.

Hahnemann began testing this theory on himself, using hundreds of substances derived from plants, minerals and animals. The experiments led to three findings that became the foundations of homeopathy: like cures like (known as the Law of Similars); the most diluted substances are the most potent (known as the Law of the Infinitesimal Dose); and illness is unique to each individual and therefore requires individualized treatment.

Today, homeopathy is sometimes used together with conventional medicine to treat common ailments such as flu and chronic illnesses such as arthritis.

Homeopathic remedies are preparations made from extremely weak dilutions of substances that otherwise bring about the symptoms they are intended to treat, a trait called the Law of Similars.

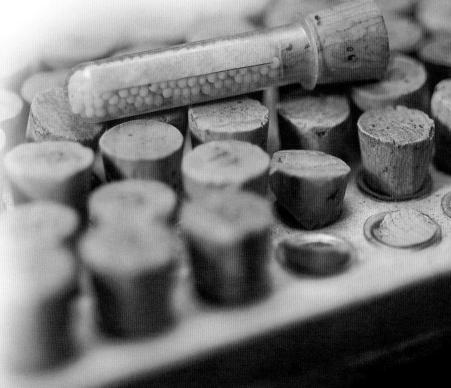

However, it is not used to treat emergencies. Its popularity is strongest in Europe. In Britain, the national health care system includes homeopathic hospitals and clinics, and homeopathy is a post-graduate medical speciality. In Germany, homeopathy is a required subject in medical school. In France, the law mandates that pharmacies sell homeopathic remedies, several of which are reimbursed by France's national health system. Homeopathic treatments are also used in India, South America, North America and Australia.

PRACTICE

Homeopathic remedies are prescribed according to an individual's symptoms. Dilutions of substances that induce those symptoms are then used to treat the ailment. This means a remedy that can create symptoms similar to a disease in a healthy person will cure that same disease. For example, *rhus toxicodendron*, a remedy made from poison ivy, is used to treat the rash caused by contact with that plant.

When being treated homeopathically, patients may get worse before they get better, a phenomenon called the 'healing crisis'. The healing crisis is considered a good sign, because it suggests that the remedy chosen to fight off the disease has adequately stimulated the body's healing forces.

TREATMENTS

There are thousands of homeopathic remedies, each of them created by diluting a substance repeatedly in water or alcohol. The potency of each remedy is identified according to its degree of dilution and the number of times it was diluted. The number of serial dilutions is labeled X (a 1:10 dilution – one part of the substance in nine parts water), C (a 1:100 dilution), and M (a 1:1,000 dilution). A remedy labeled 6X has been serially diluted and succussed (shaken) six times to a potency of 1:10; a remedy labeled 12C has

Rhus toxicodren, a homeopathic preparation made from poison ivy, is used to relieve the itching from exposure to the plant as well as back and shoulder pain.

been diluted and succussed twelve times to a potency of 1:100, and so on. The more dilute a solution and the more times it has been diluted, the more potent it is believed to be. Some remedies are so diluted the original substance cannot be measured.

An unresolved question about homeopathy – and one of the main argument critics use against it – is, why are the most dilute remedies considered the most potent? One school of thought advanced by many practitioners is that the water or alcohol used in the dilution process stores electromagnetic

CAN HOMEOPATHY HELP ME?

Although homeopathy has been used to treat virtually every illness – including some epidemics – research on its effectiveness is limited. Homeopathy should not be used in place of conventional medicine to treat serious illnesses. It does, however, show some very preliminary promise in relieving the following conditions, many of which do not respond well to conventional medicine.

- **Influenza** One of the best-known and most widely used homeopathic remedies is oscillococcinum, a highly dilute extract of duck heart and kidney that is taken to treat the flu. Duck heart and kidney are used because they are believed to harbour influenza viruses. In a study published in the *British Journal of Clinical Pharmacology* in 1989 that look at 237 flu patients, 17 percent of those who took oscillococcinum recovered after 48 hours, compared with only 10 percent who took a placebo. The remedy was not effective for patients with severe flu.

- **Respiratory allergies** Homeopathic remedies can relieve the symptoms of seasonal allergies. For example, a homeopathic nasal spray is as effective as the conventional nasal spray cromolyn sodium in relieving nasal allergy symptoms.

- **Rheumatoid arthritis** Homeopathic treatments of rheumatoid arthritis may relieve pain and stiffness and improve grip strength.

- **Diarrhoea** Individualized homeopathic treatment may speed recovery from diarrhoea.

- **Osteoarthritis** A homeopathic gel may be as effective as a gel containing a non-steroidal anti-inflammatory agent in relieving symptoms of osteoarthritis.

- **Chest pain** A homeopathic medicine along with conventional medicine for angina may reduce the recurrence of chest pain during exercise in people with ischemic heart disease (caused by constriction or blockage of the blood vessels).

- **Fibromyalgia** Homeopathic remedies may reduce pain and improve quality of life in patients with this condition. *Rhus toxidendron* can also lead to improved sleep.

- **Chronic fatigue syndrome** Homeopathic remedies may offer relief from fatigue and other symptoms of this illness.

- **Side-effects of cancer treatments** Homeopathic medicine may relieve some of the side effects of cancer treatments. For example, Traumeel S reduces the severity and duration of stomatitis (mouth sores) in people undergoing bone marrow transplants. *Belladonna* relieves radiation-induced dermatitis in women undergoing radiation therapy for breast cancer.

- **Seborrhoeic dermatitis (dandruff)** Oral homeopathic remedies have been effective in treating this condition.

- **Sprains and strains** Traumeel, a homeopathic ointment, may improve range of motion in people with sprained ankles. Marathon runners who take arnica D30 pills have also experienced a reduction in muscle pain.

- **Side-effect of haemodialysis** Homeopathic remedies may prevent the itching that often plagues people undergoing haemodialysis. This common side-effect is difficult to control with conventional medicine.

- **Mild traumatic brain injury** Homeopathic medicine may reduce the disabilities that result from mild traumatic brain injury. Persistent disabling symptoms from this kind of injury are difficult to control with conventional medicine.

signals from the original substance, and that these signals match those created by the illness being treated. So homeopathic remedies help the body heal itself by emitting electromagnetic messages to the body.

Some homeopathic doctors are sceptical about the growing practice of homeopathy in self-care. Taking packaged remedies for flu, sprains and other ailments seems to run counter to the principle that each treatment must be tailored to the individual. Some homeopathic doctors think most of these self-care remedies are not as effective as homeopathic remedies prescribed after a thorough interview and examination. The packaged medications are also typically less potent.

Anthroposophic Medicine

This holistic practice is based on the notion that each person is connected physically, mentally and spiritually with the natural world. The focus is on treating chronic illnesses (not acute conditions or emergencies) and fostering spiritual growth. Anthroposophic medicine uses conventional as well as complementary approaches, including artistic therapies (therapies that tap into a patient's creative impulses, such as painting, pottery and music) and movement therapy.

Anthroposophic Medicine employs techniques such as art and music therapy to reinforce the connection between individuals and nature. Practitioners of this system approach illness as an opportunity for personal development and growth.

HISTORY

Anthroposophic medicine was founded in 1920 by Rudolf Steiner, an Austrian scientist and philosopher, and Ita Wegman, an Austrian medical doctor. It is based on Steiner's concept of anthroposophy (Greek for 'human wisdom'), a worldview in which the spirit within each person is connected to the spirit in nature and the universe. Steiner and Wegman established hospitals for anthroposophic medicine and pharmaceutical laboratories for formulating herbal medicines in Switzerland and Germany. Today, there are anthroposophic hospitals and clinics throughout Europe, staffed by medical doctors with postgraduate training in anthroposophic medicine. It is practised elsewhere in the world, such as the United States and New Zealand, but with limited knowledge and acceptance.

PRACTICE

Anthroposophic medicine considers the human being to be made up of three functional systems, organized roughly by anatomical parts and physiological functions. Illness is an imbalance in the systems. The focus of treatment is to keep these systems in harmony. The three systems are:

- Sense-nervous system: head and spinal column.
- Reproductive-metabolic system: this consists of the limbs and digestive systems, which are parts of the body that are in constant motion.
- Rhythmic system: the heart, lungs and blood circulation; the rhythmic system connects the other two and keeps them in balance.

Illness presents an opportunity for personal growth. While practitioners aim to treat and cure disease when possible, they do not suppress symptoms because these are seen as evidence of the body's healing process. A major focus of anthroposophic medicine is to help people with terminal illnesses continue their spiritual development.

TREATMENTS

Anthroposophic medicine is practised by medical doctors who follow the anthroposophic model and add its therapies to the conventional treatments they prescribe for their patients. Treatments are customized for each patient. The treatments used depend not only on the person's symptoms or illnesses, but also their age, constitution, spiritual condition and life history.

• PERSONAL DEVELOPMENT AND SPIRITUALITY
Several treatments are intended to support personal growth and spirituality. They include artistic therapies (such as painting, pottery, and music therapy), eurythmy (described below), psychological counselling and biographical counselling.

With biographical counselling, patients record their life story and its major themes as a way of seeing their present health problems in a context and gaining insight into the meaning of their lives.

• MOVEMENT AND EXERCISE Eurythmy (the word means 'harmonious rhythm') is a type of movement therapy devised by Steiner that uses different gestures to express the sounds of speech and music. Gestures that simulate the environment by imitating its shapes, contours and textures are described as consonants. The gestures described as vowels express a patient's inner response to sounds, known as the soul response. The gestures are intensified and repeated to stimulate specific organic functions. Eurythmy is used to treat a wide range of disorders, including menstrual problems, sleep disorders, psychiatric conditions, stroke, learning and developmental problems, and digestive disorders.

• PHARMACEUTICALS AND SUPPLEMENTS Because anthroposophic medicine considers human beings to be connected spiritually with nature, it uses medicine made from natural substances – plants, minerals and animals. Some of the medicines prescribed are homeopathic remedies (pp.455–7) and others are anthroposophic formulations of herbs. The most widely prescribed anthroposophic herbal supplements are made from mistletoe and are used along with conventional medications to treat cancer. Although laboratory findings show that mistletoe extracts stimulate immune system cells, clinical studies have not shown that they reduce tumour progression or increase survival in cancer patients. There is no scientific proof that the supplements used in anthroposophic medicine can treat or cure illness.

• MASSAGE Rhythmical massage therapy (a form of light-touch massage) uses gentle rhythmic touch to correct imbalances caused by stress and illness, thereby supporting the body's healing process.

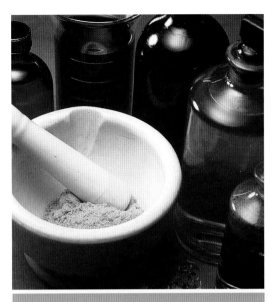

Anthroposophic medicine considers that humans are inherently connected to the natural world, and therefore recommends herbal remedies for treating illness.

CAN ANTHROPOSOPHIC MEDICINE HELP ME?

Preliminary clinical trials suggest that anthroposophic medicine may help ease the physical and psychosocial symptoms (the way individual circumstances relate to mental health) of certain illnesses and may improve the body's ability to regulate its functions. It has been studied for the following conditions.

• **Breast cancer** Adding anthroposophic care helps improve quality of life, based on the self-reporting of women being treated for breast cancer using conventional medical treatment.

• **Attention deficit-hyperactivity disorder (ADHD)** Eurythmy has helped improve attention span, coordination, and other motor skills, dexterity and social behaviour in children with ADHD.

• **Orthostatic syndrome** Using anthroposophic herbal medicine may improve the coordination of breathing and heart rate in people with this condition, in which dizziness, nausea, palpitations and other symptoms occur when a person moves from a sitting to a standing position.

• **Chronic illnesses** Anthroposophic therapies (artistic therapy, eurythmy, rhythmical massage, counselling and medication) used to treat chronic problems have lead to long-term reduction of symptoms and improved health-related quality of life, particularly in patients with psychological disorders and musculosleletal problems.

Tibetan Medicine

Tibetan medicine is an ancient system with strong ties to Buddhist thought. Like other Asian medical practices, it views health in terms of the interrelation of the mind, body, spirit and the natural world. In the Tibetan Buddhist world view, all the material in the universe can be characterized in terms of five basic elements, which are named for their most identifiable manifestations: earth, water, fire, wind and space. Combinations of these elements characterize everything in the universe, including the human body and its functions.

Tibetan Medicine, like other Asian systems of healing, views illness as the product of imbalances, some of whch can be restored with specific herbal formulations.

Tibetan medicine emphasizes behavioural therapies, such as exercise and meditation, as first-line treatments for health problems, but other therapies are also prescribed, including herbal medicines, acupuncture, massage and counselling.

HISTORY

Tibetan medicine has been practised for about 2,000 years. It is philosophically grounded in the Buddhist view that illness is related to a person's mental, emotional, spiritual and social condition. It incorporates some practices from Auyrvedic medicine, Traditional Chinese Medicine, and ancient healing traditions of Persia and Greece. Tibetan doctors are trained in schools run by the Tibetan Medical and Astrological Institute, which is based in Dharamsala, India.

Tibetan medicine is practised mainly in Central Asia, but its use is growing in Europe and North America. In recent years, practitioners have sought to educate Western doctors about Tibetan medicine by visiting medical schools in Europe and North America and assisting with clinical studies of Tibetan medicine therapies. The Dalai Lama, the head of the dominant order of Tibetan Buddhism, has personally encouraged the promotion of Tibetan medicine around the world.

PRACTICE

Tibetan medicine regards the body as composed of the following:

- Seven components: milk, blood, meat, fat, bone, marrow and essence.
- Three excreta: faeces, urine and perspiration.
- Three humours, or principles of energy: wind, bile and phlegm.

While each of the three humours is present in every individual, one or two usually predominate and define the person's overall constitution. Wind controls circulation within the body, such as blood flow, breathing, nerve impulses, speech and the swirling of thoughts in the mind. Constitutional characteristics of a person dominated by wind include creativity, high energy and changeable moods. Bile, which is related to heat within the body, controls metabolism and digestion. Constitutional characteristics of a person dominated by bile include good concentration, self-confidence and impatience. Phlegm regulates the body's functions and balances the energies. Constitutional characteristics of a person dominated by phlegm include an easygoing personality, faithfulness and slow movement.

Illness is regarded as the result of imbalances among or within the seven components, three excreta and three humours. Practitioners evaluate a patient's health by talking to the person to understand their constitution and doing a physical examination to identify imbalances. The physical examination includes observation of a urine sample, during which the practitioner notes the colour of the specimen and its odour and then, after vigorous stirring, the size, colour, amount and persistence of bubbles, and any deposits. These characteristics indicate the nature and location of the illness, and the presence or absence of infection. A practitioner will then feel the six distinct pulses at the radial artery of each wrist. These pulses indicate the movement of bodily fluids and humours, including but not limited to blood. The pulses in both arms are checked for such things as the width, depth, strength, speed and quality of the pulse. They provide information about the specific nature of the illness, its location, causes and possible complications. A practitioner may also look at the sclera of the eye, the colour, shape and coatings of the tongue, and feel for sensitivity at certain pressure points.

TREATMENTS

Because the same disease may manifest itself in different ways, depending on the person, treatments are individualized according to the imbalances observed. The first-line treatments in Tibetan medicine are behavioural, including exercise and dietary changes. Other treatments include massage, acupuncture and herbal formulas.

• BEHAVIOURAL AND LIFESTYLE CHANGES Recommended behavioural changes can include meditation, spiritual advice, counselling, exercise, and reorganizing sleep habits and eating schedules. Meditation is used to calm the mind and enhance the patient's understanding and perception of the world. It is seen as a therapeutic way of working through emotional or psychological troubles. Counselling addresses psychosocial difficulties. Yoga and other forms of regular exercise are suggested to improve overall circulation. Particular foods are suggested according to an individual's symptoms, lifestyle and environment. Dietary guidance is based on the arrangement of the five elements (described above) within each food, which influence the food's effect on the body and mind.

• HERBS, MASSAGE AND ACUPUNCTURE Herbal treatments range from simple formulas that use just three herbs to very complex ones that can include 150. Each formula is prescribed to treat a particular disease as it manifests in an individual patient. Massage (pp.468–73) and acupuncture (pp.464–5) are prescribed to balance the constituents of the body and improve overall circulation when behavioural approaches alone do not control a person's illness.

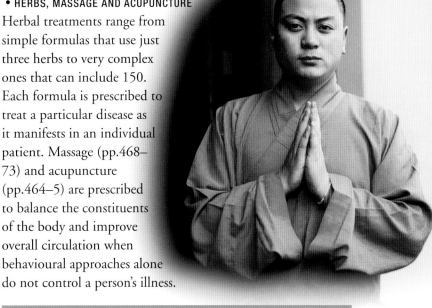

Meditation and lifestyle changes are a Tibetan Medicine practitioner's primary starting-points for patients seeking to restore the imbalances that cause illness.

CAN TIBETAN MEDICINE HELP ME?

Very little research has been published on Tibetan medicine. But small clinical and observational studies have shown it may help patients with the following chronic conditions.

- **Peripheral artery disease** Padma 28, a Tibetan herbal formula, may help people with peripheral artery disease walk farther and experience less pain.

- **Diabetes** Tibetan medical supplements (different ones are used for different patients, based on their individual signs and symptoms), used along with the American Diabetes Association's recommended lifestyle changes (increased exercise and dietary modification), may be more effective than lifestyle changes alone in controlling blood sugar in people with type 2 diabetes.

- **Constipation** Padma lax, a Tibetan herbal formula, may relieve constipation in people with irritable bowel syndrome.

- **Other conditions** Tibetan medicine helps treat rheumatism, arthritis, asthma, eczema and anxiety.

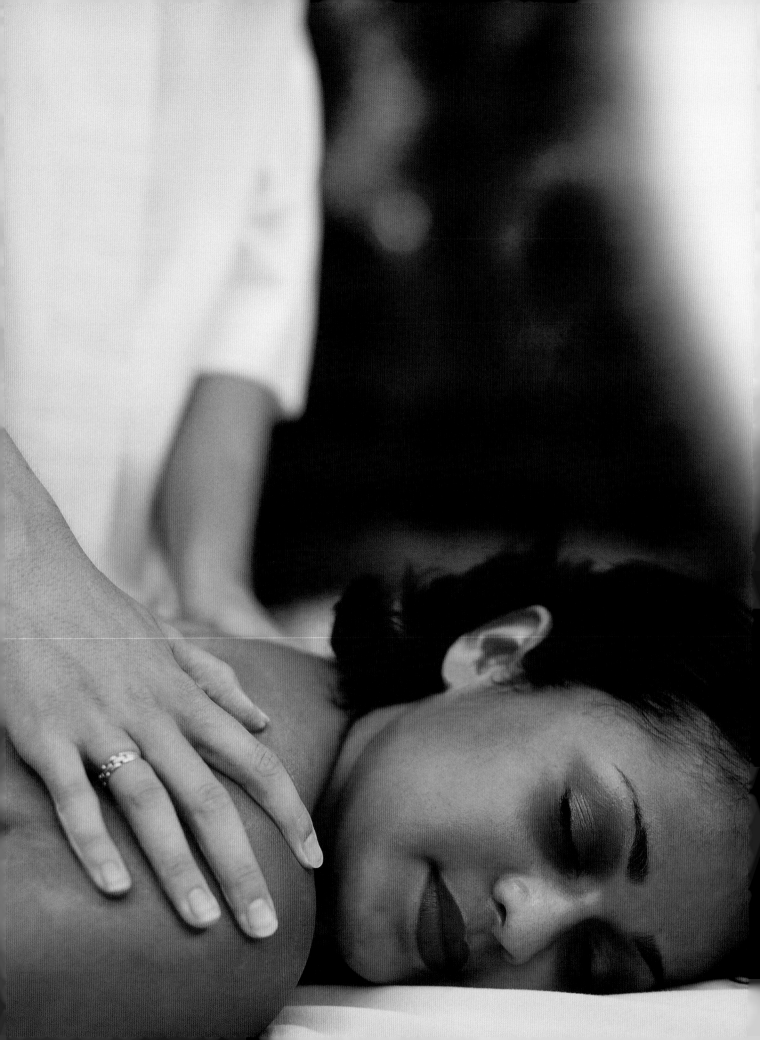

17 | THE BODY

Therapies that work with the physical body aim to affect one or more parts of the musculoskeletal system – the bones, muscles, joints, ligaments and tendons. They include manipulative therapies such as chiropractic, which works primarily with the joints of the spine; therapies that concentrate on posture, such as the Alexander technique; those that involve muscle work, including massage; those whose effects on the skull are said to influence the nervous system, such as craniosacral therapy; and systems such as yoga, which embrace the mental and spiritual alongside the physical.

Some of these techniques – yoga and progressive muscle relaxation, for instance – evoke the relaxation response, calming the sympathetic nervous system, which is responsible for the 'fight or flight' reactions to threat and danger. They also tap into the mind–body connection to reduce stress and encourage healing.

These diverse therapies have two themes in common: first, that body systems are interdependent; and second, that the body is capable of healing itself.

Acupuncture

The word 'acupuncture' is derived from the Latin words *acus,* meaning a needle, and *punctura,* meaning a prick or perforation. Acupuncture is an ancient Chinese system of medicine, now also popular in the West, that involves inserting very fine needles at specific points on the body to stimulate or balance the flow of life energy, called *qi* in Oriental philosophy.

Qi is said to flow along 14 channels called 'meridians'; the needling is targeted to about 360 specific 'acupoints' along these channels. Twelve of the channels are related to specific organs, such as lung, spleen or bladder, but the Chinese notion of their function does not exactly correspond with the Western one.

Acupuncture may be used to relieve or prevent pain – including as anaesthesia during surgery – to treat disease, and to promote health by balancing the flow of *qi.* It is generally very safe when performed by a trained practitioner using sterile, single-use, disposable needles, and has been shown to be effective in many situations, although controlled clinical trials are limited by the difficulty of providing an equivalent placebo treatment.

HISTORY

Acupuncture originated in China more than 5,000 years ago, and a 5,200-year-old mummified body, found in a glacier in the Alps, had tattoos that correspond to specific acupuncture points that relate to ailments of the joints and stomach. Having spread to Japan and Korea during the 6th century and to Europe by the 17th century, the practise of acupuncture remains key in Traditional Chinese Medicine (pp. 446–47). Since the 1960s it has been widely used in the West by both complementary and conventional practitioners.

PRACTICE

How acupuncture works is not known. The existence of meridians and *qi* is not recognized in Western medicine, nor are other of its basic tenets. These include the concept of yin and yang – opposing forces found in everything in the universe, such as dark and light, female and male, passive and active – and the notion that the universe is comprised of five elements: wood, fire, earth, water and metal. These are thought to correspond to internal organs, the meridians each connecting a particular network regulating certain bodily functions.

And yet research has revealed not only that acupuncture yields proven benefits in several medical conditions, but that it affects various brain centres, nerve fibres and chemicals – particularly endorphins, the body's internal morphine-like pain-relieving substances.

In a consultation, a practitioner usually takes a detailed medical history, concentrating on factors such as the patient's personality and lifestyle. Examination includes particular attention to the pulse – Chinese medicine

CAUTION

Acupuncture is a generally safe therapy with few adverse effects. However infection may result from improperly-sterilized needles. Very rarely, interference with pacemakers has occurred with electro-acupuncture. It is not recommended for patients with bleeding disorders.

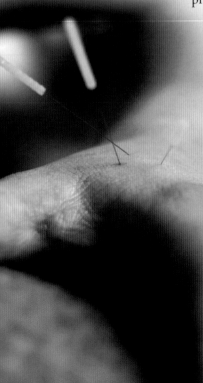

Acupuncture is an ancient Chinese system of medicine that involves inserting very fine needles at specific points on the body such as the hands.

CAN ACUPUNCTURE HELP ME?

Acupuncture is a potentially valuable treatment for a vast range of conditions. For some there is reasonably good scientific evidence of benefit; others are under investigation.

- **Nausea and vomiting** Stimulation of the P6 acupuncture point at the wrist is effective in preventing post-operative nausea and vomiting with minimal side-effects, according to a review of 26 trials by the Cochrane Collaboration in 2006.

- **Headache** Acupuncture is covered by statutory health insurance in Germany for the treatment of headache. A study of 2,022 patients showed highly significant improvements in all types of headache, with over half of all patients reporting at least a 50 percent reduction in frequency.

- **Stroke** Acupuncture is used extensively in China to treat acute stroke. However evidence from randomized controlled trials is limited and much larger studies are needed, according to a 2006 Cochrane review.

- **Childbirth** Acupuncture is often used for analgesia during childbirth. According to a study from the University of Oslo, Norway, published in 2006, its use reduces use of epidural analgesia and other drugs. As another potential application, a 2006 Cochrane review concluded that acupuncture is safe and may be effective for induction of labour, although further studies are needed.

- **Infertility treatment** A study from Denmark published in *Fertility and Sterility* in 2006 reported that acupuncture given on the day of embryo transfer significantly improves reproductive outcomes in women receiving infertility treatments.

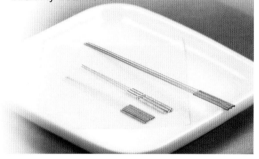

Acupuncture needles come in a variety of sizes for use on different parts of the body.

recognizes 29 different varieties; the tongue, which has 18 features; and the complexion, body type, emotions and mental state.

The practitioner's assessment governs the choice of needling locations and depths, the aim being the restoration of the flow of *qi* and the balance of yin and yang. Modern needles are ultra-fine, disposable, and made of stainless steel, copper, gold, silver or zinc. Insertion is generally painless, and the needle may be removed rapidly or left for up to 20 minutes. In some forms, needles are manually rotated or heated after insertion. In electro-acupuncture, a small electric impulse is delivered through the needle.

Practitioners often suggest repeat treatments at roughly weekly intervals; those who are Chinese herbal practitioners may also prescribe herbal remedies. Some patients experience relief after only one or two sessions, while most require six to eight treatments, followed by maintenance visits at intervals of up to six months.

In the United States, individual states may require acupuncturists to be licensed and obtain certification from the National Certification Commission for Acupuncture and Oriental Medicine. In some European countries, acupuncture can be practised only by medical practitioners. In the United Kingdom, statutory regulation is under consideration.

TREATMENTS

In addition to classical acupuncture, there are many other types, some of which include:

- AURICULAR ACUPUNCTURE Involves needling of the ear, based on the theory that points on the ear reflect various areas and functions.
- MOXIBUSTION A cone or stick of the herb moxa (mugwort or *Artemisia vulgaris*) is burned on or near an acupuncture point; it is said to strengthen *qi* and warm the blood.
- ELECTROACUPUNCTURE Passing a very weak electric current along the needle is believed to be more effective than conventional needling.

Chiropractic

The effects of the musculoskeletal system, and especially the spine, on the nervous system and the impact of this relationship on a person's overall health are the focus of chiropractic. Misalignments of the vertebrae in the spine are believed to lead to health problems because they inhibit normal nerve function. Chiropractors use hands-on manipulation techniques to correct spinal misalignments and other problems.

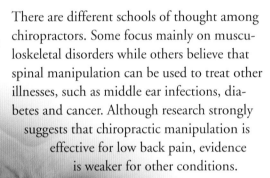

Manipulation is usually performed on a patient lying on a treatment table. The objective is to properly align the spine for optimal health.

There are different schools of thought among chiropractors. Some focus mainly on musculoskeletal disorders while others believe that spinal manipulation can be used to treat other illnesses, such as middle ear infections, diabetes and cancer. Although research strongly suggests that chiropractic manipulation is effective for low back pain, evidence is weaker for other conditions.

HISTORY

Chiropractic manipulation was developed in the late 1800s by Daniel David Palmer, an American self-taught student of anatomy. Palmer believed the body has a natural ability to keep itself healthy and that the key to this ability is normal nerve function. According to this theory, misaligned vertebrae, called subluxations, interfere with nerve function and lead to health problems. Palmer believed he could treat disorders throughout the body by using his hands to move the vertebrae into their proper positions.

For several decades, medical doctors opposed chiropractic and tried to limit its practice because they believed it had no benefits. But today chiropractic is recognized and licensed throughout the world.

PRACTICE

Chiropractors are trained at accredited colleges. They take courses in anatomy, physiology, microbiology, nutrition and other subjects related to health. Like medical doctors, their education also includes hands-on experience in treating patients. In some areas of the world, chiropractors are licensed to practise certain conventional medical techniques, including gynaecological exams, minor surgery and the setting of bone fractures.

During a visit to the workplace or home, a chiropractor will take a patient's health history and feel along the length of the spine to

CAN CHIROPRACTIC HELP ME?

The effectiveness of chiropractic manipulation has been studied for dozens of conditions. Although most of the studies have been of poor quality, they have found some benefit for the following disorders. So far there is little evidence to support the efficacy of non-manipulative practices. However, some supplements, such as glucosamine, work well.

- **Low back pain** Back pain is the reason for most visits to chiropractors and has been the focus of the majority of studies on its effectiveness. Chiropractic manipulation is comparable in effectiveness to conventional medical care.
- **Headaches** Chiropractic manipulation may help prevent tension headaches.
- **Fibromyalgia** Chiropractic manipulation may reduce pain and fatigue and improve sleep in people with fibromyalgia.

- **Asthma** Chiropractic spinal manipulation is a beneficial adjunct to conventional medicine in treating asthma in children.
- **Colic** Clinical trials that examined the effectiveness of spinal manipulation on colic have shown that the babies stop crying, indicating a reduction in their discomfort.
- **Phobias** People with phobias who receive chiropractic manipulation have a significant reduction of emotional arousal from the object of their phobias.

find misalignments. X-rays and other diagnostic tools may also be used to confirm the findings of the physical examination and check for underlying diseases such as a tumour or osteoporosis. Based on the health history and diagnostic findings, the chiropractor develops a treatment plan.

TREATMENTS

Chiropractic manipulation is the main form of treatment and there are more than 100 techniques. Many involve applying sudden force to a region of the spine to correct a subluxation or to a joint to increase its range of motion.

Manipulation usually takes place with patients lying on a Cox table – an examination table with an opening for the face, which enables the patient to lie face down. Chiropractic manipulation of the lower back is usually done while the patient is lying on their side, while manipulation of the mid and upper back is done while the patient lies face down. For cervical and neck manipulation, the patient is either lying on their back or sitting down.

Chiropractic treatment usually takes place in three phases. The first is acute care, which aims to correct misalignments of the spine and resulting nervous system impairment, and to reduce pain. Once the spine is

properly aligned, the restorative phase begins. During this, the chiropractor schedules follow-up examinations to make sure the spine stays aligned. Small adjustments are often necessary. Finally, the wellness phase consists of periodic check-ups to identify any new subluxations.

In addition to chiropractic manipulation, many chiropractors also give dietary advice, particularly as it pertains to sensible eating and weight control. They may also include as part of treatment the prescription or injection of nutritional supplements. Some chiropractors also use other holistic treatments, including homeopathy (pp.455–7), acupuncture (pp.464–5) and herbal medicine (pp.552–9).

CAUTION

Recent case reports have linked chiropractic manipulation to several serious complications. Manipulation of the neck and cervical spine appears to increase the risk of stroke, spinal fractures and nerve damage. There have also been reports of bleeding and blood clots. To reduce risk, check with your doctor before having chiropractic manipulation and, if you see a chiropractor, ensure that any underlying health problems are fully discussed before a treatment.

Massage

A wide variety of styles and techniques to manipulate muscles, ligaments, tendons and other soft tissue all fall under the heading of massage. In general, massage entails holding, moving or applying pressure to an area of the body. The aim of massage is to relieve muscle tightness and spasms, increase blood flow, stimulate or relax the nervous system, prompt the flow of lymph and other secretions, and aid in the release of toxic substances from the body, so reducing stress. There are many types of massage. Some are used for medical purposes in sports medicine, rehabilitation, pain relief and the treatment of cancer patients. Others are primarily for relaxation and the improvement of overall functioning. Massage can be practised by a therapist or other healthcare professional, or as part of self-care.

HISTORY

Massage has been used for thousands of years as a healing tool for the body and the mind. Perhaps its earliest use was in the medical systems developed in China, India and Thailand. Many more massage techniques have been devised over the last 150 years in North America, Europe and Australia. Today, massage therapy is one of the most widely practised forms of complementary and alternative medicine.

Each type of massage has a slightly different focus. Some are done to improve posture, movement and body awareness. Others aim mainly to promote relaxation, improve mood and stimulate meditation. Still other types of massage are intended to relieve muscular conditions such as strains and soreness, and to reduce swelling. Massage is also used as an adjunct to conventional therapies for reducing the severity of symptoms of a broad range of conditions, including premenstrual syndrome, labour pain, depression and cancer.

PRACTICE

Massage is carried out by massage therapists, physical therapists, nurses and other practitioners in a variety of settings, including hospitals, rehabilitation centres and spas. A massage session generally lasts about an hour. Depending on the type of massage being practised, the patient may wear loose clothing or remove some or all of their clothes. Many types of massage are done with the patient lying on a padded table with a towel or sheet covering the parts of the body that are not being massaged. The therapist may apply an oil or lotion to the body to help their hands glide over the

Clinical Query

I had a massage and I was sore afterwards. Is massage supposed to hurt?

It's not unusual to feel some muscle soreness after a deep tissue or neuromuscular massage. They involve significant pressure being applied to muscles that are sore to begin with. But the added discomfort should be mild and it should subside after a day or two. Taking a hot bath or shower helps alleviate the soreness. You should feel better than you did before the massage.

body. Music may be played to encourage the patient to relax.

Many massage techniques are easy to learn, and research has found massage practised by spouses on each other and by parents on children to be beneficial. Massage is believed to have the following physiological effects:

- Increased blood flow to the muscles that are being massaged, which warms and relaxes them.
- Increased flow of lymph fluid.
- More moist, more attractive skin due to improved functioning of the oil and sweat glands.
- Either a calmer or a more stimulated nervous system, depending on the type of massage.

TYPES OF MASSAGE

There are many types of massage. Although there is some degree of overlap, each of the following common massage styles is used for particular purposes, such as releasing tension in tight muscles, easing pain, or improving the flow of energy or fluids in the body.

To learn about other types of bodywork, see the Alexander technique (pp.488–9), Aston-Patterning (pp.486–7), osteopathy (pp.438–40), chiropractic (pp.446–7), craniosacral therapy (pp.480–1), Feldenkrais method (pp.494–5), Hellerwork (p.490), myotherapy (pp.496–7) and naprapathy (pp.498–9).

Deep Tissue Massage

This massage technique reaches the deep layers of muscle tissue in order to release tension. Slow strokes and deep finger pressure are applied to areas of muscle in the body that are tense. The hands either follow the contours of the muscles, tendons and fascia (fibrous connective tissue), or work across their grain. Deep tissue massage is often used to relieve low back pain and to loosen tight muscles.

Swedish Massage

Developed in Sweden in the 18th century, this is full body massage that uses a combination of long strokes, kneading motion and friction on the layers of muscle just beneath the skin. Friction, which is generated using circular movements that rub the underlying layers of tissue against one another, is used to increase blood flow to the area. As part of a Swedish massage session, the therapist may move some of the joints or ask that the patient moves them. Swedish massage is used to improve circulation, promote relaxation, improve flexibility and rid the tissues of waste products.

Sports Massage

Using the techniques of Swedish and deep tissue massage, sports massage focuses on the muscles used in a particular sport. The purpose is to relieve pain from an injury or to restore or maintain mobility.

Myofascial Release

This therapy focuses specifically on the fascia, the fibrous connective tissue that surrounds muscles and internal organs. Myofascial therapists use their fingers, palms and elbows to make long, stretching strokes to release tension in the fascia and muscles.

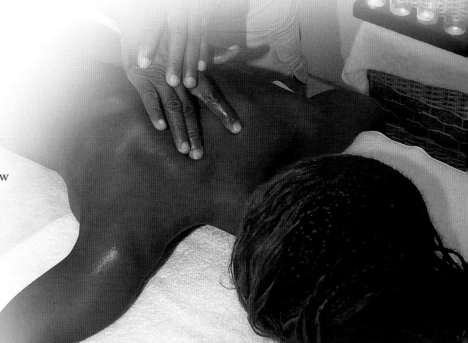

Deep tissue massage is applied to tense muscle areas. This kind of massage has been used for thousands of years around the world as a healing tool for the mind and the body.

CAN MASSAGE HELP ME?

There are many studies on the health benefits of massage, but most are small. However, research has found several types of massage to be effective for the relief of the following conditions or symptoms.

- **Nausea** Acupressure at a point above the wrist (at the P6, or neiguan, acupoint) prevents and relieves nausea due to pregnancy, anaesthesia, surgery and chemotherapy.

- **Headache** The Trager approach can relieve the symptoms of chronic headache. Self-massage can also help prevent tension headaches in people who are prone to them.

- **Post-operative pain** Acupressure is effective in relieving pain after surgery – in some cases as effective as pain medicine.

- **Low back pain** Acupressure can relieve low back pain.

- **Sports injuries** Friction massage techniques, such as Swedish massage, can help improve range of motion and reduce pain in people with frozen shoulder.

- **Premenstrual syndrome** Premenstrual women who receive massage therapy may experience less anxiety and better moods immediately after massage, and less pain and water retention in the long term.

- **Pregnancy and childbirth** Several types of massage may reduce discomfort during pregnancy and childbirth. Lymphatic reflexology, a foot massage intended to relieve swelling, can reduce both pain and foot and ankle circumference in healthy pregnant women with oedema in their ankles or feet. Massage can also decrease pain and anxiety during labour, and massage of the perineum may reduce the risk of trauma to that area from childbirth.

- **Prematurity/low birth weight** Massaging premature and low birth weight babies can lead to increased daily weight gain, as well as reduced hospital stays and reduced postnatal complications.

- **Depression and anxiety** A series of massage sessions is helpful for depression and anxiety.

- **Stress** Massage helps reduce stress in a variety of situations, including when patients are waiting for stressful medical procedures or recovering from surgery.

- **Cancer** Massage may help ease discomfort from cancer and its treatments. Manual lymph drainage relieves lymphoedema, a swelling of the upper arm associated with mastectomy and lymph node biopsy. Various types of massage therapy may

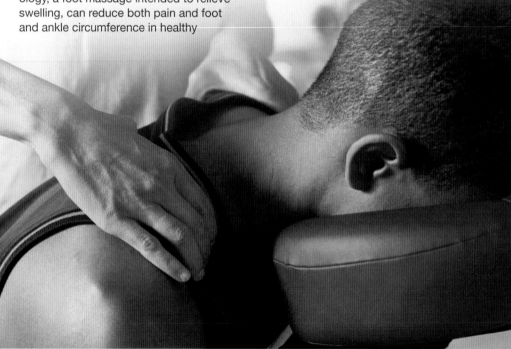

Massage therapy can help a number of conditions, including depression and anxiety as well as people suffering from cancer.

also reduce anxiety, depression, anger, hostility and fatigue, and help cancer patients increase the number of immune system cells and levels of serotonin and dopamine (neurotransmitters associated with elevated mood). Massage does not need to be performed by a therapist to be effective; massage given by a spouse can offer many of these benefits.

- **Aggression** Massage therapy may help calm people who are overly aggressive by reducing anxiety and hostility.
- **Attention-deficit hyperactivity disorder** Regular massage therapy may improve mood and classroom behaviour in children and adolescents with attention-deficit hyperactivity disorder
- **Sleep disorders** Acupressure can improve sleep quality.
- **Bedwetting** Acupressure may reduce the incidence of bedwetting in children.
- **Multiple sclerosis** Reflexology on the feet and calves may help people with multiple

sclerosis achieve more coordinated movement, less spasticity and better urinary control.

- **Autism** Nightly massage by a parent may lead to improvements in behaviour and sleep in autistic children. These improvements include more focus on tasks, better social interaction and better sleep patterns.
- **Cystic fibrosis** Children with cystic fibrosis may benefit from nightly massage by a parent. The children may experience less anxiety and better moods, as well as improved airflow readings, which are a sign of improved breathing.
- **Spinal cord injury** Massage therapy can bring about greater range of motion, improved muscle strength, and diminished symptoms of depression and anxiety.
- **Stroke** One study found that elderly people hospitalized with stroke benefit from short daily back massages. Massage may help lower blood pressure and heart rate, and enable patients to feel less anxiety and pain.

By loosening the fascia and muscles, myofascial release aims to improve posture and help people move more easily and efficiently.

Rolfing

Rolfing was developed in the 1960s by an American biochemist, Ida Rolf. Like myofascial release, Rolfing is concerned with the fascia. Fingers, knuckles and elbows are used to apply intense pressure to the fascia to make them more supple, improving the vertical alignment of the body. These changes are believed to improve flexibility and mobility.

Neuromuscular Massage

This type of massage is used to relieve muscle spasms. Fingers, knuckles or elbows are used to apply pressure for several seconds to trigger points, which are areas of the affected muscle that are in pain. Neuromuscular massage is done to stop the spasm and ultimately ease the pain by relaxing the muscle and increasing the amount of blood and oxygen that reaches it. Neuromuscular massage is usually

somewhat painful at first, but the pain should subside after a day or two.

Reflexology

This is a massage technique for the hands and feet. It is based on the theory that there are reflex points in the hands and feet that are linked to the various glands and internal organs, and that stimulating these reflex points can improve the functioning of the glands and organs. Reflexology is used to relieve stress, improve circulation, stimulate the nervous system and induce deep relaxation.

Manual Lymph Drainage

This type of massage is done to stimulate the flow of fluid in the lymphatic system, one of the main components of the immune system. Lights strokes are applied to the areas of the body where lymph nodes are clustered: the groin, the armpits and the neck. The goal is to relieve or prevent the build-up of lymph fluid in the area. Manual lymph drainage is used to relieve lymphoedema, or swelling in

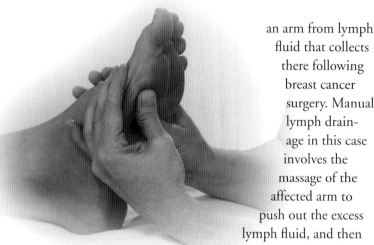

Reflexology is a massage technique based on the belief that there are reflex points on the hands and feet that are connected to other organs and glands within the body.

an arm from lymph fluid that collects there following breast cancer surgery. Manual lymph drainage in this case involves the massage of the affected arm to push out the excess lymph fluid, and then wrapping the arm with a compression bandage to prevent the fluid from returning.

Bowen Therapy

Developed in the 1950s by Thomas Bowen, a lay healer in Australia, Bowen therapy is a gentle technique that involves a series of moves that are held for several seconds and then released. To carry out these moves, the therapist pulls the skin on the back and neck away from the muscle or tendon beneath it and then applies light pressure. These moves are performed in a specific pattern. After the treatment, a patient may be instructed to drink several glasses of water and to take short, frequent walks during the day to encourage circulation and cleanse the body. Bowen therapy aims to relieve a broad range of physical and psychosocial problems, including pain, sports injuries, frozen shoulder (adhesive capsulitis, a condition characterized by pain and reduced mobility of the shoulder), gastrointestinal symptoms, fatigue, anger and depression.

Trager Approach

The Trager approach was devised by Milton Trager, an American medical doctor, over a period of 50 years from 1927 to 1980. The approach is a combination of massage, meditation and movement education. The practitioner first enters a kind of meditative state that helps them connect with the patient. In this state, they manipulate the patient's head, torso, arms and legs with soft, rhythmical pulling or rotational movements. The movements are intended to be pleasurable and to release tension, increase mobility and clear the mind. Afterwards, the practitioner outlines exercises to increase your awareness of how you move. The goals of the Trager approach are to help people move with greater ease, promote relaxation and ease neuromuscular pain.

Acupressure

This is the practice of applying pressure to acupoints, areas of the body that, in Chinese medicine, are believed to influence particular organs and their functions. Acupressure has been used for more than 2,000 years. It predates acupuncture (pp.464–5), and works in a similar way except that it uses pressure instead of needles. Acupressure is performed to relieve pain, reduce tension, increase circulation, eliminate toxins and prevent nausea.

Hot Stone Massage

This massage applies smooth, heated basalt stones to acupoints along the body. Acupoints are areas that therapists relate to particular organs or function. Hot stone massage is used to relieve tension and reduce pain. Some therapists combine hot and cold stones as a way of improving circulation.

Esalen Massage

This approach to massage blends the techniques of Swedish massage and acupressure with a more intuitive, spontaneous touch. It was developed during the 1960s at the Esalen Institute in Big Sur, California, an alternative education centre that blends Eastern and Western philosophies. Esalen is used to reduce stress and relieve muscular pain, as well as to improve body awareness, and help people cope and come to terms with crises in their lives.

CAUTION

People with certain health problems, including infections, skin conditions, bleeding disorders and serious illnesses, should check with their doctors before having any type of massage. In addition, massage should not be done over wounds or near malignancies, fractures, or inflamed joints or tissue.

Tuina

The word *tuina* means 'push-hold' in Chinese, and is a technique of TCM that uses soft-tissue massage and structural realignment to remove blockages along the meridians of the body, stimulate the flow of *qi* and blood, and to promote healing. Methods include deep pressing, tapping and kneading to massage the muscles and tendons, acupressure to directly affect the flow of *qi*, and manipulation techniques to realign the musculoskeletal structure. Massage ranges from light stroking to deep tissue work that may involve significant pressure.

Shiatsu

A Japanese adaptation of tuina, shiatsu uses firm, rhythmic pressure held on specific acupoints for several seconds. Although shiatsu is the Japanese word for 'finger pressure', practitioners also use knuckles, palms, elbows, knees and feet to apply pressure. The principal aim of shiatsu is not to work on specific muscles and joints, but on the overall energy system of the patient, unblocking the meridians and freeing up the flow of qi.

Thai Massage

Like acupressure, Thai massage is also more than 2,000 years old. It combines acupressure with other massage techniques. A practitioner applies gentle pressure to the arms, legs, hands, feet and back, and moves the body in various stretching positions. The aim is to improve flexibility, relieve muscle tension, improve the flow of energy within the body and realign the skeleton. This massage is generally done on a mat on the floor.

In hot stone massage, smooth, heated basalt stones are applied to acupoints along the body to relieve tension and reduce pain.

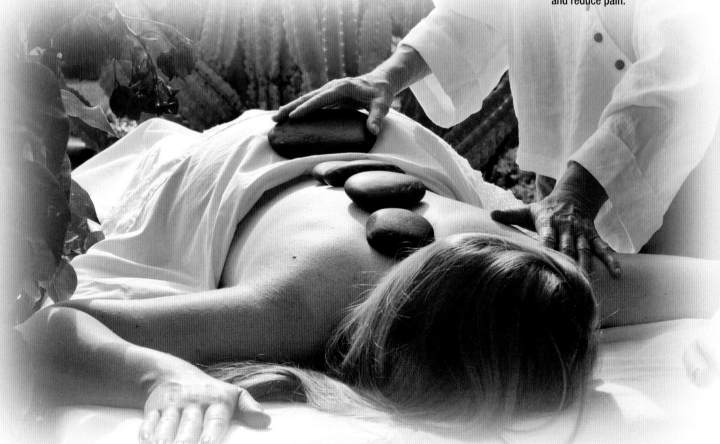

Progressive Muscle Relaxation

This technique involves sequentially tensing and then relaxing individual muscle groups in various parts of the body. It aims to increase awareness of areas that may be holding tension and to achieve progressively deeper relaxation. With practice, a person learns to distinguish states of tension and relaxation and becomes better able to prevent stress.

Relaxation lowers the activity of the sympathetic nervous system, which controls any involuntary actions, thereby decreasing heart and respiration rates and blood pressure. This, in turn, may be helpful in preventing or alleviating various stress-related conditions, such as high blood pressure (pp.236–9) and tension headaches.

HISTORY

Progressive muscle relaxation was developed by American physiologist Edmund Jacobson in the early 1920s. Jacobson was one of the first scientists to measure the electrical activity of muscles. He believed that anxiety resulted in muscle tension and that reducing this tension would lessen the body's stress response.

PRACTICE

Individual methods of progressive muscle relaxation may vary slightly. A typical routine is to lie in a comfortable, relaxed position with eyes closed and concentrate on different body areas one by one. Each major muscle group is tensed for around 15 seconds, then slowly released for about 30 seconds, inhaling on the tightening phase and exhaling with relaxation. The associated feelings should be noted. Sequences often start at the brow or eyes and work progressively down the body to the toes, until the whole body is relaxed.

TREATMENTS

Many people teach themselves this technique using books, videos or CDs. Others may prefer to learn from an experienced therapist.

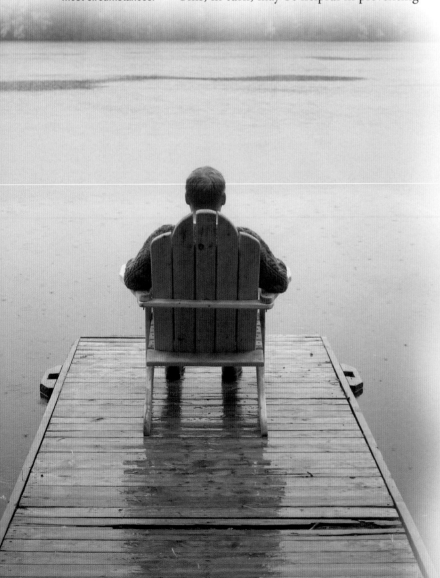

Progressive muscle relaxation can be done just about anywhere in most circumstances.

CAN PROGRESSIVE MUSCLE RELAXATION HELP ME?

Progressive muscle relaxation is used both to promote general well-being and to treat various conditions believed to be associated with or worsened by stress.

- **Psychological problems** Progressive muscle relaxation can help to alleviate anxiety, phobias, depression, insomnia and tension headaches, as well as lessening feelings of stress in people who are quitting smoking.

- **Asthma** In a 2002 study at the Department of Clinical Psychology of NIMHANS in Bangalore, India, progressive muscle relaxation along with other cognitive behaviour therapy techniques produced a significant decrease in asthma symptoms, and in anxiety and depression, compared with a control group.

- **Aggression** A study published in the journal *Stress and Health* in 2005 showed that progressive muscle relaxation is effective in treating aggression in stressed male adolescents.

- **Diabetes** A study at Duke University in North Carolina and published in 2002 in *Diabetes Care* demonstrated better blood sugar control in new diabetic patients who were taught progressive muscle relaxation.

- **Osteoarthritis** Significant reductions in pain and mobility difficulties were observed among osteoarthritis patients using progressive muscle relaxation, according to a 2004 study from Purdue University School of Nursing in Indiana.

- **Cancer Chemotherapy** Nausea and vomiting associated with cancer chemotherapy were reduced and quality of life measures increased using progressive muscle relaxation, according to a study from Korea published in the journal *Support Care Cancer* in 2005.

- **Hyperacusis** Many patients with tinnitus also complain of hyperacusis – sounds being uncomfortably loud. A small study published in the German medical journal *Laryngorhinootologie* in 2000 showed that the threshold of discomfort was raised to normal in more than half of test patients following progressive muscle relaxation training.

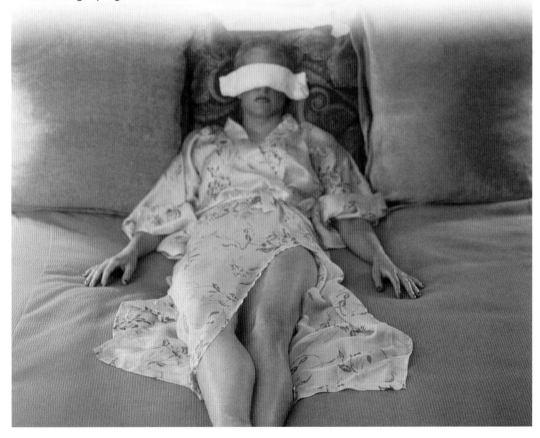

Progressive muscle relaxation can be performed sitting or lying down in a comfortable position with eyes closed and focusing on tensing and relaxing each major muscle group in turn.

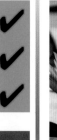

Yoga

The ancient practice of yoga has its roots in Indian philosophy. The aim of yoga is to unite body, mind and spirit or, in its more spiritual forms, the individual and the universe. This is accomplished through physical postures, controlled breathing exercises and meditation, often accompanied by chanting. The traditional discipline also includes a healthy lifestyle, good moral habits and a search for higher consciousness, although yoga is not a religion.

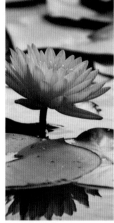

The water lily, known in yoga as the lotus flower, represent the chakras or energy centres of the body.

HISTORY

Although yoga has only relatively recently become popular in Western countries, it originated in India long before recorded history; stone carvings more than 5,000 years old apparently depicting yoga poses have been discovered during archaeological excavations. Many yoga practices were incorporated into Hinduism and other world religions, and yoga has been an important influence in Eastern cultures.

Traditionally, yoga techniques were passed down orally from teacher to student. The Sanskrit word for 'teacher' is guru, and gurus came to be seen as spiritual guides. The many forms of yoga developed from the different practices of various lines of gurus.

The eight limbs, or stages, of yoga (see p.478) that still underpin most forms of classical yoga were described in the Yoga Sutras ('yoga aphorisms'), written by the scholar Patañjali around 200 B.C.E. Hatha yoga, the most common form practised in the West, was described by Swami Swatama-rama, a guru in 15th-century India, in Hatha Yoga Pradipika.

Western forms of yoga generally take a less spiritual approach, concentrating on physical postures (asana) and breathing exercises (pranayama) to calm the physical body, along with concentration (dharana) to still the mind.

Yoga was first introduced to the Western world in the late 19th century, but was not widely known until the 1960s, when interest in Eastern philosophy spread. As the benefits of yoga for physical health and healing became apparent, it became increasingly popular and today is frequently recommended by doctors as a helpful tool for boosting fitness and reducing stress. It also serves as an adjunct to the treatment of many diseases.

PRACTICE

Yoga may be learned by taking classes, reading books, or viewing videos or DVDs, and can be undertaken at home or in a group. People may practise yoga as part of an exercise routine or a healthy lifestyle, for relaxation and stress relief, or to maintain muscular strength and flexibility. For others, it holds the hope of alleviating pain or other symptoms of illness.

Regular yoga practice reduces heart rate, breathing rate and blood pressure, increases lung capacity, improves muscle tone and boosts physical endurance. People who practise yoga often report increased energy,

CAUTION

Yoga is usually a very safe and gentle form of exercise. However, advanced yoga breathing techniques were linked in one case with a pneumothorax, and may possibly have contributed to one death from obstructed breathing. People with heart or lung disease should avoid complex yoga breathing techniques.

reduced fatigue, better sleep, lowered stress and enhanced well-being. Yoga may improve blood and lymph circulation and increase oxygenation of the blood. It may also beneficially affect brain chemicals, including the sleep hormone melatonin and the stress hormone cortisol.

Yoga is generally suitable for people of all ages and fitness levels. However people with musculoskeletal problems, recent injuries or long-term health conditions are advised to check with their doctor before taking it up.

TYPES OF YOGA

There are several hundred different types of yoga. In North America and Europe, the most common is hatha yoga. Some of the other more common forms are also described here.

Almost all forms of yoga in the West have as their main focus a sequence of postures or asanas that are either held in a static pose or moved through in a dynamic sequence, accompanied by breathing control, hand positions or meditation. Concentration is frequently accomplished by a fixed focus on an object, such as a candle or a drawing, or on a breathing rhythm or repetition of a chanted sound, called a mantra.

Ashtanga

This is a vigorous form of yoga that connects movements and breathing while performing set sequences of poses. It helps build strength, stamina and flexibility. A modern variant called power yoga has recently become popular in the United States as a form of cardiovascular workout.

Bhakti

While most forms of yoga are easily separated from spiritual influences, the exception is bhakti, or devotional yoga. Although it does not require any particular religious affiliation, it primarily involves meditation upon the idea of the existence of a divine being.

Bikram

Also known as hot yoga, bikram is practised in rooms heated to around 39° C (100°F). The aim is to sweat profusely, which loosens the muscles and tendons and promotes inner cleansing. The technique uses 26 postures in a set sequence, and may be used by both beginners and advanced yoga practitioners. People who take medication or have either chronic or acute health conditions should check with their doctor before engaging in bikram yoga.

In hatha yoga, physical postures and breathing exercises are used to promote harmony between the mind and body.

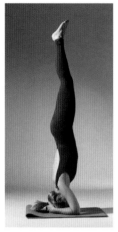

People with back or eye problems, hypertension, clotting disorders, atherosclerosis or osteoporosis should avoid inverted postures, such as headstands. In very rare cases, increased blood flow resulting from some postures may lead to a stroke.

Hatha

This most common form of yoga in the Western world has its roots in ancient tradition and is a component of ashtanga yoga as described in Patañjali's Yoga Sutras. Ha means 'sun' and tha means 'moon' in Sanskrit, so hatha represents opposing forces such as day and night, and light and dark. Hatha yoga uses physical postures and breathing exercises. Its aim is to balance the mind and body, creating harmony and promoting physical health, strength and mental calmness.

Iyengar

This is a slow, methodical form of yoga that focuses on the stillness and form of each posture that is adopted. Props such as bolsters, blocks, ropes, mats and chairs are used to enable the best possible physical alignment. This form of yoga is therefore accessible even to those with limited flexibility and fitness – yet is also undertaken by more advanced practitioners because the exercises form a carefully graded progression. It is very helpful for beginners to learn each posture very precisely.

Karma

The word karma means 'to do', and is often used to refer to the universal principle of cause and effect in Eastern philosophy. In yoga it implies working with awareness, and this form attempts to integrate yoga practice into daily life, flowing into each breath and movement. The aim is for consciousness entirely in the present moment. Meditation also plays a large role.

Kundalini

The focus of kundalini yoga is on moving energy through seven energy centres, or chakras, which enables kundalini, the life force at the base of the spine, to rise up through the body. This is a highly spiritual form of yoga, using postures with slow and deliberate movements, combined with hand positions, breathing techniques, chanting and meditation to awaken inner consciousness.

Raja

The word raja means kingly, and raja yoga is also known as the 'royal road'. It uses meditation, study, exercise and breathing to bring the mind and emotions into balance and produce a well-rounded individual.

The Eight Limbs of Yoga

The limbs, or stages of yoga first described in Patañjali's Yoga Sutras are sometimes depicted as a tree with eight branches.

Yama	Moral behaviour, restraint from vice
Niyama	Observance, healthy habits, tolerance
Asana	Physical postures
Pranayama	Breathing control
Pratyahara	Preparation for meditation: sensory withdrawal and detachment
Dharana	Concentration; focusing on a single object for a set time
Dhyana	Contemplation or meditation, being able to focus on one thing, or nothing, indefinitely
Samadhi	Higher consciousness; losing the sense of an individual self and entering a state of supreme bliss

CAN YOGA HELP ME?

The use of yoga in traditional healing has a long history – it forms an integral part of Ayurveda (pp.451–4) and there is good evidence that yoga can help relieve symptoms in a wide range of disorders.

- **Stress and anxiety** Yoga, especially forms involving meditation, has been used extensively to promote relaxation and feelings of well-being.

- **Depression** Several studies have shown useful effects in depression. For example, psychiatrists from the National Institute of Mental Health and Neuro Sciences in Bangalore, India, reported in 2000 that a type of yoga called sudarshan kriya yoga (SKY) produced significant improvements in depression scores with no side-effects. Although remission rates of 67 percent with yoga were somewhat less than rates with low-dose antidepressants (73 percent) or electric shock therapy (93 percent), they were judged sufficiently impressive to consider SKY as a first-line treatment for mild depression.

- **Attention-deficit hyperactivity disorder (ADHD)** Researchers from the University of Sydney in Australia reported in 2004 that many measures of problem behaviour improved in boys with ADHD after 20 yoga sessions. Further research is needed.

- **Hypertension** In a study reported from Mumbai, India, in 2002, 20 middle-aged patients with hypertension practised yoga for one hour a day over three months. Their blood pressure was significantly lowered, and they also experienced reduced levels of blood glucose, cholesterol and triglycerides. (Many yoga teachers recommend that patients with hypertension avoid inverted positions that may temporarily increase blood pressure.)

- **Heart disease** A study by the International Board of Yoga and published in 2004 in the *Journal of Association of Physicians of India* reported that yoga-based lifestyle modifications over one year resulted in regression of coronary artery disease, improved blood flow within coronary arteries, and significant reductions in cholesterol. (People with heart disease should talk with their doctor before starting any form of exercise.)

- **Low back pain** A 2004 preliminary study from Richard Stockton College in New Jersey found that a six-week course of hatha yoga designed to relieve low back pain was successful in treating 22 affected patients, although larger studies are needed to confirm the results.

- **Diabetes** In a 2004 study at University College of Medical Sciences in Delhi, India, 24 patients with type 2 diabetes had improved blood sugar control after doing yoga exercises for 40 days. Pulse rate and blood pressure also decreased significantly.

- **Cancer** According to a review in *Cancer Control* published in 2005, nine studies conducted with cancer patients and survivors showed overall that yoga could give modest improvements in sleep quality, mood, stress, cancer-related distress, cancer-related symptoms and overall quality of life. Yoga is not recommended as a sole treatment for cancer, but may help to deal with associated symptoms.

- **Pregnancy** Pregnant women who did yoga for one hour daily had significantly lower rates of pre-term labour, intra-uterine growth retardation, and pregnancy-induced hypertension and significantly higher birthweights, compared with a control group who just walked for an hour each day, according to a study from Bangalore, India, published in 2005 in the *Journal of Alternative and Complementary Medicine*. Yoga is generally believed to be safe in pregnancy, provided it is carried out under expert instruction. In fact, the Lamaze technique of pain control in labour is based on yoga breathing. Some yoga positions that could put pressure on the uterus are best avoided.

- **Asthma** Yoga has been claimed to improve lung function and airway sensitivity and reduce the need for asthma drugs, but the evidence is conflicting and more research is needed.

- **Epilepsy** A study published in the *Indian Journal of Medical Research* in 1996 found that patients doing sahaja yoga had a significantly reduced seizure frequency, compared with control patients. However, the number of study subjects was too small for firm conclusions to be drawn.

- **Multiple sclerosis** Regular yoga helped to relieve fatigue in people with MS, according to a small study at Oregon Health & Science University published in *Neurology* in 2004.

Craniosacral Therapy

Craniosacral therapy is a manipulation technique that involves light touch to the cranium (skull) and sacrum (base of the spine and tailbone). It is based on the theory that the movements of bones within the skull and the lower back, as well as the rhythmic flow of cerebrospinal fluid in and around the spinal cord, play a central role in the body's overall functioning. According to this theory, obstruction of these movements can contribute to a variety of problems, especially in the brain, spine and endocrine system. Craniosacral therapy is also known as cranio-occipital technique or cranial osteopathy.

HISTORY

The concept of craniosacral therapy was developed in the 1920s by Dr William Sutherland, an American osteopath. Sutherland believed the bones that make up the skull are not statically fused together. Rather, he said, where the skull bones meet (areas called sutures) there is actually the capacity for some movement – a theory that remains controversial. Anything that impedes this movement may restrict the flow of cerebrospinal fluid (the fluid that surrounds the brain and the spinal cord) and cause health problems.

Sutherland developed a system of manipulation that focuses on the sutures. The purpose of this is to identify places where bone and fluid movement are restricted and to restore proper movement as a way of helping the body to heal itself. This system of diagnosis and treatment was originally called cranial osteopathy.

In the 1970s, John Upledger, another American osteopath, assembled a team

Craniolsacral therapy is not just a head massage, although the head may be manipulated. Instead, it is intended to promote the body's natural capacity to heal itself.

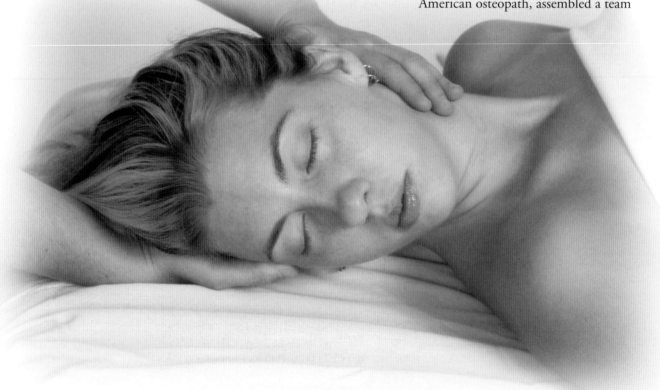

of scientists to study the craniosacral system (which includes the central nervous system, the cerebrospinal fluid, and the bones and membranes of the brain and spine). This study found that restrictions in the meninges, which are the membranes of the craniosacral system, are what cause obstructions to bone movement and the flow of cerebrospinal fluid and energy. Upledger then devised a system of manipulation that focuses on the meninges and called it craniosacral therapy.

A third type of craniosacral therapy, called the reflex approach, aims to reduce stress by stimulating the nerve endings in the scalp between cranial sutures and triggers. And yet another approach, called the sacro-occipital technique, was developed in the late 1940s by Dr Major Bertrand DeJarnette, an American chiropractor. These two techniques are both different from the original craniosacral therapy, which is an established form of osteopathic manipulation (pp.438–40). These therapies are used by massage therapists and other practitioners, who have less extensive training than osteopaths.

Today, osteopathic craniosacral therapy is used mainly in the United States and Great Britain, and to a limited extent throughout Europe, Japan, South Africa and New Zealand.

PRACTICE

Osteopathic craniosacral therapy is practised mainly by osteopathic doctors, but also by

CAUTION

The abrupt manipulation of the head and spine carries a small risk of stroke, bleeding in the skull, and other damage to the brain and spine. The more common soft adjustment typical of cranioscral therapy is unlikely to cause harm. People with recent head trauma or illnesses of the brain or spine may be at increased risk and should check with their doctor before seeing a craniosacral therapist.

CAN CRANIOSACRAL THERAPY HELP ME?

Research into craniosacral therapy for lower back pain, sports injuries, and labor and delivery has so far not found evidence that it is beneficial. However, there are anecdotal reports that it can relieve many conditions, including headache, temporomandibular joint disorder (TMJ), menstrual cramps, chronic neck and back pain, sciatica, chronic fatigue, infant colic and autism.

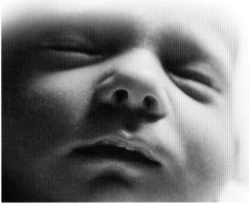

Craniosacral therapy may be able to help babies with colic, sucking difficulties, sleep problems and behavioural issues.

medical doctors, chiropractors and naturopaths. The therapist uses their hands to gently feel the motion of the craniosacral system. Sutural therapists then manipulate the sutures or where the bones meet in the skull, meningeal therapists focus on releasing restrictions of the cranial sutures and underlying membranes, and reflex therapists use manipulation to trigger the nervous system to turn off stress signals. A craniosacral therapy session usually takes 30 minutes to an hour. The practitioner applies very light pressure to the cranium and sacrum to remove restrictions to the movement of bone and the flow of cerebrospinal fluid.

TREATMENTS

Treatment has many goals: preventing illness; easing labour and delivery; enhancing the functioning of the central nervous system; and helping the body to heal or relieve a wide range of conditions, including sports injuries, ear infections, colic and menstrual pain.

Hydrotherapy

Hydrotherapy is one of the oldest and most widely used methods used to treat disease and injuries. It encompasses an array of approaches that use water of different temperatures, including baths, whirlpools, cold compresses, hot compresses, saunas, steam and enemas. Herbs and minerals are often added to the water to enhance the therapeutic effect. In its many forms, hydrotherapy is recognized throughout the world as a way of reducing inflammation from injuries and illnesses, soothing pain, relaxing the mind and body, toning the muscles and stimulating the immune system.

HISTORY

Hydrotherapy dates back thousands of years to the use of natural mineral baths, hot springs, geysers and sweat lodges by cultures around the world, including the Romans, Greeks, Egyptians, Native Americans and Chinese. Hippocrates, a Greek physician who died around 337 B.C.E., prescribed hydrotherapy to treat disorders such as rheumatism and jaundice.

Public baths were built in Europe and Asia thousands of years ago, including Greece, Rome and Japan. Today, hydrotherapy is offered at spas around the world for physical and mental rejuvenation. It is a standard approach in sports medicine, physical therapy and naturopathy. It plays a central role in self-care in such varied forms as hot and cold compresses, humidifiers, vapourizers and home spas.

PRACTICE

Hydrotherapy works on the principle that heat and cold have different effects on the

Hydrotherapy dates back thousands of years to the ancient Greeks and Romans. The mineral baths in Bath, England were built by the Romans.

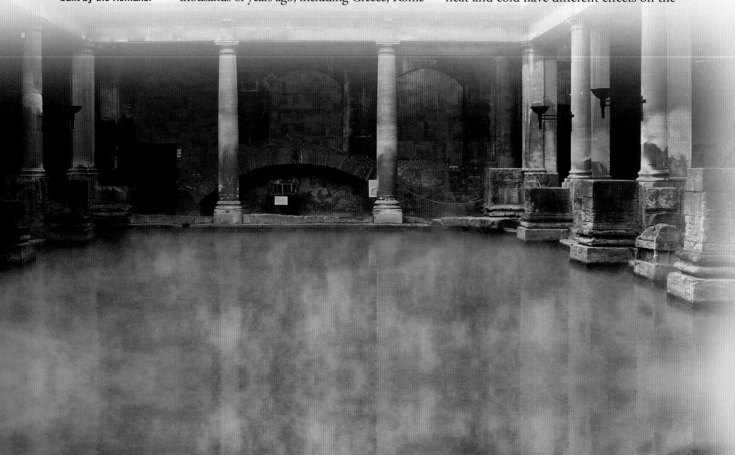

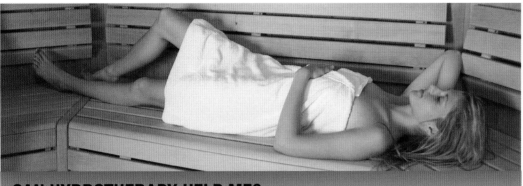

Hydrotherapy as a treatment is often available today through saunas, steamrooms and whirlpools.

CAN HYDROTHERAPY HELP ME?

Hydrotherapy is a simple, inexpensive, and safe way to relieve the symptoms of a broad range of conditions.

- **Colds, coughs and other upper-respiratory ailments** Symptoms can be relieved by hot or cool steam from a humidifier. Steam can also reduce the risk of infections by keeping the respiratory passages moist.

- **Tendonitis, sprains and muscle strains** Swelling can be decreased with ice packs applied every hour for the first day or two after the injury. After the swelling has stopped, hot compresses can relieve stiffness and soreness. The contrast of hot and cold further promotes healing of muscle injuries because it increases blood circulation.

- **Skin ailments and wounds** Hot sitz baths, in which you sit in a shallow tub of water, can help relieve the pain and itching of haemorrhoids and the discomfort of uterine cramps associated with menstrual periods. Whirlpool baths help heal skin sores and infected wounds, as well as improve the circulation of paraplegics and others who are unable to move their limbs.

body. Heat relaxes the body and helps rid it of toxic substances by inducing sweating and by dilating the blood vessels. Cold stimulates the body and constricts the blood vessels, which helps to reduce inflammation, and invigorate and tone the muscles.

TREATMENTS

There are three types of external hydrotherapy: hot water, cold water and contrast therapy, which alternates hot and cold treatments. Each type has several applications. For example, hot baths, in which the body is immersed in water above normal body temperature, are believed to help detoxify the body of harmful chemicals, such as alcohol, drugs and poisonous metals. Hot compresses can help relieve pain in specific areas – the lower back and legs for sciatica and the torso for menstrual cramps, for example. Ice packs are useful for reducing acute inflammation from sprains and strains. Constitutional

hydrotherapy is a form of contrast therapy in which first a hot compress and then a cold compress is applied to the body. It is used as a complementary therapy for a variety of ailments ranging from upper respiratory infections and asthma to irritable bowel disease and arthritis.

Medical professionals use methods of internal hydrotherapy, such as enemas and colon irrigation, to relieve constipation and to clean the bowels by stimulating elimination.

On Call

Salts, herbs and other natural substances can enhance the therapeutic effectiveness of warm baths. For example, Epsom salts promote perspiration, relax muscles and relieve joint pain. Oats help relieve itchy rashes, and soothe sunburn and other skin irritations. Chamomile also soothes the skin.

Applied Kinesiology

This is, first and foremost, a method of diagnosing and treating ailments that use muscle strength as a gauge of emotional and physical health. Applied kinesiology is based on the idea that every muscle corresponds to a particular organ or gland, and that a weakness in a muscle often indicates a problem with its related organ or gland. Upon further investigation, which builds on the knowledge of neurology, anatomy, physiology, biomechanics and biochemistry, practitioners make a diagnosis and prescribe treatment.

HISTORY

Applied kinesiology has its roots in chiropractic (pp.466–7). In 1964, George Goodheart, an American chiropractor, observed that some people have abnormal posture even when there is nothing structurally wrong with them, and that the cause can be a muscle dysfunction. He believed that by manipulating bones and muscles he could strengthen the muscles as well as their surrounding nerves.

After learning about acupuncture and its underlying principles of meridians, or energy pathways (p.464), Goodheart made acupuncture part of applied kinesiology treatment. He taught his diagnostic and therapeutic methods to other clinicians, and in 1976 the International College of Applied Kinesiology, a worldwide organization, was founded. Courses in applied kinesiology are currently being taught in Europe, North America and Australia.

PRACTICE

While most practitioners of applied kinesiology are chiropractors, other clinicians, including medical doctors, naturopaths, physical therapists and massage therapists, also

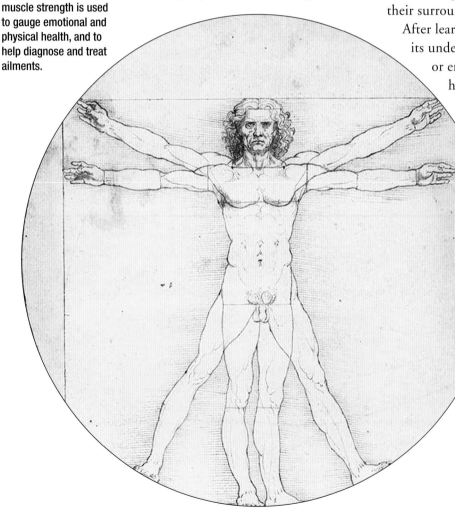

In applied kinesiology, muscle strength is used to gauge emotional and physical health, and to help diagnose and treat ailments.

use it. They all consider muscle weakness to be a sign of a number of problems, including nerve dysfunction, impaired drainage of lymphatic fluid, reduced blood supply, blockage of an acupuncture meridian or a deficiency or overabundance of certain nutrients in the diet.

The centrepiece of applied kinesiology is muscle testing. This is done by applying pressure to certain muscles, and observing how the nervous system and other systems in the body react. The practitioner then increases and decreases the pressure to see how the body adapts. The particular muscles tested and methods used vary according to each patient's symptoms, medical history and other individual characteristics. If, for example, someone who plays tennis regularly is feeling pain in a knee, diagnosis will concentrate on the muscles of the knee. If the knees are weak, treatment will focus on strengthening and stabilizing them.

Muscle testing is not the sole means used for diagnosis. Applied kinesiology is used along with a physical examination and, often, conventional diagnostic tools, such as laboratory tests and X-rays, to accurately assess a patient's condition.

Applied kinesiology is not used to treat or cure serious illnesses such as cancer, heart disease, diabetes and infections. Instead, it is part of a holistic approach, supporting conventional treatments as well as preventing health problems. Practitioners use it as a tool for diagnosing many conditions, including joint pain, arthritis, sports injuries, migraines and impotence. The goals in using applied kinesiology are to help restore normal nerve function; strengthen the

CAUTION

The use of manual stimulation or touch to diagnose nutritional problems is inaccurate and potentially dangerous.

CAN APPLIED KINESIOLOGY HELP ME?

Practitioners of applied kinesiology believe that it is effective as part of a holistic approach to diagnosing and treating some chronic conditions and neuromuscular injuries. Medical studies on the effectiveness of applied kinesiology are inconclusive.

- **Sports injuries** An evaluation at the first sign of muscle pain can identify a weak muscle early and help prevent serious injury.
- **Allergies and asthma** While applied kinesiology is not a cure, practitioners aim through its use to relieve symptoms of respiratory allergies and asthma.
- **Pain** Anecdotal evidence exists that it relieves headaches, lower back pain and carpal tunnel syndrome.
- **Nervous system illnesses** Applied kinesiology is believed to ease the symptoms of Menière's disease (a disease of the inner ear that causes deafness, ringing in the ears, and vertigo) and neuralgia (severe pain often following the course of a nerve).

immune system, digestion and other organ functions; improve the range of motion in people with conditions such as arthritis and sports injuries; and correct problems with posture and gait. To date, studies of applied kinesiology's effectiveness have been inconclusive in demonstrating the effectiveness of the procedure.

TREATMENTS

A wide range of techniques are used to manually manipulate of the spine, extremities and head. Applied kinesiology also incorporates procedures from other disciplines, including nutrition, chiropractic manipulation (pp.446–7), craniosacral therapy (pp.480–1), acupuncture (pp.464–5), osteopathy (438–40) and myofascial release (p.469).

Aston-Patterning

This is a multi-faceted programme of movement education, fitness training, bodywork and ergonomics. The goals of Aston-Patterning are to improve posture, mobility, stability and balance. Practitioners use it to relieve pain from headache, backaches and sports injuries, as well as to correct problems with posture, and increase the efficiency and effectiveness of movements.

HISTORY
Aston-Patterning was developed in the United States in the 1970s by Judith Aston, a professional dancer who also created movement education programmes for performing artists and athletes. After two car accidents left her with serious injuries that were not helped by conventional medicine, she tried Rolfing, a type of deep massage (p.471). Rolfing helped her recovery, and she then developed a programme of movement education therapy for Rolfing clients. In 1977, she separated from Rolfing and expanded her programme.

Today, practitioners can learn the techniques at Aston-Patterning training centres in the United States and United Kingdom. Clinicians certified by these training centres operate in those countries as well as in Australia and New Zealand.

PRACTICE
The underlying philosophy of Aston-Patterning is that it is healthy for the human body to move asymmetrically in the process of adapting to various activities. Practitioners acknowledge that some asymmetrical movements are negative because they inhibit the body from moving effectively.

Walking with your weight shifted to one side is an example of negative asymmetry. Pressing down on the bathroom counter with your free hand when you bend over to brush your teeth lengthens and supports the back, and is an example of adaptive asymmetry. One of the goals of Aston-Patterning is to teach people how to distinguish negative asymmetrical movements from the natural, adaptive ones.

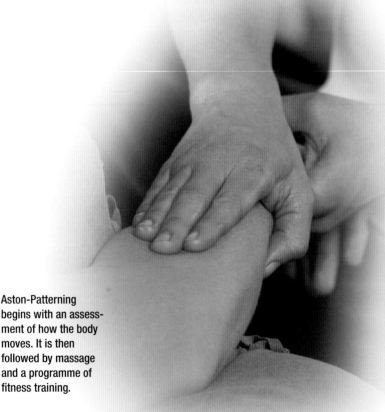

Aston-Patterning begins with an assessment of how the body moves. It is then followed by massage and a programme of fitness training.

CAUTION

The vigorous exercises and deep massage used in Aston-Patterning can be dangerous for people with heart or respiratory problems, osteoporosis, diabetes or bleeding disorders. Check with your doctor before seeing an Aston-Patterning practitioner.

CAN ASTON-PATTERNING HELP ME?

There are no studies of Aston-Patterning that establish its effectiveness. But proponents say it can improve balance and posture, aid in the recovery from injuries, and help relieve chronic back pain, neck pain and headaches.

TREATMENTS

A session begins with an assessment of the way you move and stand, followed by massage, fitness training, exercise and ergonomics.

PREVENTATIVE MEDICINE

Three kinds of massage are used to identify areas of muscular tension, decrease tension and improve movement. Aston massage is a non-compression touch that helps release muscle tension held by the nervous system. Myokinetics is a specialized type of myofascial release (p.469), a soft-tissue massage. Arthrokinetics centres on the joints and bony surfaces.

• MOVEMENT AND EXERCISE Movement education consists of instruction on ways to improve everyday movements, such as sitting, standing, walking, and bending, so that they will put less stress on the body and cause less pain. Fitness training includes cardiovascular exercises, toning and stretching, with the goal of learning healthier, more efficient ways to move.

• PHYSICAL ENVIRONMENT Ergonomics is understanding how the everyday environment affects posture, the degree of effort needed to complete tasks, and chronic pain. Modifying this environment can reduce the risk of pain and injury. Examples may include increasing the height of your desk chair so that you feel less back strain, or putting a seat cushion in your car to make driving more comfortable.

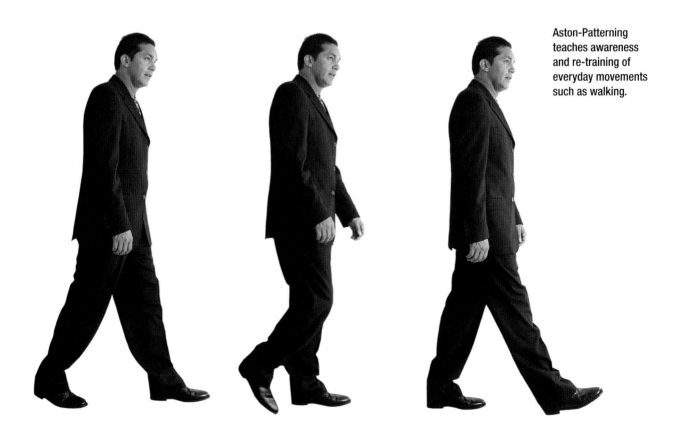

Aston-Patterning teaches awareness and re-training of everyday movements such as walking.

Alexander Technique

This instructional programme is geared towards changing habits of movement and posture that are thought to promote physical problems. The basic idea is that when the neck muscles are not overworked, the head balances lightly at the top of spine. The relationship between the head and spine is considered especially important because, when the head is balanced on top of the spine, a natural oppositional force in the torso encourages the spine to lengthen, rather than compress, with movement. This is believed to help reduce physical tension, increase energy levels, control pain and enhance physical performance. The Alexander technique is used around the world, and is especially popular with performing artists and athletes who are interested in improving their skills and in controlling pain from injuries.

HISTORY

Frederick Mathias Alexander, an Australian actor, developed this technique in the 1890s. He was searching for a cure for the laryngitis he often developed while performing. Watching himself in the mirror as he spoke, Alexander discovered that he moved his head back and forth and tensed the muscles in his neck. He concluded that these habits contributed to his laryngitis by creating excessive tension in his throat. Alexander devised a technique to improve his head and neck posture, and his recurrent bouts with laryngitis stopped. He then sought to train teachers in his method so that they could help people recognize and correct harmful postures and patterns of movement.

In 1904, Alexander moved to London and taught his technique to individuals in search of pain relief. In 1931, he began a formal three-year teacher training course, which he ran until his death in 1955. In 1958, some of his graduates founded the Society of Teachers of the Alexander Technique in London. A certification process for teachers in the United States began in 1964 with the founding of the American Center for the Alexander Technique in New York. Today, teachers of the Alexander technique practise throughout North and South America, Europe, South Africa and Australia.

PRACTICE

According to Alexander, everyone has unconscious movement habits that put undue pressure on the body. These include overusing the muscles for simple tasks such as lifting a cup and slouching when sitting. An Alexander technique teacher analyses a student's pattern of movement to identify the habits that contribute to recurring health problems, such as a bad back, neck and shoulder pain, restricted breathing, general tiredness, or limits to range of motion or general performance level. These harmful habits may include a person's characteristic way of sitting, standing and walking. The teacher then guides the student to move in a way that causes less muscular tension in the body.

TREATMENTS

The Alexander technique is taught in individual or group lessons. The teacher observes the student's posture and movement patterns in everyday activities such as going from a sitting to a standing position, walking, turning and breathing. The teacher may also gently touch the student to gather more information about their breathing and movement patterns. The teacher will then explain how movement patterns can be changed to eliminate tension, and encourage flexibility and ease of movement. Teachers also use their hands to guide students gently in the proper way to carry out the movements.

Alexander technique practitioners believe that once students understand the proper movement technique and sense what it feels like, they will be able to do it on their own and break engrained negative habits of movement. However, it can take ten or more sessions before students have internalized the Alexander technique well enough to reach this goal.

CAN THE ALEXANDER TECHNIQUE HELP ME?

The Alexander technique has been studied for the following conditions. Though some evidence suggests that it may be helpful, none of the studies were conclusive.

- **Lung function** Alexander technique may help musicians playing wind instruments breathe more easily and efficiently.
- **Balance** The technique may improve balance in people over 65 years old.
- **Back pain** Alexander technique may ease back pain and reduce related disability.
- **Temporomandibular joint disorder (TMJ)** The technique may ease chronic jaw pain caused by this disorder.
- **Parkinson's disease** People with this condition who learn the Alexander technique may experience less disability and depression.

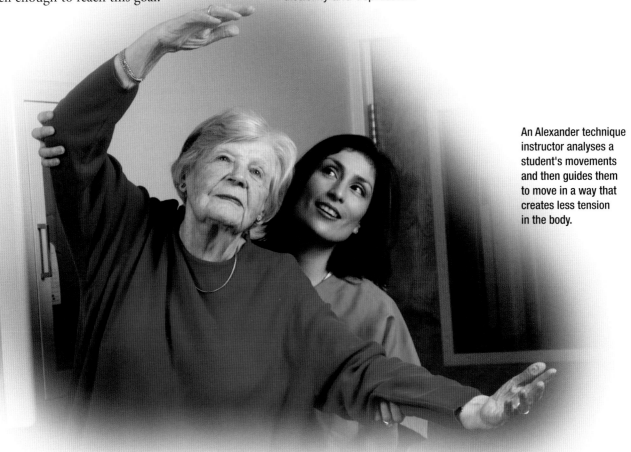

An Alexander technique instructor analyses a student's movements and then guides them to move in a way that creates less tension in the body.

Hellerwork

This is a process of improving the vertical alignment of the body and enhancing awareness of the relationship between the mind and body. It uses deep-tissue bodywork, movement education, and insight into how emotions and attitudes can cause muscle tension and impair posture. The main purpose of Hellerwork is to help the client reduce physical and emotional stress and move with greater efficiency and fluidity.

HISTORY

Hellerwork was developed in 1979 by Joseph Heller, an American aerospace engineer who became a practitioner of Rolfing (p.471), a holistic system of soft tissue manipulation that seeks to organize the whole body. Heller decided that the physical manipulation techniques used in Rolfing were not enough to put the body into proper alignment, so he added movement education, and dialogues between the practitioner and client about how thoughts and feelings can add to (or reduce) mechanical stress within the body.

Hellerwork International operates schools in North America, Europe, South Africa, Japan, Australia and New Zealand, and has a certification programme for its graduates.

PRACTICE

Hellerwork consists of several one-hour sessions – the precise number of sessions depends on the individual. It focuses on the fascia, the sheaths of connective tissue that wrap muscles throughout the body. Ideally, fascia should be loose, but they grow rigid as a result of ongoing stress from poor posture, lack of movement and emotional tension.

Each session of Hellerwork aims to improve alignment and reduce tension in a different area of the body. The first session concentrates on aligning the ribcage over the pelvis and identifying tension that is unwittingly held in the chest. This session is designed to enable patients to expand the

CAN HELLERWORK HELP ME?

Hellerwork can improve posture, movement and physical self-expression. However, the evidence for this is anecdotal – Hellerwork has not been subjected to clinical trials.

chest more fully as they inhale. Other sessions focus on the legs, knees and ankles; releasing tension in the shoulders and arms; and lengthening the spine.

TREATMENTS

The goal is to help patients achieve and sustain improvements in posture from the head down to the feet. Deep-tissue massage is used to help release tension in the fascia, improving posture, movement and balance. Movement education teaches patients how to stand, sit and carry out everyday movements (such as walking, running and lifting) with efficiency and ease. The goal is to put minimum stress on the body. Dialogues about thoughts and feelings are used to heighten awareness of the attitudes and emotions that may be contributing to physical tension.

Each session is organized around an emotional or psychological theme that relates to the area of the body that is the focal-point. For example, the theme of session 2 is Standing on Your Own Two Feet. While the physical goal is to distribute weight evenly over the legs and feet, the dialogue may delve into issues such as security, self-support, financial stability and the stability of important relationships.

Expressive Arts Therapy

This form of psychotherapy uses creative expression to help people cope with stress, chronic illness and traumatic experiences. The therapy is also designed to enhance their social and cognitive functioning. The various art forms that are part of expressive therapy include painting and sculpture, dance and movement, music, drama and writing.

HISTORY

Expressive arts therapy began to be widely used in the mid-20th century. The first of the art forms to be developed into therapies were art therapy, music therapy, dance and movement therapy and psychodrama. Psychiatrists and other mental health professionals observed that psychiatric patients benefitted from drawing, painting and talking about art, as well as from attending dance classes. Clinicians also began to use instrumental and vocal music as part of the rehabilitation process to provide emotional support and facilitate movement. Dr Jacob Moreno, a Romanian-born physician, developed psychodrama – the use of role-playing and other group dramatic techniques – to facilitate positive change in people who were in mental health programmes, as well as in business and education.

Drama therapy came into use in the 1970s, after psychotherapists, teachers and theatre professionals recognized a need for communication to help patients release the strong feelings associated with psychological, social and physical problems. Bibiolotherapy, which involves creative writing and literary discussions, became established in 1981 as a means of supporting personal growth and development, and improving coping skills. Today, expressive arts therapy is used around the world.

PRACTICE

Each of the expressive arts therapies has its own set of standards for training and practice.

• ART THERAPY Art therapists are trained in graduate-level programmes to use different art media (such as drawing, painting and clay) and in the psychological assessment and treatment of patients. They practise in a wide range of settings, including hospitals, hospices, nursing homes, mental health centres, and disaster relief centres. Art therapy involves talking about artwork and creating art as a way of increasing self-awareness, coping with physical symptoms of illness and the effects of trauma, and relieving stress.

• MUSIC THERAPY Music therapists are trained in undergraduate and graduate programmes. Training includes music theory, human development, psychotherapy and techniques of music therapy. The therapy includes singing, playing instruments, listening to music and discussing lyrics. Music therapists practise in a wide variety of settings, including hospitals, nursing homes, rehabilitation facilities and schools. The goal of therapy depends on the client, but may include reducing stress, relieving pain, improving memory, improving communication and enhancing the person's motivation to participate in rehabilitation or treatment.

Creating and analysing art is used as a way of increasing a person's self-awareness and their ability to cope with stress.

CAN EXPRESSIVE ARTS THERAPY HELP ME?

Several modes of expressive arts therapy have been studied and found beneficial as adjuncts to conventional medical treatment. Most of the studies were small and preliminary.

- **Body image** Expressive art therapy may help children cope with changes in their body image due to illness or surgery.

- **Grief** Music, art and movement therapies have enabled children suffering grief to communicate their feelings and cope with trauma and stress.

- **Alzheimer's disease** A small, brief trial comparing a group with Alzheimer's and a group with depression suggested that dance/movement therapy may benefit people with moderate-stage Alzheimer's disease. After 12 days, the Alzheimer's patients showed significant improvement in the ability to learn the dance steps, whereas the depressed patients did not.

- **Mental retardation** Dance/movement therapy may improve balance in children with mild to moderate mental retardation.

- **Rheumatoid arthritis** A therapeutic dance programme may give people with rheumatoid arthritis (pp.136–9) a greater range of motion. Dance therapy is often more enjoyable than other types of exercise, as well.

- **Pain control** Listening to music may ease pain during medical procedures. Art therapy has also been found to help children and adolescents with sickle cell disease cope with everyday pain.

- **Health and well-being in old age** A small clinical trial of elderly women compared the effects of getting together regularly and discussing artwork with the effects of simply getting together regularly. Relative to the other group, the women who discussed art showed the following improvements: better moods, lower blood pressure, fewer bouts of dizziness, less pain and less need to take laxatives.

- **Psychiatric illness** Art therapy may be beneficial for people with chronic psychiatric problems, helping to facilitate improvements in their attitudes toward themselves and enabling them to get along better with others.

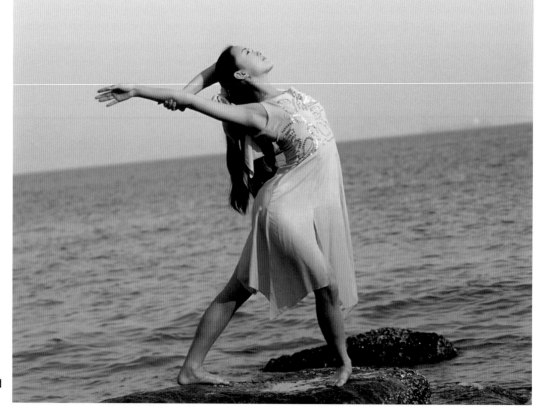

Dance therapy is used to improve social, emotional, cognitive and physical functioning.

• **DANCE/MOVEMENT THERAPY** This type of therapy is grounded in the belief that the mind and body interact to contribute to illness as well as health. Because movement is a fundamental means of personal expression, dance/movement therapists believe it is uniquely suited to be a channel that connects the mind and body to improve health. Therapists have graduate-level degrees. Dance and movement are used to improve social, emotional, cognitive and physical functioning. Clients include people with severe emotional disorders, eating disorders, autism and addiction, as well as victims of abuse. Some practitioners also believe that dance/movement therapy can help people cope with serious physical disorders such as chronic pain, high blood pressure, cardiovascular disease and breast cancer.

• **PSYCHODRAMA** This form of group therapy uses role playing and other dramatic tools. Psychodrama therapists, or psychodramatists, are trained in workshops. In a therapy session, the group first identifies a theme to explore, then brings it to life by creating a scenario centred on a problem that a protagonist must resolve. The psychodramatist guides the dramatic action and then leads a discussion about it. The goal of psychodrama is to help people make constructive changes and wiser choices in their lives. It is used in work with children, elderly people and people with mental illnesses.

• **DRAMA THERAPY** Drama therapy uses dramatic processes, props and associations for therapeutic purposes. Training involves either a graduate degree in drama therapy or a graduate degree in another field plus workshop instruction in drama therapy. In this type of therapy, a person tells an autobiographical story to gain insight into a personal problem, increase understanding of their thoughts and feelings, and achieve catharsis. Drama therapists work with children, the elderly, psychiatric patients, disabled people

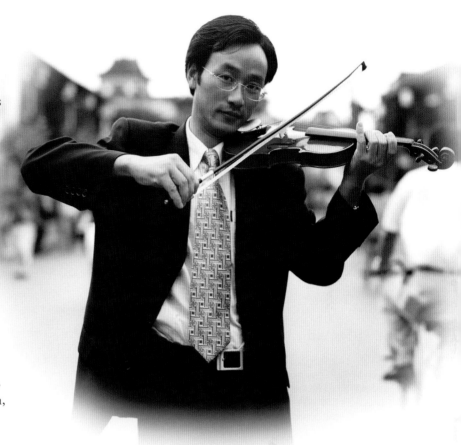

Music therapy may involve listening to, playing or discussing music. The goals range from stress reduction and pain relief, to improvement in memory and enhanced communication skills.

and people recovering from substance abuse. Therapeutic goals include reducing feelings of isolation, enhancing the quality of relationships, and improving coping skills.

• **BIBLIOTHERAPY** Bibliotherapy, also known as poetry therapy, uses creative writing and discussions about literature to foster personal growth and development, and help to control and prevent mental illness. Therapists have graduate-level degrees with training in psychology, literature, and facilitating individual and group sessions. They work in psychiatric units, mental health centres, and centres for substance abuse rehabilitation. Through the writing process and literary discussion, bibiotherapists seek to help people understand themselves better, vent their emotions, release tension, gain insights and improve coping skills.

Feldenkrais Method

The Feldenkrais method is a type of bodywork that uses movement, posture, and, in some cases, massage to improve physical functioning and psychological well-being. It is based on the view that poor posture and patterns of movement can be harmful to both body and mind. Therefore, improving posture and movement can help the body function with greater comfort and ease, which in turn can improve self-image and self-awareness and, therefore, overall health. The Feldenkrais method is used as a form of physical rehabilitation from injury or illness and as a way to enhance normal functions.

HISTORY

Moshe Feldenkrais, an Israeli physicist, mechanical engineer and judo expert, developed the Feldenkrais method in the 1940s, after he suffered a debilitating knee injury. His doctor recommended surgery, but Feldenkrais wanted to find a less invasive alternative. He studied the human nervous system and drew on his training in science and his expertise in the martial arts to devise a way to use gentle movement to help reduce his pain and increase his range of motion. He was eventually able to walk without pain.

Today, the Feldenkrais method is practised throughout the world to help relieve a wide range of health conditions, including muscle and joint pain, low back pain, anxiety and dystonia (a postural disorder characterized by spasms in the muscles of the shoulders, neck and trunk). Athletes, actors, musicians and dancers have credited the Feldenkrais method with helping them improve their performance.

PRACTICE

The Feldenkrais method is based on principles of physics and biomechanics. Practitioners guide their students through gentle movements and direct their attention to problems in how they move, with the goal of enhancing physical functioning by improving ease and range of motion, flexibility and coordination. Students eventually become more aware of their habitual neuromuscular patterns and learn new, more relaxed and efficient ways of moving. Everyday movements become more graceful and efficient.

TREATMENTS

The Feldenkrais method uses group lessons and individual therapy, either alone or in

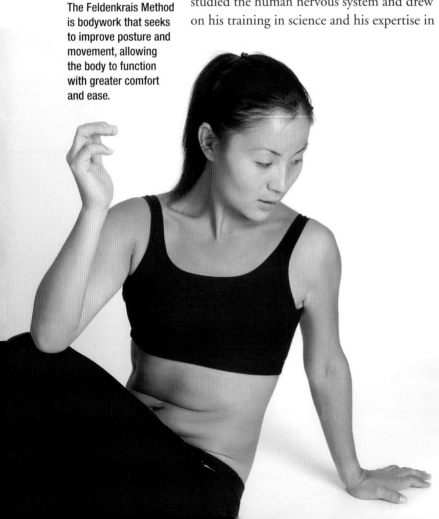

The Feldenkrais Method is bodywork that seeks to improve posture and movement, allowing the body to function with greater comfort and ease.

CAN FELDENKRAIS METHOD HELP ME?

The Feldenkrais method is used for many purposes in complementary and alternative medicine, ranging from pain relief and stroke rehabilitation to eating disorders and supportive care for cerebral palsy. But while scientific studies suggest that it is promising for some conditions, its effectiveness is, as yet, unproven.

- **Physical rehabilitation** The Feldenkrais method is useful when integrated into an overall rehabilitation programme following orthopoedic injury or surgery.
- **Musculoskeletal disorders** Feldenkrais and other forms of movement therapy are claimed to improve quality of life in people with various musculoskeletal disorders.
- **Dystonia** Feldenkrais may be an effective therapy for dystonia, a neurological movement disorder characterized by involuntary muscle contractions.
- **Muscle pain** Feldenkrais helps relieve pain in the lower back, neck and shoulders.
- **Balance problems** The Feldenkrais method can improve stability in people who have trouble walking.
- **Anxiety and mood** Awareness Through Movement sessions may reduce anxiety and improve mood.
- **Multiple sclerosis** Awareness Through Movement and Functional Integration may help people with multiple sclerosis move with greater steadiness and comfort, as

well as improve self-esteem and relieve anxiety and depression.
- **Eating disorders** Awareness Through Movement sessions may boost self-confidence in patients with eating disorders.

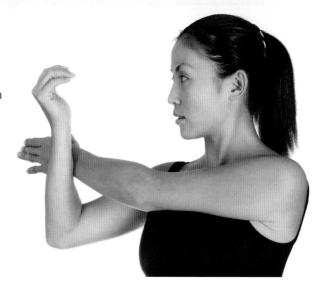

Awareness Through Movement is a series of lessons that aims to help people identify patterns of movement that are natural and comfortable.

combination. Both components are based on the philosophy that leading the body through fundamental patterns of movement can help it learn to move in ways that benefit health and conditioning, resulting in improvements in the way everyday activities are performed and in alleviating medical conditions.

• MOVEMENT AND EXERCISE Awareness Through Movement is a series of group lessons in

which Feldenkrais practitioners verbally guide a class in a slow-motion sequence of everyday movements, such as sitting or lying on the floor, standing, sitting in a chair and reaching. The purpose is to help people become more aware of how they move, identify patterns of movement that are uncomfortable, and replace them with patterns that feel better and can improve coordination and flexibility.

Private Feldenkrais lessons, which are called Functional Integration, are tailored to each student's individual needs. The practitioner guides the student's movements by gently touching them. The movements are done in sequences called manipulons. The goal is to identify patterns of movement that are natural and comfortable.

CAUTION

Tell a Feldenkrais practitioner ahead of time if you have any particular health conditions. People with muscle or bone injuries or chronic conditions such as heart disease should ask their healthcare provider before practising the Feldenkrais method.

Myotherapy

This is a specialized form of massage that applies pressure to specific muscle trigger points, which are easily irritated, tender spots that form when the muscle is traumatized. Any form of physical or emotional stress – even years later – can activate a trigger point and prompt the muscle to go into spasm, resulting in pain, soreness and stiffness. Muscle spasm itself can cause trigger points, and deep pressure massage deactivates them, enabling the muscle to relax. Stretching exercises can then be used to re-educate the muscle to maintain its optimal relaxed resting condition.

HISTORY

Myotherapy was developed by American fitness expert Bonnie Prudden in 1976, after she observed trigger point injection therapy, a technique that uses injections of saline and procaine, an anaesthetic, to ease muscle pain and spasm. Prudden found that firm pressure on a trigger point could be enough to prompt relaxation. She combined this with exercises to encourage mobility and therapeutic exercise. In 1979, Prudden opened what is still the major global training programme in myotherapy, in Arizona.

Myotherapy focuses on muscle trigger points to alleviate pain and stiffness. Once identified, practitioners apply deep pressure to them.

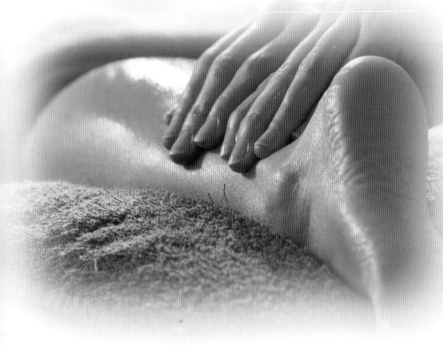

PRACTICE

Prudden claims that trigger-point pressure, plus exercise to correct muscle trauma, can alleviate 95 percent of muscular pain. Additional benefits include improved circulation, strength, stamina, flexibility and coordination, as well as enhanced energy, sleep and sports performance.

A first consultation with a myotherapist usually takes around 90 minutes, and patients are encouraged to bring a relative or friend with them because they can later help with stretching exercises. The therapist takes a detailed history, then searches for trigger points to treat. Patients wear loose clothing – only shoes need be removed.

TREATMENTS

In each treatment session, the myotherapist applies deep pressure to each painful trigger point for about five seconds, using the fingers, knees or elbows. This may be painful for a short while but it is temporary. The therapist then gently stretches the affected muscles and demonstrates appropriate exercises to do at home to maintain the benefit.

Some people are helped by simply undertaking one treatment; most require fewer than ten. Practitioners of myotherapy usually teach patients and their companions how to use the technique themselves.

CAN MYOTHERAPY HELP ME?

Myotherapy can treat a wide range of muscular problems and is used by athletes, musicians, performing artists and people in occupations such as computer work, where they are prone to repetitive movement disorders. However, despite impressive results from case studies, formal scientific evidence is lacking.

- **Muscle injuries** Among more than 1,000 workers with muscle injuries treated with myotherapy at a General Motors assembly plant in the United States over five years, 90 percent gained relief from their symptoms with only one treatment, which means less lost work time and lower medical costs.

- **Headaches** Myotherapy is used to treat all types of headaches, including migraines.

- **Fibromyalgia** This condition is regarded by practitioners as a classic example where multiple trigger points are activated.

- **Musculoskeletal disorders** Myotherapy has been used variously by practitioners to treat arthritis, carpal tunnel syndrome, tennis elbow, temporomandibular joint pain, repetitive strain injury, sciatica and whiplash, as well as shoulder, neck and back pain.

- **Dental problems** Myotherapy may help children and adults with muscle trauma or spasms that remain with them after bite misalignments (malocclusion) and other dental problems have been corrected.

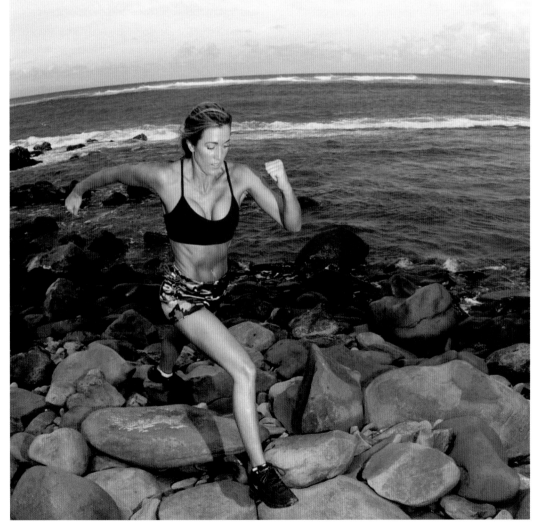

Myotherapy may improve performance in sports by aiding the participant's strength, stamina, flexibility and coordination.

Naprapathy

This is a system of manipulation aimed at mobilizing the joints and the connective tissues that hold the skeleton in place (the muscles, tendons and ligaments). Practitioners believe structural imbalances stemming from injuries, poor posture, ageing, or general wear and tear cause these tissues to lose their normal flexibility and elasticity. This impedes the flow of blood and lymph through the body, slowing nerve conduction, and leading to pain and malfunction. Because the spine is a prime site for such changes, this can cause not only back and neck pain, but also problems elsewhere if there is interference with nerves that exit from the spine.

HISTORY

The word naprapathy comes from the Czech word *napravit*, which means 'to correct', and the Greek word *pathos*, which means 'suffering'. The practice was developed in the early 20th century in the United States by Oakley Smith, one of the first chiropractors. Dissatisfied with the results of chiropractic (pp.466–7) in treating his own back pain, he focused instead on the soft tissues that surround the spine. Instead of manipulating bone, as in chiropractic, the treatment he devised uses manual techniques to heal damaged connective tissues.

PRACTICE

During a consultation, a naprapath takes a detailed medical history and performs an extensive examination to identify any sites of pain and connective tissue stiffening, particularly around the spine. Therapy involves both active and passive movements to stretch affected connective tissues. (Passive stretching means the therapist stretches the patient's muscles by manipulating the limbs.)

The major form of naprapathy in the United States is the Oakley Smith Naprapathic Method. Practitioners undertake a four-year training programme at the Chicago National School of Naprapathy to gain a Doctor of Naprapathy (DN) degree. Naprapaths in Illinois and New Mexico are granted a limited medical licence similar to those granted to dentists, optometrists and podiatrists.

Naprapathy has been used to treat carpal tunnel syndrome as well as tennis elbow, TMJ, fibromyalgia and arthritis.

CAN NAPRAPATHY HELP ME?

There is no formal evidence for the effectiveness of naprapathy, although practitioners claim impressive results in a range of conditions.

When dealing with back, shoulder and neck pain, naprapathy practitioners work with the theory that these symptoms stem from damage to the powerful ligaments supporting the spine. They also aim to relieve the symptoms of whiplash and sciatica by manipulation.

- **Headache** Release of connective tissue tension may alleviate chronic headaches, including migraines.
- **Musculoskeletal disorders** Naprapathy has been used to treat carpal tunnel syndrome, tennis elbow, temporomandibular joint (TMJ) syndrome, fibromyalgia and arthritis.
- **Digestive disorders** Nerves from the spine pass into the abdominal organs, and naprapaths aim to release trapped nerves in order to resolve various abdominal complaints.

Naprapathy is also used extensively in Scandinavia. In Sweden, it is the fourth most frequently used holistic therapy, after massage, acupuncture and chiropractic. In Finland, it is one of the most popular treatments for back pain.

TREATMENTS

The aim of naprapathy is to loosen inelastic connections in the body, free pinched nerves, improve alignment and balance, promote healing and relieve pain. Manual manipulation is usually combined with nutritional and postural advice.

In addition to manipulation, many naprapaths also use ultrasound, electric muscle stimulation (TENS, p.443), and the application of cold or moist heat to aid pain relief. They may also prescribe exercises and orthopaedic devices, such as lumbar or sacral supports and orthotics, and offer advice about postural and nutritional deficiencies.

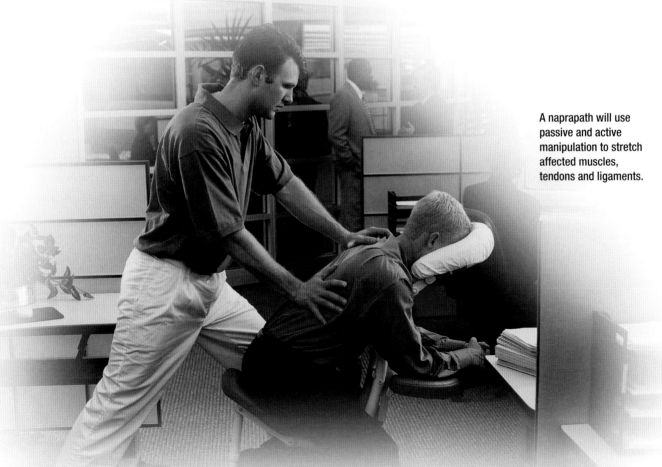

A naprapath will use passive and active manipulation to stretch affected muscles, tendons and ligaments.

Neurocranial Restructuring

Practitioners of nerocranial restructuring work toward achieving health benefits by manipulating the sphenoid, one of the bones of the skull that is located behind the eyes, between the face and the side of the head. The therapy aims to correct imbalances arising from various past traumas, including birth, falls, accidents, sporting injuries, medical procedures, and severe emotional and biochemical traumas. The sphenoid contains air spaces that are continuous with the nasal cavity, so structural reorganization of the bone is achieved progressively using an endonasal balloon – a small balloon inserted into the nostril and gradually inflated.

HISTORY

Neurocranial restructuring (NCR) was developed by American Dean Howell, a doctor of naturopathy (pp.443–5) working in Washington State, who used the technique to help himself and his patients overcome pain from injuries that were sustained in motor vehicle crashes, industrial accidents and sporting mishaps.

Its roots lie in another technique, called bilateral nasal specific therapy, developed in the 1930s, in which a latex finger "glove" was inflated inside the nostril with the purpose of realigning the nasal bones in order to treat conditions such as sinusitis.

PRACTICE

Neurocranial restructuring involves an initial series of four treatments on consecutive days. A practitioner assesses the areas that need to be manipulated and the patient is precisely positioned on the treatment table. A small endonasal balloon is inserted into the nostril, inflated for a few seconds, and then deflated and removed. The practitioner checks that this has achieved the intended movement of the sphenoid bone. Repeat

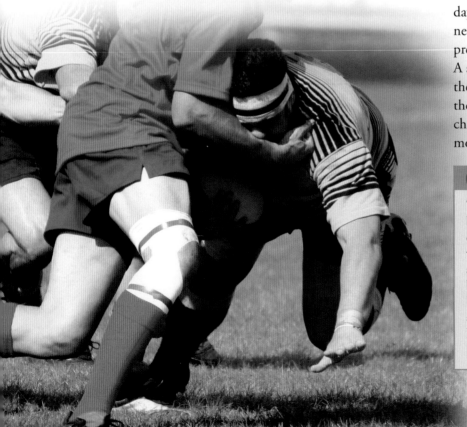

Neurocranial restructuring claims to correct problems that stem from various traumas including head and sports injuries, such as those that may occur in a rugby scrum.

CAUTION

The technique on which NCR is based, bilateral nasal specific therapy, has caused one death. In 1983, a baby was asphyxiated when the latex finger glove slipped from the syringe used to inflate it and lodged in the baby's windpipe. The practitioner responsible was convicted of manslaughter. In 2003, a case of fracture of the nose resulting from NCR was reported in the journal *Archives of Otolaryngol Head and Neck Surgery*.

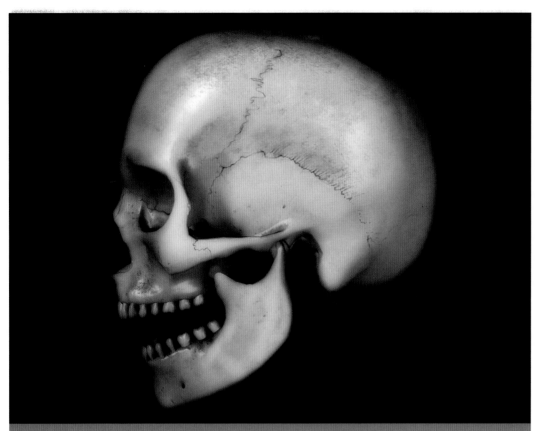

Practitioners of neuro-cranial restructuring believe that manipulation of the sphenoid bone (coloured red) helps correct imbalances caused by past traumas, such as birth, accidents, sporting injuries and medical procedures.

CAN NEUROCRANIAL RESTRUCTURING HELP ME?

NCR is claimed to be able to treat an astonishing range of medical conditions and to have remarkable cosmetic benefits. However, it is difficult to present a scientific rationale for moving the sphenoid bone, and there is no evidence to support any of these claims.

- **Mental and emotional problems** NCR claims to help attention-deficit disorder, hyperactivity, dyslexia, autism, depression, anxiety, aggression, phobias, psychosis and schizophrenia.

- **Musculoskeletal problems** Scoliosis, whiplash, fibromyalgia, sciatica, bursitis, arthritis and rheumatism may benefit.

- **Head problems** Headache, sinus problems, ear infections, balance problems, tinnitus, deviated nasal septum, temporomandibular joint (TMJ) syndrome, dental problems

and glaucoma may lessen or disappear.

- **Neurological conditions** NCR claims to help Alzheimer's disease, amyotrophic lateral sclerosis, multiple sclerosis, cerebral palsy, concussion, Lou Gehrig's disease, Parkinson's disease, concussion, seizures and strokes.

- **Miscellaneous conditions** Lymphoma, osteoporosis, polio, migraine, relationship difficulties, Down's syndrome, deafness and muscle spasms are also claimed to benefit from NCR.

treatment series may be suggested at one- to six-month intervals.

Howell originated his own training and certification programme in neurocranial restructuring. In 2005, there were 18 certified NCR practitioners worldwide, most of them in the United States.

TREATMENTS

NCR involves controlled release of stored connective tissue tensions that may accumulate from physical or emotional trauma. By manipulating the sphenoid bone, practitioners say they enable the body to return to its original design.

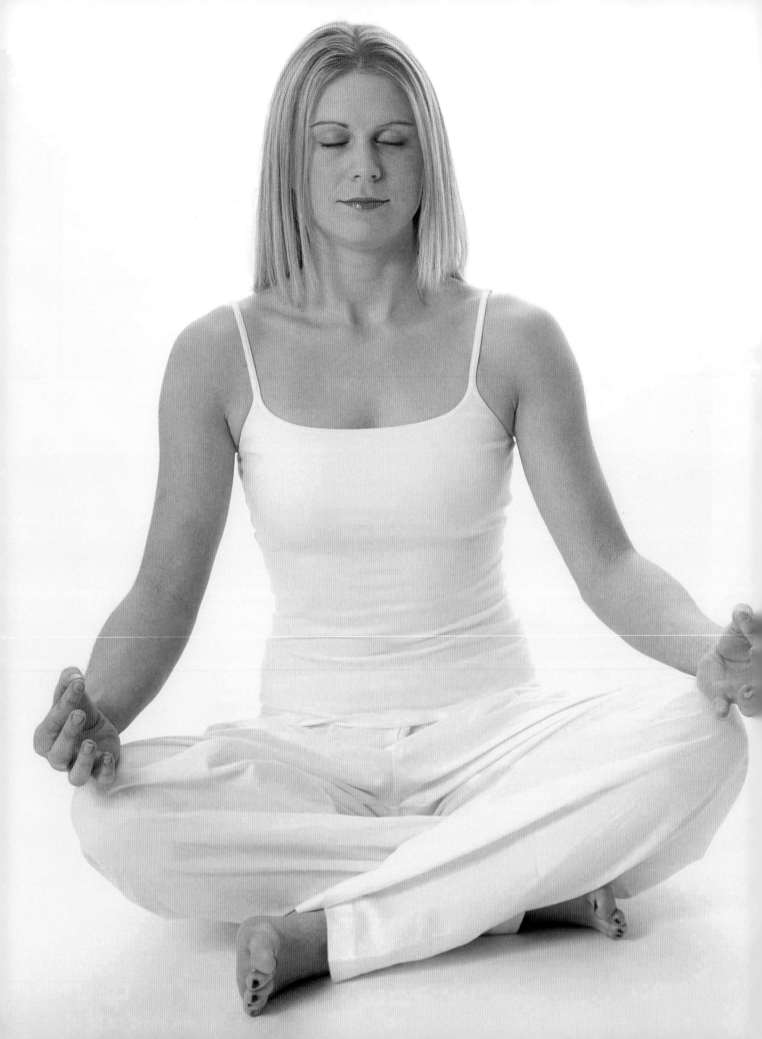

18 | THE MIND

Therapies that tap into the mind–body connection to promote health or healing demonstrate the powers of the human psyche and its ability to influence bodily functions – even those that are thought to be below the level of conscious awareness. These powers – whether deliberately harnessed or accessed incidentally – have the potential to affect virtually any body system, with outcomes that include reducing blood pressure, easing conditions such as heart disease and symptoms such as joint pain, and altering brain wave patterns and hormone release. The effects may even be responsible for the occasional anecdotal reports of spontaneous healing in people with serious diseases.

Although science cannot always explain such effects, evidence from clinical studies continues to mount, demonstrating the links between the mind and physical function. Psycho-neuroimmunology – the scientific study of the interactions of the emotions, the brain, and the immune system – is just one new area of study. It is revealing not only the links between mind, hormones, immunity and other physical functions, but also that physical phenomena affect emotions.

Biofeedback

We are usually not aware of most of the physiological processes that take place in the body, such as blood circulation and heartbeat, and generally have no control over them. However, we may be able to consciously control them through biofeedback, a technique that provides direct information about these physical functions. Being able to intentionally regulate these functions offers many possibilities for relief of symptoms of various conditions, stress reduction and performance enhancement.

In biofeedback, electronic instruments measure involuntary physiological activities. By monitoring this information, people can learn to alter their physiological responses to stress and other conditions.

To help people learn to achieve this control, sensitive electronic instruments are used to measure physiological activities such as pulse rate, skin temperature, muscle tension and brain wave activity. The machine provides a signal, either on a display or via sound, as changes occur. The instruments usually take measurements (often processed through a computer) from the surface of the skin.

Under the guidance of a therapist, people pay attention to these signals and gradually learn to alter their responses. This decreases stress responses and increases relaxation responses, improves autonomic nervous system balance, and controls automatic functions such as blood pressure. Biofeedback is an increasingly popular way of dealing with a variety of health problems without drugs.

HISTORY

Biofeedback was developed in the 1960s as a result of interactions among researchers in medicine, psychology, neurophysiology and cybernetics. Developments contributing to the emergence of the therapy include physiologist Edmund Jacobsen's work on progressive muscle relaxation

(pp. 474–5) and psychiatrist and neurologist Johannes Schultz's autogenic training in the 1930s. Research into feedback and brain wave patterns in the 1950s by Joe Kamiya, a University of Chicago psychologist, was also important, as was the work of American psychologist B. F. Skinner and others in the 1960s on operant conditioning (the process of reinforcing desired responses to increase the likelihood of their being chosen in the future) and behaviour modification. Other influences include studies of relaxation, imagery and awareness by psychologist Les Fehmi at the State University of New York at Stony Brook in the 1960s and 1970s and, around the same time, animal and later human experiments by psychologist Neal Miller and colleagues at Rockefeller University in New York into how operant conditioning can be used to affect internal physiology.

Research conducted between 1950 and the 1980s by Canadian biofeedback pioneer John Basmajian showed that electrodes placed over muscles could enable people to consciously control individual components of muscle activity that are normally beneath awareness. When someone decides on a particular movement, it is carried out by an interplay of many hundreds of bundles of muscle fibres, each bundle known as a 'motor unit'. Basmajian showed that individuals could learn to control the activity of individual motor units even

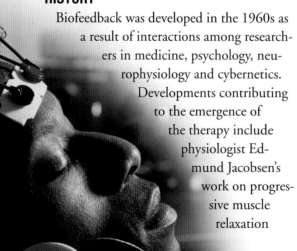

though they were not normally aware of them as separate entities) – a technique that eventually played an important role in physical therapy and rehabilitation, and gave credibility to biofeedback principles.

Beginning in the 1960s, physicist and biopsychologist Elmer Green and his wife, psychologist Alyce Green, and their colleagues at the Menninger Clinic in Topeka, Kansas, USA, investigated states of consciousness and brain wave patterns, especially the alpha brain waves that are associated with relaxation, and used biofeedback techniques to study individuals with exceptional abilities of mind–body control, such as Swami Rama, an Indian yogi.

Since then, overwhelming evidence has shown that people can learn to self-regulate physiological functions and control internal processes using feedback about their bodily states. In 1969, the Biofeedback Research Society (later the Association for Applied

Psychophysiology and Biofeedback) was founded in California, and by the mid-1970s biofeedback protocols had been deemed effective treatments for disorders including high blood pressure (pp.236–9) and bedwetting.

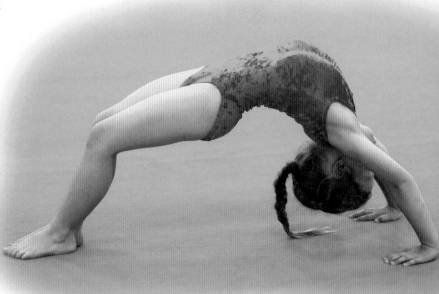

Biofeedback can enhance physical ability and concentration, and is employed by many professional and amateur athletes.

Clinical Query

Is it true that peak performance training can help make my workouts more effective?

As well as its use in healthcare, biofeedback has been used to enhance physical or mental abilities, such as improving attention and concentration, and enhancing gymnastic and other types of athletic performance. This is known as 'peak performance training'.

For example, galvanic skin response (GSR) biofeedback training has been used by the United States Rhythmic Gymnastics team. The gymnasts typically use the equipment in conjunction with guided imagery (pp.520–2) while mentally rehearsing their routine. Biofeedback enables them to identify anxiety-provoking cues that could impair performance. It is also used to enhance concentration and impart confidence

and a sense of self-control. Such techniques have widespread applications and may be useful for all kinds of athletes and performers, from figure skaters to sharp-shooters.

A study conducted at Imperial College, London, and published in 2003 in *Neuroreport* reported that, when music students were given brain feedback training in attention and relaxation, their musical performance under stressful conditions improved.

In another small study, also conducted at Imperial College, London and published in 2005 in *Applied Psychophysiological Biofeedback*, it was demonstrated that both brain feedback and heart rate variability (HRV) biofeedback training produced significantly enhanced performance among ballroom and Latin dancers, whereas no improvements were seen among dancers in a control group. (For more information on HRV, see Heart Coherence on pp.528–9).

CAN BIOFEEDBACK HELP ME?

Impressive evidence supports the effectiveness of many biofeedback applications to treat different conditions, including the following.

- **Pain** Biofeedback is often used to help headaches, including migraines and childhood headaches, as well as back pain and temporomandibular joint (TMJ) syndrome (pp.84–5). It may help phantom limb pain. As well as techniques aimed at controlling blood flow and muscle activity, researchers from Stanford University in California reported in 2005 that people watching their own brain activity while inside a magnetic resonance imaging (MRI) scanner could learn to alter their brain responses to pain. Subjects were shown real-time MRI scans of a brain area thought to be responsible for processing pain, and taught mental exercises to affect the activation of this area. They were able to deliberately affect their responses to a pain stimulus. Patients suffering from various types of chronic pain who learned the techniques reported

reductions in their levels of ongoing pain after the training.

- **Incontinence** The United States Agency for Health Care Policy and Research practice guidelines for adult urinary incontinence (1992) recommend biofeedback accompanied by Kegel exercises as a first-line treatment to help women gain awareness and control of their pelvic muscles. Biofeedback has also been used, sometimes with exercises and electrical stimulation, to train people with faecal incontinence to control the anal sphincter, although insufficient evidence exists to assess its usefulness.

- **Bedwetting** This effective alarm is a basic biofeedback device that helps children learn to self-monitor and self-regulate nighttime urine output.

- **High blood pressures** According to an analysis of 22 studies of 905 patients

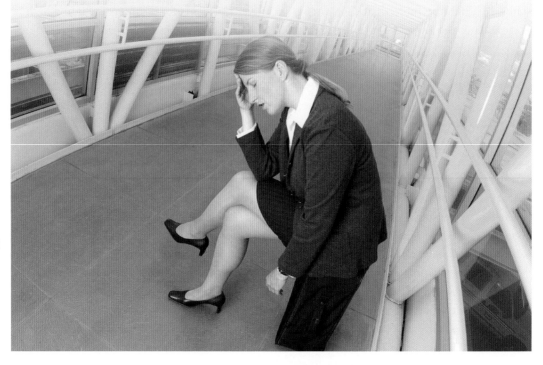

Headaches, including migraines and childhood headaches, are just two conditions that can be effectively treated with biofeedback. People using the technique can also learn to reduce their response to stress.

No regulations currently govern training or practice for biofeedback therapists. In the United States, many biofeedback professional hold a certificate from the Biofeedback Certification Institute of America (BCIA).

PRACTICE

People may seek biofeedback themselves or be referred by a doctor. At a first consultation, the practitioner usually discusses the patient's medical history, explains what physiological

published in *Hypertension Research* in 2003, biofeedback combined with relaxation techniques produces significant reductions in blood pressure (pp.236–9) in patients with hypertension.

- **Raynaud's disease** Biofeedback training aimed at warming the hands may help Raynaud's disease (p.243), a condition in which blood vessel constriction in response to low temperatures causes the extremities to become cold and painful. However according to a 2001 study from the Medical University of South Carolina, USA, only about one in three patients successfully learned to produce the desired response.

- **Tinnitus** This disorder (pp.72–3), characterized by an intensely annoying ringing in the ears, is notoriously difficult to treat. According to a 2005 study at the Institute for Psychosomatic Medicine in Munich, Germany, patients undergoing short-term EEG biofeedback training were able to alter brain-wave patterns and experienced a

significant reduction in the annoyance of tinnitus by the end of the training.

- **Stress** People using biofeedback can learn to reduce stress responses, including those occurring in anxiety and panic disorders (pp.354–5).

- **Epilepsy** A small randomized, controlled trial at the Institute of Neurology in London, published in 2004 in *Epilepsy & Behaviour,* showed that GSR biofeedback training significantly reduced the frequency of seizures in ten patients with drug-resistant epilepsy (pp.176–7).

- **Attention Deficit Hyperactivity Disorder (ADHD)** Brain feedback may be an effective non-pharmacological treatment for children with ADHD, according to a study at Eberhard-Karls-University in Tübingen, Germany, reported in 2003 in *Applied Psychophysiological Biofeedback.* A three-month EEG feedback programme produced improvements in tests of attention and in behaviour as rated by both parents and teachers.

changes are desirable, and sets up biofeedback equipment to measure relevant function. This may involve sensors attached over specific muscles, the scalp, the fingertips or toes. The equipment allows patients to see their various responses. With time and motivation, they can learn to consciously control them. The therapist will usually suggest specific exercises to practise at home between sessions.

TREATMENTS
Several types of measurements are used in biofeedback. Galvanic skin response (GSR), also known as skin conductance or electrodermal activity, measures electrical changes on the surface of the skin during activity of the sympathetic nervous system, which controls the 'fight or flight' response. It is often used to assess stress responses as an adjunct to psychotherapy or behaviour therapy.

Surface electromyography (EMG) measures the electrical activity in muscle fibre; it may be used to train muscle functions or to alleviate muscular pain and headaches.

Thermal feedback measures skin temperature, usually at a fingertip, giving an assessment of blood flow. It may be used to promote relaxation or to alleviate conditions such as Raynaud's disease (p.243), hypertension (pp.236–9) and migraines (pp.166–7).

Brain biofeedback, also known as neurofeedback or 'brain training', uses electroencephalograph (EEG) recordings of brain-wave activity. It has become popular to treat depression (pp.364–5), anxiety, attention-deficit hyperactivity disorder (pp.362–3), migraines and seizures (pp.176–7).

Other tests used in biofeedback can include pneumograph recordings of respiratory rate and pattern; photo-plethysmograph measurements of heart rate and blood pulse volume; and perineometer measurements of vaginal muscle contraction, used in combating urine leakage and with exercises to enhance vaginal muscle tone, known as Kegel exercises because they were devised by the inventor of the perineometer, California gynecologist Arnold Kegel (p.507).

Hypnotherapy

A hypnotized person enters a state of altered consciousness, known as a trance. They may enter this state because of suggestions made by another person or by self-hypnosis. When a person willingly enters this state for therapeutic purposes, it is called hypnotherapy.

Trance is a specific altered state of consciousness. Its major characteristics are absorption (the ability to selectively focus attention on a single theme or focal-point), intentional alteration of attention, dissociation (the ability to maintain the trance experience separate from conscious awareness) and suggestibility (an increased capacity to respond to suggestions and instructions). A person under hypnosis experiences changed sensations, perceptions, thoughts or behaviour, that may affect subsequent physical or psychological function, or social experience.

Hypnotherapy is often used to alter counterproductive behaviour or habits, to treat emotional and psychological problems, to aid in the relief of pain, or to alleviate symptoms of various medical conditions, such as hay fever and eczema.

Hypnosis has been shown to lower heart rate and blood pressure and affect skin temperature, intestinal secretions and immune responses. Brain wave changes occur similar to those seen in other forms of deep relaxation. Hypnosis is also believed to affect the brain's emotional centres and pathways that control hormone release.

HISTORY

The word hypnosis comes from the Greek *hypnos,* meaning 'sleep'. Trance-like states were used in most early human cultures, including those in ancient Egypt, Greece, India, China, Africa, North America, and northern Europe. They were written about in China in 2600 B.C.E., described in Greek mythology, and are mentioned in the Bible, the Talmud, and the Hindu Vegas. Shamans have used trance states for healing in native cultures for thousands of years.

In the 18th century, hypnotherapy was popularized throughout Europe by Austrian physician Franz Mesmer, who proposed that illness was due to imbalances of magnetic body fluids. He said that these imbalances could be corrected by transferring 'animal

Clinical Query

Can people be hypnotized to do something against their will?

The altered consciousness achieved during hypnosis is not unique. Similar altered states may occur during guided imagery, meditation and even daydreaming. Most hypnotherapists say that people cannot be induced under hypnosis to do anything that their personal moral code would normally forbid. Hypnotized people remain under their own control; indeed, it is sometimes argued that all hypnosis is really self-hypnosis and hypnotherapists merely facilitate the process.

However, occasional adverse outcomes have been reported, including exacerbation of disturbing memories in people with post-traumatic stress disorder, or worsening of psychotic symptoms. Some people believe that there is a risk of false memories arising in some types of hypnotic regression. It is therefore sensible to consult only a properly trained and accredited hypnotherapist.

magnetism' from another person. The medical establishment was hostile to the concept of 'mesmerism', as it came to be known.

It was revived in the 19th century by several British physicians, including Scottish surgeon James Esdaile, working in Calcutta, India. He performed more than 2,000 operations over seven years, including major surgery such as amputations, using only hypnotherapy for anaesthesia. After the discovery of chloroform, hypnotherapy for major surgery was largely abandoned – although it was later noted that it also reduced the risk of surgical shock. Another Scottish surgeon, James Braid, studied the phenomenon scientifically and coined the term hypnotism.

In the late 19th century, prominent French neurologist Jean Charcot speculated that hypnosis was a form of hysteria. Later, his pupil Sigmund Freud based his theories of psychoanalysis on his observations of patients under hypnosis.

Frenchman Charles Poyen introduced mesmerism to the United States. This led to advances in psychology and influenced

psychologist William James' work on mystical experiences. Psychiatrist Milton Erickson studied medical applications of hypnosis, and became the best-known American hypnotherapist of the 20th century.

By the mid-20th century, hypnotherapy was accepted as a medical procedure by the American Medical Association, British Medical Association and American Psychological Association. In 1995, it was endorsed by the National Institutes of Health in the United States to alleviate chronic pain.

Some physicians, dentists and accredited psychologists use hypnotherapy, although there is no standard licensing system, and considerable variation in training and certification exists. The American Society for Clinical Hypnosis (ASCH) and the Society for Clinical and Experimental Hypnosis are academically recognized certifying bodies.

PRACTICE

A session typically begins in the pre-suggestion phase, with deep relaxation, often using guided imagery (pp.520–2) or concentrated

One technique in hypnotherapy is time and body disassociation, in which a person imagines being in a pleasant and peaceful place. This disassociation can be useful in the management of pain.

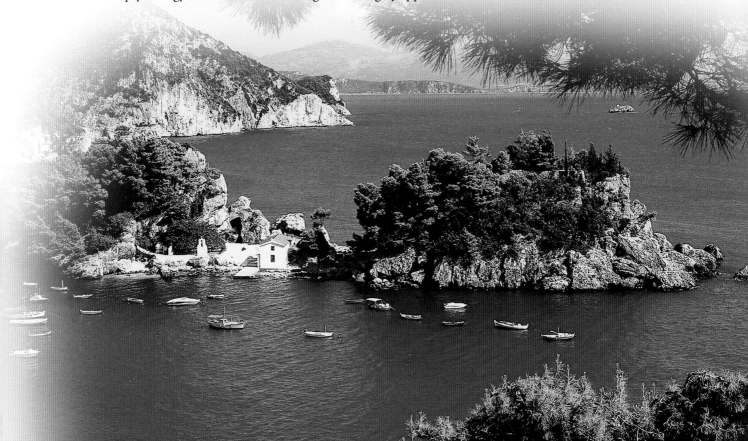

CAN HYPNOTHERAPY HELP ME?

Hypnotherapy has been used to treat many different conditions, often with solid evidence of its effectiveness.

- **Childbirth** Hypnosis may ease childbirth and promote satisfaction with pain management in labour, according to a 2005 *Cochrane Review* of three trials that included 189 women.

- **Eczema** A trial at Oxford University in England found that autogenic training was more effective than standard medical care or an intensive skin education programme in improving symptoms and reducing the use of steroid skin creams.

- **Hay fever** Patients who are taught to use self-hypnosis experience significant improvements in hay fever symptoms, according to a study at University Hospital Basel, Switzerland, published in 2005 in *Psychotherapy and Psychosomatics.*

- **Headache** Autogenic training, followed by regular practice for four months, resulted in a significant reduction in headache frequency among 25 women sufferers with migraines, tension headaches or mixed headaches, according to a study published in *Headache* in 2003. This was accompanied by reduced use of migraine drugs, analgesics and medication for anxiety.

- **Infertility** Some forms of infertility are associated with psychological stress, and autogenic training has been claimed to yield improved hormone levels and, possibly, increased conception rates.

- **Irritable bowel syndrome** Hypnotherapy consistently produces significant improvements in irritable bowel symptoms in the majority of patients, according to a 2005 review from Baylor College of Medicine in Houston, Texas.

- **Multiple sclerosis** A pilot programme of autogenic training for people with multiple sclerosis reported in *Behavioural Medicine* in 2005 that after 10 weekly sessions, patients reported they had more energy and vigour than the control group, and found physical and emotional problems less limiting.

- **Smoking cessation** Though useful to some individuals, conflicting results among published trials means there is insufficient evidence to show whether hypnotherapy is truly effective in attempts to quit smoking, according to a 2005 *Cochrane Review.*

- **Surgery** Hypnotherapy may alleviate anxiety, provide anaesthesia and pain relief, and speed recovery in a variety of procedures, especially removal of skin lesions and cosmetic procedures. A study at the University of Rennes, France, published in 2005 in *Paediatric Anaesthesia,* demonstrated that hypnosis was superior to standard drugs for pre-medication in children.

- **Weight control** A *Cochrane Review* published in 2005 concluded that hypnotherapy may improve weight loss, although evidence is insufficient. Any benefit is likely to be small, according to a 2005 comparative review done at the universities of Exeter and Plymouth in England.

focus on an object to still the conscious mind and allow access to the unconscious. During the suggestion phase, the hypnotherapist may ask questions or present statements to alter perceptions, suggest goals or explore memories. Finally, the person is returned to the post-suggestion phase, or normal consciousness, when physical, mental, emotional or behavioural changes may occur.

Some people achieve lasting change after a single session of therapy, while others need regular sessions to maintain the benefit.

Some hypnotherapists teach patients to use self-hypnosis, and some people learn through learning materials such as books or video tapes, CDs or DVDs.

People vary in their susceptibility to hypnotic suggestion, and recent neuroimaging studies suggest that this may be because of differences in brain structure. Generally, people are more 'hypnotizable' if they believe in the process, and hypnotic induction is more successful when labelled as such, rather than when viewed as simple relaxation.

TREATMENTS

In addition to offering pain relief and an alternative to anaesthesia, hypnotherapy is helpful in overcoming fear and anxiety before surgery and in reducing post-operative pain and complications. It is often used in conjunction with other techniques, including meditation (pp.514–19), guided imagery (pp.520–2), neurolinguistic patterning (pp.524–5) and autogenic training (below).

Hypnotherapy is sometimes used along with cognitive behaviour therapy (therapy intended to revise counterproductive thought patterns and perceptions). It is also used to help victims or witnesses of crimes recall events, although this is controversial. Individuals may access memories under hypnosis that they are unable to recall consciously, but there is no guarantee that these memories are real. In fact, it is also true that therapists can implant memories in the minds of patients, even accidentally, by making suggestions; this phenomenon has been dubbed 'false memory syndrome'.

A treatment related to hypnotherapy is autogenic training. It was developed in the 1930s by German psychiatrist and neurologist Johannes Schultz as a technique for balancing the autonomic nervous system (or damping the sympathetic nervous system, which is responsible for 'fight or flight' reactions to perceived danger). Later, repetitive therapeutic suggestions were added to the technique.

The technique is said to lower stress and increase the capacity for self-healing. It includes auto-suggestion, which is similar to self-hypnosis, combined with visual and verbal cues, to achieve a state of deep relaxation. The person imagines being in a restful place and mentally focuses on different physical sensations, moving progressively from feet to forehead. These sensations may include heaviness and warmth in the limbs, control of the heartbeat and breathing, warmth in the upper abdomen and coolness in the forehead.

Providing autogenic training requires professional training, commitment and an ability to focus intensively. It may be particularly useful for people with medical problems such as hypertension.

Sudden, sharp increases or decreases in blood pressure have been reported in some people doing autogenic exercises. Anyone with blood pressure abnormalities or heart problems is advised to seek medical advice before undertaking autogenic training.

Hypnotherapy may alleviate anxiety, provide anaesthesia and pain relief, and speed recovery in a variety of procedures, including surgery and dental work.

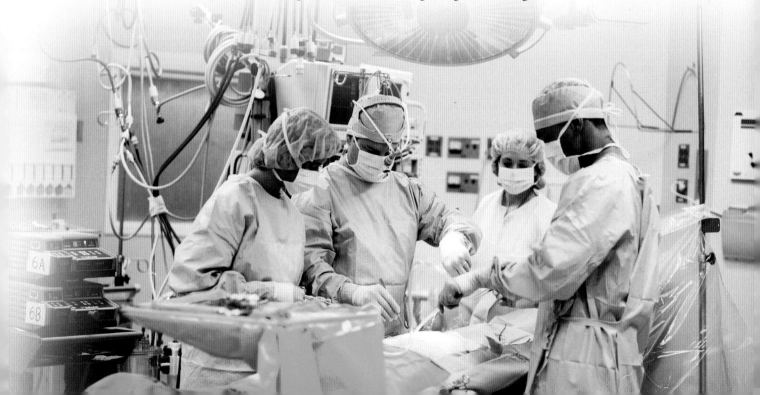

Sophrology

The goal of sophrology is to achieve harmony between body and mind through understanding and conscious awareness of the interplay between, and functions of, both. The practice involves controlled breathing, deep relaxation, concentration and visualization; attention to posture, balance and movement are also key. It may be used to reduce stress, alleviate symptoms of disease and enhance performance, or as prophylaxis against pain and anxiety from medical or surgical procedures and childbirth.

Sophrology can be helpful in facing fears, anxieties and living in the present moment.

The technique is based on the study of how physiological changes can modify consciousness. Sophrology also embraces a philosophy that includes health awareness, harmonious living and expanded consciousness.

The term sophrology derives from three Greek words: *sos,* meaning harmony, serenity, balance and freedom from disease; *phren,* meaning the diaphragm and emotional heart, and implying consciousness or spirit; and *logos,* science or study. Sophrology is thus the science of harmonious consciousness.

HISTORY

Sophrology was developed during the 1960s by Alfonso Caycedo, a Colombian neuro-psychiatrist working in Spain, who wanted to bridge Western and Oriental approaches. It combines Western techniques derived from therapeutic hypnosis (pp.508–13), progressive muscle relaxation (pp.474–5), autogenic training (p.511) and phenomenology (a philosophy that seeks to extract the essence of everyday phenomena from intuitive or conscious experience of them), with Eastern elements of Indian rajah yoga, Tibetan Buddhist meditation and Japanese Zen.

Sophrology is a popular relaxation method in France and is recognized as a medical therapy in several Western European countries. It is also used in Japan and South America, and has recently been introduced to the United States. Institutes offer practitioner training in France and Switzerland; the Foundation Alfonso Caycedo in Andorra, still run by Caycedo, trains master practitioners. A branch in Columbia focuses on social sophrology, which aims to enhance collective awareness to promote a better society.

PRACTICE

Although intended as a life skill, sophrology must first be learned from a practitioner. Many practitioners are physicians, other healthcare professionals or complementary therapists.

A sophrology session can be conducted individually or in groups and may last between 15 and 60 minutes. It usually takes about five sessions to master the basic technique, and those sessions are generally followed by further training to become proficient.

When working with individuals, the practitioner first discusses specific needs and goals so that the session can be tailored for them. When working with groups, the practitioner usually begins by explaining the techniques and the sensations participants may expect. They are encouraged to record their experiences for further practice at home.

There are four levels through which participants may progress; classes offered in health and sports clubs sometimes focus on the first level, deep bodily relaxation to release stress. In the second and third stages, participants learn to visualize and become aware of parts of the body, then to meditate, focus on specific goals, release negative emotions and live in the present moment. The fourth stage involves increasing spiritual awareness.

TREATMENTS
Stage One
• **DYNAMIC RELAXATION** This is the underlying state needed for all subsequent work, and involves physical relaxation accompanied by a state of consciousness enabling concentration. While standing or sitting in an upright posture, participants are guided by the practitioner into a state of complete bodily relaxation, releasing muscular tensions and breathing rhythmically from the abdomen.

• **BODY READING** Participants focus on one body area at a time, working from head to toe, to become aware of it separately and ensure total relaxation. Awareness is then expanded to embrace the whole body.

• **MEDITATION** Next, participants learn to meditate on an object that arouses no emotions to clear the mind of background thoughts and feelings. After stage one, participants have enhanced body awareness and a sense of well-being. This is useful to cope with stress, improve body image and release tension.

Stage Two
While in a state of deep relaxation, participants turn attend to internal organs and concentrate on achieving inner peace. The practitioner guides them to visualize a personal goal, such as developing a more positive attitude. Participants are encouraged to visualize activating their energies and capabilities in their chosen situation. This may be used to help overcome an addiction, become more

CAN SOPHROLOGY HELP ME?

There is little formal research on the effects of training in sophrology. It was first used as an adjunct to medical treatment, to enable patients to cope better with fear and anxiety, and reduce pain or nausea, for example after surgery. It has also been used to help alleviate symptoms in conditions such as skin disease, ulcers, asthma, depression, insomnia and addictions. When used for health purposes, it is intended to supplement but not replace conventional medical treatment. The techniques are also now used in stress management and personal development.

confident about a forthcoming trial such as an examination or interview, or improve sporting, dramatic or musical accomplishments.

Stage Three
In the next stage, still in the relaxed state and breathing with hands crossed over the lower abdomen, participants learn to deal with negative emotions. As well as visualization and meditation, they are guided to correct posture, balance and movement to remove negativity from the body. The aim is to face, accept and release feelings of tension, anxiety and insecurity, while learning to live in the present moment.

This can be useful to overcome physical or psychological pain and trauma from past or anticipated events in the future. It may help to treat phobias or prepare people for surgery or childbirth, easing anxiety and pain. It can also help athletes control apprehension, reduce injury, enhance motivation and have a positive attitude, even when they are losing.

Stage Four
The most advanced stage of sophrology aims for emotional and spiritual awareness through meditation on humanity, society and the universe, and attempts to experience emotion and sensation fully in the present moment.

Meditation

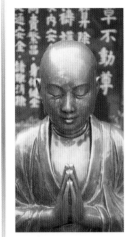

Meditative techniques are the product of diverse cultures and peoples around the world; many are rooted in the traditions of the world's great religions.

The ancient human activity of meditation involves the self-regulation of attention, an awareness that arises with attention, and subsequent insight and understanding of inner and outer experiences. There are thousands of ways to meditate, and it can be practised in any posture, whether a person is still or moving. The purposes of meditation are best defined by the context, and may differ significantly between religious or spiritual contexts and contemporary health settings. Experiences common to practically all meditation methods include physical relaxation and quieting of the mind.

HISTORY

Various forms of meditation have been used for millennia in different religious and cultural practices, but primarily in those of Asia. Meditation is a prominent part of practices as varied as yoga, the martial arts and Buddhism. Most techniques aim to help the practitioner achieve understanding, inner peace, and enlightenment, often with a spiritual component.

Meditation was a predominantly Eastern practice until the 1960s, when it became part of pop culture in the West, partly through the enthusiasm of The Beatles, the enormously popular group. In the West, it is more often used without any religious context, although contemplative prayer has been called a form of concentrative meditation.

In the 1960s and 1970s, scientists began to study what appeared to be the extraordinary abilities of some experienced meditators to control physical functions previously assumed to be outside awareness, such as heart rate, blood pressure and the production of stress hormones.

Meditation came to the attention of influential physicians such as Herbert O. Benson, professor of medicine at Harvard University. Benson called the physiological changes produced during meditation 'the relaxation response', and demonstrated that this

occurred regardless of technique or underlying religious belief. Similar responses occur in other practices that induce deep relaxation.

In 1979, a mindfulness-based stress reduction programme began at the University of Massachusetts Medical Center, and during the 1990s, programmes there and at Harvard University began to use meditation to accompany conventional medical treatments.

Benson has used magnetic resonance imaging (MRI) to study the brains of people meditating and found increased activity in sites associated with attention and control of the autonomic nervous system (which controls automatic functions such as digestion

CAUTION

One small study has suggested that meditation may increase the risk of seizure. Those findings have been disputed, however; anyone with a tendency to epilepsy or seizures should consult their doctor before starting a meditation programme. A sudden drop in blood pressure during meditation is very rare, but those with a tendency toward the problem should seek medical advice before starting meditation. Patients with borderline personality disorders or psychotic illnesses should carefully follow the guidance of a doctor before and during a meditation programme.

and blood pressure and is usually beneath conscious awareness). Other studies have found increases in blood flow in areas of the brain associated with cortical activity, and altered brain chemistry. Meditation has even been linked with changes in brain structure; recent evidence shows that certain cortical areas are thicker in those people who meditate regularly.

Meditation is becoming a well-accepted technique, as increasing evidence emerges of its benefits in healthcare and disease prevention. Regular meditation is associated with changes in brain wave patterns, as shown on an electroencephalogram (EEG), and particularly with increased alpha wave activity, associated with many forms of relaxation. It has been shown to produce a shift in brain activity away from regions associated with stress and fear responses to those that are active when a person is calm.

Meditation is now a popular form of relaxation and stress reduction, a path to personal development and an adjunct to medical treatment. No regulation or certification system exists for practitioners and teachers, although individual forms of meditation, such as transcendental meditation (TM) do have requirements for training and issuing credentials.

PRACTICE

Meditation is simple to learn, requires no special equipment or clothing, and can be done by anyone, whatever their level of fitness. Once learned, it can be used independently at home or in almost any setting: experienced meditators can learn to 'tune out' external distractions, and meditate even in noisy or crowded environments.

Practitioners say that regular meditation leads to enhanced concentration, alertness, mental efficiency and productivity. Other reported benefits include lowered blood pressure and heart and breathing rates; increased

skin resistance (a measure of lowered arousal) as a result of reduced activity of the sympathetic nervous system (which is responsible for reactions to stress and threat); reduced levels of stress hormones such as epinephrine and cortisol; and increased levels of melatonin, a hormone involved in regulating sleep–wake cycles. Lipid peroxidation in arteries – fatty changes linked with the development of atherosclerosis and cardiovascular risk – is reduced. Beneficial effects on the immune system suggest that meditation may help the body's own powers of disease resistance and healing.

Meditation is often now taught in health care and spiritual settings. It may be taught in individual or group sessions. It is also possible to learn through books and audiovisual material, or even over the Internet. Some techniques cost nothing to learn; others, such as TM, may be fairly expensive to study. Although TM claims superior results, research comparing meditation forms is in its infancy.

However, once learned, meditation has no costs, making it an accessible lifelong – and possibly life-prolonging – habit.

Some evidence has suggested the possibility of suffering harm from intense meditation practices. One small study published in the *International Journal of Psychosomatics* in 1992 reported 17 of 27 meditators experienced at least one adverse effect after attending a meditation retreat, although generally significantly more positive than negative effects were reported.

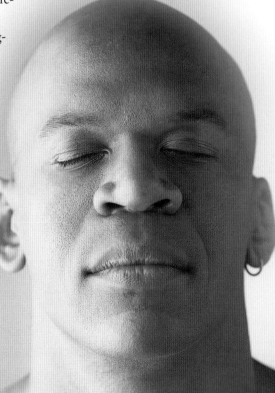

Most forms of meditation can be divided into one of two broad categories: those that focus attention on an object or idea, and those that allow all experiences to come into awareness.

CAN MEDITATION HELP ME?

Accumulating scientific evidence suggests that meditation may help improve numerous medical and psychological conditions.

- **Stress** Meditation is an important component of many stress reduction and relaxation programmes, and produces measurable physiological effects in a short time. Mindfulness-based stress reduction emphasizes developing awareness of patterns of stress reactivity and replacing them with healthier patterns of conscious response. Relaxation techniques support this awareness focus.

- **Anxiety** Psychiatrists at the University of Massachusetts Medical Center showed that mindfulness meditation used to promote stress reduction produced statisti-cally significant improvements in symptoms among 22 patients with an anxiety disorder. A follow-up study of 18 patients showed that most were still meditating three years later, with continued benefits. This suggests that long-term beneficial effects of meditation may be gained from relatively short-term intervention.

- **Depression** The meditation practice that is part of the ancient system of Kundalini yoga has been adapted to specific purposes, including the treatment of depression. It has also been found to help combat the mental fatigue and low energy associated with depression in cancer patients. However, further research is needed before definitive conclusions can be drawn. Mindfulness-based stress reduction approaches have also been reported to reduce depression and risk of depression in a variety of patients, including those with cancer, chronic pain and relapsing depression.

- **Fatigue** Regular meditation is said to boost alertness and energy levels and to relieve subjective fatigue.

- **Insomnia** Practitioners say meditation helps regulate sleep cycles and alleviates symptoms of insomnia, although this has not been shown empirically.

- **Addictions** Transcendental meditation (TM) is said to reduce the need for alcohol and tobacco. Mindfulness meditation may reduce the incidence of relapse in addiction treatment and recovery.

- **Aging** According to studies at the Maharishi International University in Fairfield, Iowa, the practice of TM among 73 residents of homes for the elderly improved learning, cognitive flexibility and mental health. Favourable changes in blood pressure, ratings of behavioral flexibility and ageing

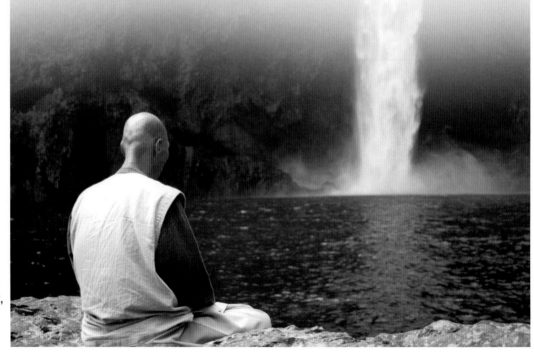

Vipassana, sometimes called mindfulness, is a type of meditation that encourages becoming deeply aware of the present moment, and fully experiencing what happens in the here and now.

effects were also observed. Participants' three-year survival rate was 100 percent, compared with 87.5 percent in a similar group of older people who underwent a mental training programme that did not include TM.

- **Gastrointestinal disorders** Stress reduction through meditation practice may improve symptoms of some gastrointestinal complaints, including constipation, diarrhoea, gastritis, stomach ulcers and chronic nausea, but more research is needed. A small study from the State University of New York, published in 2002 in *Psychosomatic Medicine,* reported that meditation aimed at engaging the relaxation response produced significant reductions in symptoms of abdominal pain, diarrhoea, flatulence, and bloating among ten patients with irritable bowel syndrome; benefits lasted for one year after the original intervention.

- **Psoriasis** A study in *Psychosomatic Medicine* in 1998 reported that patients with psoriasis who were given audiotape instruction on mindfulness meditation for stress reduction had faster clearance of skin lesions while undergoing ultraviolet light therapy, compared with patients who did not meditate.

- **Asthma** Early studies suggested TM's positive effect on asthma; additional research is required.

- **Hypertension** Meditation-related blood pressure reductions have been observed even among students with blood pressure in the normal range. The effects of TM on high blood pressure have been extensively studied, but a review published in the *Journal of Hypertension* in 2004 concluded that many trials used poor methodology and were potentially biased. Therefore, definitive conclusions about the cumulative effects of TM on hypertension cannot be drawn.

- **Stroke** TM is claimed to lower blood cholesterol levels and reduce build-up of fatty plaque, a major contributor to coronary disease, in arterial linings. A study published in *Stroke* in 2000 reported that carotid artery lining thickness, a secondary measure of coronary atherosclerosis, was reduced after TM practice for six to nine months among 60 hypertensive African-Americans, a group that suffers disproportionately high cardiovascular disease mortality.

- **Heart disease** According to a study of 21 patients with documented coronary artery disease at the State University of New York in Buffalo, an eight-month TM programme produced increases in exercise tolerance and maximal cardiac workload, and reductions in worrying electrocardiograph (ECG) changes on exercise. A small study from Texas Tech University published in *Family and Community Health* in 2003 found that mindfulness-based stress reduction may reduce anxiety in women with heart disease.

- **Heart failure** Researchers from São Paulo University Medical School in Brazil reported in the *Journal of Alternative and Complementary Medicine* in 2005 that twice-daily meditation for twelve weeks significantly improved quality of life in 19 elderly people, even though they were already receiving optimal pharmacological treatment for congestive heart failure.

- **Arthritis** Meditation is said to reduce inflammation and so help to relieve arthritis pain and associated symptoms, such as anxiety, stress and depression. Research is needed to document these assertions.

- **Fibromyalgia** A ten-week mindfulness meditation-based stress reduction programme improved well-being, pain, fatigue and sleep disturbances related to fibromyalgia, according to a study of 77 patients at Newton Wellesley Hospital, Massachusetts.

- **Chronic pain** According to a study done at Duke University and reported in the *Journal of Holistic Nursing* in 2005, a type of Buddhist meditation called loving-kindness meditation, which aims to transform anger into compassion, produced significant improvements in 43 patients with persistent low back pain after eight weeks. Meditation also reduced feelings of anger and psychological distress. Early evidence in the 1980s indicated that mindfulness-based stress reduction produced relief from chronic pain that lasted up to 48 months after training.

- **Menstrual symptoms** Relaxation techniques, including meditation and yoga, may help ease menstrual cramps.

- **Transplantation** Researchers at the University of Minnesota reported in Progress in Transplantation in 2005 that meditation significantly improved symptoms of anxiety, depression and insomnia that commonly plague recipients of organ transplants.

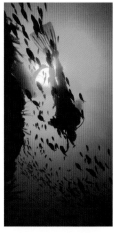

Transcendental meditation, or TM, views the mind like an ocean; the busy, active everyday level of thinking is on the surface; quieter feelings and wisdom lie in the depths. TM encourages diving into the ocean to experience the mind in its silent, wakeful state, where all creativity, intelligence and happiness lie.

Types of Meditation

There are many forms of meditation, most of which involve a focus on detaching the mind from everyday ruminations through the use of mental concentration, allowing non-judging awareness and physical relaxation.

Meditation practices can be divided into two broad categories: those that involve concentration and the steadying of attention, and those that involve allowing all experiences to come into awareness. In either case, the effect is to quiet the often negative 'running commentary' that goes on in people's minds much of the time. This quieting results in the achievement of calm, mental clarity and an awareness – and acceptance – of the present moment. Both external stimuli and intrusive thoughts and feelings are simply allowed to pass, or just to exist, without the person feeling concerned about them.

Most types of meditation also involve elements in addition to mental concentration. Some techniques, such as Vipassana and Zen, have a spiritual component. Meditation also plays an integral role in yoga (pp.476–9). And similar concentrated mental focus is involved in techniques including visualization and guided imagery (pp.520–2). In forms of yoga and meditation that involve focus on the breath, there may be a deliberate attempt to control patterns of inhalation and exhalation (see Breath Work, pp.526–7).

Following are some common contemporary examples of meditation practices used in or associated with healthcare settings.

Mindfulness

This state is an awareness that arises out of paying attention without judging what comes into focus. Mindfulness lies at the heart of the mainstream traditions of Buddhism, and has been introduced to Western health care largely through the techniques of mindfulness-based stress reduction (MBSR) and dialectical behaviour therapy (DBT). MBSR was developed as an approach to illness, involving stress reduction and management of negative emotions. DBT is a technique used to treat people who suffer from borderline personality disorder, who tend to react abnormally to emotional stimulation but lack the skills for coping

Clinical Query

How can I tell what type of meditation would be best for me?

It depends on your goals and your general outlook on life. All forms of meditation engage the relaxation response, which is known to have several benefits, including stress reduction and cardiovascular health.

You may feel more comfortable with the idea of focusing on a particular object, or on bodily rhythms such as breathing, or just allowing thoughts to flow past. Posture is important in certain types of meditation, such as Zen and yoga meditation, and for some people this may either appeal or be beyond their physical abilities. People who include their meditation as part of the yoga practice can expect tangible physical benefits as well, particularly in promoting and maintaining agility and flexibility.

Zen meditation may be most suitable for people seeking a spiritual dimension and self-awareness, as well as other benefits. TM also has a spiritual component, and its health benefits have been particularly well-researched, though many of the studies have been carried out by those in the field, so they may be biased. It is also relatively expensive to learn.

Mindfulness-based stress reduction (MBSR) was specifically developed for people who wish to take a more active role in their own health and healing process. The meditation and yoga practices taught require no particular faith or religious view, and are easily available to anyone willing to practise them.

with these sudden, intense surges of emotion. DBT aims to teach these skills.

Recent research has demonstrated the benefits of mindfulness meditation practices in treating specific health problems, including addiction, chronic pain, binge eating, depression, anxiety and skin disorders.

Vipassana

In the Theravada tradition of Buddhism, the term often used for mindfulness meditation is Vipassana. One way to practise Vipassana meditation is to focus attention on a physical sensation, such as breathing, and then allow awareness to expand to include other physical sensations, thoughts and emotions. Through increasingly sensitive, non-judging, allowing attention, the meditator dwells more clearly in the present moment. Buddhists believe such attention and present moment awareness reveal the true nature of reality. Healthcare providers have found that it can reveal unconscious habits of mind–body interaction and reactivity.

Transcendental Meditation

This technique, often abbreviated as TM, was brought to the West by Maharishi Mahesh Yogi in the late 1950s; it became popular among many pop culture icons, including The Beatles. TM is now a worldwide organization (and a registered trademark). The technique involves repetition of a single sound – called a mantra – either aloud or in one's head, with the goal of achieving a state of relaxed awareness and altered consciousness. The mantra is a meaningless word or phrase that is said to have a particular vibratory effect, and is specifically chosen by the teacher for each individual student. Any thoughts that arise are simply allowed to pass and attention is returned to the mantra.

It has been claimed that Transcendental Meditation can lead to a state of 'pure awareness'. Some adherents assert that advanced TM practitioners can alter the mental state and

emotions of other people, producing positive changes for society, and that TM can increase IQ and reduce propensities towards violence. Some practitioners are even said to perform a sort of levitation known as 'yogic flying'. Such claims have led to calls for TM to be classified as a religion or cult. However, TM's health benefits have been documented, and are similar to those of other types of meditation.

Zen Meditation

The most common form of meditation in Zen Buddhism is called zazen, from the Japanese words *za*, meaning 'sit', and *zen*, meaning 'absorption'. Strict instructions for posture, breath and attention are part of zazen, which aims to integrate body, breath and mind by assuming a seated pyramid structure (like the Buddha), combined with focusing on deep, abdominal breathing and counting breaths. If the attention wanders, the count is started again. Ultimately, this intense concentration is said to lead to samadhi—single-pointedness of mind.

In its purest form, zazen is not directed at any particular object and has no content. The practitioner dwells in a state of thought-free, alertly wakeful attention. Zen meditation offers zazen as the shortest, but perhaps most challenging path to the understanding of the self.

One variation of Zen meditation is kinhin meditation, also known as walking meditation. In this practice, which is sometimes used during long periods of zazen, participants walk clockwise around a room, attending to the feeling of the earth beneath one's feet.

Zazen is a particular kind of meditation unique to Zen Buddhism.

Guided Imagery

Using the imagination in a directed way – which is the essence of guided imagery – harnesses the power of the mind to bring about beneficial physical, psychological and emotional changes. Mental imagery, whether guided by another or self-guided, can be used to open the door to feelings and personal insights. It can also reduce stress and help people cope with health conditions and symptoms that are emotionally and physically taxing. Guided imagery has been proven to provide several positive effects, including diminishing perception of pain, lowering blood pressure and helping to control anxiety. Because of its demonstrated benefits, this is one of the most widely used complementary treatments in the world.

HISTORY

Guided imagery emerged as a complementary therapy in the 1970s, following the discovery that emotions and thoughts can have a profound effect on physical and mental health. For example, feeling stressed can depress immune function, anger can increase the risk of heart disease, and feeling relaxed and in control can improve overall well-being and even promote healing.

As a result of that realization, several techniques have been developed to help patients visualize images that enable them to experience beneficial emotional states, gain important insights into the nature of their illness and their reactions to it, cope better with pain and disease, and make difficult decisions related to their health.

Today, guided imagery is one of the most widely used and accepted forms of complementary therapy. It is beneficial for any condition or symptom that has an emotional component, including anxiety, pain, insomnia and addiction, as well as for end-of-life care. As an adjunct to conventional medical treatment, guided imagery can help improve

Many physiological responses are provoked by the mind as well as by external stimuli. Imagining biting a citrus fruit, for instance, stimulates saliva flow; and thinking about lying in the sun increases skin blood flow.

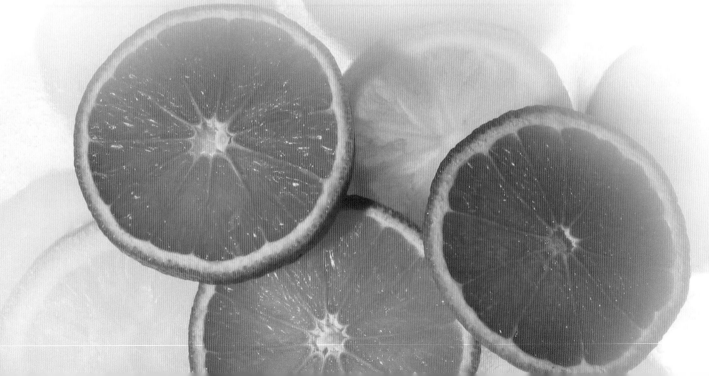

CAN GUIDED IMAGERY HELP ME?

Research shows that guided imagery may be helpful in many ways.

- **Arthritis** In a pilot study published in *Pain Management Nursing* in 2004, listening to guided imagery tapes, plus progressive muscle relaxation twice a day for twelve weeks, significantly reduced pain and mobility problems associated with osteoarthritis.

- **Asthma** Imagery targeted at biological functions significantly reduced symptoms, including wheezing and anxiety, and improved disease management among 70 asthma patients in a study published in the *Journal of Alternative and Complementary Medicine* in 2005.

- **Smoking cessation** According to a study from the University of Akron in Ohio, published in 2005 in the *Journal of Nursing Scholarship,* smoking abstinence rates were more than twice as high in people who practiced guided imagery daily, compared with standard education and counselling.

- **Pain relief** It can help relieve headaches, neck and back pain. A pilot study published in *Orthopaedic Nursing* in 2004 showed trends towards better pain relief, reduced anxiety and decreased hospital stay following joint replacement surgery among patients given guided imagery audiotapes, compared with music audiotapes.

- **Medical procedures** Guided imagery, when used just prior to having a biopsy or undergoing chemotherapy, can ease the pain and soothe the nausea, and other side-effects that are often experienced with these procedures.

- **Chronic conditions** When used with conventional medical treatments, it can help relieve symptoms of asthma and arthritis by controlling pain and relaxing muscles.

- **Anxiety** Guided imagery can help people suffering from anxiety recognize situations that provoke anxiety attacks, reducing their fear and their tendency to avoid difficult situations.

- **Heart disease** When used with conventional treatments, guided imagery has been shown to improve survival in people with heart disease by lowering blood pressure, and reducing stress and anger.

- **Pregnancy** Guided imagery has been used to help reduce birthing complications by enabling women in labour to relax deeply and fully, thus easing the birth process and lowering the need for Caesarean sections. It can also help reduce the perception of pain during childbirth.

- **Brain injury** In a randomized controlled trial of 46 stroke patients, rehabilitation experts at Hong Kong Polytechnic University found that mental imagery produced better relearning of both trained and untrained (new) tasks, compared with conventional functional training.

quality of life and health for people suffering from serious illnesses such as cancer, heart disease, and brain injury such as stroke.

PRACTICE

Creating images and exploring their meaning has several therapeutic effects. It can help change physiological functions in positive ways. Research using brain imaging technology shows that the parts of the brain that are active when people physically engage in tasks are also active when people visualize engaging in the tasks. Some of the areas of the brain involved in imagination also control the body's vital functions, such as breathing, heart rate and digestion. Therefore, the act of imagining can help influence these functions – for example, by lowering blood pressure and regulating heart rate.

Guiding the imagination, either with the help of a professional or on one's one, can direct its power to influence the body. When athletes are injured, for example, they can conjure images of themselves going through their training sessions as a way of reinforcing the neurological sequences of their performance. If someone is tired, closing their eyes and imagining themselves taking a nap or getting a massage can help them to feel refreshed.

Guided imagery can also improve mental outlook. The process of creating images and exploring their meaning helps provide insights and perspective that can be used to better understand a physical condition. Because the images people conjure are often emotionally meaningful, guided imagery can help them understand and modify their emotions, which in turn can help decrease the many health problems associated with emotional distress, including pain, anxiety, gastrointestinal upset and heart disease.

Visualization, sometimes called creative visualization or creative imagery, is a type of imagery that emphasizes visual sensations.

TREATMENTS

Many health professionals use guided imagery, and it is easy to learn the basic techniques with the help of books and videos. Those who prefer the support of a guide can attend a few sessions to learn the basics before engaging in guided imagery on their own.

The steps of guided imagery are usually as follows. The first is to take a few moments to relax. Next, the patient is asked to visualize images that relate to their health condition. This might be something that represents a

symptom being felt. Questions could be asked directly about that feeling, such as why it is there, what it needs, and what can be learned from it. If there is pain, an inner sanctuary might be pictured, where there is no pain and where it is possible to meet with an inner advisor – an image of a being who can help cope with the pain and explore ways to relieve it.

Mental imagery can also be used, when emotions or strong thoughts arise, by an individual alone or with a professional. For example, if one suddenly feels a wave of fear, it might be useful to use a crayon or pen to draw what the fear feels like. Once an image or scribble is at hand, it can be examined. This process of approaching difficulties as learning opportunities can yield rich rewards.

Figuring out what the images are, what they mean and why they are important can become a path to any number of resolutions: sorting out emotional conflicts, making decisions related to healthcare, feeling less frightened by an illness, or making changes in attitudes or health habits that can enhance the healing process.

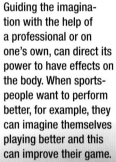

Guiding the imagination with the help of a professional or on one's own, can direct its power to have effects on the body. When sportspeople want to perform better, for example, they can imagine themselves playing better and this can improve their game.

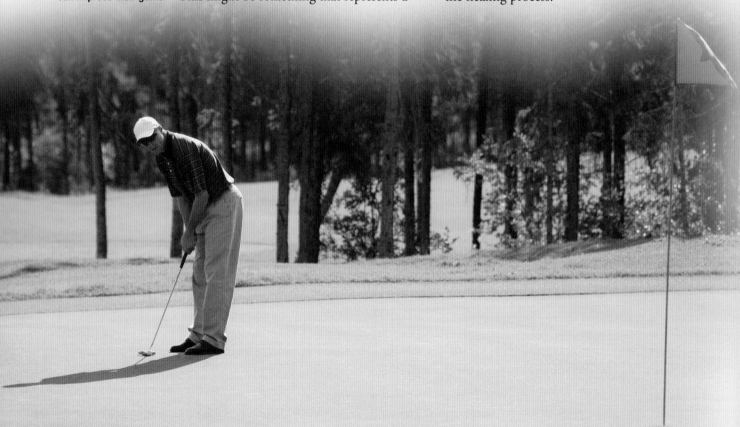

Flotation Therapy

Isolating the mind and body from external sensations can induce deep relaxation. In flotation therapy, a person floats in a soundproofed tank of warm salt water kept at body temperature, with sufficient salt concentration to give enough buoyancy to float without effort.

HISTORY

Flotation therapy was developed in the 1950s by American neurophysiologist and psychoanalyst Dr John Lilly. His experiments with sensory deprivation revealed that being effectively weightless and without external sensory cues produced a state of deep relaxation and improved imagination and problem-solving abilities.

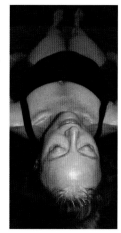

Isolating the mind and body from external sensations can induce deep relaxation. In flotation therapy, a person floats in a soundproofed tank of body temperature warm water, with sufficient salt concentration to allow buoyancy without effort.

CAN FLOTATION THERAPY HELP ME?

The therapeutic effects of flotation therapy have not been well studied, but may benefit the following conditions.

- **High blood pressure** One study has shown significantly greater blood pressure decreases after a relaxation programme in a flotation tank than after the same programme in a normal environment.

- **Stress and anxiety** Flotation may reduce levels of stress hormones immediately after a session and after regular sessions have ended. One study found that four sessions of flotation therapy produced significant decreases in muscle tension, anxiety, depression, heart rate and blood pressure.

- **Chronic pain** Flotation therapy can help to reduce tension headaches and perhaps rheumatoid arthritis symptoms. One study showed that flotation therapy lessened pain intensity among people with chronic neck and back muscle pain while in the water. Patients also had lower levels of stress hormones, less anxiety or depression, increased optimism, and reported falling asleep more easily at night.

Flotation therapy is a Restricted Environmental Stimulation Technique (REST), a term that originated in the 1970s and refers to relaxation techniques in which external sensory inputs such as touch, noise, and light are minimized. It also includes dry REST, where a thin polymer membrane separates the person from the water.

Flotation tanks have become increasingly popular in health clubs in the United States and Europe. Practitioners say flotation may improve problem-solving ability and other mental skills, and it is claimed to increase scientific creativity, and musical, artistic and sports performance. More research is needed to document these claims.

PRACTICE

Most flotation tanks are about 2.5 m (8 ft) long by 1.25 m (4 ft) wide and contain 25 cm (10 in) of water. A flotation session may last two hours can trigger the release of endorphins, the body's own morphine-like pain-killing and pleasure-inducing chemicals.

TREATMENTS

The flotation tank is usually enclosed and dark; earplugs may be worn for complete silence, or the person may listen to relaxing music, instructions on guided imagery (pp.520–2), or educational material.

Because of the extreme isolation of the tank, flotation therapy is not advised for those who suffer from claustrophobia or serious mental disorders.

Neurolinguistic Patterning

The goal of neurolinguistic patterning (NLP) is to model excellence in human achievement. The techniques are designed to enable people to manage their thought processes, feelings and behaviour more effectively, communicate better, change unhelpful beliefs, respond to circumstances with more flexibility, understand their own motivations, develop empowering beliefs and a sense of purpose, identify personal goals, tap into their true potential, improve performance and generally achieve greater success in life.

Some people create a sense of confidence, empathy and responsiveness that encourages effective communication by 'mirroring' the other person – their posture, gestures, eye contact, tone, rate of speech and even breathing patterns.

Neurolinguistic patterning studies human functioning, and offers a model for the subjective processing of experience and communication, together with techniques to reprogramme behaviour. The term comes from its goals of accessing and integrating the sensory and physiological reactions of mind and body (neuro), language-processing (linguistic), and thought and behaviour patterns.

NLP has been used in therapy and counselling, sports, performing arts and commerce to improve outlook and performance. Although well described, empirical studies of its effectiveness are limited.

HISTORY

NLP was conceived in the 1970s by mathematician and psychologist Richard Bandler and linguist John Grinder at the University of California in Santa Cruz. Through their study of excellence, they analysed the techniques of renowned therapists such as hypnotherapist Milton Erickson, Gestalt therapy founder Fritz Perls and prominent family therapist Virginia Satir. They were also influenced by British anthropologist Gregory Bateson's work on communication and systems theory. This led to an attempt to devise a model of how people think and perceive subjective experience and interactions.

Bandler and Grinder ceased collaboration, but their books helped popularize NLP, as did seminars and workshops developed by adherents, including motivational speaker Anthony Robbins, who rapidly became a media personality. NLP in various forms is now used all over the world by thousands of practitioners.

In addition to benefits in outlook, performance and communication, some NLP practitioners say it can help alleviate disease by changing beliefs about one's prospects for recovery. Improvements have been claimed in conditions such as arthritis, allergies, migraines, Parkinson's disease, AIDS and cancer. No validated studies support these claims.

Today, numerous NLP training and certification organizations exist, but there is no formal oversight or registration of practitioners.

PRACTICE

A fundamental precept of NLP is that our experience of the world is affected by our sensory perceptions and mental representations or constructs – neurolinguistic maps – and these, not objective reality, are what frame people's understanding and behaviour. Recognizing how people create their unique internal world can enable re-programming of limiting beliefs to create more effective representations and more successful behaviour.

People are taught to access these representations through body language and speech cues, and use techniques to change limiting beliefs, create inner resources, produce more useful behaviour and move people to their desired state. NLP techniques may be useful in therapy to aid personal development, improve communication skills, enhance creativity or performance, and accelerate learning.

People may consult an NLP practitioner individually or attend a course, group seminar or workshop, or use books or audiovisual material. Practitioners claim that some people experience dramatic changes in as little as a single session, while others may require a series of consultations. Many NLP techniques, once learned, can be used for self-help.

TREATMENTS

Rapport, the way successful people create a sense of confidence, empathy, and responsiveness for effective communication, is key in NLP. Rapport can be learned by 'mirroring' another person – copying their posture, gestures, eye contact, tone, rate of speech, even breathing patterns. NLP practitioners use mirroring to create rapport, enabling them to pace and lead an interaction.

Eye accessing cues (eye movements) give practitioners vital information about how people prefer to have material presented to them: visually, through hearing, or through feeling (kinesthetically) – and whether they are accessing memories or mental constructs.

One way to alter beliefs is to presuppose that a background belief is true. A practitioner may make a statement or ask the person to act 'as if' an outcome was inevitable or

CAN NEUROLINGUISTIC PATTERNING HELP ME?

Very few formal studies of NLP exist and there is no scientific evidence to support its theories or its effectiveness. However, practitioners claim numerous benefits.

- **Communication** NLP is frequently used as a business and sales tool to create rapport with customers and tailor sales pitches to their underlying goals. It is also commonly used to create rapport between therapists and their clients.
- **Phobias** Practitioners say NLP can cure most phobias. Only anecdotal support exists for this claim.
- **Lifestyle changes** Ample anecdotal evidence suggests that NLP helps efforts to stop smoking, change one's diet and lose weight.
- **Performance** Athletes and creative performers have used NLP to overcome blocks and enhance their performance.

already true. Some presuppositions used generally in NLP include the belief that every behaviour has a positive intention, conscious or not, and so represents the best choice the person could make at the time; that undesired outcomes represent feedback, not failure – a chance to act differently next time; and that people have all the inner resources they need.

Reframing, or changing the internal representation, meaning or context of a problem or unwanted behaviour to achieve a desired change, is a key NLP tool. The technique involves finding the underlying intention behind an unwanted behaviour and coming up with new ways to fulfill the same purpose.

In NLP, a stimulus that is linked to and triggers a particular physiological or emotional state is known as an 'anchor'. Resource anchoring involves evoking a positive, resourceful state and associating it with a simple anchor, like a particular touch or gesture. The anchor can then be used to call up a resourceful state when needed.

Breath Work

Also known as 'intentional control of breathing' or 'conscious breathing', breath work is a term that covers several techniques. These techniques are used to promote physical healing and induce emotional changes, as well as impart a sense of spirituality and well-being.

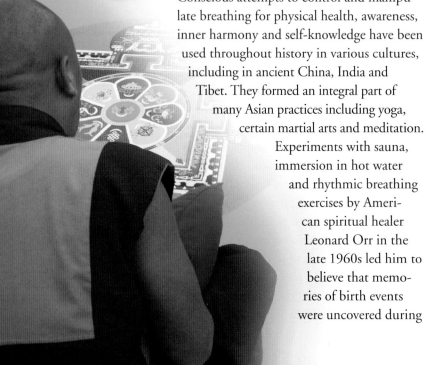

In holotropic breath work, participants may be encouraged to make mandala drawings, ancient circular patterns said to develop from unconscious inspirations. Mandalas are sometimes used in art therapy to help people integrate their experiences.

Controlled breathing plays a role in visualization and guided imagery (pp.520–2), meditation (pp.514–19), progressive muscle relaxation (pp.474–5), hypnotherapy (pp.508–11) and yoga (pp. 476–9). Breath work is most often used to induce the relaxation response and to focus on the relationship between breathing and emotion. It may also be used to induce altered states of consciousness that some practitioners believe can offer access to the unconscious, enabling people to recover early memories, interpret past experiences, and resolve hidden conflicts stored in both mind and body. Breath work may be used along with various forms of psychotherapy and spiritual healing.

HISTORY

Conscious attempts to control and manipulate breathing for physical health, awareness, inner harmony and self-knowledge have been used throughout history in various cultures, including in ancient China, India and Tibet. They formed an integral part of many Asian practices including yoga, certain martial arts and meditation. Experiments with sauna, immersion in hot water and rhythmic breathing exercises by American spiritual healer Leonard Orr in the late 1960s led him to believe that memories of birth events were uncovered during the altered states these practices produced. He called his refined breathing techniques 'rebirthing'. This developed into a type of breathing therapy performed on a mattress, that became popular in the 1970s.

Similar forms of breath work expanded to encompass childhood problems and current life issues. In the late 1970s, therapists Stanislav and Christina Grof developed holotropic breath work (see below) as a way of inducing psychedelic states without drugs.

Breath work techniques aimed at inner transformation now take many forms and are used by practitioners of both psychological and body therapies. Practitioners claim improvement for emotional conditions including:

- **Emotional conflict** Breath work is claimed to promote peace of mind and resolve emotional issues by enabling awareness, acceptance, and healing of repressed problems.
- **Relationship and sexual problems** Because these may stem from emotional issues, practitioners believe breath work can help.
- **Low self-esteem** To the extent that low self-esteem results from poor self-image stemming from childhood events, breath work may uncover and resolve conflicts.
- **Spirituality** Some people use breath work to try to achieve higher consciousness.

PRACTICE

Breath work may be conducted as individual or group therapy, and may be combined with psychotherapy or bioenergetics (p.569). Once learned, the techniques may be used for self-help. Facilitators often begin by getting everyone to take a short time to become calm and comfortable, with attention focused on the present, before being guided to become consciously aware of their breathing, and often deliberately adoptspecific breathing patterns. This is sometimes undertaken in pairs, with one member consciously breathing and the other supporting in turn.

Most forms of breath work involve concentrating on breathing more deeply, to avoid common but unhealthy patterns of shallow breathing that may be a response to stress and a way of avoiding uncomfortable emotions. A common technique is circular or connected breathing – inhaling and exhaling without the usual pause between breaths. After a time this is said to allow stored memories and repressed feelings to surface, possibly promoting emotional release, deeper understanding of personal issues and enhanced spiritual awareness. Some practitioners believe this breathing can lead to regression to earlier experiences, including those experienced before birth.

Sessions may last an hour or two; some are open-ended to allow issues to be fully explored. The experience can be cathartic; facilitators may need psychotherapeutic skills to deal with deep emotional issues that may surface, so it is advisable to undertake more intense forms of breath work only under the guidance of a highly trained professional.

TREATMENTS

There are several types of breath work. In holotropic breath work, breathing cycles are focused to flow with rhythmic music to induce altered consciousness. Practitioners also use trans-personal psychology, whose goal is to develop a sense of connectedness with the universe or higher forces outside the self. They may incorporate energy therapy techniques to encourage the release of negative emotions stemming from past traumas, and encourage people to make mandala drawings – ancient circular forms said to

CAN BREATH WORK HELP ME?

Almost any form of controlled breathing exercise may promote relaxation, relieve tension, reduce physiological responses to stress, and enhance energy. There has been little formal study of breath work and no evidence so far to support its effectiveness in psychological therapies.

develop from unconscious inspirations and often used in art therapy to help people interpret their experiences.

Rebirthing, also known as 'intuitive breathing', aims to allow memories of birth trauma to surface and be released.

The goal of Middendorf is breathing without interfering with its natural rhythm, to allow the essence of 'self' (the sense of one's unique qualities, place and purpose) to unfold.

Vivation uses continuous, circular breathing and 'unconditional love' (complete and unconditional positive acceptance of oneself and any emotions that arise) to relieve pain, stress and negative emotions.

Radiance breath work aims at emotional release through breath work, sometimes combined with various forms of bodywork, particularly massage.

Optimal breathing, also known as 'advanced working breath', uses exercises that are based on enhancing breathing mechanics and respiratory capacity to boost energy, optimum health and, it is claimed, longevity.

CAUTION

Some people experience effects such as tingling of the hands and feet, sleepiness or dizziness, and may even faint during intense breath work. People with asthma or other respiratory complaints, epilepsy and those with severe emotional disturbances or mental health problems are advised to consult their physician or mental health provider before undertaking breath work.

Heart Coherence

The interval between successive heartbeats normally varies because of the continual feedback between the sympathetic nervous system (responsible for the 'fight or flight' reactions), which increases heart rate, and the parasympathetic system, which reduces it. This heart rate variability (HRV) is a physiological mechanism that enables the body to adapt to changing circumstances – greater variability means more flexibility of response, so a high HRV is generally healthy. Reduced HRV has been linked with ageing, trauma and various disease states, and has been found to predict a higher risk of death after a heart attack.

Heart rate variability is also highly sensitive to emotions. Positive emotions, such as love, appreciation, compassion, and gratitude may enhance HRV, revealing the heart's ability to modulate its frequency as needed. This phenomenon is shown on heart monitoring equipment as a regularly undulating wave pattern that represents the smooth ebb and flow between the sympathetic and parasympathetic systems – practitioners refer to this state as 'coherence'.

In contrast, negative emotions, such as anger, frustration, insecurity, anxiety and depression reduce the variability between successive heartbeats. This represents reduced synchronization between sympathetic and parasympathetic systems and is shown on monitoring equipment as erratic peaks and troughs—a state in which the heart is less able to adapt flexibly to demands placed upon it, and that practitioners call "chaos."

Heart coherence uses biofeedback (pp.504–7) to teach people how to control their HRV and maintain the best pattern. In turn, this ability can cause physiological changes in the nervous system and hormone balance. Benefits of heart coherence are claimed to include enhanced mental clarity, stress reduction, lowered blood pressure, improved immunity and better overall health.

Practitioners of heart coherence say it can lead to enhanced mental clarity, reduced levels of stress and decreased blood pressure.

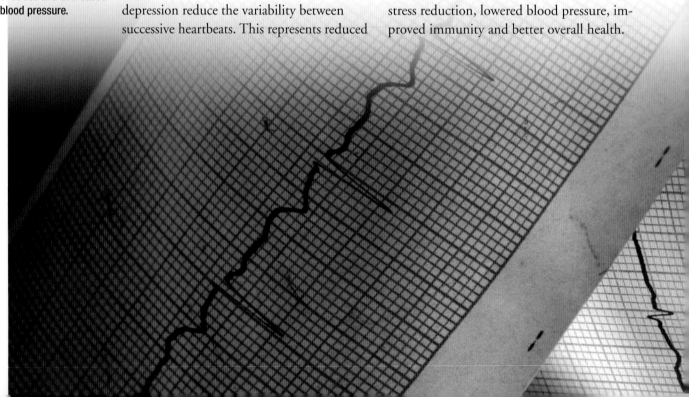

HISTORY

The use of HRV as a measure of health dates to the 1960s, when it began to be employed during delivery to monitor the health of newborns. Today, HRV is well accepted as an indicator of overall health. For instance, when people are exposed to pollution, their HRV drops. The HRV of people suffering from work-related stress improves while they are on vacation. In fact, HRV is now considered to be the best, most powerful predictor of mortality after heart attack—or from any disease.

In addition to positive emotions, other factors that can help improve HRV include (but are not limited to) a healthful diet, exercise, yoga (pp.476–9), accupuncture (pp. 464–5), and healthy sleep patterns.

The concept of heart coherence was first described in 1992 by physicist Dan Winter, and then popularized by the Institute of HeartMath, a nonprofit research organization in Boulder, Colorado. HeartMath researched practical applications of heart coherence and developed testing equipment to measure HRV and record its wave patterns. Its work has been further developed by others, including Dr Alan Watkins in the United Kingdom. Heart coherence has also been demonstrated extensively by cognitive neuroscientist David Servan-Schreiber, Professor of Psychiatry at the University of Pittsburgh.

Practitioners say heart coherence can benefit people with a variety of conditions, both physical and psychological. However, few specific studies of its effects on emotional well-being have been conducted. Stress, depression, anxiety, panic disorder, post-traumatic stress disorder and attention-deficit hyperactivity disorder are said to improve when the technique is practised, but empirical evidence is still needed to support this assertion. The techniques are also said to improve examination and sports performance, but this, too, needs to be better studied.

CAN HEART COHERENCE HELP ME?

Recent conventional medical research has linked low HRV with hypertension, heart disease, and mortality from all causes, lending support to some claims of heart coherence.

- **Stress-related conditions** Much like qigong (p.450) and meditation (pp.514–19), to which it is related, heart coherence may be effective alongside conventional treatments for sleep disorders, fibromyalgia, chronic fatigue syndrome, hypertension and asthma.
- **Psychological issues** Stress, depression, anxiety and panic disorder, are said to improve; more empirical support for this is needed.
- **Performance** The techniques are said to improve examination and sports performance; more research is needed.
- **Congestive heart failure** In one study, heart coherence, when taught to people suffering heart failure, reduced symptoms of depression and increased functional capacity measured by how far patients could walk in six minutes.

PRACTICE

Heart rate variability can be monitored using a standard ECG, or from pulse wave recordings from a fingertip or earlobe. Computer software converts heartbeat intervals to the HRV waveform. At a session, practitioners demonstrate how changes in thoughts and emotions alter the HRV waveform pattern, and then teach people biofeedback techniques that can alter their mental state to create coherence instead of chaos.

TREATMENTS

Breathing sequences accompanied by a focus on the heart and positive emotions are used to move the HRV waveform toward heart coherence. Once people learn to alter the waveform pattern during monitoring, they can use the techniques at any time to maintain coherence and counteract negative emotions.

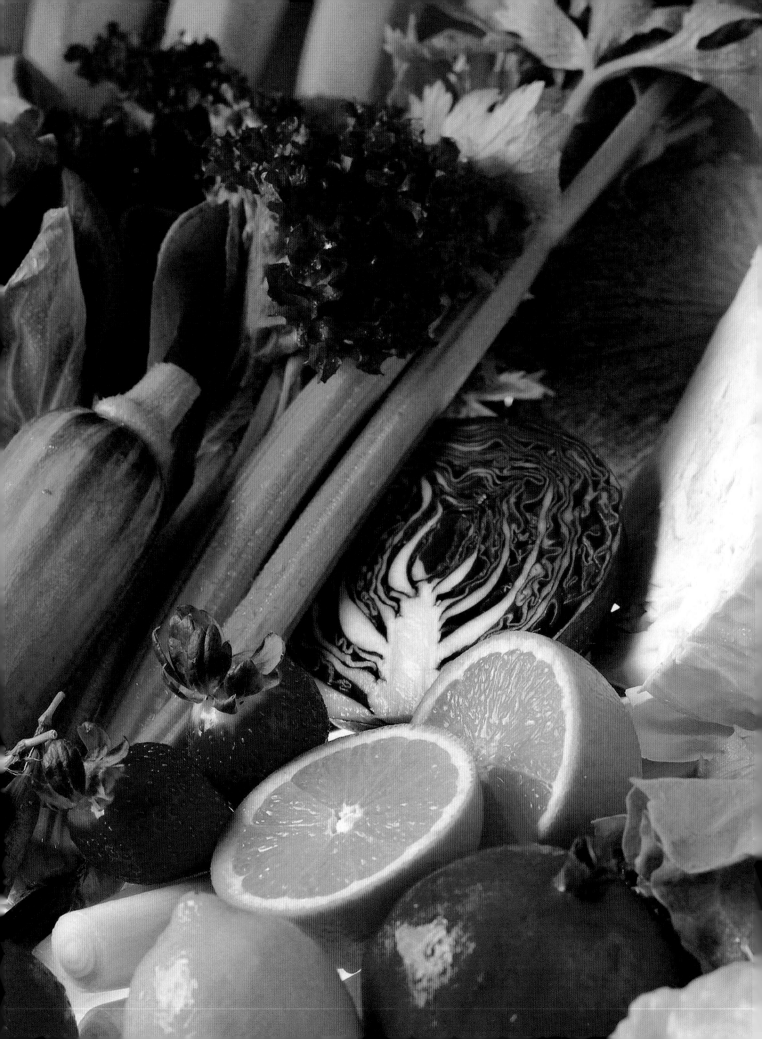

THE NATURAL WORLD

19

People have been aware of the therapeutic powers of plants since long before recorded history. The healing traditions of herbalism and other botanical therapies have been written about for millennia. They form the basis of much conventional medicine, and still play a vital role in many systems of complementary and alternative medicine.

In parallel with the vast technological progress occurring in other areas, the 20th century saw an explosion of knowledge about body chemistry, including the discovery of vitamins – vital ingredients in foods that are necessary for normal functioning and for staving off disease. The ability to supplement both our diets and our foods with vitamins and minerals has played a crucial role in eliminating many diseases that were formerly common, debilitating and frequently fatal.

At the same time, holistic ('whole person') health systems began to look for more subtle influences that could be attributed to plants, in the form of aromatherapy and flower essences, and later developed the idea of using concentrated juices to obtain even greater health benefits from fruits and vegetables.

The ability to use these natural influences to benefit our health is a primary component of integrative medicine.

Supplements, Vitamins & Minerals

Any product that contains ingredients intended to add a nutrient to the diet is a supplement. Supplements include vitamins, minerals, herbs and other botanicals (pp.552–9), amino acids, enzymes (pp.542–53), organ tissues, glandular extracts, metabolites (substances produced in the metabolism of an original substance), extracts and concentrates – substances extracted from a plant, body fluid or tissue, or concentrated from them.

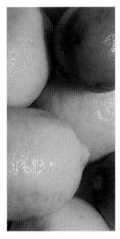

In 1747, Scottish naval surgeon James Lind noted that scurvy could be prevented by consuming citrus fruits. Another 40 years passed before British naval rations began to be supplemented with lemon and lime juice.

Vitamins are substances derived from foods that are required for health but cannot be manufactured in the body. The exceptions are vitamin D, which is produced in the skin when it is exposed to sunlight, and niacin, small amounts of which can be synthesized in the liver. Vitamins perform numerous functions that are vital to digestion, metabolism, growth, resistance to infection, and healthy functioning of muscle, nerves and other body tissues.

Of the 13 vitamins currently recognized, four – vitamins A, D, E and K – are fat-soluble. This means they require bile to be absorbed by the body and that any excess over the body's immediate requirements is stored in the liver and in fatty tissue. Therefore, they do not necessarily need to be consumed every day. If these vitamins are taken in excess, they can accumulate in the body to potentially toxic levels. If non-digestible fats are present in the intestines, this may prevent the absorption of fat-soluble vitamins and eventually lead to a deficiency. Such problems can occur if mineral oil is used extensively (for example, to treat constipation). Another concern is the use of fat substitutes in food, which also inhibit the absorption of fat-soluble vitamins.

The other nine vitamins – eight B vitamins plus vitamin C – are water-soluble. They are not stored in the body in significant amounts (with the exception of folate and vitamin B_{12} in the liver), so they need to be ingested regularly. Any extra beyond what the body requires is simply excreted in urine, However, large excesses may still result in toxic side effects (see the chart on pp.516–17).

As with vitamins, minerals also often occur naturally in food. Minerals form major components of the skeleton and teeth, provide important structural elements in cells and contribute to the make-up of some enzymes. Their presence helps regulate fluid balance and nerve impulses, and some minerals play an important role in cellular respiration, helping to convey oxygen to cells and carry away carbon dioxide waste.

Some minerals are required in relatively large quantities (more than 250 mg daily), including calcium, magnesium, phosphorous, sodium, chloride, potassium and sulphur. Others, known as trace minerals, are needed only in tiny amounts; these include copper, iron, zinc, iodine, fluoride, chromium, selenium, manganese and molybdenum.

In addition to vitamins and minerals, other dietary components used as supplements include essential fatty acids (EFAs), which are present in fish oils, and essential amino acids, as well as many plant-based supplements (pp.552–9), and a profusion of others not originally from nutritional sources, such as shark cartilage, coral calcium and the hormone melatonin. The vast range of available supplements comes in many forms, including tablets, capsules, powders, granules, lozenges and liquids.

A healthful, balanced diet remains the best source of most of the vitamins and minerals the body needs. A healthy diet also provides other ingredients vital to good health, such as dietary fibre, antioxidants (substances that keep in check potentially harmful free radicals – unstable molecules produced in many metabolic processes), and phytochemicals (substances found in fruits and vegetables that protect the body against diseases such as heart disease, diabetes, high blood pressure and cancer). In addition, many vitamins and minerals are best assimilated from foods, which typically contain a range of nutrients whose combinations and proportions may be better matched to the body's needs.

However, many people do not eat the types and variety of foods necessary to get optimum levels and balances of vitamins and minerals, even with modern Western diets in which food is generally plentiful. To make up any deficiencies, and for certain therapeutic purposes, it may be sensible for some people to take supplements.

HISTORY

The idea that food components are linked with health and disease has been recognized for millennia. The ancient Egyptians knew 3,500 years ago that night blindness (now known to be due to deficiency of vitamin A) might be alleviated by eating foods such as liver. Such knowledge has probably always been part of the folklore and traditions of herbal medicine, although much of it was lost during the Middle Ages.

In 1747, Scottish naval doctor James Lind noted that scurvy (which at the time killed more British sailors than those who

died in enemy action) could be prevented by eating citrus fruits, although the nutrient responsible, vitamin C, was then unknown. (Scurvy causes spontaneous bleeding, loose teeth, joint pain, fatigue, diarrhoea, impaired wound-healing, skin-thickening and seizures, and can be fatal.) It took another 40 years, and the death from scurvy of another 100,000 sailors, before naval rations began to be supplemented with lemon and lime juice, from which came the phrase 'limeys' to describe the sailors, and later, Britons in general.

In 1889, Dutch physician Christiaan Eijkman was sent to the Dutch East Indies to investigate beriberi, a disease that causes nerve damage, muscle weakness, heart failure, movement abnormalities and brain dysfunction. We now know it is caused by a vitamin B_1 deficiency, but at the time the disease was believed to be an infection. He found, by chance, that chickens developed a similar condition when fed polished rice (rice grains with the husks removed), and that it was cured when their diet was changed back to unpolished rice, which he

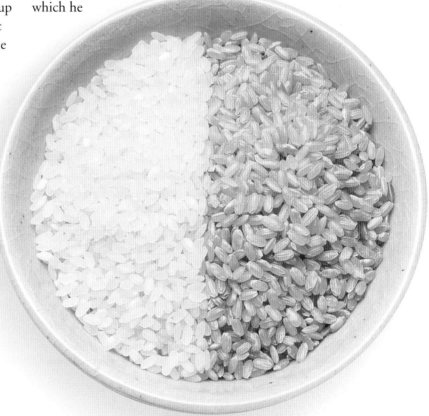

In 1907, an English doctor, William Fletcher, proposed that polished rice, either directly or indirectly, caused beriberi. In fact, it was the lack of vitamin D in polished rice that caused the disease.

suggested contained some 'anti-beriberi' factor that could prevent the disease in humans. His work led to the discovery of vitamins.

Similar experiments were carried out in 1905 by a British doctor, William Fletcher, among asylum inmates in Kuala Lumpur, Malaysia. Almost a quarter of those eating polished rice developed beriberi, compared with less than 2 percent of those given unpolished rice. In a report published in the medical journal *The Lancet* in 1907, Fletcher proposed that polished rice either directly or indirectly caused beriberi.

In 1906, a British biochemist called Sir Frederick Gowland Hopkins proposed that, along with their main constituents such as proteins and carbohydrates, foods contained 'accessory factors' that were vital to body functions. In recognition of the importance of their discoveries, Eijkman and Hopkins shared the Nobel Prize in Medicine in 1929.

Meanwhile, in 1911, Kazimierz (often Anglicized to Casimir) Funk, a Polish chemist working at the Lister Institute in London, read Fletcher's work and set about isolating the anti-beriberi substances in rice husks. He coined the term vitamines (meaning 'vital amines'), in the mistaken belief that these factors were amines (derived from ammonia). The spelling was changed to vitamin in 1920 when it became clear that not all vitamins are amines.

Hopkins and Funk now jointly formulated the vitamin hypothesis of deficiency disease, which says that a deficiency of vitamins causes disease, and it soon became apparent that other diseases, including pellagra

(a disease that causes scaly skin and depression) and xerophthalmia (a condition in which the cornea and conjunctiva of the eye dry out), were also due to vitamin deficiencies.

As more and more vitamins were discovered, isolated in their pure chemical forms and subjected to chemical analysis, researchers sought ways to produce them in larger quantities. Vitamin C was the first to be synthesized, in the 1930s, with commercial production starting soon afterward. By the end of the decade, vitamin supplements had become both popular with the public and profitable for manufacturers.

Vitamins and minerals also gained considerable public health attention in this period with the introduction of fortified foods – foods to which vitamins and minerals have been added. These include iodine in salt, vitamin D in milk and margarine, and B vitamins and iron in flour and bread. The additions lead to a dramatic decline in rickets (a disease in which the bones do not harden) and virtually eradicating pellagra and riboflavin deficiency. Other foods, including yogurt, milk and even water, are often fortified with minerals, vitamins and other supplements.

In the 1940s, a Canadian doctor, Evan Shute, began to use supplements to treat conditions other than deficiencies – in this case, vitamin E to treat cardiovascular disease. Soon such uses were being extensively investigated. In 1954, physician Denham Harman proposed that free radicals were responsible for cell damage, disease, and aging, and that antioxidants, such as vitamins C and E, could neutralize them. In the 1960s, another Nobel Prize-winning scientist, Linus Pauling, popularized the idea that eating certain foods could maintain health and treat disease.

Since then, vitamins and other supplements have increasingly been investigated for functions beyond their nutritional value, for example in lowering cholesterol, treating arthritis and even preventing cancer.

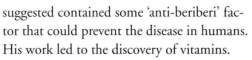

Folic acid is a vital nutrient for woman before they become pregnant and once they are pregnant to prevent birth defects from spina bifida.

CAN SUPPLEMENTS HELP ME?

Some of the many conditions for which dietary supplements are used include:

- **Arthritis** Strong evidence suggests that fish oil supplements can ease symptoms, especially in rheumatoid arthritis, and that chondroitin and glucosamine can benefit osteoarthritis. Some botanical therapies (pp.552–9) may also be helpful.

- **Heart disease** Antioxidant vitamins have been suggested to lower the risk of coronary artery disease (CAD). According to a report in the *American Journal of Clinical Nutrition* in 2004, any protective effect of vitamin E or carotenoid supplements is small; however, people taking a supplement containing more than 700 mg of vitamin C daily reduced CAD risk by about a quarter. Some research also suggests that omega 3 fatty acids (pp.252–3) are more effective than statins in reducing mortality from CAD.

- **Osteoporosis** Calcium supplements do not build bone, but they can reduce bone mass loss that occurs in women after menopause; this may reduce the incidence of fractures.

- **Colds** Very little evidence supports the belief that consuming high doses of vitamin C prevents or treats cold symptoms, but other supplements may help. In 2005, scientists from the Federal Research Centre for Nutrition and Food in Kiel, Germany, found that taking a dietary supplement containing probiotic bacteria plus vitamins and minerals for at least three months in the winter and spring reduced the duration, frequency and severity of common cold symptoms in otherwise healthy adults.

- **Multiple sclerosis** Increasing evidence suggests that MS is, in part, a vitamin D-deficiency disease. Vitamin D supplementation seems to be associated with a reduced incidence of MS, although the effect on established disease is less certain, according to a review from the University of Heidelberg, Germany, published in 2005. Others believe that there is a defect in fat metabolism in MS, and a diet very low in saturated fat, perhaps with supplements of polyunsaturated oils such as fish oils, flaxseed or evening primrose oil, may help.

- **Cancer** Research suggests that various supplements might influence cancer risk, but results are largely inconclusive. In a large trial among nearly 30,000 men in Finland, vitamin E or beta-carotene supplements failed to reduce the incidence of lung cancer in smokers. Beta-carotene increased lung cancer risk in smokers, but decreased risk for colon cancer in non-smokers. Vitamin E seemed to offer some protection against prostate cancer, but it also increased the risk of stroke.

- **Vision loss** According to two Cochrane reviews published in 2005, taking antioxidant vitamin and zinc supplements may slow progression of age-related macular degeneration (pp. 40–1); however, their use in prevention is less certain; more research is needed.

- **Birth defects** Folic acid taken during pregnancy, and preferably from three months before conception, can reduce a woman's risk of having a baby with neural tube defects (NTD) such as spina bifida. Since folic acid was added to cereal grains in the United States in 1998, NTD rates have fallen by around 50 percent, according to one government study published in 2004.

- **Premenstrual symptoms** Premenstrual mood disturbances may be reduced by taking supplements of calcium, magnesium, vitamin B6 (deficiency of which has been linked with premenstrual symptoms) or L-tryptophan, according to a review published in the medical journal *Psychoneuroendocrinology* in 2003.

- **Measles** Vitamin A deficiency is common in developing countries and has been linked with more severe infection in children who have measles. An analysis of five trials in Africa published in the *Journal of Tropical Pediatrics* in 2002 showed that vitamin A supplementation may reduce mortality in severe cases, especially among children under two years old given two doses of 200,000 international units (IUs).

- **Alzheimer's disease** According to a study published in *The Archives of Neurology* in 2004, people over age 65 who took both vitamins C and E in combination substantially reduced their risk of Alzheimer's disease, whereas taking either vitamin without the other made no significant difference.

PRACTICE

Many nutritionists and healthcare practitioners advocate taking vitamin and mineral supplements, often along with dietary and other lifestyle changes. As well as asking extensive questions about diet and eating habits, some practitioners may ask the patient to keep a food diary and perform tests to determine whether any deficiencies exist.

Supplements are widely available in chemists and supermarkets, and many people take them on their own initiative. Estimates suggest that 40 percent of the United States population, and up to 50 percent of children, take at least one dietary supplement. In one survey in the United Kingdom, 40 percent of women and 29 percent of men were taking supplements, with the highest use (55 percent) among women ages 50 to 64. Another study in the United States revealed that, ironically, the people who were most likely to consume plenty of fruit and vegetables were also those who took the most vitamin supplements.

In the United States, dietary supplements are regulated by the Food and Drug Administration (FDA), although that agency has limited power to regulate supplements compared with those it exercises over prescription drugs. Manufacturers are responsible for determining the safety of their products and do not require FDA approval before marketing them, unless they contain a novel ingredient that is not present in existing foods. Supplements must be labelled with their ingredients and nutritional content, and manufacturers must not claim that a product is a treatment, prevention or cure for a specific disease or condition. However, they may draw attention to the relationship of dietary components to health and disease (for example, 'Diets high in calcium may reduce the risk of osteoporosis') or to bodily structure and function (for example, 'Calcium builds strong bones'). The FDA can stop manufacturers from making false or misleading claims, and has the power to ban products believed to pose unreasonable risks.

In the United Kingdom, all food supplements must comply with the general safety, description, and labelling rules for foodstuffs. In addition, since 2003, European Union regulations set down a list of permitted vitamins and minerals, all others being prohibited, plus additional labelling requirements.

Consumers should treat supplements with as much caution as they do pharmaceutical drugs. Supplements should be stored in a locked cupboard out of the reach of children. Iron supplements can be especially dangerous in excess; iron is a leading cause of childhood poisoning deaths in the United States.

Some supplements may interact with prescription drugs or herbal medicines, and some may affect the results of medical tests. Vitamins E and K affect blood clotting and may cause bleeding, especially among patients taking warfarin and other anticoagulant drugs. People taking dietary supplements should inform their doctor, herbalist or other healthcare practitioner.

CAUTION

Generally, it would be hard to take too much of a vitamin or mineral just by changing your diet. The exception is the possibility of consuming toxic levels of vitamins A and D, which are concentrated in certain organ meats. So pregnant women are advised not to eat liver due to the risks that excess vitamin A could pose to the foetus. More commonly, it is overconsumption of supplements that leads to rare cases of vitamin overload, usually of the fat-soluble vitamins, because the excess is stored in the body.

TREATMENTS

There is a bewildering array of supplements available, with single or combined ingredients, believed to be useful for particular purposes.

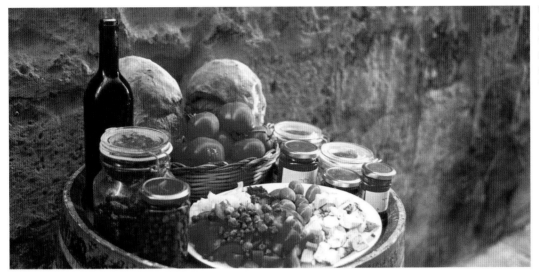

Vitamins and other supplements should be taken in addition to consuming a balanced diet, and not as a substitute for eating healthfully.

Clinical Query

Should I take a daily multivitamin?

Yes – at least according to the American Medical Association (AMA), which in 2002 reversed a previous position and advised all adults to take a multivitamin supplement. However, taking a supplement is not a substitute for a healthy diet. If you are over age 50, overweight, pregnant, breastfeeding, trying to conceive, have any illness or take prescribed medication, it is wise to first discuss supplements with your doctor.

Choose a supplement that provides near to the recommended daily allowance (RDA) of each vitamin and mineral. Note, however, that most will not provide 100 percent of the daily allowance of calcium, as the tablet would be too large. Products in the United Kingdom must clearly state the RDA of each vitamin and mineral, in line with the Food Labelling Regulations. Pharmacists should always provide advice on vitamin supplements and remind people that eating vitamin-fortified food could increase cumulative vitamin intake above levels that are safe. In 2002, the Expert Group on Vitamins and Minerals set safe upper limits for nine vitamins and minerals.

There are some groups of people at higher risk of nutritional deficiencies who may benefit most from taking a multivitamin supplement.

• Anyone who consumes fewer than 1,200 calories per day
• People on a restricted diet
• Vegetarians or vegans, who may be deficient in vitamin B$_{12}$
• People with lactose intolerance or those who avoid dairy produce for other reasons
• People who regularly skip meals or mainly eat fast food or junk food
• Adolescent girls and pre-menopausal women, who may need extra iron and folate
• Post-menopausal women, who may benefit from extra calcium and vitamin D for bone strength and to prevent osteoporosis
• Elderly people, who may have poor diets, spend much of their time indoors, and sometimes have reduced ability to absorb vitamin B$_{12}$ because of changes in gastric secretions
• Anyone who does not get much exposure to the sun, either because of the local climate or because of clothing habits that cover most of the body
• People with chronic illnesses, who take regular medications, or are recovering from an accident or surgery
• Smokers, because smoking interferes with vitamin C absorption
• People with a high alcohol intake, which may interfere with vitamin B absorption.

PART 2: COMPLEMENTARY AND ALTERNATIVE THERAPIES   537

	Chemical name(s)	Food sources	Main effects in the body	
Vitamin A	Retinoids Retinol Beta-carotene	fish oils; liver; kidneys; eggs; dairy products; dark green, leafy vegetables; yellow vegetables; carrots; pumpkin	vision; cell growth; teeth, bone and skin formation	
Vitamin B_1	Thiamin Thiamine aneurine	beef, beans, brewer's yeast, milk, nuts, pork, beans, oranges, wheat, soy products	heart, nerve, and muscle function; carbohydrate metabolism; digestion	
Vitamin B_2	Riboflavin Riboflavine	milk, eggs, meat, liver, green vegetables	cell function and growth; red blood cell production; releases energy from carbohydrates	
Vitamin B_3	Niacin Nicotinic acid Nicotinamide	meat, poultry, fish, milk, eggs, green vegetables, yeast, grains	nerve function, digestion, energy production; may lower cholesterol	
Folate	Folic acid (synthetic version)	green, leafy vegetables; peas, chickpeas, brown rice, oranges, bananas, mushrooms, liver	DNA synthesis; red blood cell formation	
Vitamin B_6	Pyridine Pyridoxamine Pyridoxal phosphate	pork, poultry, cod fish, cereals, carrots, eggs, peanuts, potatoes, soy products	red blood cell formation; neurotransmitter and myelin production; skin metabolism	
Biotin Vitamin H	Biotin Vitamin H	fish, milk, egg yolks, cereal, cabbage, broccoli, potatoes, dried fruits	fat and carbohydrate metabolism; hormone and cholesterol synthesis	
Vitamin B_5	Pantothenic acid Dexpanthenol	chicken, beef, fish, milk, eggs, cereals, cabbage, broccoli, potatoes	protein and carbohydrate metabolism; hormone and cholesterol synthesis	
Vitamin B_{12}	Cobalamin Cyanocobalamin Hydroxocobalamin	meat, eggs, milk, poultry, salmon, cod fish, algae	metabolism; red blood cell formation; nervous system functioning	
Vitamin C	Ascorbic acid Ascorbate	citrus fruits, berries, tomatoes, green vegetables, potatoes	bone, cartilage, muscle, and blood vessel formation; maintains teeth and gums; iron absorption; wound healing; antioxidant	
Vitamin D	Ergocalciferol (D2) Cholecalciferol (D3)	cheese; butter; fish; oysters; eggs; also made in the skin on exposure to sunlight	bone formation; promotes calcium absorption and regulates levels of calcium and phosphorus in the blood	
Vitamin E	Tocopherol	wheatgerm; nuts; seeds; green, leafy vegetables; vegetable oils; olives	antioxidant; red blood cell formation; metabolization of vitamin K	
Vitamin K	Phytomenadione Menaquinone	cabbage; cauliflower; spinach; soy products; also made by bacteria in the gut	blood clotting; bone strength	

Deficiency	Cautions	U.S. RDA*
progressive eye problems (including night blindness, xerophthalmia, keratomalacia, and blindness); skin disorders, diarrhea; (all rare in the Western world, but common in developing countries)	excess causes liver damage and weakens bones in women	Men: 900 mcg (3,000 IU) Women: 700 mcg (2,300 IU); 750–770 mcg (2,500–2,600 IU) if pregnant; 1,200–1,300 mcg (4,000–4,300 IU) if breastfeeding
beriberi	allergic reactions (rare); large doses may cause drowsiness; alcoholics are at risk for deficiency	Men: 1.2 mg Women: 1.1 mg; 1.4 mg if pregnant or breastfeeding
ariboflavinosis (fatigue, sore mouth, skin irritation, anaemia)	none	Men: 1.3 mg Women: 1.1 mg; 1.4 mg if pregnant; 1.6 mg if breastfeeding
pellagra, dermatitis, dementia, diarrhoea	serious allergic reactions (rare), skin flushing; other side-effects and inter-actions are common; alcoholics are at risk for deficiency; excess causes liver damage	None DRI** for adults: 16–18 mg
spina bifida in unborn children	excess may mask vitamin B_{12} deficiency	Men: 400 mcg Women: 400 mcg; 600 mcg if pregnant ; 500 mcg if breastfeeding
skin problems, mouth soreness, nerve damage (rare), convulsions (rare)	drug interactions are common; excess causes skin problems, nausea, headaches, and nerve damage	None
skin and tongue soreness, hair loss, impaired digestion, impaired nerve function	excess causes baldness, eye problems (rare); in children, excess causes retarded development and immune deficiencies	Men: 300 mcg Women: 300 mcg
headache, fatigue, abdominal pain, tingling in the extremities (all extremely rare)	excess causes diarrhoea, nausea, heartburn	None
anaemia, movement and gait disturbances, psychiatric symptoms, muscle weakness, vision problems	drug interactions are common; vegetarians and people with pernicious anaemia are at risk for deficiency	Men: 2.4 mcg Women: 2.4 mcg ; 2.6 mcg if pregnant; 2.8 mcg if breastfeeding
scurvy	excess causes diarrhoea, nausea, abdominal cramps, kidney stones	None DRI** Men: 90 mg Women: 75 mg; 85 mg if pregnant; 120mg if breastfeeding
weak bones, rickets, osteomalacia	drug interactions are common excess causes high blood calcium levels, bone loss, impaired kidney function	None Adequate intake: 5–10 mcg (200–400 IU)
nerve damage, blindness, heart rhythm disturbances, dementia (all rare)	excess causes increased bleeding, and rarely, diarrhoea, headache, blurred vision	Men: 15 mg (22.5 IU) Women: 15 mg (22.5 IU); 19mg (28.5 IU) if breastfeeding
reduced blood clotting, uncontrolled bleeding (all rare)	drug interactions, especially with warfarin; excess causes liver damage	None

*RDA: Recommended Daily Allowance, the daily dietary intake of a nutrient considered sufficient by the U.S. Food and Nutrition Board of the National Academy of Sciences to meet the requirements of nearly all healthy individuals in each life-stage.

**DRI: Dietary Reference Intake, determined by the Standing Committee on the Scientific Evaluation of Dietary Reference Intakes of the Food and Nutrition Board, Institute of Medicine, National Academy of Sciences, with help from Health Canada.

For information on plant-based supplements, including herbs, see Botanicals Therapy, pp.554–9; Probiotics, pp.550–1; and Omega-3 Supplements, pp.252–3.

Vitamins

Many vitamins are still popularly known by their original letter classifications, which were given before their chemical structure was understood. There are actually eight B vitamins: B_1, B_2, B_3, folate, B_5, B_6, biotin and B_{12}. Numbering gaps exist because some substances were discovered not to be vitamins.

Minerals

Many different minerals are present in foods. Some of those required by the body include:

• **CALCIUM** Vital for strong bones and teeth, this mineral also regulates muscle and heart contractions and helps with blood clotting. It is found in dairy foods, green leafy vegetables and the tiny edible bones of fish such as sardines. Calcium requires vitamin D for absorption. Adults need between 1,000 and 1,300 mg daily. Low intake may lead to osteoporosis (pp.146–7). Excess doses may cause abdominal pain, diarrhoea, or kidney stones.

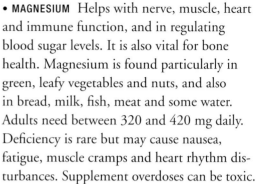

Fish oils, such as those found in salmon, have numerous health benefits including alleviating joint pain and reducing the risk of heart attack and stroke.

• **MAGNESIUM** Helps with nerve, muscle, heart and immune function, and in regulating blood sugar levels. It is also vital for bone health. Magnesium is found particularly in green, leafy vegetables and nuts, and also in bread, milk, fish, meat and some water. Adults need between 320 and 420 mg daily. Deficiency is rare but may cause nausea, fatigue, muscle cramps and heart rhythm disturbances. Supplement overdoses can be toxic.

• **IRON** Vital to the function of red blood cells in transporting oxygen around the body, iron is found in red meats, fish, poultry and legumes (lentils and beans). A deficit leads to iron-deficiency anaemia, which the World Health Organization (WHO) rates as the most common nutritional disorder in the world. Pre-menopausal women (because of menstrual blood loss and pregnancy) and children (because of high requirements) are most affected. Anaemia causes fatigue and impaired immunity in adults, and retardation of physical and intellectual growth in children. The RDA ranges from 8 mg daily in adult men to 27 mg per day for pregnant women. Excess iron, however, can be extremely toxic.

• **ZINC** This mineral plays many vital roles in the body, including growth, wound healing and immunity. It is found particularly in oysters and also in red meat and poultry. The RDA for adults ranges from 8 to 12 mg daily, and deficiency may result in growth retardation, delayed sexual maturation and impotence. Excess intake can affect iron and copper levels in the body, decrease immunity, and lower levels of HDL cholesterol (the beneficial variety).

Other Supplements

A vast array of nutritional and other supplements is now available. Some of the most popular and promising include:

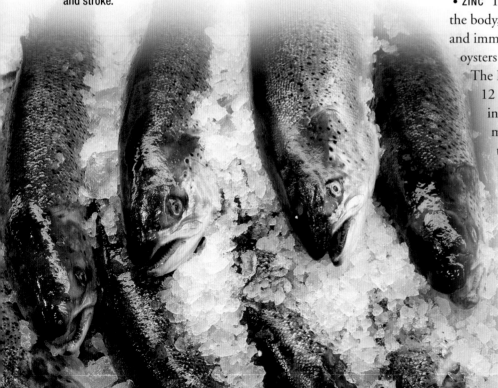

• **COENZYME Q10** This chemical is regarded by some nutritionists as a vitamin, even though it is manufactured in the body. Levels decrease with age and also, some nutritionists believe, in the presence of various chronic diseases, including high blood pressure, congestive heart failure, Alzheimer's disease, angina and breast cancer. However, there is so far little evidence of benefits from taking coenzyme Q_{10} supplements.

• **FISH OILS** The lack of heart disease among the Inuit people of Greenland, despite their enormously high fat intake, led to investigations of the protective effects of the high polyunsaturated fatty acid content of cold-water fish. Scientists found that oily fish contain two essential fatty acids (EFAs): eicosapentaenoic acid (EPA) and docosahexaenoic acid (DHA). These omega-3 fatty acids (pp.252–3) have many health benefits, including reducing heart attacks and strokes, and alleviating joint pain and inflammation. They are believed to be essential for brain growth and development in foetuses and babies. Fish oils, among the leading supplements sold in Europe, are usually obtained from the livers of white fish, typically cod or halibut, or from the flesh of oily fish such as sardines and salmon, which contains even higher amounts of EPA and DHA.

• **CHONDROITIN** A major constituent of joint cartilage, it is often taken as a supplement to relieve symptoms of arthritis, frequently in conjunction with glucosamine.

• **GLUCOSAMINE** Produced naturally in the body, glucosamine assists in the formation of joint cartilage. Good evidence suggests that patients with osteoarthritis in the knees may be able to take fewer anti-inflammatory drugs if they regularly consume glucosamine supplements.

• **MELATONIN** This hormone is produced naturally by the pineal gland in the brain in response to darkness, and is believed to be important in regulating the daily rhythms of bodily functions. It has been used to treat jet lag and sleep disturbances.

Fortified and Enriched Foods

Once it was recognized that many common diseases were due to vitamin or mineral deficiencies, it was a short step to attempting to correct or prevent nutritional shortcomings in the population as a whole by adding supplements to staple foods. A wide variety of common foods are now fortified, and in future, the practice may extend to measures to prevent the chronic degenerative diseases now so prevalent in Western societies, such as heart disease, osteoporosis and even cancer.

Many developing countries are now also adopting food fortification programmes to make up for poor nutrition among their populations. The minerals iron and iodine and vitamin A and iodine – the most common deficiencies – can be added to staple foods very cheaply. A programme to fortify sugar with vitamin A has been highly successful in Guatemala, for example, while in Venezuela cornflour is fortified with both vitamin A and iron.

The practice of supplementing foods with ingredients that are not present naturally is called fortification, while restoring nutrients lost during food processing is known as enrichment, although the distinction is not always recognized. Supplements are also sometimes used to standardize nutrient contents that can vary significantly due to seasonal fluctuations or different processing methods (for example, with vitamin C in orange juice), or to give alternative products similar nutrient values (for example, adding vitamins normally present in butter to margarine, or calcium to soy milk).

In addition, some foods have extra ingredients added to provide specific health benefits – for example, margarine-type spreads containing plant sterols and stanol esters, which lower cholesterol levels and so may help prevent heart disease. The amounts added are substantially higher than concentrations found naturally in plants.

Enzyme Replacement Therapy

A substance that speeds the rate of a biological reaction without being used up itself is called an enzyme. Enzymes are proteins produced throughout the body that facilitate many processes of metabolism and digestion. They are biological catalysts. Because all foodstuffs were once living tissue – meats or plants for example – they contain enzymes. These enzymes are responsible for fruit ripening, grain sprouting and meat ageing – and, ultimately, all of these things spoiling.

Practitioners of enzyme replacement therapy believe that modern techniques of food processing, storage and cooking remove or destroy the natural enzymes in food, just as they do many vitamins and minerals. They recommend eating more raw foods, and also taking replacement enzymes as supplements to improve digestion, and prevent or help treat a variety of chronic illnesses.

Papain, an enzyme derived from papaya is often used as a digestive aid and has been shown to have anti-inflammatory effects.

HISTORY

American physician and biochemist Edward Howell is known as the 'father of food enzymes'. His research in the 1930s and 1940s led him to believe that food enzymes are essential nutrients for digestion, but are destroyed by cooking and food processing. Typical Western diets lead to enzyme deficiencies, impaired digestion, nutritional imbalance and susceptibility to degenerative diseases.

In 1932, Howell started the National Enzyme Company, which remains the leading global supplier of digestive enzyme replacement products from its base in the United States.

Products may be obtained from various natural medicine clinics, some staffed by physicians, and from other practitioners, including some nutritionists and chiropractors, or purchased for self-treatment from outlets such as healthfood stores or the Internet.

PRACTICE

Enzymes that digest foods include proteases that digest protein, lipases that digest fats and amylases that digest carbohydrates. These enzymes initiate digestion in the mouth and stomach. For example, amylases in saliva begin digesting carbohydrates while they are

On Call

Food enzyme supplements are different from the single replacement enzymes used in conventional medicine to correct the few rare, usually hereditary disorders that are due to specific enzyme deficiencies. Enzyme replacement is also used to treat disorders such as chronic pancreatitis, where disease results in deficiency of normal enzyme output from the pancreas, and cystic fibrosis, in which pancreatic ducts become blocked by thick mucus so that vital pancreatic digestive enzymes cannot reach the intestines.

being chewed, and hydrochloric acid and pepsinogen, secreted in the stomach, initiate the protein digestion. However, the various enzymes needed for complete digestion of food are secreted in the small intestines, farther down the digestive tract. These digestive enzymes are also found in raw food, and while food is held in the stomach, the enzymes in that food can help start the process of digestion and reduce the body's need to produce digestive enzymes.

When these natural enzymes in foods are lacking, food is not properly digested and nutrients are not fully absorbed, leading to bloating and indigestion. Consequences include low energy, fatigue, mental slowness, poor circulation, impaired immunity, susceptibility to allergies and infections, degenerative diseases and a reduced life span.

Practitioners say enzyme supplements can offer increased vitality and youthfulness, strengthen immunity, ease weight loss, and alleviate fatigue, mood swings, depression, insomnia and sexual dysfunction. Patients with arthritis, fibromyalgia, acne, sinus problems, acid reflux and irritable bowel syndrome, heart disease, high cholesterol, low or high blood pressure, arteriosclerosis, osteoporosis, diabetes and colon cancer are also said to benefit.

TREATMENTS

In a consultation, a practitioner takes a detailed history of general health and dietary habits, and may do laboratory tests on blood or urine samples. Replacement digestive enzymes are selected according to the patient's profile and are sometimes combined with vitamins, minerals, fatty acids and other supplements. Some practitioners also advocate a raw food diet or juicing (p.544).

Supplementary enzymes are derived from plants, animals or microbes and may include proteases, lipases, amylases and glycases (for the digestion of sugars).

CAN ENZYME REPLACEMENT THERAPY HELP ME?

Only scant scientific evidence exists to support enzyme therapy. There is also no evidence that the amount of enzymes in foods affects the amount produced by the body, nor of any effect of enzyme production on life span.

- **Lactose intolerance** Lactase in some enzyme preparations may help people with lactose intolerance, an inability to digest milk sugar.

- There is little evidence that enzymes intended for digestive support have health benefits, but scientists have been investigating other specific enzymes, often derived from plants, for possible therapeutic actions.

- **Arthritis** Bromelain, a protease in pineapples, has anti-inflammatory properties that may ease osteoarthritis (pp.136–9). A study done at the University of Reading in Britain and published in *Phytomedicine* in 2002 showed that pain, stiffness, and physical function were significantly improved in 77 patients with mild acute knee pain who took bromelain. They also reported enhanced overall psychological well-being.

- **Rheumatic diseases**. A preparation containing bromelain, trypsin (an enzyme secreted by the pancreas) and rutoside (a flavonoid antioxidant found in several plant species), is as effective as the non-steroidal anti-inflammatory drug (NSAID) diclofenac in reducing pain and joint-swelling in patients with osteoarthritis, according to a study published in 2001 in the *Journal of the Association of Physicians of India*. In Herne, Germany, analysis of records of 2,139 patients with various rheumatic diseases treated over two years revealed that those given this preparation were more likely to experience symptom relief and had far fewer side-effects than those treated with a conventional NSAID.

- **Burns** According to a study published in *Burns* in 1999, papaya pulp, a traditional burn dressing in many parts of Africa, is effective in treating even serious burns in children, helping to speed healing, prevent infection and promote a wound surface that is suitable for skin grafting.

Juice Therapy

The theory behind juice therapy, also known as juicing, is that breaking down much of the fibre in fruit and vegetables allows the body to more efficiently extract the vitamins, minerals and other nutrients in these healthy foods. As well as avoiding the nutrient losses that can occur when food is processed and cooked, juicing raw or 'live' fruit and vegetables concentrates nutrients and enables easy absorption and rapid entry into the bloodstream. Juice therapy is said to promote general health and fitness, boost immunity, aid weight loss, and prevent or contribute to healing many diseases.

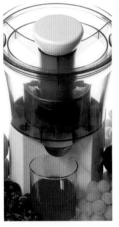

There are several types of juicer. Get advice from a local healthfood store about the best model for your purposes.

HISTORY

The health benefits of consuming fruit and vegetable juices have been known for centuries, and juicing is often advocated by naturopaths and other practitioners who give dietary advice. Juicing was popularized again in the early 1990s, with the publication of many books on juicing. Since then, juice extractors have become increasingly common in many households and juice bars have sprung up in many areas.

PRACTICE

Juicing helps the body absorb all the nutrients from fruits and vegetables. It also enables people to eat more vegetables than they might in a normal diet. Practitioners recommend mixing the pulp produced by juicing back into the juice and consuming it, to make sure the diet has sufficient fibre.

TREATMENTS

Juice must be freshly prepared from raw, organic fruit and vegetables, because commercially processed juices do not offer the same benefits. Almost any fruit or vegetable may be juiced. Popular ingredients include wheat grass, carrot, banana, citrus fruits and berries. Specific juices may be recommended to treat or prevent specific health problems (see *Can Juice Therapy Help Me?*).

CAN JUICE THERAPY HELP ME?

As well as general benefits, some juices have individual therapeutic effects, some of which have been validated by medical studies.

- **Fasting** A juice fast is often advocated leading into and after a total fast. Juice fasts may yield a very low calorie diet, promoting weight loss, and are also believed to detoxify the body, promoting healing from a variety of ailments. No significant research demonstrates any benefit from fasting or that detoxification occurs; more research is needed. (If you have a pre-existing condition or take medications, a medical practitioner should be consulted before fasting.)

- **Cardiovascular disease** Tomato juice and other tomato products, such as tomato sauce, may help prevent cardiovascular disease.

- **Stomach ulcers** Researchers from Johns Hopkins University in Baltimore, Maryland, reported in 2002 that compounds from broccoli and brussel sprouts may help to eliminate *H. pylori* bacterium, which causes ulcers (p.276).

- **Urinary infections** Cranberry juice is helpful in preventing and perhaps in treating urinary tract infections (page 302–3).

- **Cancer** Pomegranate juice may prevent or slow the growth of prostate cancer (pp.430–1); further studies are needed.

Flower Essences

The idea of flower essences is that diseases of the body come about as a result of negative emotional states. Remedies that are made from flowers are believed to contain the energy of plants and act to restore inner balance and harmony, thus enabling the body to heal itself. They are often used to treat psychological problems or physical problems made worse by stress and anxiety, or mental shock following traumatic physical or emotional events.

HISTORY

The use of flower essences has a history as long as that of botanicals therapy (pp.552–9). The current remedies were developed in the 1930s by Edward Bach, a British doctor, bacteriologist and homeopath. Each of the 38 Bach Flower Remedies he described is intended to deal with a particular emotional state or personality pattern. Bach's work is still being taught and practiced at the Dr Edward Bach Centre in England.

The flowers are picked at their peak of vitality, and are then left in the sun or boiled. The extracted essence is then filtered and diluted with spring water, and preserved with brandy to make a mother tincture.

Bach's remedies are based on English flowering plants; other flower essences have since been developed that use plants in other parts of the world. Richard Katz, a herbologist who founded the Flower Essence Society in California in 1979, added North American plants. There is also a range of Australian flower essences.

PRACTICE

Flower essences do not treat physical complaints directly; rather, each treats a particular emotional imbalance. They can be used alone or in combination.

A practitioner selects essences after talking with a patient. Both their current emotional state and general personality are considered.

Up to six remedies may be taken at once. The mixture is diluted in mineral water and placed on the tongue, or mixed into a beverage.

TREATMENTS

The best-known flower essence is Rescue Remedy, a combination of five other Bach flower remedies (impatiens, rock rose, clematis, cherry plum and star of Bethlehem) that are intended for emergencies, to alleviate the after-effects of shock following acute physical or mental trauma. This may be taken either diluted in water, to be sipped at intervals or, in an acute crisis, dropped directly from the stock bottle onto the tongue.

CAN FLOWER ESSENCES HELP ME?

There are no data from rigorous clinical trials that show the efficacy of flower essences. However, conditions in which flower essences may be used include:

- **Anxiety** A study of 61 people in Germany published in the *Journal of Anxiety Disorders* in 2001 found that levels of anxiety reduced significantly in their test subjects, but this was the same as the result for a control group.

- **Psychological problems** The flower essences are said to help improve a range of negative mental states and personality traits, such as nervousness, indecision, despair, irritability, guilt and the inability to cope.

Orthomolecular Medicine

A branch of nutritional medicine, orthomolecular medicine focuses on manipulating the body's biochemistry through nutrition, particularly by taking large quantities of vitamin supplements to maintain optimal health and equip the body to fight disease.

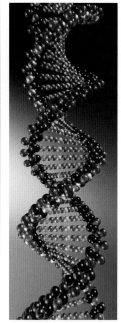

Orthomolecular medicine focuses on the manipulation of the body biochemistry through nutrition.

Practitioners of orthomolecular medicine believe a person's internal biochemical environment is partly determined by genetics and partly influenced by the environment, and varies considerably among between individuals. Specific biochemical imbalances may cause or contribute to many chronic conditions. The prefix ortho means 'straight' and the term orthomolecular means the therapy corrects these imbalances at a molecular level, returning the body's internal environment to an optimal state.

This is generally achieved using supplements of substances that are normally found in the body – vitamins, minerals, enzymes, amino acids and essential fatty acids. Practitioners may also use other natural substances, such as shark cartilage. In addition, some treatments may involve restricting the diet or removing toxins from the body.

Although some treatments that are used in orthomolecular medicine are regarded as unorthodox, its principles form the mainstay of conventional treatment for a variety of deficiency diseases and metabolic disorders.

CAUTION

Although popularly perceived as natural and free from side-effects, large quantities of vitamin supplements may have toxic effects – especially vitamins A, D and E and, to a lesser extent, vitamin C and nicotinic acid. High doses should only be taken under strict medical supervision.

HISTORY

The term 'orthomolecular' was coined by double Nobel laureate Dr Linus Pauling in the article 'Orthomolecular Psychiatry', published in *Science* in 1968. Pauling had previously contributed to discovering the cause of sickle-cell anaemia, the first condition to be described as a molecular disease. He later became interested in molecular influences on mental function, and subsequently in the biochemistry of nutrition. He defined the broader discipline of orthomolecular medicine as "the preservation of good health and the treatment of disease by varying the concentration in the human body of substances that are normally present in the body."

Pauling was particularly fascinated by the properties of vitamin C (ascorbic acid). His book, *Vitamin C and the Common Cold,* published in 1970, became a best-seller and did much to popularize vitamin supplementation. He began to examine the potential protective effects of high doses of vitamin C against conditions, including influenza, cardiovascular disease and ageing. In 1979, he and his colleagues published an article in *Cancer Research* examining its possible anti-cancer properties.

The Linus Pauling Institute of Science and Medicine was founded by Pauling and his colleagues after his retirement from Stanford University in 1973, to conduct research of and provide education about orthomolecular medicine. He continued to work there until 1992. Although Pauling believed that orthomolecular medicine should constitute an important part of standard medical practice,

CAN ORTHOMOLECULAR MEDICINE HELP ME?

The quality of evidence available in support of orthomolecular treatments varies considerably, with research results showing a definite benefit for some supplements, while others are more controversial. Treatments for cancer and schizophrenia, for example, have not been scientifically proven to be effective.

- **Osteoarthritis** Supplements of glucosamine and chondroitin (normal constituents of joint cartilage) are effective in relieving symptoms of osteoarthritis.

- **Diabetes** A study conducted at the University of Puerto Rico and published in 2004 in *Puerto Rico Health Science Journal* found that an orthomolecular supplement combination of vitamins, minerals and herbs taken for 30 days successfully reduced fasting blood glucose levels in 15 patients who had uncontrolled type 2 diabetes. Preliminary results from Japan have found that tungstate, a natural supplement, may also effectively regulate diabetes.

- **Autism** According to a review of 12 studies published in the *Journal of Autism and Developmental Disorders* in 1995, a majority of the studies reported favourable results from taking supplements of vitamin B$_6$ and magnesium in patients with autism.

the public enthusiasm for vitamins and other micronutrients was not always matched by the medical profession.

PRACTICE

Orthomolecular medicine is offered by a variety of healthcare professionals, including nutritionists, naturopaths, some chiropractors and some doctors. The nature of a consultation varies accordingly, and usually includes detailed questions about medical history, symptoms and diet. Blood, urine, and hair samples may be taken for testing.

Some practitioners recommend immediate supplementation and dietary changes, to be adjusted as necessary when the test results

come back. Practitioners usually recommend that patients follow a high-protein, low-carbohydrate diet in addition to whatever supplements are recommended. Follow-up assessment after a couple of months is usually advised. The aim is generally to achieve levels of vitamins, minerals and their derivatives in the body that are comparable with those found in healthy young people.

Many people take supplements on their own, without consultation (see Supplements, Vitamins & Minerals, pp.532–41), but orthomolecular medicine is practised under the guidance of a healthcare professional.

TREATMENTS

Supplements are tailored to the patient's individual biochemical profile and to any current health problems, with the aim of correcting any imbalances in vitamins, minerals and other body constituents – usually with doses in excess of those recommended as standard nutritional intake. Practitioners may also recommend other supplements, such as glucosamine for joint pain. If patients are found to have an excess of certain components, or evidence of vascular disease, treatments such as chelation therapy (pp.576–7) may be recommended to clear the bloodstream.

Many people take supplements on their own initiative, without any consultation. For more information, see Supplements, Vitamins & Minerals (pp.532–41).

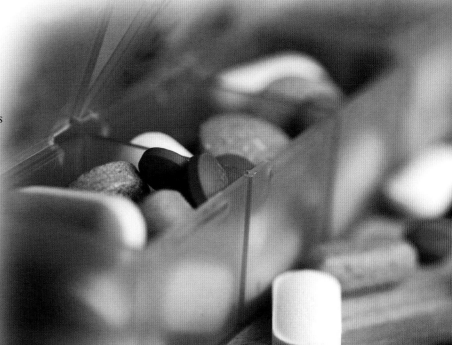

Aromatherapy

The use of aromatic plants and plant extracts, called essential oils, to promote health and well-being is known as aromatherapy or aromatic medicine. This therapy works primarily through smell, one of the oldest and most primitive of our senses because it is closely linked with the limbic system—the brain's emotional centre.

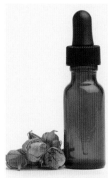

Essential oils are very concentrated and therefore require large quantities of plant material to make.

Aromatherapy has been used to aid relaxation, improve mood, reduce stress and anxiety, and alleviate symptoms of various diseases. In addition, essential oils applied to the skin may be absorbed and have physical effects in the body, and they are often used in massage therapy (pp.468–73).

Commercial oils are usually produced by steam distillation and require huge quantities of plant material – about 2,000 kg (4,400 lb) of rose petals is needed to produce 1 kg (2.2 lb) of rose oil, for example – which is why the pure oils are very expensive. Because they are so concentrated, oils are almost never used undiluted, but are mixed into a carrier oil, usually a simple vegetable oil.

HISTORY

Plant oils have been used for their healing powers for thousands of years and are an integral part of many traditional systems of medicine, including Ayurveda (pp.451–4) in India and Traditional Chinese Medicine (pp.446–50). Essential oils were used by healers in ancient Egypt, Greece and the Roman Empire. In medieval Europe, they were used to ward off plague, and in World War I to help treat burns and skin infections in the pre-antibiotic era.

The word 'aromatherapy' was introduced in the early 20th century by a French chemist, René-Maurice Gattefossé. It comes from the Greek words *aroma* (which means 'pleasant smell') and *therapeia* ('healing'). Gattefossé accidentally burned his arm while working in a perfume factory, and drenched the burn in lavender oil that happened to be nearby. He was so impressed by the resulting pain relief and rapid healing that he began studying the therapeutic potential of essential oils. His book was *Gattefosse's Aromatherapy*, first published in 1937, which is still in print today.

PRACTICE

Essential oils are volatile, which means that they evaporate easily – hence the ready transmission of fragrance to the nose. Their precise mode of aromatherapy action is not entirely understood, but signals from the nose travel directly to two structures deep in the brain, the amygdala and the hippocampus, that are intimately involved in emotional memory and may influence alertness, hormone release and other key pathways in the body.

A aromatherapy consultation will typically last at least an hour and include detailed questions about general health. Usually therapy is carried out as part of a massage, using a blend of oils selected to match the patient's needs.

CAUTION

Essential oils can be poisonous; they should not be taken internally, and should be stored well out of the reach of children. In addition, some essential oils, such as peppermint and eucalyptus, can cause skin rashes or chemical burns if applied undiluted. Always consult a qualified healthcare practitioner before using essential oils and follow directions carefully before applying to the skin.

CAN AROMATHERAPY HELP ME?

Many of the suggested uses of aromatherapy are unproven, and much research is preliminary. However mounting evidence suggests that aromatherapy may be effective in alleviating the symptoms of a variety of conditions and that its beneficial effects on mood and relaxation can often help people cope with the effects of serious illness.

- **Stress, anxiety and insomnia**. Lavender oil may aid insomnia and relieve stress and anxiety.
- **Arthritis** A blend of essential oils may decrease pain and depression in patients with arthritis.
- **Bronchitis** Aromatherapy significantly improves mucus clearance for up to an hour after treatment in patients with chronic bronchitis.
- **Fungal infection** Lemongrass oil suppresses fungal growth in the laboratory, supporting its use as a treatment for candida (thrush) infections.
- **Alopecia** Daily scalp massage with essential oils may improve the patchy hair loss characteristic of the autoimmune disease alopecia areata.
- **Infections** Researchers from Britain's Manchester University reported in 2004 that certain essential oils could kill a wide range of bacteria and fungi, including types of bacteria that are resistant to antibiotics. In future, these essential oils could be blended into formulas such as soaps or shampoos to help counteract dangerous hospital-acquired infections.
- **Constipation** In a small study at the College of Nursing Keimyung University in Korea, published in 2005, abdominal massage with rosemary, lemon, and peppermint oils produced significantly greater improvement in constipation in elderly patients than massage alone.
- **Epilepsy** Aromatherapy has been used in conjunction with hypnosis (pp.508–13) to teach people to associate a particular scent with relaxation. Some people with epilepsy are able to prevent a seizure from developing by sniffing their chosen essential oil at the first warning signs.
- **Immunity** Massage with various essential oils may boost lymphocyte count, one measure of immunity.
- **Cancer** Aromatherapy massage can reduce anxiety in cancer patients and perhaps lessen some physical symptoms, although more research is needed.
- **Childbirth** Aromatherapy has been reported to reduce the number of interventions required in childbirth and increase satisfaction with the experience of labour.
- **Dementia** Aromatherapy, especially combined with massage, may reduce agitation and disturbed behaviour, and promote sleep among people with severe dementia.
- **Menopause** Aromatherapy has been reported to produce significant improvements in menopausal symptoms.

At home, essential oils can also be applied to the body, chest, stomach, or temples, or they can be inhaled, diffused in a vaporizer, or a few drops can be added to bathwater.

TREATMENTS

Of the enormous number of essential oils available, some are especially popular. For instance, the herb chamomile has been used traditionally for centuries, especially to promote relaxation, aid sleep, ease infant colic, and help skin conditions. Other oils thought to promote relaxation include geranium, lavender and jasmine.

Peppermint and its menthol extract are well-known as digestive aids. They are also stimulating, as is eucalyptus oil, which is traditionally used to ease breathing and reduce the congestion caused by upper respiratory infections; it is a common ingredient in over-the-counter cough and cold remedies.

Lemon, vanilla and rosemary oils are considered revitalizing; tea tree oil has antiseptic properties.

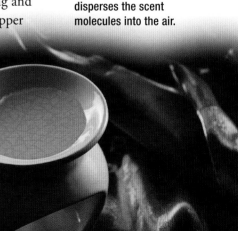

In a diffuser, a small candle heats a mixture of water and a herb's essential oil. The heat disperses the scent molecules into the air.

Probiotics

Many of the bacteria that naturally live in the human gut aid digestion and protect the intestinal lining. These 'friendly bacteria', or probiotics, may also stimulate the immune system and may help to keep potentially harmful microorganisms in check, both through simple competition for a limited supply of nutrients and possibly by producing substances that inhibit the growth of other organisms.

HISTORY

Health claims for foods such as fermented milk date back to biblical times. With the discovery of microorganisms in the late 19th and early 20th centuries, microbiologists came to realize that the range of intestinal microflora (tiny organisms present in the gut) of healthy people was different to that of those who were ill. Giving the ill people some of the bacterial cultures they were missing was found to be helpful in treating symptoms such as diarrhoea, and such effects began to be attributed to alterations in the balance of intestinal flora and enhanced resistance to disease.

The term 'probiotic' (meaning 'for life') was first used in 1965 to refer to substances secreted by one microorganism that stimulate the growth of another. Over time, its meaning was broadened to encompass any product that contains live microorganisms that alter the microflora of a host animal and are beneficial for health.

PRACTICE

Disturbances in the intestines can reduce the population of some probiotic bacteria and cause the overgrowth of others, along with inflammation, infection and digestive disturbances. These consequences may be prevented or alleviated by taking probiotics from outside sources. Probiotics are found in foods including cultured milk products such as yogurt, and can be taken as supplements in capsule, tablet, powder or liquid form. Some probiotics are inserted into the vagina (usually to treat yeast infections) or applied to the skin.

Probiotic organisms feed on undigestible carbohydrates called prebiotics, stimulating the growth and activity of beneficial bacteria of the intestinal flora. Prebiotics include complex sugars and foods such as raw milk, bananas, garlic, miso and tempeh. Prebiotics stimulate the growth of probiotics and suppress the growth of potentially harmful organisms. Supplements that combine prebiotics and probiotics are called synbiotics.

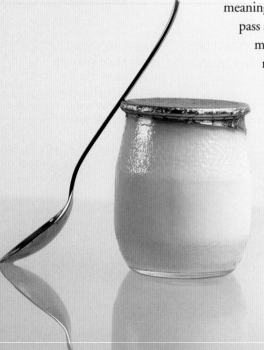

Probiotics are found in some foods, especially cultured milk products such as yogurt, and can be taken separately as supplements in capsule, tablet, powder or liquid forms. Sometimes probiotics are inserted into the vagina (primarily to control yeast infections) or put on the skin.

On Call

By killing off beneficial microorganisms as well as disease-causing ones, antibiotic treatment may have detrimental effects on the body's microflora balance. In particular, they may promote conditions such as diarrhoea and vaginal candida (yeast) infections. Probiotics have been suggested as a way to counteract this by repopulating the intestinal tract and other areas with 'good bacteria'. In addition, they may have helpful effects in fighting infections when antibiotics do not work because bacteria have become resistant to them.

CAN PROBIOTICS HELP ME?

Probiotics and prebiotics have been tested in an increasing range of conditions.

- **Allergies** According to a study from the Academy of Sciences of the Czech Republic published in 2003 in *International Archives of Allergy and Immunology,* premature infants given a probiotic *Escherichia coli* strain to colonize the intestine after birth had a significantly reduced incidence of repeated infections and allergies (p.262) 10 years later. Another group of full-term infants were shown to have a lower incidence of allergies after 20 years.

- **Bottle-feeding** Supplementing infant formulas with a prebiotic mixture of GOS and FOS to stimulate intestinal bifidobacteria and lactobacilli produces changes in stool characteristics of bottle-fed infants, making them more like those of breast-fed infants, according to a review from the University of Ferrara, Italy, published in 2005 in *Acta Paediatrica, Supplement.* These prebiotics appear to have beneficial effects on intestinal flora and immune function similar to those provided by human breast milk.

- **Eczema** Administration of a lactobacillus strain to at-risk newborns reduces the incidence of atopic eczema (pp.102–3) up to age four, according to a trial at the University of Turku, Finland, published in *The Lancet* in 2003.

- **Dental cavities** Just as they exert beneficial effects on microflora in the intestinal tract, probiotics may play a role in combating dental disease. Preliminary evidence suggests that some species of lactobacilli and bifidobacteria may inhibit mouth bacteria such as streptococci, which may be involved in cavity formation (pp.86–7).

- **Diarrhoea** There is good evidence that probiotics reduce diarrhoea (p.268) associated with antibiotic treatment, rotavirus infection and chemotherapy, and some evidence that they help in preventing or reducing the duration of traveller's diarrhoea.

- **Stomach ulcers** There is some evidence that probiotics reduce the incidence of *Helicobacter pylori* infection, which causes the majority of gastric ulcers (p.276).

- **Gastrointestinal disorders** According to a review in the *Journal of Clinical Gastroenterology* in 2003, controlled clinical studies have demonstrated the efficacy of probiotics in maintaining remission of ulcerative colitis (pp.266–7), and in treating Crohn's disease (pp.266–7). More research is needed to definitively establish the role of probiotics in the treatment of irritable bowel disease (pp.270–1).

- **Colon cancer** Preliminary evidence suggests that probiotics not only stimulate immunity but also reduce levels of potentially cancer-causing chemicals in the colon.

- **Rheumatoid arthritis** Probiotics may help in rheumatoid arthritis (pp.136–9), possibly due to their beneficial effects in reducing inflammation and boosting immunity.

- **High blood pressure** According to Japanese research published in the *Journal of the American College of Nutrition* in 2005, people with hypertension who took tablets of powdered fermented milk containing a lactobacillus species experienced blood pressure reductions after four weeks' therapy, although more research is needed.

Naturopaths, nutritionists and some conventional physicians may recommend probiotics. Many food manufacturers promote products containing probiotics, especially live cultures in yogurts. Probiotic foods and supplements are popular as self-help measures.

TREATMENTS

Many different species of bacteria have been found to have probiotic properties, including acidophilus, lactobacillus bulgaricus, bifido- bacteria and lactobacilli, and the yeast saccharomyces. Even some strains of E. coli – often a harmless component of gut flora but that is sometimes associated with infection – have been noted to be probiotic.

In addition, prebiotic mixtures of fructo-oligosaccharides (FOS) and galacto-oligo-saccharides (GOS) stimulate the growth of intestinal bifidobacteria and lactobacilli and reduce the growth of potentially harmful microorganisms, improving colon function.

Botanicals Therapy

Using plant-based remedies to maintain health and cure disease may be the oldest healing practice in the world. Botanicals therapy is a substantial component of most traditional healing systems, and there is a custom of 'folk medicine' in most societies, with knowledge of healing herbs handed down through the generations. Botanicals therapy encompasses herbal medicine (herbalism), eating plant foods that have medicinal value, and taking dietary supplements (pp.532–41) intended to give the benefits of specific food components, such as vitamins and minerals. Foods with therapeutic powers are sometimes called functional foods, or nutraceuticals.

Although herbal remedies are now often regarded as alternative medicines, the modern drug industry owes its origins to attempts to isolate and purify the compounds in plants that are responsible for their healing properties. Many modern medicines – aspirin, morphine, quinine and the heart drug digitalis among them – were derived directly from plants. Many more are the result of the synthesis of chemical ingredients first taken from botanical sources.

As modern medical science developed over the past century, it became heavily dependent on the growing pharmaceutical industry and attention paid to the original sources of many drugs waned. But now that there is growing scientific evidence of the efficacy of plant-based remedies, there has been renewed interest in herbalism.

Estimates suggest that there are between a quarter and half a million flowering plant species on the planet, of which fewer than 1 in 100 have been subjected to detailed chemical analysis. It is believed that only a tiny fraction of the potentially therapeutic plants have so far been identified. Researchers are increasingly curious about the possibilities of novel medicines developed from the active ingredients – called phytochemicals – of both known and as-yet-undiscovered plant sources.

In addition, there is growing general awareness of the importance of nutritional influences in the genesis of illness and in maintaining good health. Studies both between and within populations have shown dramatic differences in the incidence of various diseases that appear to be related to dietary factors.

In addition to the use of botanicals therapy to treat specific symptoms – for example, headache or depression – many herbs and plant-based foods are being shown to have properties that are potentially useful for treating or preventing illness, especially

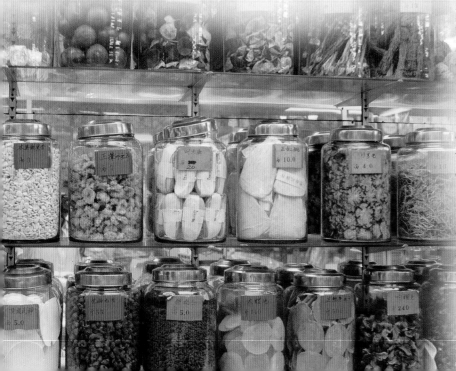

Botanicals therapy has existed for millennia in virtually every human culture. Traditional Chinese Medicine dates back over five thousand years ago.

Clinical Query

How can I tell whether an herbal medicine has been approved as safe to use?

Generally, you do not have the same level of assurance for herbal medicines as you do with prescription drugs – for which, in most countries, extensive evidence of safety and efficacy must be presented before the drug is allowed onto the market.

In the United States, herbs and other botanicals are now defined as dietary supplements, which means the FDA has only limited powers of regulation. Responsibility for determining safety lies largely with manufacturers, but the FDA can take action if the manufacturers make false or misleading claims, and has the power to ban products believed to pose unreasonable risks. For example, in 2004 it prohibited the sale of products containing the herb ephedra *(Ephedra vulgaris)*. (For more information on regulations governing dietary supplements, see pp.538–9).

In Europe, the European Union Directive on Traditional Herbal Medicinal Products requires that all herbal medicines for sale must be regulated for safety and quality, although existing manufacturers have a seven-year transition period (starting in 2005) in which to submit data for registration approval to the Medicines and Health care Products Regulatory Agency (MHRA). Similar regulations are being put in place in all European Union countries.

HISTORY

Botanicals therapy has existed for millennia in virtually every human culture, and even some animals have been observed seeking out healing plants. It is the oldest form of healing known, probably dating to prehistoric times when early humans learned through trial and error that some plants were edible while some were poisonous, and noted that some were helpful in alleviating injuries and ailments. Healing plants formed the basis of most medical systems before the development of modern pharmaceuticals.

The medicinal properties of plants were written about in Mesopotamia (now Iraq) more than 5,000 years ago. Archaeological excavation has uncovered clay tablets written by the ancient Sumerians describing the use of healing herbs.

Traditional Chinese Medicine (TCM, pp.446–50), which includes a large body of herbalist knowledge, dates back to around the same period. Possibly the first book on the subject, the *Pen Tsao Ching* (*Divine Husbandman's Materia Medica*), attributed to the emperor Shen Nung, described 365 medicinal minerals, animals and plants, including ma huang (ephedra), from which the drug ephedrine (commonly used as a decongestant) is derived.

About 4,000 years ago, medicinal herbs were described in the sacred scripts of ancient India, called the *Vedas*. Herbalism is also a primary component of traditional Indian medicine, Ayurveda (pp.451–4), and there is evidence that by 800 B.C.E., practitioners were using more than 500 healing plants.

The ancient Greeks were also familiar with botanical medicine. The Greek physician Hippocrates (ca. 460–375 B.C.E.), who is sometimes regarded as the father of modern medicine, advocated the use of willow bark for rheumatism (many centuries later, scientific analysis of the active ingredient, salicylic acid, led to the development of aspirin).

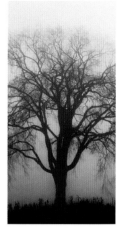

Hippocrates advocated the use of willow bark for rheumatism. Many centuries later, scientific analysis of the active ingredient led to the invention of aspirin.

the chronic degenerative diseases that plague modern civilizations. For example, the consumption of fruit and vegetables appears to play a strongly protective role against heart disease (pp.230–3), stroke (pp.168–9), hypertension (pp.236–9), high cholesterol, diabetes (pp.338–41), diverticulitis (p.285), cataracts (pp.34–5), macular degeneration (a common cause of vision loss, pp.40–1), as well as various cancers.

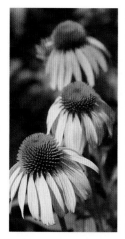

Echinacea is used as an ingredient in many cold preparations because it stimulates the immune system. It may also help combat urinary and vaginal yeast infections, and is often used topically to treat wounds.

CAN BOTANICALS THERAPY HELP ME?

As well as thousands of years of experience in many different healing systems, there is increasing scientific evidence that many botanical treatments are effective.

- **Headache and migraine** Feverfew has become increasingly popular as a migraine, preventative, although evidence from formal trials is inconclusive. In one German study published in *Cephalalgia* in 2005, treatment for 16 weeks produced significant reductions in migraine attack frequency, on average by almost two attacks per month, with few side-effects.

- **Depression** In a study at Massachusetts General Hospital in Boston, published in 2005 in the *Journal of Clinical Psychopharmacology,* St John's wort proved to be significantly more effective than the antidepressant fluoxetine, while a review in *Evidence Based Mental Health* in 2005 showed it to be at least as effective as the drug paroxetine.

- **Dementia** Gingko biloba has been found to improve brain function in Alzheimer's almost as much as conventional medication, but with fewer side-effects. According to one analysis published in *Pharmacopsychiatry* in 2003, ginkgo extract produced significant improvements in cognitive function in patients with early Alzheimer's and multi-site dementia.

- **Arthritis** According to a 2005 Cochrane Collaboration review, convincing evidence exist that unsaponifiables, active ingredients in avocados and soybeans, have beneficial effects on pain, functioning, and the number of non-steroidal anti-inflammatory drugs (NSAIDs) required by patients with osteoarthritis, without serious side-effects. In addition, devil's claw *(Harpagophytum procumbens)* has been found to be as effective as NSAIDs in treating arthritis pain.

- **Claudication** A review of multiple clinical trials published in *Atherosclerosis* in 2005 concluded that *ginkgo biloba* is an effective treatment for intermittent claudication due to peripheral vascular disease.

- **Respiratory infections.** Some limited evidence supports the use of echinacea to ease symptoms of the common cold.

- **Eczema** Chinese herbal medicines have received considerable publicity for their beneficial effects on eczema (pp.102–3). According to a review by the Cochrane

Database published in 2005, one mixed herbal preparation called Zemaphyte improved skin damage, redness, and itching, and helped ease sleep disturbance in patients with atopic eczema, although further trials were recommended. However, the product is no longer manufactured.

- **Prostate problems** According to two reviews published in the Cochrane Database in 2005, both saw palmetto *(Sarenoa serrulata)* extract and pygeum *(Pygeum africanum)* have beneficial effects on urinary tract symptoms that may accompany prostate enlargement in older men. The benefits of saw palmetto are comparable with those seen with the prescription drug finasteride, with fewer adverse effects.

- **Childbirth** Raspberry leaf *(Rubus idaeus)* tea is said to make childbirth easier and swifter if drunk in increasing doses in the later stages of pregnancy. There is little supporting research, but two small studies from Australia, published in *Australian Collective of Midwives Inc.* journal in 1999 and in 2001 in the *Journal of Midwifery and Women's Health,* found some evidence to support beneficial effects. The first showed that women taking raspberry leaf products had shorter labours, with no adverse effects for either mother or baby. Raspberry leaf also reduced the likelihood of pre-term and post-mature labour, and women taking it were less likely to have artificial rupture of the membranes, caesarean section, or forceps or vacuum deliveries than women in the control group. The other study found that raspberry leaf tablets shortened only the second stage of labour, but did result in a lower rate of forceps intervention.

- **Menopause** Several herbal and nutritional products contain ingredients that act like the female hormone oestrogen, and so are known as phytoestrogens. Although research is limited, soy-based foods and extracts, which are phytoestrogenic, and herbs such as black cohosh *(Cimicifuga racemosa),* not a phytoestrogen, are frequently recommended to alleviate symptoms such as hot flushes. According to a review from the Department of Obstetrics and Gynecology at the University of Illinois College of

Medicine, published in 2005 in the *Journal of Women's Health,* black cohosh is safe and effective in reducing menopausal symptoms, primarily hot flushes and possibly mood disturbances; phytoestrogen extracts such as soy and red clover *(Trifolium pratense)* seem to have only minimal effects. St John's wort was also effective for menopause-related mood changes.

- **Stroke** *Ginkgo biloba* promotes the increase of brain blood flow and uptake of glucose, and there is limited evidence that it may help in the treatment of acute ischemic stroke (pp.168–9). Further research is needed into its use in recovery after a stroke has ended.

- **Cancer** Many herbs and dietary supplements are said to have cancer-preventing or therapeutic effects. There is increasing interest in investigating botanical agents for their potential anti-cancer value, and several are believed to have proven merit. The drug Taxol, for example, is a synthetic version of a compound originally derived from the Pacific yew tree *(Taxus brevifolia),* and is now used to treat ovarian and advanced breast cancer. Other botanicals attracting interest include the following:

    Maitake mushroom *(Grifola frondosa)* is often used in Japan and is increas ingly popular among cancer patients in the West. An ingredient called beta glucans is believed to have anti-tumor properties, and limited evidence suggests it may induce tumor regression in some patients with breast, lung, or liver cancers.

    Shiitake mushroom *(Lentinus edodes)* is popular as a health food in Japan, and may stimulate cellular immunity and inhibit tumor growth. However there is little evidence of efficacy in patients, and many people have allergic reactions to it.

Mistletoe *(Viscum album)* has been used medicinally since antiquity. It contains ingredients that may stimulate the immune system to fight cancers. It has been tested on several types of cancer but results are inconclusive.

Turmeric *(Curcuma longa)* is a spice that has been associated with a lower risk of colon cancer among individuals who consume it regularly. The effect is believed to be due to the pigment curcumin, which gives turmeric its yellow colour.

Propolis is a resinous substance collected from tree buds by bees. It may have protective effects against inflammation and skin damage due to radiation, and against heart muscle damage from chemotherapy. There are currently investigations into the anti-cancer properties of propolis to test whether it can enhance the effects of radiation treatment of cancer in humans.

Cabbage and other cruciferous vegetables such as broccoli, contains chemicals called isothiocyanates that may have anti-tumour effects. According to a study published in *The Lancet* in 2005, regular consumption – at least once a week – can cut lung cancer risk for people with particular genetic patterns found in about 70 percent of the population.

Astragalus *(Astragalus membranaceous),* used in Traditional Chinese Medicine, it is said to have immune stimulating and anti-cancer properties. There is little scientific support for this.

Hippocrates believed in the importance of diet, fresh air and proper rest in helping the body harness its 'life force' to heal itself. He wrote, "Let food be thy medicine, and medicine be thy food."

In the first century C.E., Pedanius Dioscorides, a Greek physician, compiled his famous *De Materia Medica* (*On Medical Matters*), five volumes that list more than 500 healing plants. It remained an important reference work on herbs for 16 centuries and was one of the earliest works to be produced in book form following the invention of the printing press in the 15th century.

Herbalism was extensively practised in the monasteries of medieval Europe. Monks were often called upon by local people to heal the sick, frequently maintained their own herb gardens, and preserved the knowledge of many earlier manuscripts on herbalism by copying out the texts. Folk medicine also thrived in the villages, with

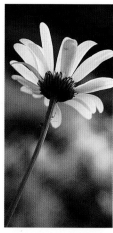

Chamomille is included in many cold preparations for its actions in stimulating the immune system. It may also help combat urinary and vaginal yeast infections, and has been used topically to treat wounds.

many 'wise women' who were knowledgeable about healing plants eventually becoming the target of witch-hunts. Between the 15th and the 17th centuries, many other 'herbals' (guides to the medicinal use of herbs) were printed, and traditional knowledge on the subject became more widely available. The first English volume was *Grete Herball,* by an unknown author, in 1526. Nicholas Culpeper's classic, *The English Physician Enlarged,* was published in 1653 to considerable hostility from traditional physicians for its blend of herbalism, folklore, magic and astrology. It nevertheless became extremely popular and is still available today.

Early European settlers in North America not only imported their own folk medicine, but also integrated it with the extensive herbal traditions of Native American shamans to create American folk medicine, some components of which were returned to Europe. Some Native American remedies, like those of European folk medicine, have now been demonstrated to have a scientific basis. For example, mashed yucca root was commonly used as a topical treatment for arthritis, and yucca has now been shown to have anti-inflammatory properties.

In the 19th century, even as conventional medicine came increasingly to be dominated by chemistry and the refinement of synthetic drugs, the system of naturopathy (pp. 443–5) developed in Europe. It used a regime of fresh air, sunshine, a healthy diet, fasting and exercise along with herbal remedies to promote the body's self-healing powers. Naturopathy was brought to the United States at the turn of that century, and helped to preserve herbalist traditions in the face of increasingly technological medicine.

Today, as the value of plant-derived remedies is increasingly being recognized again, scientists are once more looking to plants as potential sources of healing medications.

PRACTICE

A herb can be any part of a plant, including its bark, leaves, roots, seeds, or flowers, or even single-celled plants such as algae. A fundamental tenet of herbalism is the importance of using the plant part as a whole; although the individual actions of its multiple chemical constituents may not be understood, together they form a natural balance that is responsible for the herb's effects. Some of the chemical constituents of a herb act in concert, enhancing each others' effects (a process known as synergy), while in other herbs, one constituent may counteract possible detrimental effects of others. Many herbalists believe that, unlike a drug formulated from a single component or a chemical copy of an active plant ingredient, herbal medicines are less likely to produce harmful side-effects.

Botanicals therapy plays an important role in many healing systems, and is usually one element in a holistic approach. A consultation with a practitioner will therefore take

CAUTION

Despite the popular perception of botanicals as 'natural' and therefore safer than pharmaceutical drugs, they are still powerful and need to be treated with the same caution and respect as pharmaceuticals. Many preparations have potentially harmful side-effects. In particular, many plant foods and herbal remedies contain substances that may interfere with blood-clotting and interact, possibly dangerously, with anticoagulant drugs such as warfarin.

In addition, there have been instances of adulterated and contaminated products offered for sale, for example, allegedly 'herbal' preparations that actually contain drugs such as steroids and benzodiazepines. Some remedies have been found to be contaminated with heavy metals, including lead and arsenic. Because the sale of herbal products is poorly regulated in most countries, what is written on the label may not always be what is inside the package.

different forms, depending on the system in which the therapist is operating. Most will ask detailed questions about the patient's current problems, medical history, diet and lifestyle during a first consultation, which generally takes about an hour. Several subsequent shorter sessions may be required.

Generally, herbalists do not attempt to diagnose illness but rather assess a patient's overall physical and emotional health in the context of their environment and lifestyle. In continental Europe, however, some herbalists are also medical doctors and may combine a herbal approach with orthodox medical diagnosis and treatment.

As well as prescribing herbs, a practitioner may recommend dietary changes, supplements and other treatments, depending on his or her orientation. For example, a practitioner of Traditional Chinese Medicine may combine botanicals therapy with acupuncture.

Most herbal and nutraceutical preparations are taken orally, usually as tablets or capsules, sometimes as freeze-dried herbs, tinctures, decoctions or teas. Some botanicals may be used topically on the skin as a poultice or made into an ointment.

As well as consulting trained practitioners, many people self-treat with botanical therapies at home. It has been estimated that between a third and a half the population in the United States uses some form of herbal dietary supplement, the most popular being echinacea *(Echinacea angustifolia),* ginseng *(Panax quinquefolium),* ginkgo *(Ginkgo biloba),* St John's wort *(Hypericum perforatum)* and garlic *(Allium sativum).*

In many other countries, herbal medicine forms a mainstay of available treatment. The World Health Organization (WHO) estimates that herbal remedies are the primary medicines for two-thirds of the world's population.

TREATMENTS

There is a vast range of herbs and nutraceutical products in common use in the West, as well as a profusion of foods believed to have therapeutic properties. They include:

• FEVERFEW (CHRYSANTHEMUM PARTHENIUM) The active ingredient, parthenolide, inhibits production of prostaglandins (hormone-like substances) that cause inflammation; the herb also has a long history of use treating raised temperature and arthritis. It has more recently been used to prevent migraine headaches.

• ECHINACEA Included in many cold preparations for its actions in stimulating the immune system, this herb may also help combat urinary and vaginal yeast infections, and has been used topically to treat wounds. Echinacea should not be taken by people with autoimmune conditions, such as rheumatoid arthritis and multiple sclerosis.

• ST JOHN'S WORT This herb's active ingredients, hypericin and hyperforin, influence neurotransmitters in the brain and may boost levels of serotonin, a feel-good chemical that, unfortunately, may also promote migraines. St John's wort has been used to calm nerves for centuries and is now widely taken for

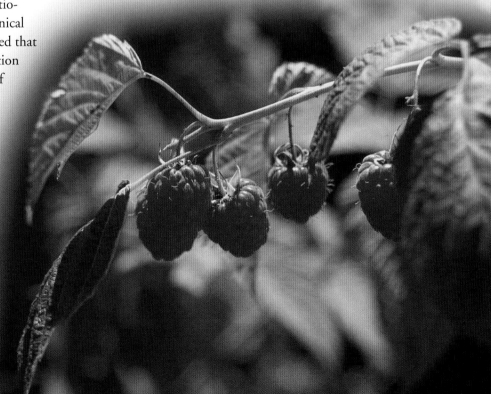

If drunk in increasing doses in the later stages of pregnancy, raspberry leaf tea is a traditional herbal medicine said to make childbirth easier and swifter.

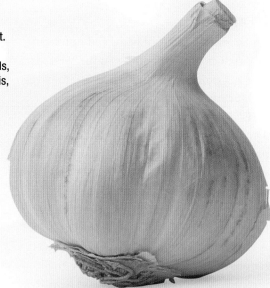

Garlic is commonly taken as a supplement. It may help to reduce blood cholesterol levels, prevent atherosclerosis, and lower blood pressure.

its antidepressant effects. In Germany, it is a licensed medication, and is prescribed more often than antidepressant drugs. It may also ease anxiety, panic attacks, premenstrual symptoms, fibromyalgia and alcoholism. Its antibacterial and antiviral properties are used in ointments for wounds, burns, haemorrhoids, and cold sores.

• GINKGO *(Gingko biloba)* This herb may help conditions in which blood flow to the brain is impared, including stroke (pp.168–9), peripheral vascular disease and Alzheimer's disease (pp.178–9). Gingko is widely used in Germany and France to enhance memory and concentration. It has also been used for premenstrual symptoms, altitude sickness, ringing in the ears (tinnitus, pp.72–3) and peripheral claudication (pain in the legs when walking due to insufficient blood flow). The use of ginkgo may lead to bleeding, so the herb must be used with caution by people who suffer from bleeding disorders, those taking anticoagulant treatments, and patients who are having surgery or dental treatment.

A much-used herb in Chinese medicine, ginseng has abundant purported benefits, including enhanced mental and exercise performance, lowered fatigue, reduced blood sugar levels in type 2 diabetes, and alleviation of heart and lung disease.

• GARLIC The active component, allicin, is believed to inhibit platelet function, reducing the risk of blood clotting. Garlic is often taken as a supplement and may help decrease blood cholesterol levels, prevent atherosclerosis and decrease blood pressure. It may also have anti-cancer properties, based on comparisons of cancer incidence in populations that tend to consume a lot of garlic in their diet and populations that do not.

• KAVA KAVA *(Piper methysticum)* Despite the extensive use of kava to treat anxiety and insomnia, kava has been withdrawn in many European countries and in Canada due to its toxic effects on the liver. Cases of complete liver failure have been reported. It is still available in the United States, but the FDA has issued warnings about its use.

• GINSENG *(Panax ginseng)* Valued in Chinese medicine, its purported benefits include enhanced mental and exercise performance, lowered fatigue, reduced blood sugar levels in people with type 2 diabetes (pp.338–41), and alleviation of heart and lung disease. Some evidence supports enhanced learning, but generally results are inconclusive.

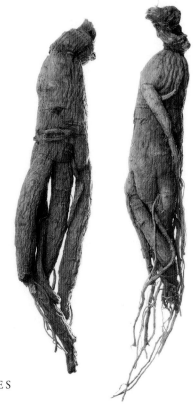

On Call

Many interactions between herbal medicines, foods and pharmaceutical drugs have been reported. They include the following.

• St John's wort may reduce the effectiveness of a number of agents competing for the same metabolic pathways in the liver. These include: digoxin, warfarin, oral contraceptives, immuno-suppressive agents such as cyclosporin, and some drugs used to treat AIDS. St John's wort may interact with other antidepressants and should not be taken together with any serotonin re-uptake inhibitor (of the Prozac family).
• Feverfew, *ginkgo biloba*, garlic, ginseng, turmeric and arnica (*Arnica montana*) all may promote bleeding and should be used with caution if taken with aspirin, anticoagulants such as warfarin or heparin, anti-platelet drugs such as clopidogrel, non-steroidal anti-inflammatory drugs (NSAIDs) such as ibuprofen or naproxen, or with other herbs that promote bleeding
• Liquorice (*Glycyrrhiza glabra*) extracts some-times taken to relieve peptic ulcers or cold sores, among other uses, may raise blood pressure and counteract the effect of anti-hypertensive drugs. Liquorice can also boost absorption of many drugs, possibly increasing their side-effects, so it should be taken with a one- to two- hour gap before and after any other medication. Liquorice may also reduce the efficacy of the oral contraceptive pill.
• Wild yam (*Dioscorea villosa*) is sometimes used to treat menstrual and menopausal symptoms, and to lower blood cholesterol. It may lower blood sugar levels, so caution is advisable in people taking insulin for diabetes. It may also have hormonal effects that could increase side-effects of the oral contraceptive pill or hormone replacement therapy. There is some evidence that it could reduce the effect of indomethacin and perhaps other anti-inflammatory drugs.
• Grapefruit (*Citrus paradisi*) fruit and the juice may have beneficial effects in lowering blood pressure and cholesterol levels, and seem to reduce the risk of developing kidney stones. But grapefruit interacts with many drugs, including heart and blood pressure medication, lipid-lowering statins, anticoagulants, some antibiotics, and hormone preparations. Effects include reducing the efficacy of some drugs and increasing the side-effects of others.
• Sweet almond (Rosaceae family) is sometimes used to lower cholesterol levels. It may also lower blood sugar levels, so should be used with caution in patients on insulin.
• *Kava kava* may have sedative effects, and so may magnify the effects of alcohol and sedative drugs, increasing the risks of accidents when driving or operating machinery. Its toxic effects on the liver mean it should not be used with drugs that affect the liver, such as acet-aminophen, isoniazid and methotrexate. It may also interfere with drugs taken for Parkinson's disease (p.181), and reportedly prolongs the effects of anaesthetics. Due to reported cases of liver failure, *kava kava* is not recommended for any reason.
• Ginseng may lower blood sugar levels, and so may heighten the effects of diabetic drugs. It interacts with the monoamine oxidase (MAO) inhibitor type of antidepressant drug to produce unpleasant side-effects, including headaches, tremors, insomnia and mania, and may alter the effects of heart and blood pressure medica-tions. It also interferes with the analgesic effects of opiate drugs.

• **EVENING PRIMROSE OIL** This essential oil, derived from *Cenothera biennis,* has beneficial effects on joint inflammation; some people with rheumatoid arthritis (pp.136–9) report it is superior to fish oils for easing aching joints. The active ingredient is an omega-6 essential fatty acid, gamma-linolenic acid (GLA). It has also been used to treat cyclic mastalgia (breast pain linked with the menstrual cycle) and atopic eczema (pp.102–3). It may enhance any tendency to have seizures and should not be taken by people with epilepsy.

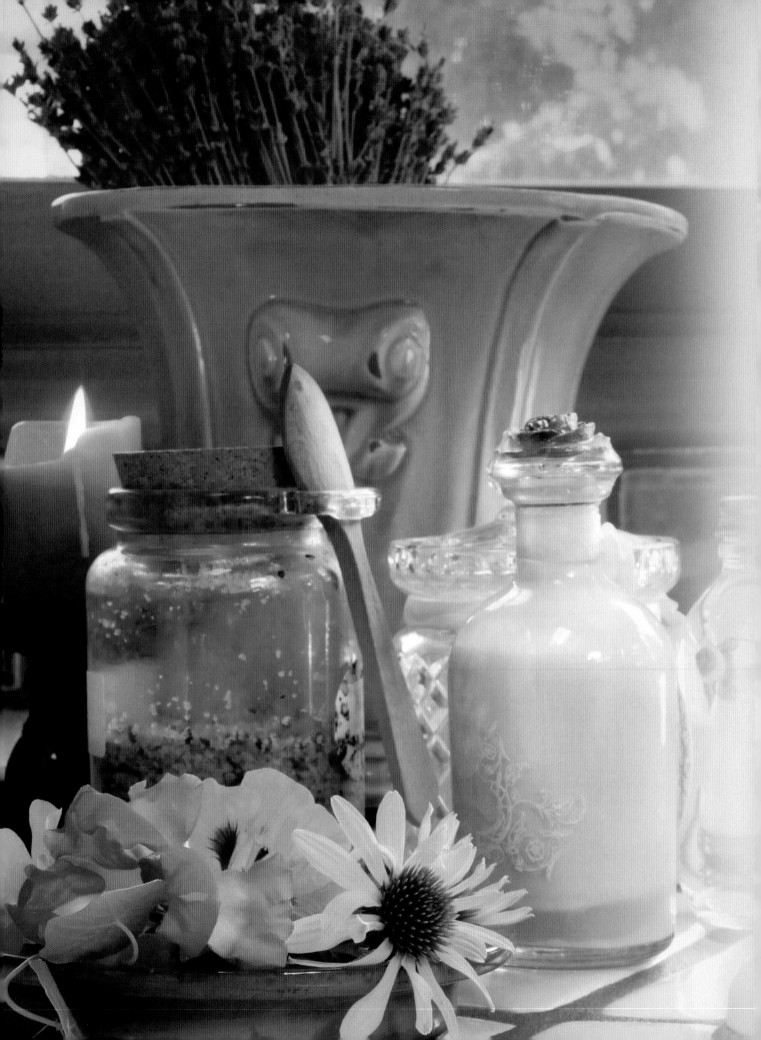

20 | ENERGY THERAPY

- Healing Touch
- Aura-Soma Therapy
- Polarity Therapy
- BioAcoustic Therapy
- Bioenergetics
- Chakra Balancing
- Light Therapy
- Magnet Therapy
- Reiki
- Radionics
- Sound Therapy

Healing therapies based on energy medicine may be broadly divided into two types, according to the form of energy that underlies their therapeutic effects. The first type is energy that exists in measurable wavelengths and frequencies, such as light, sound, magnetism and radiation. The second involves subtle energy fields – those believed by many ancient systems of medicine to flow through and surround the body. In various cultures this life energy has been given different names, including qi (in China) and prana (in India). It may be described as flowing through channels called meridians or concentrated in energy centres called chakras.

Although this bioenergy has as yet not proved measurable with conventional scientific equipment, it is the basis of many ancient medical systems, including Traditional Chinese Medicine (pp.446-50) and Ayurveda (pp.451-4). Many therapists believe they can detect, channel or influence it in order to promote optimum health or effect healing of symptoms that may be the result of disturbances in this energy flow.

Healing Touch

The aim of healing touch is to affect the energy field that is said to be in and around body to promote health and healing. The term healing touch covers a number of techniques. As well as the touch itself, practitioners consider the relationship between patient and healer to be extremely important. The idea is for both to work together as equals to facilitate healing. Therapeutic touch (TT), a related therapy, uses the power of touch to promote health and healing. Practitioners usually do not actually touch the patient, but bring their hands 10–18 cm (4–8 in) from the body, at which distance they believe they can detect a patient's energy field and correct any imbalances. This therapy is mainly used by nurses.

HISTORY

Healing touch was developed in Denver, Colorado, in 1980 by nurse Janet Mentgen. The American Holistic Nurses' Association began certifying training courses in 1993, and it is now an endorsed programme. Since 1996, Healing Touch International, a certification and educational institution in Lakewood, Colorado, has trained nurses and other healthcare professionals and now certifies practitioners and runs courses in the United States, Canada, Mexico, Australia, Europe, South Africa and South America.

Therapeutic touch was developed by nurse Delores Krieger and holistic healer Dora Kunz in the early 1970s. The training organization for therapeutic touch practitioners, Nurse Healers–Professional Associates International, in Warnerville, New York, teaches a standardized technique. The therapy's mode of action is not amenable to conventional scientific explanation, and its use of the concept of life energy has caused some opposition to its use in nursing practice. But it has become increasingly popular, especially for children; several studies suggest positive results, particularly for pain and anxiety.

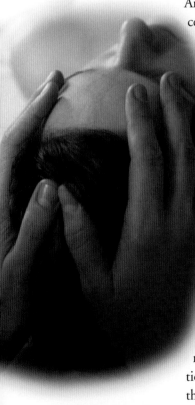

Healing touch and therapeutic touch may reduce levels of pain and anxiety, especially in children.

PRACTICE

Healing touch providers use gentle, non-invasive touch to influence and support the human energy system within and surrounding the body. Practitioners first ascertain the patient's state and symptoms, then centre and attune themselves by standing calmly and breathing deeply. They place hands on the patient's shoulders and scan the body for energy field imbalances, which are corrected with sweeping motions of the hands. In the case of serious energy blockages, therapists may leave their hands on the body for a while to promote release.

A therapeutic touch session may last between 5 and 30 minutes, and typically consists of four steps.

• **CENTERING** With an intention to help, the practitioner focuses attention on the patient and tries to promote mental calmness.
• **ASSESSING** With hands placed close to the patient's body, the practitioner evaluates his or her energy field and searches for imbalances.
• **INTERVENTION** The practitioner attempts to correct the patient's energy flow with hand movements.
• **EVALUATION/CLOSURE** After checking that the energy flow has been adjusted, the practitioner brings the treatment session to an end.

CAN HEALING TOUCH HELP ME?

Healing touch has become an increasingly popular adjunct to conventional treatment. However, it is difficult to distinguish whether the reported benefits of healing touch are due to energy balancing or to the general therapeutic effects of attention and caring.

- **Paediatrics** Healing touch is widely used to help ease pain, stress and anxiety among hospitalized children. A review from Wake Forest University School of Medicine in Winston-Salem, North Carolina, and published in 2004 in *Pediatric Annals,* found that it does produce an enhanced sense of well-being (among practitioners and patients). More research is needed to explain why.

- **Cardiac procedures** A study at Duke University published in the *Lancet* in 2005 showed that patients receiving music, imagery and touch therapy during angiograms or other cardiac procedures were 65 percent less likely to die in the following six months than patients who received no such intervention.

- **Cancer** In a study from the University of Minneapolis published in 2003 in *Integrative Cancer Therapies,* healing touch was found to lower blood pressure, heart and breathing rates, fatigue, mood disturbance and pain ratings among patients receiving chemotherapy. Results were better than those seen with standard care alone or with the added presence of a therapist without healing touch.

CAN THERAPEUTIC TOUCH HELP ME?

Despite some encouraging studies, little formal evidence for the effectiveness of therapeutic touch exists. One controversial study, published in the *Journal of the American Medical Association* in 1998, cast doubt on its premise when it seemed to show that blindfolded practitioners could not detect the experimenter's energy fields.

- **Fibromyalgia** A study in *Holistic Nursing Practice* in 2004 reported that six therapeutic touch treatments resulted in significantly reduced pain and increased quality of life in patients with fibromyalgia.

- **Osteoarthritis** Significant improvements in pain and functioning in 25 patients with osteoarthritis of the knee who received therapeutic touch was reported in a study in the *Journal of Family Practice* in 1998.

- **Dementi** Therapeutic touch produced significant reductions in behavioural symptoms of dementia, particularly restlessness and inappropriate vocalization, in a study of 57 nursing home residents published in 2005 by the University of Arkansas for Medical Sciences.

- **Chemical dependency** Pregnant women receiving therapeutic touch for 20 minutes daily over 7 days had significant reductions in anxiety scores during treatment for chemical dependency, compared with standard management, according to a 2004 study at British Columbia Women's Hospital in Canada.

TREATMENTS

There is no specific healing touch technique, in fact, healing touch uses more than 20 different techniques from a variety of sources. Some practitioners put their hands on the patient, while others place their hands very close to the body.

In therapeutic touch, the practitioner conducts a holistic assessment of the client and then chooses the best method or combination of methods based on the assessment. Advanced practitioners use what they call 'higher sense perception' and intuitive gifts to assess cues about the patient's energy state. By manipulating the body's external energy field, therapeutic touch practitioners can affect different systems within the body, depending on the patient's symptoms. The autonomic nervous system, involved in control of automatic functions such as blood pressure, is believed to be particularly sensitive. Practitioners say they can also affect internal mechanisms and thereby help resolve disorders of blood and lymphatic circulation, the musculoskeletal system, and hormonal control in women.

Aura-Soma Therapy

The meaning and therapeutic properties of colour are used in aura-soma therapy to promote self-healing, connection with inner feelings and personal growth. Aura refers to the subtle life energies that are said to radiate out from a person; soma means the physical body. The vibrational powers of colour are said to harmonize mind, body and spirit; impart the sensation of being balanced and energized; instill a sense of inner peace; and improve health.

The technique involves choosing from an array of richly-coloured bottles. Both the colours chosen and the order of selection are believed to convey information about aspects of the self and the purpose in life.

HISTORY

The use of colour to affect mood has a long history. Its application as aura-soma therapy was developed in London in the mid-1980s by holistic healer Vicky Wall, who was blind. When she lost her sight, she claimed that her psychic powers were enhanced, enabling her to see people's auras. She described being guided by an inner voice to make her first series of 'equilibrium bottles', without knowing their exact purpose. Later she realized that the oils, essences, and other extracts they contained were able to enhance perception and self-knowledge.

Aura-soma therapy is frequently offered in spas and health resorts in Europe, and is becoming increasingly popular in the United States. There is no regulation or formal certification of practitioners.

PRACTICE

In a consultation, a client is shown a back-lit display of about 100 vibrantly-coloured equilibrium bottles. Some bottles are of a single colour, but most have two colours, created by a layer of coloured oil on coloured water, which is said to balance the watery and oily

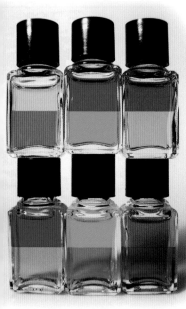

In aura-soma therapy, the colors of bottles, as well as the order in which they are chosen, offers clues to a person's life purpose.

CAN AURA-SOMA THERAPY HELP ME?

There has been little formal study of aura-soma therapy, although the effects of environmental colour on mood are well-recognized.

- **Self-realization** Therapy is said to enable a person to see clearly into their personal depths and enhance communication with the higher self.
- **Spiritual growth** Colour vibrations are said to promote soul consciousness, love and wisdom.
- **Transformation** Aura-soma therapy is said to alleviate fear and suffering.

aspects of various plants. The client is invited to choose four bottles. Choices are believed to represent needs and feelings at a deep level, and to demonstrate one's purpose in life, past issues, current circumstances and future prospects. Practitioners say working with the colours imparts knowledge of the inner self and enables cognitive understanding of the intuitive and emotional insights gained.

TREATMENTS

As well as contemplating the chosen colours, aura-soma therapy may involve shaking the bottles and applying the mixtures to the skin, sometimes with massage. Light, crystals and natural aromas may also be used during a session. Aura-soma therapy is one method of chakra balancing (p.570).

Polarity Therapy

A form of subtle energy balancing, polarity therapy is based on the belief that life energy flows through the body and that it can be detected and influenced by movements of the practitioner's hands. It integrates aspects of Ayurveda (p.451–4), hermetic philosophy, chakra balancing (p.570), and the notion of yin and yang that is central to Traditional Chinese Medicine (pp.446–50).

Energy flows through the body along five pathways, enabled by positive and negative poles of body cells. Five energy centres along the spine represent the five elements of Ayurvedic tradition (space, air, fire, water and earth), each with certain physical functions. Energy must be balanced and flow freely to maintain health. Practitioners aim to correct disturbances and enable optimal physical, emotional and spiritual functioning.

HISTORY

Polarity therapy was developed in the 1940s by Randolph Stone, an American chiropractor, osteopath and naturopath who worked in Chicago. Stone sought to integrate the traditional healing systems of India and China with modern understanding of electromagnetic fields. His work continued in the 1970s by his students, especially naturopath Pierre Pannetier. In 1984, a group of practitioners founded the American Polarity Therapy Association in Colorado, USA, an organization for practitioners, teachers and students.

PRACTICE

Before a consultation, patients are usually asked to remove their shoes and jewellery and other metal objects, such as keys, which are believed to interfere with energy flow. The client lies down and the therapist takes a medical history and then moves their hands over the patient's body, seeking any energy blockages or imbalances.

Practitioners use three levels of contact: placing the hands near the body (to detect energy fields), light touch and deep massaging touch. Using the positive and negative polarities of their hands, therapists strengthen and balance the patient's energy currents. Each treatment lasts 60 to 90 minutes; up to eight weekly treatments are usually recommended.

TREATMENTS

Practitioners also teach polarity yoga exercises, stretching routines believed to balance the energy field. A cleansing diet and drinking plenty of fluids are recommended. Counseling includes ways to increase self-awareness, self-esteem, and to release negative emotions and mental energy blocks.

Ether, air, fire, water, and earth are the five elements of the Ayurvedic tradition represented by the five energy centres located along the spine.

CAN POLARITY THERAPY HELP ME?

More formal study of polarity therapy is needed. Initial reports show the following:

- **Stress** Most patients report deep relaxation after treatment; many experience emotional release.

- **Pain** Polarity therapy and exercise may lessen pain and increase flexibility.

- **Caregivers** The U.S. National Institutes of Health is conducting a trial to assess whether polarity therapy is more effective than taking breaks in reducing stress, anxiety and depression, and improving health and quality of life among Native American carers of dementia patients.

BioAcoustic Therapy

All humans have unique vocal frequencies that reflect their state of health, according BioAcoustic therapy. Each person emits a unique 'signature sound' that represents the vibrational energies of the body and its functions. Altered vibrations due to distress or disease may be detected through computerized analysis of the voice and regularly listening to one's own corrected sound frequencies harmonizes the body's energy field, enabling healing.

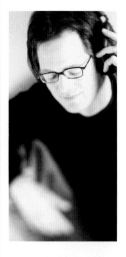

According to BioAcoustic therapy, distress and disease can be detected in the sound frequency of a voice.

The therapy is said to help predict sports performance and injuries; identify nutritional imbalances, toxins and pathogens in the body; and diagnose and treat disease.

HISTORY

BioAcoustics as a therapeutic approach was developed by American Sharry Edwards in 1982, after she realized she could hear unusually high frequencies and mimic people's unique voice frequencies. Her research led her to formulate the concept of signature sounds and the idea that distortions due to pain, emotional stress and disease could be detected via a voice print, and corrected with frequency-specific sounds.

Human BioAcoustic Vocal Profiling was developed by the Ohio-based Sound Health Research Institute as a form of energy or vibrational medicine. Edwards says she has trained thousands of people, including doctors and relatives of chronically ill patients, to use bioacoustic techniques and equipment. There are bioacoustics facilities in six other countries.

PRACTICE

All animals emit sound frequencies that vary with their physical and emotional state. These are affected by a combination of genetic and environmental influences, as well as inner functioning. Bioacoustics equipment detects these frequencies in people through voice analysis.

CAN BIOACOUSTIC THERAPY HELP ME?

There is little scientific validation of either the principles or the therapeutic powers of bioacoustic therapy. Practitioners claim good results in treating a wide range of conditions, including arthritis, emphysema, epilepsy, heart disease, high blood pressure, multiple sclerosis, allergies and Down's syndrome.

Patients speak into a microphone for about 45 seconds as a computer captures a voice sample. The analysed sample reveals data about of their musculoskeletal system, hormonal state, biochemistry, emotional state and exposure to infectious agents or environmental toxins. This vocal profile is used to create a sound protocol that corrects distortions in the person's pattern of vibrational energy. The sounds are stored in a portable tone box, and the patient listens to this protocol daily through headphones, with the aim of achieving balance.

TREATMENTS

Sound Health produces a programmable Self-Management Auditory Device for practitioners, and portable computerized diagnostic systems for home use. Bioacoustics has been used as a component of sports medicine, massage, physical therapy, music therapy and nutritional therapy.

Bioenergetics

This form of mind–body psychotherapy is based on the idea that the body stores negative emotions as 'cellular memories'. These memories cause muscle tension and stiffness, inhibit self-expression and spontaneity, and reduce vitality. Practitioners say they can 'read' patients' past experiences from their posture, movements, breathing, tone and emotional expression, and use these patterns to diagnose physical and psychological problems.

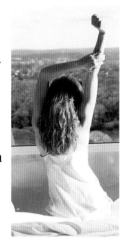

Bioenergetics uses movement as a way for patients to gain relaxation and a mode of self-expression.

The aim of therapy is to release trapped emotions and return the body to a state of health and balance, through therapy that encourages actions such as crying, screaming and kicking, combined with relaxation techniques and gentle touch to relieve muscle tension.

HISTORY

Scientists use the word to bioenergetics to describe cellular energy. As a holistic technique, it was developed in the 1950s in New York by psychiatrist Alexander Lowen, a proponent of the theories of therapist Wilhelm Reich (himself a student of Sigmund Freud). Reich postulated that repressed emotions are held by the body as muscle tension and rigidity, which he called 'body armour'.

Lowen trained with Reich and developed bioenergetic analysis for himself and his patients. He set up the International Institute for Bioenergetic Analysis in New York in 1956. It now has headquarters in Zurich, with branches around the world.

Bioenergetics is a form of psychotherapy, but some practitioners claim it can relieve side-effects of cancer treatment and perhaps boost the ability to fight disease. However, no scientific evidence support these claims.

PRACTICE

During a consultation, the psychotherapist assesses the patient's posture, expression, muscular patterns and energy levels. These suggest exercises to help overcome patterns of constriction, explore the origins of repressed emotions and encourage their release. The aim is the conscious integration of mind and body. Treatment may require psychotherapy in individual, couple or group sessions.

TREATMENTS

Bioenergetics uses many techniques to release traumatic memories: body awareness focuses attention on such elements as muscular tension and restricted breathing; physical exercise promotes relaxation and self-expression; and emotional expression encourages understanding and the integration of difficult or traumatic experiences into present understanding, and the enhancement of emotional awareness.

CAN BIOENERGETICS HELP ME?

There has been little independent study of bioenergetics and, because most practitioners are psychotherapists, its effects are difficult to distinguish from those of psychotherapy in general.

- **Emotional problems** Bioenergetics may benefit people with depression, anxiety, self-esteem and sexual abuse issues.

- **Relationship difficulties** The therapy may intensify feelings for others – either positive or negative – promote healthier and more satisfying relationships, and help patients deal with loss and grief.

Chakra Balancing

The chakras are seven energy centres along the middle of the body, from the base of the spine to the top of the head. Chakra balancing, also known as chakra healing, chakra therapy and chakra work, includes any form of therapy with the stated aim of facilitating the flow of life energy – known as prana or *qi* in Asian medical systems – through these centres.

HISTORY

The concept of the body having chakras dates back thousands of years. The word *chakra* means 'circle' or 'wheel' in Sanskrit. Chakras are an integral part of ayurveda (pp.451–4), the ancient Indian healing system, and of the belief system associated with yoga (pp.476–9). More recently, growing Western interest in various forms of energy medicine has prompted renewed interest in the possible benefits of chakra balancing.

Each of the chakras is said to correspond to particular organs of the body, and so to specific ailments that may result from energy blockages in that centre. The chakras are also associated with colours, elements and emotions. The basics may vary among systems and individual practitioners.

Some healing systems use crystals to balance the chakras. Each chakra is associated with a specific colour. Crystals of corresponding colours help balance the chakra.

PRACTICE

Many practitioners of widely varying approaches may draw on the concepts of life energy and chakras. In addition, many people adapt these beliefs to their own forms of self-help and personal development through such modes as meditation (pp.514–19), visualization, and practices such as yoga.

Although there is no single technique of chakra balancing, most of these modes have as a common theme an intense concentration on the physical regions of the body in which the chakras are located, and on the characteristics of each.

CAN CHAKRA BALANCING HELP ME?

The existence of chakras is not accepted by conventional Western science, so there has been little research into their effects on health. Practitioners say chakra balancing can help people with the following illness.

- Heart disease. Attention to the heart chakra is said to relieve heart enlargement, although a full cure may take many months.
- Headaches. Energizing and decongesting the head is said to produce rapid resolution of headaches.
- Respiratory infections. Weakness of the throat chakra is said to lead to coughs, colds, sore throats, and tonsillitis. Strengthening it may speed healing.
- General well-being. Maintaining the flow of body energy through the chakras is said to promote health, vitality, and a strengthened immune system.

TREATMENTS

Chakra balancing may be carried out through a number of healing systems. These include yoga, therapeutic touch (p.562), acupuncture (pp.464–5), polarity therapy (p.567), reflexology, Indian head massage, aromatherapy (pp.548–9), and crystal and colour therapy (p.564). Each technique has its own technique and vision of healing.

Light Therapy

In conventional and complementary medicine, light therapy has become popular for treating depression and sleep problems. Compensating for lack of natural sunlight is especially helpful in treating seasonal affective disorder (SAD) or 'winter blues', a type of depression. By synchronizing circadian rhythms (the roughly 24-hour cycle of physiological processes), light may also help people with insomnia and jet lag, and those doing shift work.

Sunlight can affect levels of melatonin and seratonin, hormones that regulate sleep and mood respectively.

HISTORY

Sunlight's healing powers have been recognized since ancient times, but the therapeutic use of artificial light has emerged only recently. The study of natural biological rhythms in the 1970s and 1980s led to an increasing realization that lack of light can have detrimental physical and emotional effects.

Today, some complementary practitioners use light to treat infections and pain. Light treatment (phototherapy) is sometimes used in conventional medicine for certain skin diseases and in the treatment of some cancers.

CAN LIGHT THERAPY HELP ME?

Light therapy may be helpful for:

- **Depression** Light therapy is as effective as drugs in treating SAD (Seasonal Affective Disorder), according to a review in the *American Journal of Psychiatry* in 2005. Most patients notice significant mood improvement within a week. Light therapy has also been used to treat depression associated with premenstrual symptoms, childbirth and eating disorders.

- **Sleep disorders** Insomnia and other sleep problems, including those associated with shift work and jet lag, may respond to light therapy.

- **Dementia** Bright light therapy may be effective in managing sleep, and behaviour and mood disturbances associated with dementia. More research is needed.

PRACTICE

Light therapy is believed to work by affecting the secretion of melatonin, a sleep-regulating hormone, and serotonin, a mood-elevating hormone. These chemicals also influence body temperature, blood pressure, blood-clotting, pain sensitivity, appetite, digestion and immunity, all of which can be affected by light.

Light therapy may be recommended by doctors, physical therapists, psychologists or other healthcare practitioners. Many people purchase light boxes or other devices for treatment at home.

TREATMENTS

Light therapy most often involves sitting in front of a light box for 30 minutes to 2 hours each morning. Other products available include bulbs for room lighting that simulate natural daylight, and dawn-simulating devices, which very gradually increase light levels in the early morning.

Several forms of light are used in this type of therapy. Bright light provides high light intensity to compensate for the lack of natural light. Full-spectrum light mimics the frequencies of natural sunlight, although most products eliminate potentially harmful ultraviolet (UV) rays.

Cold light, also called soft or low-level laser therapy, focuses a beam of low-intensity laser light to treat pain, inflammation and wounds, and may stimulate healing.

Magnet Therapy

Both permanent magnets and pulsed electromagnetic fields are used to treat a variety of ailments, especially pain. The therapeutic effects are not fully understood, but there are several theories. The magnetic field may increase blood flow and oxygen in tissue, alter the ability of nerves to conduct impulses and so block pain, prevent fluid retention, relax muscles, counteract inflammation, stimulate immunity, prompt the release of endorphins or stimulate acupuncture points.

HISTORY

The ancient Greeks and Egyptians used magnetic rocks (called lodestones) to relieve pain. In the 4th century B.C.E,. Hippocrates, considered the father of Western medicine, advocated the use of magnets. In the 3rd century C.E., Greek physicians were treating arthritis with magnetic rings. By the 18th and 19th centuries, magnets were widely sold to treat a variety of diseases, including headaches, burns and inflammation of the bowels.

PRACTICE

Conventional and complementary practitioners use magnetic therapy. In clinical settings, treatments may last a few minutes to two hours, and usually require repeat visits. Magnets are also recommended for home use, and are widely available for self-treatment. Magnets may affect the functioning of some medical equipment, and should be avoided by people with implanted devices such as pacemakers, defibrillators or insulin pumps.

TREATMENTS

Magnetic therapy is usually used on specific body parts, such as painful joints. Permanent magnets may be laid over the body part, or, in the case of pulsed electromagnetic fields,

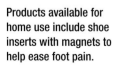

Products available for home use include shoe inserts with magnets to help ease foot pain.

CAN MAGNET THERAPY HELP ME?

Magnet therapy may help the following.

- **Pain** A study in the *Journal of Alternative and Complementary Medicine* in 2005 reported that static magnets offer relief for many types of pain. Electromagnets may be even more effective.

- **Osteoarthritis** Wearing a magnetic bracelet for 12 weeks reduces hip and knee pain from osteoarthritis, according to a 2004 trial in the *British Medical Journal*.

- **Fractures** Pulsed electromagnetic fields can assist healing of broken bones that fail to mend properly.

- **Parkinson's disease** A study in 2005 in *Movement Disorders* suggested that repetitive transcranial magnetic stimulation improves gait in Parkinson's patients.

- **Depression** Repetitive transcranial magnetic stimulation may be as effective as electroconvulsive therapy (ECT) in treatment-resistant depression. Additional research is needed.

a coil is placed around the body part and a power source generates a current. Transcranial magnetic stimulation, aimed at the brain, has recently been tested to treat several neurological and psychiatric conditions.

Products for home use include wrist bands and wraps, self-adhesive strips and foils, shoe insoles, mattress and pillow pads, magnetic jewellery, and even magnetized water.

Reiki

A form of energy medicine also known as 'energy healing', reiki is an ancient Tibetan Buddhist practice in which practitioners serve as conduits for universal life energy by systematic placement of their hands. The word comes from the Japanese words *rei,* meaning 'universal spirit' and *ki,* meaning 'life energy'. In traditional Chinese medicine (pp.446–50), this life energy is called *qi.*

Reiki is used to reduce stress, improve health and quality of life, and heal physical and emotional ailments. Its spiritual aspect is believed to promote harmony, self-awareness, creativity and mental clarity. At times, reiki is also used to impart a sense of peace to the dying.

HISTORY

Reiki is mentioned in the Tibetan sutras (religious texts) and may have originated about 2,500 years ago. It was revived in the 19th century by Japanese physician and Buddhist monk Hichau Mikao Usui, and introduced to the West in 1930 by a Japanese Hawaiian, Hawayo Tokata. Today, reiki is often used by nurses and has growing acceptance as an adjunct to conventional treatments in the United States and Europe, particularly in hospices.

There are three levels of reiki certification: introductory, practitioner techniques and the reiki master, who is qualified to teach. There is no formal regulation, but members of the International Association of Reiki Professionals pledge to uphold its code of ethics.

PRACTICE

Practitioners use 12 to 15 specific hand positions, each held for a few minutes on or near the patient's clothed body. Patients may experience heat or tingling and feel a sense of peace and serenity. Sessions last 30 to 90 minutes; the number of treatments needed varies. Some practitioners claim the treatments can be effective even over long distances.

TREATMENTS

Practitioners treat their clients with no expectations about outcome; they simply intend to heal by allowing life energy to flow through them and into the patient's body. The patient is believed to receive only the amount of energy needed for the body to heal itself.

CAN REIKI HELP ME?

Formal scientific evidence to support reiki is minimal, but it has been used to treat a growing number of conditions.

- **Pain.** Cancer patients had increased pain control and quality of life when reiki was added to standard medications, according to a preliminary study done at the University of Alberta, Canada, reported in 2003 in the *Journal of Pain & Symptom Management.*

- **Fibromyalgia** Reiki may relieve pain and improve psychological well-being in patients with fibromyalgia. The U.S. National Institutes of Health is currently conducting trials.

- **Depression** A study in 2004 in *Alternative Therapies in Health & Medicine,* reported that patients treated with reiki experienced significant reductions in psychological distress, compared with those given placebo treatment; the difference was maintained after one year.

- **Prostate cancer** Following inconclusive results elsewhere, the U.S. National Institutes of Health is undertaking a pilot study to discover whether reiki affects disease progression and anxiety in newly diagnosed prostate cancer patients.

Radionics

Radionics is based on the theory that stress, pollution and disease produce weaknesses in the subtle energy fields of living tissues, that these weaknesses parallel physical anatomy, and that they can be detected in tissue samples or even non-biological characteristics unique to a person, such as a signature.

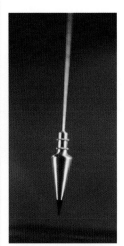

Radionics practitioners use a combination of diagnostic techniques, including a pendulum for dowsing, to detect 'vibrational energies' from the patient.

Radionics practitioners use a combination of extrasensory perception (ESP), a form of dowsing (using an instrument to detect hidden water or mineral deposits underground, or to find missing people or diagnose disease), and an instrument called a black box, which they believe can detect vibrational energies from an item closely associated with a patient, which is called a 'witness'. The box records a series of coded numbers called 'rates', which represent the energy states required for healing. The healing energy is then transmitted back to the patient, either via the box or through the practitioner's intention.

HISTORY

Radionics was developed in the early 20th century by California neurologist Albert Abrams, who believed disease represents an electron imbalance that is detectable in a person's radiated energy. Initial experiments involved tapping the abdomen of a healthy volunteer holding a wire connected to a sick patient or vial of diseased tissue. Abrams later placed a variable potentiometer (a bit like a volume control) in the wire. He believed its settings could be adjusted to correlate with various health conditions, like the rates read off the black box that is used today. Abrams subsequently decided that no physical contact with the patient was required.

CAN RADIONICS HELP ME?

There is no evidence to support either the theory or the usefulness of radionics.

The techniques were adapted by a California chiropractor, Ruth Drown, who claimed to have established ideal rates that could be used to detect deviations from normal. The perfect settings could then be fed back to the patient to enable remote healing or prompt treatment recommendations. The use of radionics on humans is illegal in the United States; it is legal in Canada and the United Kingdom. The Radionics Association in the UK trains and maintains a register of qualified practitioners.

PRACTICE

A consultation may take place by mail or over the telephone. The patient completes a health questionnaire and provides a sample of blood or hair. This is placed in the radionics box and rates are obtained to diagnose the problem. The box may be said to send the treatment directly to the patient, or to focus the healing thoughts of the practitioner.

Pratitioners say radionics is particularly helpful in conditions where conventional medicine has little to offer. For example, it is said to produce benefits in patients with chronic physical, mental and emotional conditions. Some practitioners claim also to be able to ease a person's passing after death.

TREATMENTS

Practitioners may recommend various holistic treatments, including homeopathy (pp.455–7), chiropractic (pp.446–7), colour therapy (p.564), dietary changes, or herbs and supplements (pp.432–41).

Sound Therapy

Unlike forms of energy medicine based on subtle ideas of a life energy that is not measurable, sound therapy uses a known energy source with specific, measurable wavelengths and frequencies. Sometimes called sound healing, or vibrational or frequency therapy, it encompasses any form of treatment that uses sound vibrations, which may be felt as well as heard.

Some practitioners believe specific sound frequencies resonate with specific organs of the body, creating physiological effects that can stimulate mental and physical healing. Sound vibrations are claimed to affect heart and breathing rates and brain wave patterns. Music, particularly, has been shown to promote relaxation and release of endorphins, the body's natural pain-killers.

HISTORY
Sound has been used to promote health and relieve pain for millennia. Music therapy has been studied since the 1920s, when music was found to affect blood pressure. Modern variants have been developed using complex electronic modifications of sound and feedback loops to create various physical effects.

PRACTICE
While all sound therapy involves listening to specific sounds, there is no typical approach. Rather, it is used in a variety of settings as an adjunct to conventional healthcare, as a form of healing, or in work to effect personal growth. It may be applied as short-term intervention, for example during surgery, or as an ongoing therapy to assist physical or emotional problems.

TREATMENTS
In addition to music and voice, other sound sources for therapeutic effects include wind chimes, tuning forks, Tibetan singing bowls, drums, gongs and Australian didgeridoos.

CAN SOUND THERAPY HELP ME?

Good evidence suggests that music therapy has physiological and emotional effects; other uses of sound therapy have been less well studied.

- **Pain** A trial involving 75 patients and published in the *European Journal of Anaesthesiology* in 2005 found that, music played during or after surgery may reduce postoperative pain, anxiety, and morphine consumption.
- **Childbirth** Women who listen to their choice of music during labour are less likely to need anaesthesia. Music increases satisfaction with caesarean delivery.
- **Palliative care** Music therapy may ease pain, fatigue and anxiety, and boost mood and quality of life among hospice and palliative care patients, according to a review in 2005 in *Evidence-Based Complementary and Alternative Medicine.*
- **Gait disturbances** Muscle activity may become more regular and efficient when synchronized with music with embedded metronome pulses helps stroke and Parkinson's patients walk with better stride, cadence and foot placement.
- **Mental skills** Various specialized forms of sound therapy, such as the Tomatis method (which involves modified auditory feedback), have been used to help children with dyslexia, learning disorders, autism and attention deficit disorder. The feedback helps them modify behaviour.
- **Geriatrics** Music therapy can enhance well-being and ease agitation, anxiety, depression and neuro-degenerative disease symptoms in nursing home residents.

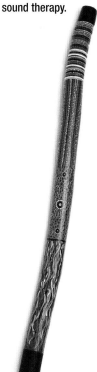

Instruments as diverse as wind chimes and Australian didgeridoos can be used in sound therapy.

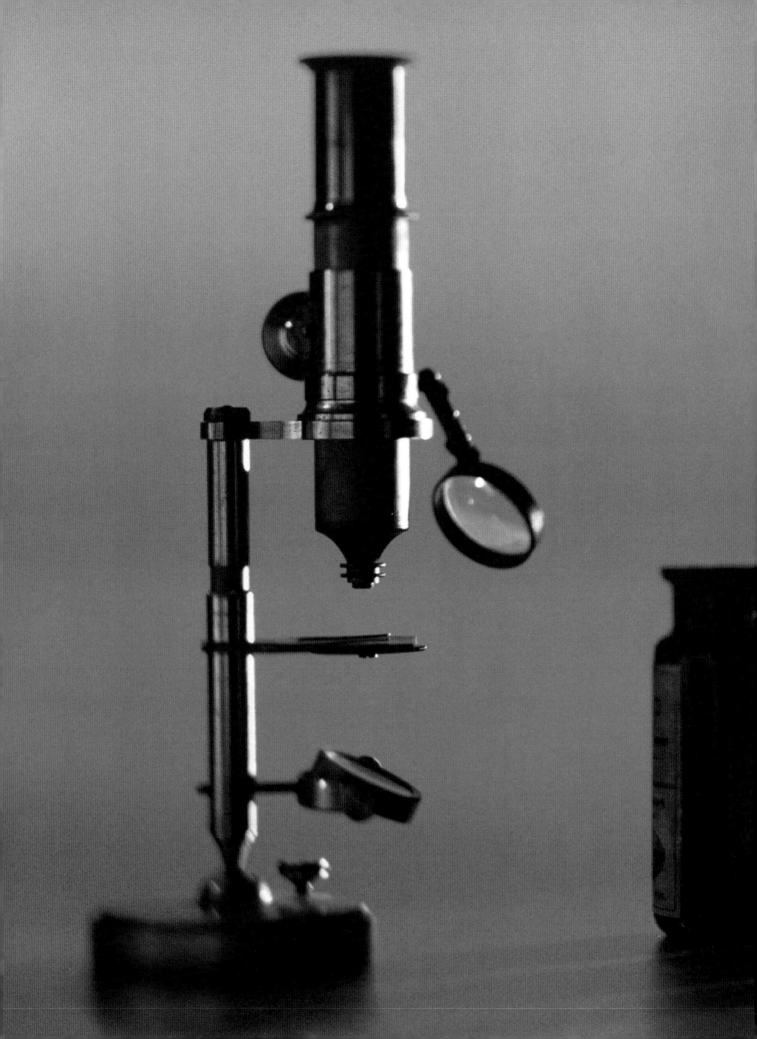

21 OTHER APPROACHES

There is an eclectic collection of other therapies, not mentioned in the previous sections, that, to a greater or lesser extent, defy categorization. These other approaches range from largely diagnostic methods such as iridology, which is said to be able to detect the condition of the body from clues within the eye and about which orthodox medicine is largely unenthusiastic, to chelation therapy, a treatment that involves infusing chemicals directly into the bloodstream and that is currently the subject of a large trial being conducted under the auspices of the prestigious United States National Institutes of Health to test its efficacy in treating cardiovascular disease.

While there is no common theme to these approaches, all hold to the basic principles of complementary and alternative medicine, including approaching the patient as a whole person. Their broad scope reflects the complexity of the workings of the human body and the correspondingly varied approaches that may be adopted in the attempt to harness its healing forces.

Chelation Therapy

This orthodox medical treatment for heavy metal poisoning is being increasingly used by holistic practitioners to treat atherosclerotic disease (hardening of the arteries). In this condition, cholesterol-laden plaques clog the inner linings of arteries, making them narrow and inflexible and impairing normal blood flow. Eventually, reduced flow can lead to pain, heart attacks, strokes and cramping in the legs when walking caused by the inability of the arteries to pump enough blood to cope with the demands of exercise.

Chelation therapy uses a synthetic amino acid called ethylene diamine tetra-acetic acid (EDTA) to remove metals, toxins and other harmful substances from the blood. It is believed to clear out the arteries, halt the progression of atherosclerosis (pp.230–3), and sometimes even reverse it.

The term chelation is also sometimes used to refer to treatments that involve other chemicals (called chelating agents) that have a similar action of binding with a substance in the body with the purpose of removing it.

HISTORY
Chelation therapy was originally developed in the 1950s as a treatment for heavy metal poisoning, for example with lead, iron, mercury or copper. For instance, a person with lead poisoning may be given chelation therapy to bind and remove the excess lead from their body before it can cause damage.

CAUTION

Very rarely, side-effects have been reported after chelation therapy, including phlebitis (vein inflammation) at the infusion site, a sudden drop in blood pressure, lowered blood calcium levels, kidney damage, heart rhythm abnormalities, interference with blood clotting, and bone marrow supression. This therapy is only advisable under qualified medical supervision.

In addition to treating toxicity caused by accidental exposure, chelation therapy has also been used to treat conditions such as thalassemia, in which repeated blood transfusions lead to iron overload; high blood calcium levels; and the calcium deposits in tissues that can occur in some advanced cancers.

It was noticed early on that chelation treatment appeared to be associated with a reduction in angina (chest pain caused by heart problems), and that it had favourable effects on cholesterol metabolism.

Some physicians began to propose that chelation therapy might be helpful in treating atherosclerotic diseases – which, at the time, were thought to be caused by calcium deposits. Many thousands of patients have now been treated with chelation for heart and arterial disorders, as well as a variety of other conditions. However results have not been consistent, and the understanding of how the therapy works in heart disease is still limited.

PRACTICE
EDTA is usually given by an infusion into a vein rather than orally, because it is poorly absorbed from the gut. EDTA is mostly excreted by the kidneys into the urine – more than 95 percent is removed from the body after 24 hours. Because is not metabolized in the body, side-effects from chelation therapy are rare. However, there may be a burning

CAN CHELATION THERAPY HELP ME?

Chelation therapy is accepted as an orthodox medical treatment for metal toxicity. Its use in atherosclerotic and other diseases, however, has limited scientific proof.

- **Heart disease** A review published in *Alternative Medicine Review* in 1998 concluded that chelation could be a viable alternative or adjunct to heart bypass surgery. However, most of the studies that have been carried out on coronary artery disease have been too small or failed to meet the scientific criteria required to draw firm conclusions. To remedy this, a major trial of chelation therapy for heart disease is under way in the United States, sponsored by the National Institutes of Health, and a report is expected in 2009. This should help to answer some of the remaining questions and give better evidence as to the efficacy and safety of chelation for this condition.

- **Claudication** Chelation has been reported to improve symptoms of claudication and increase walking distance.

- **Cerebrovascular disease** Narrowing of the arteries that supply the brain with blood can lead to a variety of mental symptoms, including stroke (pp.168–9). Although improvements in brain blood flow after chelation therapy have been reported, again, there is insufficient formal evidence to draw firm conclusions.

- **Metal toxicity** Lead exposure from old paint, soil and other residues remains a serious problem in children and has been linked with low educational achievement. A study published in the *New England Journal of Medicine* in 2001 reported that treatment with the chelating agent succimer succeeded in lowering raised blood lead levels in children. However, this made no difference to their scores on learning tests, suggesting it may not be able to reduce damage already done.

- **Kidney disease** Improved kidney function may result from chelation therapy, and it has been used to slow the progression of kidney failure.

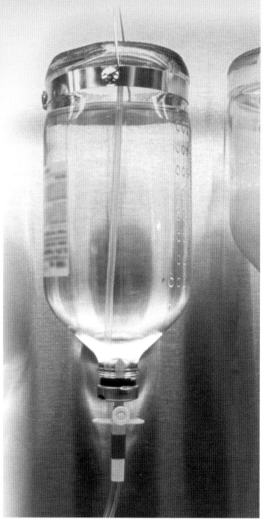

In chelation therapy, the chelating agent EDTA is generally given intravenously. A treatment generally takes around three hours and may be repeated weekly.

sensation at the site of the injection and patients often feel tired after treatment. Some experience transient temperatures, headaches, nausea, vomiting or diarrhoea after treatment.

TREATMENTS

A typical chelation infusion session takes approximately three hours and patients usually undergo a primary course of weekly treatments for a duration of two or three months. Afterwards, it may be recommended that they have infusions every few months to maintain the benefits. High-dose vitamin supplements taken orally are usually also recommended, partly for their own benefits to the arterial system and partly to compensate for vitamins that may be removed from the body by the chelation infusions.

Cell Therapy

The attempt to replace diseased human cells with healthy animal ones is known by names including cell, cellular, cellular suspension, fresh cell, live cell, embryonic cell, glandular, metabolic or organo therapy. It involves injecting cells, or sometimes other components, derived from animal tissue, often taken from the foetuses of those animals, to treat many diseases.

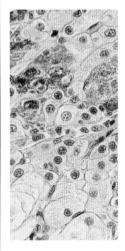

In cell therapy, healthy animal cells are injected into a patient to promote regeneration and healing.

Such techniques are distinct from medically approved therapies that are also described as 'cell' or 'cellular' therapy, such as bone marrow transplants, skin grafting using cultured cells, laboratory manipulation of a patient's own cells or stem cell technology.

HISTORY

Cell therapy was started by physician Paul Niehans in Switzerland in the 1930s, but is related to the ancient idea that because the organs of humans an animals operate in

CAUTION

Cells from animals cannot normally replace those of humans. People have suffered fatal immunological reactions after cell therapy, and severe allergic reactions and serious disease have also been reported, including three fatal cases of gas gangrene. In 1984, the United States Food and Drug Administration (FDA) banned all imports of cellular extracts for injection.

almost the same ways, the cells of healthy animal organs can treat disease in the corresponding human organs. The technique became popular among celebrities as a form of rejuvenation therapy. It is controversial and is not legally available in the United States, but Niehan's Clinic La Prairie in Clarens-Montreux, Switzerland, still operates today.

PRACTICE

When injected or, sometimes, taken orally, cellular preparations are said to travel to the corresponding organ in the patient's body to promote regeneration and healing. Some practitioners give multiple preparations at once.

TREATMENTS

Animal-derived substances used in cell therapy include whole embryos and tissues from brain, heart, liver, kidney, pancreas, spleen, intestine, spinal cord, bone marrow, eye, ovary and testis, and the pituitary, thyroid, adrenal, thymus and salivary glands.

CAN CELL THERAPY HELP ME?

There is no accepted scientific evidence that cell therapy is effective, but proponents claim it can treat many conditions.

- **Ageing** Clinic La Prairie claims that cellular rejuvenation occurs in laboratory samples and that patients experience improved physical and mental capacity, and relief from tiredness, headaches, cramps, impotence and menopause.

- **Skin disorders** Embryo skin extracts are said by proponents to help psoriasis, eczema and vitiligo.

- **Cancer** Practitioners claim that tumours regress after treatment. The American Cancer Society strongly advises patients against this kind of treatment.

- **Down's syndrome** A study in the *Australian Paediatric Journal* in 1987 showed no evidence that cell therapy was effective.

- **Other conditions** Practitioners claim that cell therapy can treat epilepsy, AIDS, asthma, arthritis, chronic fatigue syndrome, diabetes and osteoporosis.

Oxygen & Ozone Therapies

The ozone molecule (O_3) has three oxygen atoms (oxygen in the air has two). Ozone tends to form in the upper atmosphere, playing an important role in protecting the earth from harmful solar radiation. At ground level it is regarded as a pollutant and has been linked to diseases such as asthma. However, ozone also has anti-microbial properties, and oxygen therapy with ozone or hydrogen peroxide, has been use to treat many conditions.

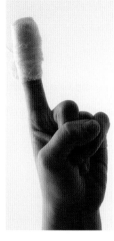

Ozone, when mixed with liquids such as water or vegetable oil is sometimes used to treat skin infections, burns and insect bites.

HISTORY

Ozone was discovered in Germany in 1840; it has been used medicinally since the late 19th century. It was used to treat wounds, trench foot and poison gas exposure during WWI. In the 1930s, German physician and Nobel Prize-winner Otto Warburg proposed that increasing oxygen levels in the body could fight cancer. The theory was later discredited, but it prompted increased use of oxygen therapies.

PRACTICE

Oxygen and ozone therapies may be proposed by a variety of holistic practitioners and, in some countries, by medical doctors. They may be used alone or as part of a more extensive regimen of therapies for specific symptoms.

TREATMENTS

There are numerous ways of introducing ozone into the body, generally mixed with water, air or oxygen. Liquid ozone may be applied to the skin, swallowed, or

CAUTION

Insufflation of gases into body cavities may cause damage, such as rupture of the eardrum or bowel. Ozone can cause various cardiovascular complications, including breathing and heart problems, and stroke. Auto-haemotherapy has been linked with the transmission of viral hepatitis, blood count reductions and death from gas embolism.

CAN OZONE THERAPY HELP ME?

Some small studies of ozone therapy have been done, but most reports are anecdotal.

- **Arthritis** Ozone-enriched water may be injected into joints to relieve pain.

- **Cardiovascular disease** A technique called auto-haemotherapy involves removing blood from a patient, combining it with ozone outside the body, and then re-injecting it into the patient. According to a 1995 study conducted in Cuba and published in *Free Radical Biology and Medicine*, this may reduce harmful blood cholesterol levels.

- **AIDS** Studies published in the journal *Blood and Antiviral Research* in 1991 showed that ozone can deactivate the AIDS virus in laboratory samples, but there is no evidence that ozone treatment of blood helps treat the disease itself. However, one small study in 1993 of five patients in San Francisco suggested that rectal insufflation of ozone and oxygen may alleviate AIDS-associated diarrhoea.

introduced into a body cavity. As a gas, it can be introduced into room air, inhaled, insufflated (pumped into a body cavity, such as the ear, vagina or colon) or used to surround the body – except the head – in a technique known as bagging. Water or blood that has been enriched with ozone may be injected into the bloodstream or joints.

Iridology

Studying the iris, the coloured part of the eye, can reveal information about a person's health, according to iridology practitioners. They say that body parts, internal organs and functions are mapped on the iris, the pattern of which can reveal the person's general state of health and any underlying diseases.

HISTORY

The iris has been studied since ancient times, but modern iridology was developed in the 19th century by Hungarian physician Ignatz von Pezcely and Swedish clergyman Nils Liljequist, both of whom published iris 'maps' that were very similar. In the mid-20th century, iridology was popularized by American chiropractor Bernard Jensen, who produced detailed iris diagrams that are still used today.

PRACTICE

Today, the iris is studied with the naked eye, magnified photographs, and sometimes microscopes or computer imaging. Practitioners examine colour, patterns, pigmentation, fibres, rings and marks in the iris, and sometimes the sclera (white of the eye) and pupil. Iridologists have not been shown to be consistent in describing such features or in the conditions they identify as a result.

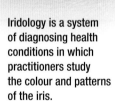

Iridology is a system of diagnosing health conditions in which practitioners study the colour and patterns of the iris.

TREATMENTS

Iridology is a system of diagnosis, not treatment, but iridologists may prescribe herbs or dietary supplements to correct the conditions they diagnose. Problems arise from inaccurate diagnoses. In a classic study in the *Journal of the American Medical Association* in 1979, iris photographs of 143 patients with kidney disease and 95 control subjects were reviewed by three iridologists who knew nothing about the patients. The iridologists were no more accurate in their diagnosis than would be expected by chance. And there was little correlation among the iridologists' ratings.

Another well-known study, in the *British Medical Journal* in 1988, involved five Dutch iridologists who were asked to examine 78 eye slides of people with or without gallbladder disease (said to be readily recognized by eye changes). Again, results were little better than chance and there was little agreement among the iridologists.

A review published in the journal *Allergy* in 2004 concluded that iridology was not useful in diagnosing allergies, and in fact could lead to inappropriate diagnosis and delays in proper treatment.

CAN IRIDOLOGY HELP ME?

Iridology is used by many complementary practitioners worldwide, especially in naturopathy (pp.443–5). There is almost no scientific evidence to support its use.

- **Hypertension** The appearance of the iris has strong hereditary influences, and brown eye colour is linked with the development of high blood pressure. Researchers at Kyung Hee University in South Korea studied hypertensive and non-hypertensive subjects classified according to iridology features. The results, published in 2004 in the *Journal of Alternative and Complementary Medicine,* showed that a significantly more patients with hypertension had a neurogenic constitution, and this iris pattern increased the risk of hypertension in subjects with specific genetic profiles. However, larger studies are needed to confirm the finding.

Prolotherapy

The 'prolo' in prolotherapy is short for 'proliferate'. With this therapy, harmless irritants, such as dextrose (sugar), are injected into soft tissues to stimulate the formation of new connective tissue and promote healing. This therapy can often reduce pain associated with such conditions as arthritis, back problems and sports injuries.

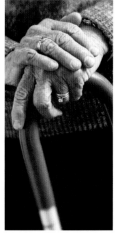

Prolotherapy is used to ease pain caused by arthritis, back problems and sports injuries.

HISTORY

Prolotherapy is a development of sclerotherapy, which uses sclerosing (hardening) injections to treat conditions such as haemorrhoids and hernias. In the 1930s it was applied to joint injuries in an attempt to stimulate connective tissue repair.

The term prolotherapy was coined in 1956 by George S. Hackett, an insurance company doctor in Ohio, USA. Today, prolotherapy is offered by medical doctors, osteopaths and naturopaths who are trained to perform the technique.

PRACTICE

Prolotherapy injections induce an inflammatory reaction by causing the proliferation of fibroblasts, the specialized cells that make collagen (the protein that is the main component of connective tissue). This promotes the formation of new, stronger collagen in ligaments, tendons and joint tissues.

TREATMENTS

A prolotherapy practitioner may use touch, X-rays or thermography (heat imaging) to locate painful points. The area around them is then injected with a solution, using a very fine needle. The solution, which may contain the natural sugars glucose or dextrose, often also contains local anaesthetic, producing immediate pain relief. Repeat treatments are usually recommended at two- to six-week intervals, with between six and thirty sessions needed altogether, depending on the problem.

CAN PROLOTHERAPY HELP ME?

Clinical studies of prolotherapy have often been promising, but results have not been consistent and vary with the injection technique used. Most formal studies have used injections of saline (a weak salt solution) as the placebo control (a treatment that is supposed to be harmless but ineffective), and this often works just as well as active prolotherapy.

- **Low back pain** According to a study of 177 patients in Alberta, Canada, in 2004, up to 90 percent of patients with chronic back pain may experience relief with prolotherapy. However, in the same year, researchers from the University of Queensland in Australia reported that pain and disability were reduced equally regardless of whether the solution injected was glucose plus local anaesthetic or normal saline.

- **Osteoarthritis** A trial at Bethany Medical Center in Kansas City, published in 2000 in *Alternative Therapies in Health and Medicine,* found that dextrose prolotherapy in established osteoarthritis of the knee yielded significant reductions in pain, swelling and frequency of knee buckling, with an increase in flexibility and improved X-rays.

- **Headache** Prolotherapy to the neck area may alleviate chronic headaches.

- **Childbirth** Injections of saline around the lumbar area may reduce labour pains. However, sterile water, which is extensively used in Scandinavia, may work even better – suggesting that the benefit may come from the injection itself.

Colonics

Various forms of colonic irrigation, also known as colonic lavage, are types of hydrotherapy related to enemas. They use water to flush out the lower bowel to remove waste material and aid detoxification.

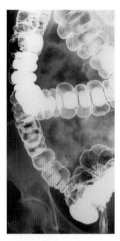

Colonics are used to eliminate toxins from the body and restore normal muscular activity in the colon.

HISTORY

Ancient Egyptians, who associated faeces with bodily decay, used colonic cleansing, as did the people of ancient Greece, China, and India. The modern use of colonics began in the late 19th century, when European spas promoted them to clients who were keen on 'regularity' of bowel movements. The advent of germ theory boosted the idea that the colon contained toxic products. The practice was further popularized in the 1920s and 1930s, partly due to alternative cancer treatments.

PRACTICE

The theory of 'autointoxication' proposes that poor digestion causes waste to accumulate in mucosal folds lining the colon, where toxins may be absorbed into the bloodstream. A variety of complementary practitioners offer colonic irrigation to relieve autointoxication and promote general well-being. In the procedure, the patient lies on the treatment table undressed except for a gown. The

CAUTION

Colonic irrigation should be administered only by trained practitioners. There are reports of infections from inadequately sterilized equipment and even perforation of the bowel, which can be fatal. Repeat treatments may lead to excess water absorption, causing disturbances of body chemistry that may cause vomiting, heart failure, or rhythm disturbances and coma. Colonics should not be used in people with gastrointestinal disorders, tumours, haemorrhoids, or heart or kidney disease.

CAN COLONICS HELP ME?

Colonics are used to promote general health and alleviate a wide variety of conditions including chronic fatigue, arthritis, gastrointestinal disorders, headaches and skin disorders such as psoriasis. However there is no significant formal evidence of benefit in such conditions and increasing concern about risks. In conventional medicine specialized forms of colonic irrigation may be used in stoma care and sometimes before or during bowel surgery.

therapist passes a speculum through the anus about 50 mm (2 in) into the rectum. A thin tube from a feeder tank uses gravity to introduce warm, purified water, sometimes containing herbs, probiotics (pp.550–1) or coffee. A wider tube removes water and waste material expelled by natural bowel contractions. In a 'high colonic', a longer plastic tube is passed into the colon. The procedure takes 30 to 60 minutes.

In the United States there is no specific regulation of practitioners, but equipment is regulated by the Food and Drug Administration (FDA), so its use should be supervised by a licensed physician. In Europe, most colonic therapists have trained at approved colleges, are registered, and their premises regularly inspected.

TREATMENTS

Practitioners usually also advise on dietary changes and may recommend herbal and other supplements for colon cleansing between colonic treatments, and sometimes supervised fasting to aid detoxification.

Biological Decoding

The notion that disease is a response to emotional trauma lies at the heart of biological decoding, which views symptoms as messages representing the body's attempts to deal with psychological conflict. Biological decoding, also known as 'total biology' (*biologie totale* in France), is hailed as a novel paradigm for 'new medicine', a new way of looking at disease.

The underlying notion is that the brain cannot distinguish perception from reality – people salivate imagining the flavour of food, or hearts are set racing by watching a horror movie. The brain responds to both physical and psychological stimulii with an internal biological programme aimed at repair. Since repair cannot occur in the case of unresolved emotional trauma, symptoms appear.

Individuals vary in the emotional weight given to similar events, which in turn evoke different brain programmes and bodily responses. The connection between specific diseases (such as cancer) and underlying emotional events may not be obvious, so decoding is needed. Once the origins are uncovered, symptoms may resolve.

HISTORY

Biological decoding was developed by French physician Claude Sabbah in the late 1970s, who observed that patients responded differently to illness, some recovering with no medical help, while others resisted all treatment. Sabbah also proposed that symptoms could stem from ancestral experiences, and be transmitted down the generations.

CAN BIOLOGICAL DECODING HELP ME?

Although there are anecdotal reports of the cure of many physical and psychological ailments, there is no formal evidence to support benefits from biological decoding.

CAUTION

There is a significant and life-threatening danger in choosing psychologically based therapies in place of other treatments with clear documented evidence for effectiveness. It is important to thoroughly review treatment options and the evidence for effectiveness with a medical practitioner.

His theories were taken up by German physician, Ryke Geerd Hamer, in the early 1980s. He suggested that biological dysfunction resulted from short-circuits in the brain following severe emotional shock, that these could be seen on brain scans and that the individual's response affected the nature of symptoms. His German New Medicine® is now a prominent form of biodecoding.

PRACTICE

Rather than seeking a physical cause for a particular symptom, practitioners look for its symbolic meaning to uncover the original emotional trauma and the belief behind it. When this happens, symptoms lose their purpose and healing becomes possible. Training and certification in biodecoding is available in Europe and North America, although there is no regulation of practitioners.

TREATMENTS

Practitioners may use relaxation (pp.474–5), hypnosis (pp.508–13), or NLP (pp.524–5) as part of their therapeutic techniques.

Nambudripad's Allergy Elimination Techniques

The idea that allergies are due to a form of energy blockage underlies this therapy, popularly known as NAET. It uses a combination of applied kinesiology (pp.484–5), acupressure (p.472), acupuncture (pp.464–5), chiropractic (pp.446–7), and nutritional changes (pp.586–97). Practitioners also believe that most illnesses are caused by undiagnosed allergies, and that these can be cured or substantially alleviated by NAET techniques.

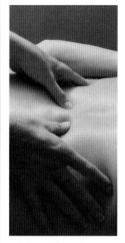

NAET uses a combination of therapies, including acupressure, to diagnose and then eliminate allergies.

HISTORY

NAET was developed in 1983 by Devi Nambudripad, an Indian doctor living in California. (Because her degree is from a university in Antigua, a qualification not recognized in California, she has also been represented as a nurse, acupuncturist, chiropractor and kinesiologist.)

Nambudripad had suffered from multiple ailments since her childhood. She attributed these health problems to a wide range of food, drug, and environmental allergies. She lived on rice and broccoli for three and a half years before coincidentally giving herself acupuncture while in contact with some carrots, and discovered that she was no longer allergic to them. After finding similar results in others, she set about developing a system to reprogramme the brain's response to allergy-provoking substances. According to Nambudripad, more than 7,500 practitioners worldwide have trained in her methods.

PRACTICE

A consultation with a NAET practitioner involves muscle testing (kinesiology) to discover what substances prompt allergic reactions. The patient holds the suspected substance while the practitioner presses on the arm. Weakness in the arm is believed to demonstrate an allergic reaction. Then, with the patient again holding the substance, acupressure (or, in severe cases, acupuncture) is applied to spinal points in order to stimulate the central nervous system and reprogramme the brain. The patient must avoid the culprit substance for 25 hours after the treatment.

TREATMENTS

The NEAT procedure treats one allergen at a time, so some people may need just one visit. However most need 15 to 20 sessions to desensitize them to multiple food and environmental allergens.

CAN NAET HELP ME?

The NAET Web site claims that 80 to 90 percent of patients experience complete relief from allergic symptoms to treated substances, and that studies to prove the effectiveness of NAET are under way. However, independent patient reports are more variable, and there is currently no scientific evidence to support the theory or the therapy.

- **Pain** The Nambudripad's Allergy Elimination Technique Web site claims that various painful conditions, including headaches, back aches, joint pains, indigestion, cough and body aches; sensitivites to heat and cold; as well as addictions and premenstrual symptoms, are actually caused by allergies.

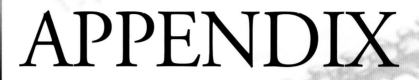

APPENDIX

Health & Healing For Women Nutritional Guidelines

Developing a healthy and balanced nutritional pro-gramme is a cornerstone for attaining optimal health. These guidelines detail nutritional recommendations for overall health, and provide specific research-based recommendations for the prevention of breast cancer, heart disease and osteoporosis. Traditional Western diets containing excessive amounts of processed foods can contribute to the development of disease and impede the healing process. The key aspects of this programme will be to create a sustainable diet rich in antioxidants and other healthy nutrients, and to target specific nutrients that are important to the process of building and maintaining health.

NOTE: Use this information in light of other health issues you may have, foods that you like and that are agreeable to you, and any more specific recom-mendations provided by your doctor.

1.INCREASE FRUIT & VEGETABLE INTAKE

Goal: To eat at least 7 servings of fruits and vegetables daily and increase variety.

Fruit: 1 serving = ½ banana, 1 medium fruit, 12 cl (4 fl.oz) juice, 2 tbsp raisins

Vegetables: 1 serving raw vegetables, ½ serving cooked vegetables

- INCLUDE DARK GREEN VEGETABLES DAILY: broccoli, spinach, kale, collards, cabbage, brussel sprouts, mustard greens, salad mix
- INCLUDE ORANGE FRUITS AND VEGETABLES DAILY: sweet potato, carrots, carrot juice, winter squash, melon, dried apricots
- INCLUDE ANTIOXIDANT-RICH FRUITS AT LEAST WEEKLY, including: prunes, raisins, blueberries, strawberries, raspberries
- EAT LYCOPENE-RICH FOODS REGULARLY (4 + servings weekly), if well-tolerated: cooked tomato sauce, salsa, tomatoes, watermelon, red grapefruit (1 serving = 100 g (4 oz) cooked tomato sauce or spaghetti sauce)
- INCREASE GARLIC AND ONION CONSUMPTION (3+ servings weekly), if well-tolerated. Add to stir fries,

soups and pasta sauce. Eat chopped with salsa on crackers or toast.

Overall Health

The dark green cruciferous vegetables contain indole-3-carbinol, a substance that facilitates the re-moval of cancer-causing substances by stimulating liver detoxification enzymes. Eat dark greens raw or lightly steamed because cooking destroys this potent com-pound. The crucifers are also rich sources of folic acid, calcium, vitamin K, beta-carotene, lutein, vitamin C and fibre, all of which have been shown to be protec-tive against an array of diseases.

Dark greens, red, orange and yellow vegetables contain carotenoids, a family of over 600 phytochemi-cals, including beta-carotene and lutein. Many of the carotenoids and other antioxidants found in fruit and vegetables protect DNA from free radical damage (a process that leads to ageing and disease), may prevent heart disease by inhibiting LDL oxidation (a process that increases heart disease), enhance the immune system, and may be protective against cancers of the oesophagus, lung, stomach, colon, breast and cervix.

Greens are a great source of lutein, a carotenoid that may lower colon cancer risk. Calcium from greens may also lower colon cancer risk by binding to bile salts and other carcinogens in the intestine. NOTE: Garlic exhibits anticoagulant properties. If you are taking blood-thinning supplements, such as vita-min E, gingko biloba, fish oil, or aspirin or are taking warfarin or other medications, consult a doctor before adding large amounts to your diet.

Heart Health

A study of 84,251 women (Nurses Health Study), aged 34 to 59 years, found that a single serving of dark green vegetables consumed daily reduced the risk of coronary heart disease by 23 percent. In the same study, among 68,782 women, those consuming 28 g (1 oz) fibre (from fruit, vegetables and cereals) had a

19 percent reduced risk of developing heart disease than women consuming 10 g (0.3 oz) of fibre. The crucifers are a rich source of folic acid, calcium, potassium, beta-carotene, vitamin C and fibre, all of which have been shown to be protective against heart disease.

Bone Health

Greens are an excellent source of absorbable calcium and vitamin K, a nutrient that is essential for the manufacture of proteins found in bones. A study of over 72,000 women found that those consuming the least vitamin K had a 30 percent increased risk of hip fracture compared to those consuming at least 109 mcg daily (see chart below), or the amount in ½ serving of frozen spinach. Greens are also a rich source of folic acid, vitamin B_6, vitamin C and an array of phytochemicals important to maintaining healthy bones.

Food (1 serving cooked)	Calcium (mg)	Vitamin K (mcg)	Folate (mcg)
Spring greens	360	370	130
Spinach	270*	280	262
Turnip greens	250	106	170
Kale	180	360	18
Broccoli	178	240	78
Mustard greens	150	270	104
Cabbage	50	180	30
Lettuce (green), raw	38	112	28

* Calcium absorption from spinach is low (5 percent) due to high oxalic acid content.

Breast Health

Over 35 studies have shown a statistically significant inverse relationship between tomato intake or blood lycopene level and the risk of cancer. In a case-control study of 289 women with confirmed breast cancer and 442 controls, those in the highest intake of lycopene intake had a 36 percent reduced risk of breast cancer, even after factoring out six other nutrients known to affect breast cancer risk.

Orange, red, yellow and dark green fruit and vegetables are excellent sources of alpha-carotene, beta-carotene, beta-cryptoxanthin, lutein and zeaxanthin. Serum levels of these specific carotenoids may have

an inverse relationship to breast cancer risk. A case-control study (270 cases, 270 controls) found that individuals in the lowest quarter of total carotenoid intake had a 231 percent increased risk for breast cancer. Indole-3-carbinol has been shown in laboratory tests to inhibit breast cancer cell growth. Broccoli contains sulforaphane, a substance that has also shown cancer-suppressing properties in laboratory tests. The crucifers are also rich sources of the nutrients, folic acid, vitamin C and fibre, which are associated with a reduced risk of overall cancer.

Garlic and onions contain diallyl sulphide, a potent tumour suppressor, as well as other beneficial sulphur-containing compounds. Cooking destroys some of the beneficial properties of garlic and onion.

2. BUILD THE DIET AROUND HEALTHY FATS

- REDUCE SATURATED FATS to no more than 0.7 oz (20 g) daily: these include cheese, red meat, butter, ice cream, whole-milk and processed foods

Food	Saturated Fat
Ice cream (1 portion vanilla – 16% fat)	15 grams
Hamburger (100 g regular)	8 grams
Hotdog (1 regular beef)	7 grams
Cheese (30 g)	6 grams
Whole milk (1 glass)	6 grams
Butter (1 pat)	3 grams

- REPLACE POLYUNSATURATED OILS AND SATURATED FATS with monounsaturated oils at restaurants.
  Request that dishes be prepared with olive oil or rapeseed oil instead of butter, soybean or corn oils
  Request extra-virgin olive oil and balsamic vinegar/lemon juice for salads instead of salad dressings made from unhealthy vegetable oils
  Use olive oil instead of butter on bread
- BUY QUALITY OILS FOR HOME USE
  Extra-virgin olive oil, organic (non-genetically modified) rapeseed oil, high-oleic sunflower oil, high-oleic safflower oil, and light olive oil for higher temperature cooking
  Sesame oil, grapeseed oil, virgin coconut oil (use in small amounts)

• EAT HEALTHY FATS:

Plant fats: nuts and nut butters, seeds (pumpkin, sesame, flaxseed and sunflower seed) and seed butters (tahini), olives, avocado

Goal: To eat at least five servings weekly. Serving = small handful nuts, 2 tbsp nut and seed butters, 1 tbsp ground flaxseed, 10 olives, ¼ avocado

NOTE: Because flaxseed contains phyto-oestrogens (weak oestrogens), women with hormone-sensitive conditions such as breast, uterine cancer or endometriosis should consult a doctor before adding flaxseed.

Omega-3s: salmon, sardines, bluefish, light tuna, herring, mackerel

Goal: To eat at least one serving, 425 g (15 oz) weekly, Farmed salmon can contain higher levels of PCBs (polychlorinated biphenyls) and other contaminants. Limit farmed salmon to monthly on average. Choose wild salmon instead. Most canned salmon products are made from wild Alaskan salmon. Chum, sockeye and pink salmon are all wild varieties.

Fish and omega-3 content	Per 100 g (3.5 oz) serving
More than 1.0 gram	Anchovies, bluefish, herring, Spanish mackerel, king mackerel*, salmon, sardines, lake trout*, bluefin tuna*, albacore tuna*
0.5 grams–0.99 grams	Striped bass*, sea bass*, rainbow trout*, blue mussels, oysters, flounder, halibut*
Less than 0.5 grams	Carp, catfish, clams, crab, cod, grouper*, lobster*, perch, mahi mahi, mullet, orange roughy*, pike, red snapper*, scallops, sea trout*, shrimp, sole, squid, sturgeon, swordfish*, canned light tuna (not albacore)

*CAUTION: Fish possibly containing higher concentrations of mercury, PCBs and dioxin

Omega-3s: organic 'designer' eggs (see label) that contain omega-3s. Four DHA-rich eggs have the same omega-3 content as 100 g (3.5 oz) of salmon

Goal: Aim to eat four eggs per week. Eggs from free-running chickens contain more vitamin E, higher levels of beneficial carotenoids and less saturated fat.

• AVOID TRANS-FATTY ACIDS (foods containing hydrogenated oil): hard margarine, fried potato/tortilla chips, french fries and other fried foods, bought pastries and baked goods, commercial cookies
• AVOID FRIED FOODS: french fries, fried chicken, fried fish.

Overall Health

Fats are essential for the proper functioning of cells, the synthesis of beneficial hormone-like substances called prostaglandins, the absorption of fat-soluble nutrients, such as vitamins A, D, E and K, for improving the taste of food, and overall satisfaction. While fat is a concentrated source of calories, an adequate intake of healthy fats makes it easier to lose and sustain a lower weight.

Saturated fats, in excess, increase total and LDL cholesterol (a heart disease risk factor) and are associated with an increased risk of several types of cancers. Excessive amounts of Omega-6 polyunsaturated fats (corn oil, sunflower oil, soybean oil, animal fat from non-organic sources) also contribute to inflammation and possibly to allergic reactions.

Monounsaturated fats and polyunsaturated fats in plant foods lower total cholesterol and LDL levels, maintain HDL levels, and are not associated with an increased risk for cancer. Omegas-3s, a class of polyunsaturated fats, promote the synthesis of PG3 prostaglandins that exert an anti-inflammatory and blood-thinning effect. These fats are being investigated for their role in reducing heart disease, cancer, rheumatoid arthritis, depression and other diseases.

Trans-fats (from hydrogenated oils) increase total and LDL cholesterol, lower beneficial HDL cholesterol levels and interfere with the metabolism of omega-3s. Because trans-fats malfunction when incorporated into cell membranes, they may increase the risk of cancer. Fried foods contribute excessive fat calories and fried oils contain higher levels of damaging free radicals. Most commercially fried foods, such as fast-food french fries, are cooked in partially hydrogenated oils (and contain trans-fats).

Heart Health

A study (Nurses Health) of 80,082 women (34–59 years old) with no known heart disease conducted over a 14-year period found that replacing 5 percent of energy intake from saturated fat with an equal amount of monounsaturated or polyunsaturated fat would reduce the risk of heart disease by 42 percent. In other words, if the average woman reduced her daily saturated fat intake from 26 g to 15 g (1 oz to 0.5 oz) by substituting a healthier fat, she would reach this goal.

Bone Health

Long-term observational studies positively correlate vitamin D intake with reduced hip fracture rate. A 100 g (3½ oz) serving of salmon, tuna or sardines provides 200 IU–400 IU, the same amount found in 2–4 glasses of fortified milk.

Breast Health

Several studies have shown that women who consume more olive oil (but not necessarily more fat) have more than a 30 percent reduced risk of developing breast cancer. Olive oil contains numerous compounds that have anti-cancer potential. A case-control study using body fat stores of trans fatty acids was conducted on 698 women with post-menopausal incident cases of primary breast cancer. Women with trans-fat stores in the highest 25 percent had an increased risk of post-menopausal breast cancer 40 percent greater than women with trans-fat stores in the lowest 25 percent. Omega-6 polyunsaturated fatty acids stimulate the growth of mammary tumours when fed to animals, whereas monounsaturated fatty acids do not exhibit tumour-promoting effects. The polyunsaturated omega-3 fats found in oily fish and flaxseed may inhibit tumour growth. A large study in Japan found that women consuming more omega-3s had a significantly lower risk of breast cancer.

3. SHIFT THE PROTEIN SOURCES IN YOUR DIET

- REDUCE RED MEAT CONSUMPTION, less is better: hamburgers, steak, roast beef, pork, bacon, sausage
- AVOID CURED OR SMOKED FOODS that contain nitrates/nitrites: hotdogs, sausage, bologna and other luncheon meats
- CHOOSE LOW-FAT ANIMAL PROTEIN: chicken breast, turkey breast, fish, egg whites and organic low-fat dairy (yogurt, cottage cheese and milk)
- EAT AT LEAST ONE OMEGA-3-RICH TYPE OF FISH every

week (aim for 425 g/15 oz per week). See description under fats.
- REPLACE AT LEAST THREE SERVINGS OF ANIMAL PROTEIN each week with a plant-based meal: ethnic vegetarian dishes (Indian, Thai, Chinese, Mexican, Ethiopian), pasta with vegetables, beans and rice, vegetable stir-fries, vegetable stews, whole bean burritos, hummus sandwiches; soy-based veggie burgers, soymilk, edamame, soy-based breakfast meats, tofu, tempeh (One serving = 1 glass soy milk, 1 soy veggie burger, 4 tbsp roasted soy nuts, 100 g/4 oz tofu, 100 g/4 oz tempeh).

Soy-based food	Serving size	Soy protein	Isoflavones
Texturized soy protein (dry)	4 tbsp	6 grams	94 mg
Soy nuts (dry roasted)	4 tbsp	10 grams	84 mg
Green soybeans (Edamame)	8 tbsp	11 grams	70 mg
Tempeh	100 g	19 grams	60 mg
Tofu	100 g	13 grams	38 mg
Soy yogurt	100 g	4 grams	26 mg
Soy milk	16 tbsp	4–10 grams	20 mg
Soy-based veggie burger	1 patty	12–18 grams	5–20 mg
Other soy meats	25 g	4–10 grams	5–20 mg

NOTE: Because soy products contain phyto-oestrogens (weak plant oestrogens), women with hormone-sensitive conditions such as breast or uterine cancer or endometriosis should consult a doctor before adding to the diet. Avoid concentrated soy isoflavones, such as found in soy protein powders.

Overall Health

Red meat is a significant contributor of saturated fat in the Western diet. Excess saturated fat is associated with heart disease and inflammation. Avoid cured or smoked foods that contain nitrites because they can form cancer-causing compounds called nitrosamines in the stomach. Low-fat animal protein choices reduce saturated fat intake. A regular beef hotdog contains half the recommended intake of saturated fat for the day.

Fish intake is correlated to a lower incidence of disease, particularly heart disease and cancer. Increasing the percentage of plant-based protein sources will increase the levels of beneficial plant nutrients in the diet, including antioxidants and fibre.

Heart Health

Among 84,688 women followed for 16 years, those that ate fish once a week had a 31 percent reduced risk of heart disease compared to those eating fish less than once a month. While a recent review found that regular soy consumption may not confer the heart benefits as previously thought, soy products may still offer a significant benefit for those with elevated cholesterol levels, particularly when soy is consumed in place of higher fat animal products. Soy products are a source of dietary protein that is low in saturated fat and rich in nutrients known to support cardiovascular health, such as fibre.

Bone Health

While the jury is still out on the role of soy and bone health, several studies have shown that the isoflavones in soy products may stimulate bone formation and suppress bone breakdown. A study of twenty-three healthy perimenopausal women provided with either an isoflavone supplement (62 mcg) or a placebo found a significant reduction in the excretion of bone resorption markers (indicating favourably bone metabolism) in the isoflavone group.

Eating less animal protein may reduce the risk of fracture. The Nurses Health Study found a 20 percent increased risk of forearm fractures for women eating a 'high-normal' amount of protein versus moderate protein intake (95 g/3.4 oz of protein daily versus 68 g/2.4 oz). No relationship to fracture rate was found with vegetable protein. Another study of 1,035 women (65 years and older) found a significantly increased risk of hip fracture rate for those eating a higher ratio of animal protein to vegetable protein.

4. INCREASE FIBRE-RICH FOODS

- EAT BEANS AT LEAST FOUR TIMES A WEEK: black bean burritos, hummus, garbanzo, kidney, pinto and other beans in salads and soups, rice and beans, vegetarian 'pork and beans', bean-based ethnic dishes.
- EAT WHOLE-GRAIN BREADS: select those with at least 2 g (0.1 oz) of fibre per slice: whole wheat, spelt, kamut, rye, sprouted grains
- EAT HIGHER-FIBRE CEREALS: select those with at least 4 g (0.2 oz) of fibre per serving
- REDUCE REFINED, LOW-FIBRE CARBOHYDRATES: bagels, white breads, juices, white pasta, white rice
- GREATLY REDUCE EMPTY CALORIE CARBOHYDRATES: pastries, soft drinks, cakes, sweets, biscuits, baked goods, ice cream.

Overall Health

Fibre intake plays a key role in slowing the absorption of dietary sugars, maintaining intestinal regularity (primarily insoluble fibre), reducing cholesterol levels (soluble), as well as a possible role in reducing the risk of colon cancer. Fibre-rich foods, including whole grains, are excellent sources of vitamins (vitamin E, folic acid), minerals (selenium, magnesium and zinc), antioxidants and phytochemicals (isoflavones, lignans, phytates and flavonoids) that are associated with reducing overall disease risk.

The refining process removes the wheat bran and wheat germ, sources of essential nutrients that play a significant role in bone health. Whole-wheat flour contains twice as much calcium and copper than white flour, three times more potassium, four times more zinc and fibre, five times more manganese, six times more magnesium, and eight times more vitamin B_6.

It is still not clear whether fibre reduces the risk of colon cancer. However, there are many reasons (such as to lower cholesterol, improve blood sugar regulation, lower C-reactive protein, regularity, etc.), for your diet to contain at least 25 g (1 oz) fibre each day.

Heart Health

A study of 9,632 men and women followed over an average of 19 years found that those consuming beans four times or more per week compared with less than once a week had a 22 percent lower risk of developing coronary heart disease. A study of 75,521 women aged 38–63 years (Nurses Health) with no previous diagnosis of cardiovascular diseases was followed for ten years. Those eating a diet comprised of more high-glycaemic foods (a marker for more refined carbohydrates) had a 98 percent increased risk of developing heart disease compared to those eating foods lower on the glycaemic index.

Recent findings of a large observational study found that fibre intake is independently associated with C-reactive protein. Those eating more fibre had significantly lower levels of this inflammatory marker. The lowest C-reactive protein was found among those consuming 32 g (1.2 oz) of fibre or more each day. In addition, those that reach the RDA for magnesium each day by consuming magnesium-rich foods such as whole grains and beans, have a significantly lower C-reactive protein level than those that do not reach the daily RDA of 310 mg–420 mcg.

Among 68,782 women in the study, a 5 g (0.17 oz) per day increase in cereal fibre was associated with a 37 percent reduced risk of heart disease. This amount is found in one serving of most whole-grain cereals.

The FDA permits the following label: 'Three grams of soluble fibre in a diet low in saturated fat and cholesterol may reduce the risk of heart disease.' Increase overall fibre intake and foods that are good sources of soluble fibre (see chart below).

Goal: To eat at least 25 g (1 oz) of total fibre daily (ideally 30–45 g/1–1½ oz a day):

Food	Fibre Content	Soluble Fibre
Kidney beans (8 tbsp)	6.6 grams	1.6 grams
Black beans (8 tbsp)	6.1 grams	2.4 grams
Most beans (8 tbsp)	4–6 grams	0.8-2.4 grams
Spinach (16 tbsp cooked)	4.5 grams	1.0 grams
Oat bran (8 tbsp)	4.5 grams	2.2 grams
Pear (1 medium)	4.3 grams	1.1 grams
Raspberries (8 tbsp)	4.2 grams	0.45 grams
Baked potato with skin (150 g)	4.2 grams	1.0 grams
Oatmeal (8 tbsp dry)	4 grams	2.2 grams
Popcorn (48 tbsp)	4 grams	0.1 grams

Fibre-rich foods, including whole grains, are excellent sources of vitamins (vitamin E, folic acid), minerals (magnesium, copper, manganese), antioxidants, and phytochemicals (isoflavones, flavonoids) that are associated with reducing overall heart disease risk.

Bone Health

Researchers are discovering that the body needs more than calcium, vitamin D and vitamin K to maintain healthy bones. Many required nutrients are those that are lost when we choose refined grains instead of whole grains. Magnesium, for example, is a mineral that activates vitamin D, increasing calcium absorption. Copper is a mineral that slows the rate of bone loss. Zinc, another nutrient lost in the refining process, supports osteoblasts, specialized cells that develop bone minerals.

Breast Health

Fibre intake, although the research is unclear, may play a role in preventing breast cancer. Fibre-rich foods, including whole grains, are excellent sources of vitamins (vitamin E, folic acid), minerals (selenium) antioxidants and phytochemicals (isoflavones, lignans, phytates and flavonoids) that independently are associated with reducing overall cancer risk.

Eating more fibre (29 g/1 oz in one study) has been shown to significantly reduce oestrogen levels (serum estradiol) which may reduce breast cancer risk. It is advisable to continue to eat a diet with many different high fibre plant foods.

- EAT NUTS AND SEEDS

Goal: Aim to eat five servings of unsalted nuts and seeds weekly and increase variety: almonds, almond butter, Brazil nuts, macadamias, peanuts, natural peanut butter, pecans, pine nuts, pistachios, pumpkin seeds, sunflower seeds, walnuts. Serving = 30 g (1 oz) or 150–200 calories (4 tbsp of nuts or seeds or 2 tbsp nut/seed butters)

Overall Health

While it is true that nuts and seeds are high-fat foods, the predominant type of fat is the healthier monounsaturated type. Nuts and seeds provide a source of nutrients that are lacking in many diets. Eat appropriate servings (a handful) of unsalted nuts to avoid excessive fat and calorie intake. Make nuts and seeds part of a snack or add them to cooked dishes and salads.

A large case control study found that women consuming nuts regularly (5+ servings per week) had a 30 percent less risk of colon cancer compared to those consuming no nuts or seeds. This preliminary finding was not observed in men.

Heart Health

Studies have found that 5+ servings of nuts weekly may reduce the risk of heart disease by as much as 30–50 percent. Nuts and seeds contain many heart-healthy nutrients, including: vitamin E, folic acid, copper, magnesium, potassium and arginine. The body uses arginine to create nitric oxide, a potent vasodilator that helps to relax arteries.

5. SUNBATHE EARLY OR LATE IN THE DAY

It is good to expose your skin to the gentle morning or late-afternoon sun, without sunscreen, for 10–15 minutes at a time only. Be warned though that excessive exposure to the sun can be harmful and should be avoided.

Overall Health

Direct sunlight triggers the synthesis of vitamin D, a nutrient that is necessary for calcium absorption. Although vitamin D is fat-soluble and is stored for months, conscious sunbathing is necessary for those who have less exposure to the sun or those living in northern climates. A large study in Norway found that sunlight exposure during the diagnosis and treatment of breast and colon cancer increased the prognosis of these cancers.

Bone Health

Long-term observational studies positively correlate vitamin D intake (and not total calcium or milk intake) with reduced hip fracture rate. In addition to 10–15 minutes of direct sunlight, consume oily fish, fortified dairy products and a multivitamin to ensure adequate levels.

Breast Health

Vitamin D regulates cell growth and promotes differentiation in a number of cell types, a step that reduces the risk of cancer. A study of 190 women with incident breast cancer from a cohort of more than 5,000 found evidence that sunlight and the dietary vitamin D reduce the risk of breast cancer. A case-control study of breast cancer over an 11-year period in 24 U.S. states also found an inverse relationship between sunlight exposure and the risk of breast cancer.

6. MODERATE ALCOHOL INTAKE

- DEFINED AS ONE DRINK OR LESS per day for women: 35 cl (12 fl.oz) beer, 18 cl (6 fl.oz) glass of wine, 4 cl (1¼ fl.oz) of distilled spirits

Overall Health

Excessive alcohol intake (more than 2 drinks daily for women) increases the risk for physical dependence, malnutrition and cirrhosis, as well as cancers of the mouth, pharynx, larynx, oesophagus and liver and may contribute to colon, rectum and breast cancer. Excessive alcohol increases the risk for all-cause mortality, ischaemic stroke and hypertension. Alcohol is a source of empty calories and can contribute to excess body weight. Red wine is a source of potent antioxidants called polyphenols. Other sources include red grapes, blueberries, cherries and green tea.

Women with a higher alcohol intake (more than one drink per day) and a low folate intake (less than 180 mcg per day) had a significantly higher risk for colon cancer. The risk was not seen when folate intake was high (400 mcg). Women are advised to take a multivitamin containing 400 mcg folic acid and eat a diet rich in folate (beans, greens, nuts and oranges).

Heart Health

A meta-analysis of 42 studies comparing the relationship between alcohol intake and heart disease markers consistently showed one drink daily was beneficial. Researchers estimate that one alcoholic drink daily would cause an estimated reduction of 24.7 percent in risk of coronary heart disease.

Bone Health

The consensus on alcohol intake at this time is that two to four drinks daily for women can increase hip fracture rate by 44 percent. Among 489 elderly women (65–77 years of age), those who had 1–2 alcoholic drinks per week had significantly higher spine (10 percent), total body (4.5 percent), and midradius (6 percent) bone mineral density than did non-drinkers.

Breast Health

A pooled analysis of six prospective studies conducted in Canada, the Netherlands, Sweden and the United States of 322,647 women for up to 11 years, including

4,335 participants with a diagnosis of incident invasive breast cancer found a linear relationship between alcohol intake and breast cancer risk. For women consuming ¾ drink–1 drink per day, risk was increased by 9 percent compared to non-drinkers. For those consuming 2–5 drinks per day, the adjusted relative risk was increased 41 percent versus non-drinkers.

7. INCREASE WATER INTAKE

Goal: To drink at least 1.5 litres (48 fl.oz) daily. An adequate intake of water reduces the incidence of kidney stone and gallstone formation, facilitates waste elimination and improves overall immune function. Invest in a simple filter that removes lead, fluoride, chlorine and other contaminants. Choose water that is distilled, purified by reverse osmosis, or purified by carbon filtration when purchasing bottled water.

8. DRINK 1–3 CUPS OF GREEN TEA DAILY (CAFFEINATED OR DECAFFEINATED)

Green tea contains powerful antioxidants called polyphenols. It is theorized that these polyphenols, similar to those found in red wine, act to prevent LDL oxidation and possibly reduce the risk of heart disease. Epidemiological studies show a correlation between green tea intake and significantly lower total cholesterol, triglycerides, LDL and higher HDL levels. One of the phenols, EGCG, is being investigated for its anti-carcinogenic properties. Preliminary research in animals suggests that regular tea consumption is protective against cancers of the stomach, lung, oesophagus, duodenum, pancreas, liver and colon. Drinking at least half a cup of green or Oolong tea has also been associated with a reduced risk of high blood pressure.

To make decaf green tea, simply steep the tea for 45 seconds in hot water and then pour off the liquid. Then add hot water and steep in the manner you would normally use to brew a cup of that tea. As up to 80 percent of the caffeine will be released into the brief infusion of water, the subsequent infusions will have minimal amounts of caffeine.

9. AVOID EXCESSIVE CAFFEINE

A study of 489 elderly women (65–77 years of age) found that a daily intake of 300 mg of caffeine or more significantly increases the rate of bone loss from the spine. The study found an even greater relationship among women with a genetic susceptibility (vitamin D receptor polymorphism) to osteoporosis. This amount of caffeine equals about 0.5 litre (18 fl.oz) strongly brewed coffee daily or 6 glasses of soft drinks or tea.

Caffeine stimulates the central nervous system and can cause insomnia, nervousness, gastric irritation, nausea and vomiting. It can shorten the stress response, increase heart rate, increase blood pressure, raise homocysteine levels, quicken the respiratory rate and in great excess, cause tremors and convulsions.

Drink	Caffeine (milligrams)
Brewed coffee (227 g)	60–120 mg
Instant coffee (227 g)	90–110 mg
Espresso (28 g)	45–100 mg
Black tea (227 g)	50 mg
Green tea (227 g)	30 mg

10. CHOOSE QUALITY ANIMAL PRODUCTS WHEN POSSIBLE

• FREE-RANGE, HORMONE-FREE CHICKEN AND TURKEY
• EGGS FROM FREE-RANGE, UNMEDICATED CHICKENS
• ORGANIC DAIRY PRODUCTS

Choose quality animal products to avoid the potentially damaging effects of hormones (including steroid-like compounds), medication (including antibiotics) and other chemicals used by the industry to increase production. Eggs from free-running chickens contain higher levels of omega 3 fats, vitamin E and carotenoids, such as beta-carotene.

11. CONSIDER ADDING THE FOLLOWING REGULARLY

• EAT ORGANIC LOW-FAT YOGURT (4+ pots a week) or soy yogurt with live cultures.

Live cultures in yogurt such as *Lactobacillus acidophilus* and *Lactobacillus bulgaricus* are beneficial bacteria that help maintain healthy intestinal flora of the digestive tract.

Health & Healing For Men Nutritional Guidelines

In a recently published study of 44,875 men (aged 40–75), with an eight-year follow-up, those eating the healthiest 'prudent pattern' diet which contained a high intake of vegetables, fruit, legumes, whole grains, fish and poultry had only half the risk of developing heart disease as those eating the 'Western pattern' diet, characterized by high intake of red meat, processed meat, refined grains, sweets and desserts, french fries and high-fat dairy products.

These guidelines detail nutritional recommendations for overall health, and provide specific research-based recommendations for the prevention of heart, prostate and colon disease. Traditional Western diets containing excessive amounts of processed foods can contribute to the development of disease and impede the healing process. The key aspects of this programme will be to create a sustainable diet rich in antioxidants and other healthy nutrients, target specific nutrients that are important to the process of building and maintaining health, and provide supplement recommendations to support optimal health.

NOTE: Use this information in the light of other health issues you may have, foods that you like and that are agreeable to you and any more specific recommendations provided by your doctor.

1.INCREASE FRUIT & VEGETABLE INTAKE

Goal: To eat at least 7 servings of fruits and vegetables daily and increase variety:

Fruit: 1 serving = ½ banana, 1 medium fruit, 12 cl (4 oz) juice, 2 tbsp raisins

Vegetables: 1 serving = 1 serving raw vegetables, ½ serving cooked vegetables

- INCLUDE DARK GREEN VEGETABLES DAILY: broccoli, spinach, kale, collards, cabbage, brussel sprouts, mustard greens, salad mix
- INCLUDE ORANGE FRUITS AND VEGETABLES DAILY: sweet potato, carrots, carrot juice, winter squash, melon, dried apricots
- INCLUDE ANTIOXIDANT-RICH FRUITS at least once a week, including: prunes, raisins, blueberries, strawberries, raspberries
- EAT LYCOPENE-RICH FOODS REGULARLY (4+ servings weekly): cooked tomato sauce, salsa, tomatoes, watermelon, red grapefruit
- INCREASE GARLIC AND ONION CONSUMPTION if well tolerated. Add to stir fries, soups and pasta sauce. Eat chopped with salsa on crackers or toast.

Overall Health

Fruit and vegetables provide an array of beneficial nutrients and eating seven servings daily 'displaces' less healthy snack foods and helps with weight control. The dark green cruciferous vegetables contain indole-3-carbinol, a substance that facilitates the removal of cancer-causing substances by stimulating liver detoxification enzymes. Eat dark greens raw or lightly steamed because cooking destroys this potent compound. The crucifers are also rich sources of folic acid, calcium, vitamin K, beta-carotene, lutein, vitamin C and fibre.

Dark greens, red, orange and yellow vegetables contain carotenoids, a family of over 600 phytochemicals, including beta-carotene and lutein. Many of the carotenoids and other antioxidants found in fruit and vegetables protect DNA from free radical damage (a process that leads to ageing and disease), may prevent heart disease by inhibiting LDL oxidation, enhance the immune system, and may be protective against cancers of the oesophagus, lung, stomach and colon. NOTE: Garlic exhibits anticoagulant properties. If you are taking blood-thinning supplements, such as vitamin E, gingko biloba, fish oil, or aspirin or are taking warfarin or other medications, consult a doctor before adding to the diet.

Heart Health

A survey of 22,071 men in the Physicians' Health Study, found that those who had consumed 2.5 servings of vegetables daily had a 23 percent reduced risk of heart disease compared to those eating less than one vegetable daily over a 6-year period. An eight-week DASH diet (Dietary Approaches to Stopping Hypertension), that consists of nine servings of fruit and vegetables, as well as other dietary changes that reduce total fat and saturated fat, has been shown to significantly reduce blood pressure and cholesterol levels, both risk factors for heart disease.

Prostate Health

Over 35 studies have shown a statistically significant inverse relationship between tomato intake or blood lycopene level and the risk of cancer. Consumption of 6 mcg a day or more of lycopene (best absorbed from cooked tomato products and with a small amount of fat, such as olive oil) is linked with a reduced incidence of prostate cancer in large population studies. An 24 cl (8 fl.oz) cup of tomato juice provides about 23 mcg of lycopene. A study of more than 47,000 men found that those who ate at least two meals a week containing tomato products lowered their risk of prostate cancer by 24–36 percent compared to those eating tomato products less than once a month. A good reason to eat tomato-based products instead of lycopene supplements is that other carotenoids in tomatoes, such as phytofluene and zeta-carotene, reduce prostate cancer cell viability in laboratory tests.

Garlic and onions contain diallyl sulphide, a potent tumour suppressor, as well as other beneficial sulphur containing compounds. In a case-control study, men who ate garlic two or more times weekly had a 44 percent reduced risk of developing prostate cancer compared to men that never consumed garlic. Cooking destroys some of the beneficial properties of garlic and onion.

Colon Health

Greens are a great source of lutein, a carotenoid that may lower colon cancer risk. Calcium from greens may also lower colon cancer risk by binding to bile salts and other carcinogens in the intestine.

2. BUILD THE DIET AROUND HEALTHY FATS

• Reduce saturated fats to less than 15 g (½ oz) daily, including: cheese, butter, ice cream, whole-milk, beef, processed foods

Food	Saturated Fat
Ice cream (1 portion vanilla – 16% fat)	15 grams
Hamburger (100 g regular)	8 grams
Hotdog (1 regular beef)	7 grams
Cheese (25 g)	6 grams
Whole milk (1 glass)	6 grams
Butter (1 pat)	3 grams

• REPLACE POLYUNSATURATED OILS AND SATURATED FATS with monounsaturated oils at restaurants.
Request that dishes be prepared with olive oil or rapeseed oil instead of butter, soybean or corn oils
Request extra-virgin olive oil and balsamic vinegar/lemon juice for salads instead of salad dressings made from polyunsaturated oils
Use olive oil instead of butter on bread
Buy quality oils for home use
Extra-virgin olive oil, organic (non-genetically modified) rapeseed oil, high-oleic sunflower oil, high-oleic safflower oil and light olive oil.
Sesame oil, grapeseed oil, virgin coconut oil
• EAT HEALTHY FATS:
Plant fats: nuts and nut butters, seeds (pumpkin, sesame and sunflower) and seed butters (tahini)
Goal: Eat at least five servings weekly.
Omega-3s: salmon, sardines, bluefish, albacore tuna, herring, mackerel
Goal: Eat at least one serving, 425 g (15 oz) a week

Fish and omega-3 content	Per 100 g (3.5 oz) serving
More than 1.0 gram	Anchovies, bluefish, herring, Spanish mackerel, king mackerel*, salmon, sardines, lake trout*, bluefin tuna*, albacore tuna*
0.5 grams - 0.99 grams	Striped bass*, sea bass*, rainbow trout*, blue mussels, oysters, flounder, halibut*
Less than 0.5 grams	Carp, catfish, clams, crab, cod, grouper*, lobster*, perch, mahi mahi, mullet, orange roughy*, pike, red snapper*, scallops, sea trout*, shrimp, sole, squid, sturgeon, swordfish*, canned light tuna (not albacore)

*CAUTION: Fish with higher concentrations of mercury.

Omega-3s: Organic 'designer' eggs (see label) that contain omega-3s

Four DHA-rich eggs have the same omega-3 content as 100 g (3.5 oz) salmon

Goal: Aim to eat four eggs per week

- Avoid trans fatty-acids (foods containing hydrogenated oil): Hard margarine, fried potato/tortilla chips, french fries and other fried foods, store-bought baked goods, commercial cookies
- Avoid fried foods: French fries, fried chicken, fried fish

Overall Health

Fats are essential for the proper functioning of cells, the synthesis of beneficial hormone-like substances called prostaglandins, the absorption of fat-soluble nutrients, such as vitamins A, D, E and K, for improving the taste of food, and for overall satisfaction. While fat is a concentrated source of calories, an adequate intake of healthy fats makes it easier to lose and sustain weight.

Saturated fats, in excess, increase total and LDL cholesterol and are associated with an increased risk of several types of cancers. Saturated fats increase the synthesis of PG1 prostaglandins, hormone-like compounds that support the inflammatory response.

Polyunsaturated oils are more readily oxidized, a step associated with heart disease progression and cellular damage. Monounsaturated fats and polyunsaturated fats in plant foods lower total cholesterol and LDL levels, maintain HDL levels, and are not associated with an increased risk for cancer. Omegas-3s, a class of polyunsaturated fats, promote the synthesis of PG3 prostaglandins that exert an anti-inflammatory and blood-thinning effect. They help reduce heart disease, cancer, rheumatoid arthritis and depression.

Trans fats (from hydrogenated oils) increase total and LDL cholesterol and lower beneficial HDL cholesterol levels. Because trans-fats malfunction when incorporated into cell membranes, they may increase cancer risk. Most commercially fried foods, such as fast-food french fries, are cooked in partially hydrogenated oils (and contain trans-fats).

Heart Health

A six-year follow-up study of 43,757 male health professionals free of heart disease found that those consuming 32 g (1 oz) of saturated fat daily had a 121 percent increased risk of developing fatal coronary heart disease compared to those consuming less than 16 g (½ oz) of saturated fat.

Prostate Health

Animal fats are consistently associated with an increased risk of prostate cancer. A case series analysis of prostate cancer cases found a 215 percent increase in advanced prostate cancer risk among those consuming the most saturated fat. The relationship in this study increased significantly with saturated fat intake.

NOTE: In a Harvard study, alpha-linolenic acid (ALA) intake increased the risk of presenting with more advanced prostate cancer. Because flaxseed is a concentrated source of ALA, men with prostate cancer or strong family history of prostate cancer should avoid flaxseed until further research is conducted.

Colon Health

While there is little data to support an adverse relationship between trans-fat intake and colon cancer, an ecological study that examined the adipose tissue from eight European countries and Israel found a relationship between trans fat intake and colon cancer.

3. SHIFT THE PROTEIN SOURCES IN YOUR DIET

- Reduce red meat consumption. Less is better: hamburgers, steak, roast beef, pork, bacon, sausage
- Avoid cured or smoked foods that contain nitrates/nitrites: hotdogs, sausage, bologna other luncheon meats
- Choose low-fat animal protein: chicken breast, turkey breast, fish, egg whites, low-fat yogurt, low-fat cottage cheese, low-fat milk
- Eat at least one omega-3 rich type of fish every week (aim for 425 g/15 oz a week)
- Replace at least three servings of animal protein each week with a plant-based meal: ethnic vegetarian dishes (Indian, Thai, Chinese, Mexican, Ethiopian), pasta with vegetables, beans and rice, vegetable stir-fries, vegetable stews, whole bean burritos, hummus sandwiches. Soy-based veggie burgers, soymilk, edamame, soy-based breakfast meats, tofu, tempeh

Overall Health

Red meat is a significant contributor of saturated fat to the Western diet, and is associated with heart disease and cancers of the lung, colon, rectum and prostate. Avoid particularly cured or smoked foods that contain nitrites because they can form cancer-causing compounds called nitrosamines in the stomach. Low-fat animal protein choices help to minimize saturated fat intake. A regular beef hotdog contains half the recommended intake of saturated fat for the day.

Soy products may offer a significant benefit for those with elevated cholesterol levels, particularly when soy is consumed in place of higher fat animal products. Soy products are a source of dietary protein that is low in saturated fat and rich in nutrients known to support cardiovascular health, such as fibre.

Fish intake is correlated to a lower incidence of disease, particularly heart and cancer. Vegetarian protein sources eaten more often will increase the levels of beneficial plant nutrients in the diet, including antioxidants and fibre.

Heart Health

Consumption of one to two servings a week of fish oils from dietary sources appears to reduce the risk of coronary heart disease death by 25 percent. Replacing animal protein with soy protein increases LDL particle size to a better pattern, lowering heart disease risk.

Prostate Health

Red meat is a significant contributor of total fat and saturated fat in the American diet, both of which have shown a correlation to an increased risk of prostate cancer. The dietary habits of 20,316 Hawaiian men were studied and dietary correlations were established between red meat intake and the 198 prostate cancer cases that developed in the following 15-year period. Those in the highest third of beef consumption had a 60 percent increased risk of prostate cancer compared to those in the lowest third. A study of 51,529 health professionals found a 50 percent increased risk of metastatic prostate cancer among those eating the most red meat, after controlling for the effects of saturated fat.

A study of 225 incident cases of prostate cancer in 12,395 California Seventh-Day Adventist men found that consumption more than once a day of soy milk

was associated with a 70 percent reduction of the risk of prostate cancer. It is unclear whether soy products are beneficial in the treatment of prostate cancer.

The essential omega-3 oils play an important role in producing hormone-like compounds called prostaglandins that exert anti-inflammatory, blood-thinning properties and in animal experiments, anti-tumour effects. A study of 6,272 men over 30 years found that those eating no fish had a 2–3 times higher risk of prostate cancer compared to those consuming fish regularly.

Colon Health

One large study found that a higher intake of red meat and processed meats over time increases the risk for colon cancer by more than 50 percent compared to those consuming more poultry and fish.

4. INCREASE FIBRE-RICH FOODS

- EAT BEANS AT LEAST FOUR TIMES PER WEEK: black bean burritos, hummus, garbanzo, kidney, pinto and other beans in salads and soups, rice and beans, vegetarian 'pork and beans', bean-based dishes
- EAT WHOLE-GRAIN BREADS: select those with at least 2 g (0.1 oz) fibre per slice: whole wheat, spelt, kamut, rye, sprouted grains
- EAT HIGHER-FIBRE CEREALS: select those with at least four grams of fibre per serving
- REDUCE REFINED, LOW-FIBRE CARBOHYDRATES: bagels, white breads, juices, white pasta, white rice
- GREATLY REDUCE EMPTY CALORIE CARBOHYDRATES: pastries, soft drinks, cakes, sweets, biscuits, baked goods, ice cream

Overall Health

Fibre intake plays a key role in slowing the absorption of dietary sugars, maintaining intestinal regularity (primarily insoluble fibre), reducing cholesterol levels (soluble), as well as a possible role in reducing the risk of colon cancer. Fibre-rich foods, including whole grains, are excellent sources of vitamins (vitamin E, folic acid), minerals (selenium, magnesium and zinc), and antioxidants and phytochemicals (isoflavones, lignans, phytates and flavonoids).

The refining process removes the wheat bran and wheat germ, sources of essential nutrients that play a significant role in prostate health. Whole-wheat flour contains twice as much calcium and copper than white flour, three times more potassium, four times more zinc and fibre, five times more manganese, six times more magnesium and eight times more vitamin B$_6$.

Heart Health

In a six-year follow-up of 43,757 male health professionals free from heart disease, those consuming 29 g (1 oz) of fibre daily had a 41 percent reduced risk of having a heart attack compared to those consuming 12 g (½ oz) of fibre daily (the average intake for an American male). Of the three main contributors to fibre intake (vegetable, fruit and cereal), cereal was most strongly associated with a reduced heart attack risk.

Recent findings of a large observational study found that fibre intake is independently associated with C-reactive protein. Those eating more fibre had significantly lower levels of this inflammatory marker. The lowest C-reactive protein was found among those consuming 32 g (1¼ oz) of fibre or more each day.

Increase overall fibre intake and foods that are good sources of soluble fibre (see chart below).

GOAL: To eat at least 25 g (1 oz) of total fibre daily:

Food	Fibre Content	Soluble Fibre
Kidney beans (8 tbsp)	6.6 grams	1.6 grams
Black beans (8 tbsp)	6.1 grams	2.4 grams
Most beans (8 tbsp)	4–6 grams	0.8-2.4 grams
Spinach (16 tbsp)	4.5 grams	1.0 grams
Oat bran (8 tbsp)	4.5 grams	2.2 grams
Pear (1 medium)	4.3 grams	1.1 grams
Raspberries (8 tbsp)	4.2 grams	0.45 grams
6 oz. Baked potato with skin	4.2 grams	1.0 grams
Oatmeal (8 tbsp dry)	4 grams	2.2 grams
Popcorn (48 tbsp)	4 grams	0.1 grams

Fibre-rich foods, including whole grains, are excellent sources of vitamins (vitamin E, folic acid), minerals (magnesium, copper, manganese), antioxidants and phytochemicals (isoflavones, flavonoids) that are associated with reducing overall heart disease risk.

A study of 9,632 men and women followed over an average of 19 years found that those consuming beans four times or more per week compared with less than once a week had a 22 percent lower risk of developing coronary heart disease.

Recent findings found that fibre intake is independently associated with C-reactive protein. Those eating more fibre had significantly lower levels of this marker. The lowest C-reactive protein was found in those consuming 32 g (1¼ oz) of fibre or more a day.

Prostate Health

A case control study found that men consuming a diet with a greater percentage of high glycaemic index foods (more refined carbohydrates) have as much as a 57 percent increased risk of prostate cancer.

Colon Health

Fibre-rich foods, including whole grains, are excellent sources of vitamins (vitamin E, folic acid), minerals (selenium) antioxidants and phytochemicals (isoflavones, lignans, phytates and flavonoids) that independently are associated with reducing overall cancer risk.

5. EAT NUTS AND SEEDS

Goal: Aim to eat five servings of unsalted nuts and seeds weekly and increase variety: Almonds, almond butter, Brazil nuts, filberts, macadamias, peanuts, peanut butter, pecans, pine nuts, pistachios, pumpkin seeds, sunflower seeds, walnuts. Serving = 28 g (1 oz) or 150–200 calories (4 tbsp of nuts or seeds or 2 tbsp nut/seed butters).

Overall Health

While it is true that nuts and seeds are high fat foods, the predominant type of fat is the healthier monounsaturated type. Nuts and seeds provide a source of nutrients that are lacking in many diets. Eat appropriate servings (a handful) of unsalted nuts to avoid excessive fat and calorie intake. Make nuts and seeds part of a snack or add them to cooked dishes and salads.

Heart Health

Studies have found that 5+ servings of nuts weekly may reduce the risk of heart disease by 30–50 percent. Nuts and seeds have many heart-healthy nutrients, including: vitamin E, folic acid, copper, magnesium, potassium and arginine. The body uses arginine to create nitric oxide, a potent vasodilator that helps to relax arteries.

6. MODERATE ALCOHOL INTAKE.

• DEFINED AS TWO DRINKS OR LESS per day for men. 35 cl (12 fl.oz) beer, 18 cl (6 fl.oz) glass of wine, 4 cl (1¼ oz) of distilled spirits.

Overall Health

Excessive alcohol intake (more than 3 drinks daily for men) increases the risk for physical dependence, malnutrition, cirrhosis as well as cancers of the mouth, pharynx, larynx, oesophagus and liver and may contribute to colon and rectum cancer. Excessive alcohol increases the risk for all-cause mortality, ischaemic stroke and hypertension. Alcohol is a source of empty calories that can contribute to excess body weight.

Heart Health

An analysis of 42 studies comparing the relationship between alcohol intake and heart disease markers consistently showed one alcoholic drink daily was beneficial. Researchers estimate that one alcoholic drink daily would cause an estimated reduction of 24.7 percent in risk of coronary heart disease. Red wine is a source of potent antioxidants called polyphenols.

Colon Health

A study of nearly 48,000 male health professionals found that those consuming more than two alcoholic drinks per day who also had a low intake of folate had a three times greater risk for developing colon cancer. However, those with a high intake of folate had no increased risk for colon cancer. Men are advised to take a multivitamin containing 400 mcg folic acid and eat a diet rich in folate (beans, greens, nuts and oranges).

7. INCREASE WATER INTAKE

Goal: Drink at least 1.5 litre (48 fl.oz) daily. An adequate intake of water reduces the incidence of kidney stone and gallstone formation, facilitates waste elimination, and improves overall immune function. Invest in a simple filter that removes lead, fluoride, chlorine and other contaminants. Choose water that is distilled, purified by reverse osmosis or purified by carbon filtration when purchasing bottled water.

8. DRINK 1-3 CUPS OF GREEN TEA DAILY

Green tea contains powerful antioxidants called polyphenols. It is theorized that these polyphenols, similar to those found in red wine, act to prevent LDL oxidation and possibly reduce the risk of heart disease. One of the phenols, EGCG, is being investigated for its anti-carcinogenic properties. Preliminary research in animals suggests that regular tea consumption is protective against cancers of the stomach, lung, oesophagus, duodenum, pancreas, liver and colon.

9. AVOID EXCESSIVE CAFFEINE

Caffeine stimulates the central nervous system and can cause insomnia, nervousness, gastric irritation, nausea and vomiting. It can shorten the stress response, increase heart rate, increase blood pressure, raise homocysteine levels, quicken the respiratory rate and in great excess, cause tremors and convulsions.

Drinks	Caffeine (milligrams)
Brewed coffee (227 g)	60–120 mg
Instant coffee (227 g)	90–110 mg
Espresso (28 g)	45–100 mg
Black tea (227 g)	50 mg
Green tea (227 g)	30 mg

10. CHOOSE QUALITY ANIMAL PRODUCTS WHEN POSSIBLE

• FREE-RANGE, HORMONE-FREE CHICKEN
• EGGS FROM FREE-RANGE, UNMEDICATED CHICKENS
• ORGANIC DAIRY PRODUCTS

Choose quality animal products to avoid the potentially damaging effects of hormones (including steroid-like compounds), medication (including antibiotics) and other chemicals used by the industry to increase production. Eggs from free-running chickens contain higher levels of omega 3 fats, vitamin E and carotenoids, such as beta-carotene.

11. CONSIDER ADDING THE FOLLOWING

• EAT ORGANIC LOW-FAT YOGURT (4+ pots a week) or soy yogurt with live cultures.

Live cultures in yogurt such as *Lactobacillus acidophilus* and *Lactobacillus bulgaricus* are beneficial bacteria that maintain the intestinal flora of the digestive tract.

GLOSSARY

abortion A procedure in which a developing foetus is removed from the uterus before it is able to survive on its own.

abscess A swollen and inflamed cavity formed as a result of an infection. An abscess is filled with pus or a yellowish–white substance composed of dead white blood cells.

ace inhibitor Angiotensin converting enzyme (ACE) inhibitors are medications that lower blood pressure by slowing the production of angiotensin II, a blood vessel constrictor.

acetaminophen A medication that works to relieve pain and reduce a fever. Unlike aspirin, this drug does not produce an anti-inflammatory response.

acidosis A condition in which the bloodstream contains an elevated amount of acid.

acromegaly A disorder in which the pituitary gland produces excess growth hormone resulting in bone thickening and cartilage growth. It is often characterized by an enlargement of the nose, ears, jaw, fingers and toes.

acupoint Contraction of 'acupuncture point', a site of needle insertion for acupuncture, located along one of several meridians.

adaptive asymmetry Imbalance of posture or movement between the two sides of the body of a form regarded as helpful in Aston-Patterning (contrast negative asymmetry).

addiction Compulsive behaviour due to physical or psychological dependence on drugs or other substances.

adenoid Tiny glands located behind the nose that capture and filter out germs entering the body as well as produce antibodies needed to fight off infection.

adenoma A typically benign tumour that is composed of glandular tissue such as from the breast, thyroid, lung, pancreas or colon.

adenovirus A type of virus that can cause infections in the upper respiratory tract, the gastrointestinal tract, bladder and the eye.

adhesive capsulitis Inflammation of the shoulder joint causing pain and restricted movement, 'frozen shoulder'.

adrenal gland An endocrine gland located near the kidneys that produces sex hormones, stress hormones and steroid hormones. It plays a key role in the regulation of blood pressure and the heart rate.

aldosterone A corticosteroid hormone that is secreted by the adrenal gland. Aldosterone regulates the balance between salt and water within the kidneys.

allergy/allergen A substance that causes the immune system to overreact.

alternative medicines Substances used to treat disease outside the remit of orthodox medicine

amenorrhoea A period of time in which a woman does not experience her menstrual cycle. It can occur as a result of pregnancy, breastfeeding, birth control, hormonal imbalances or stress.

amino acid A biochemical substance used to form a protein. There are 20 amino acids which can join together in various sequences to create a protein.

anabolic steroids A class of hormones that promote the growth of tissues resulting in the development of muscle enhancement, bone size and strength. Testosterone is an example of an anabolic steroid.

anaesthesia A drug that produces the loss of feeling in a specific area of the body or a loss of consciousness. Anaesthesia blocks pain impulses from nerve endings thus preventing the sensation of pain.

analgesic A type of medication used to relieve pain. These compounds work by lowering one's sensation to pain.

angina Pain in the chest due to insufficient oxygen reaching the heart muscles when blood supply is inadequate.

anorexia nervosa An eating disorder in which a person has an altered body perception causing the development of an aversion to food. Those with this disorder suffer from extremely low body weights.

antenatal A term used to describe the period of time before a pregnant woman gives birth.

antibiotic A class of drugs capable of destroying bacteria.

antibody A protein produced by B cells that can recognize, attach to, and destroy harmful substances within the body. These are a major part of the immune system and trigger the initiation of the body's self-defence strategies.

anticoagulant A substance that prevents the formation of blood clots.

anticonvulsant A drug that can prevent or decrease the severity of seizures.

antifungal A substance that inhibits the growth of fungi.

antihistamine A medication that inhibits the action of histamine within the body's tissues. This class of drugs is used to treat allergic reactions.

antihypertensive A medication that lowers blood pressure.

anti-inflammatory A substance that reduces inflammation, the body's natural response to injury.

antioxidants Substances that inhibit oxidation and so counteract the effects of free radicals in the body. Also known as free radical scavengers.

antipsychotic A medication that produces a calming effect and that is used to treat psychotic disorders.

antiseptic A drug that can be applied to damaged tissue to prevent the growth of microorganisms. It is used to prevent the development of infection in a wound.

antiviral A substance used to treat a viral infection. These medications prevent the multiplication of viruses and can destroy them.

aortic valve Located between the left ventricle of the heart and the aorta, the aortic valve regulates blood flow from the heart into the aorta and prevents the back flow of blood.

apnoea A condition in which breathing is temporarily suspended. During an episode of apnoea, the muscles that control respiration do not move, and the volume of air within the lungs remains constant.

arnica A plant-derived medicine applied as a salve to treat bruising and pain, and also used in homeopathy.

aromatic medicine Alternative term for 'aromatherapy'.

arsenic A poison at one time used in medicine to treat syphilis and parasites.

arthokinetics Gentle joint manipulation aimed at releasing tension in Aston-Patterning.

asana A physical posture in yoga.

aspirate The inhaling of fluid or foreign matter into the lungs. Also defined as the removal of fluid, usually from a cyst, through the use of suction.

assisted reproduction technology (ART) Procedures that aid an infertile couple in achieving pregnancy. Examples include in vitro fertilization, gamete intra-fallopian transfer and intracytoplasmic sperm injection.

astringent A substance used to stop bleeding, close the pores and contract skin tissues.

autogenic training A relaxation technique using a form of self-hypnosis.

autohaemotherapy One technique of ozone therapy in which blood is removed, mixed with ozone and reinjected.

autoimmune A condition in which the body's immune system attacks its own healthy tissues.

bacteria A type of microorganism that is composed of a single cell.

beneficial bacteria Bacteria that live in harmony within the body and help to keep harmful microorganisms at bay.

benign A word used to describe a non-cancerous tumour. Benign tumours are not life-threatening and cannot invade surrounding tissues.

beriberi A nutritional disease caused by a deficiency of Vitamin B_1 (thiamin).

beta-2 agonist A drug that relaxes the muscles surrounding the airways thus increasing the passage of airflow during an asthma attack or a condition called chronic obstructive pulmonary disease.

beta-blockers A class of drugs with the ability to reduce blood pressure and decrease the heart rate thereby reducing the workload of the heart.

beta-carotene A carotenoid chemical naturally present in yellow- or orange-coloured fruit and vegetables that is used in the body to manufacture Vitamin A.

bibliotherapy The use of literature in psychological therapies.

bilateral nasal specific therapy Manipulation of the nasal bones using pressure inside the nostril. A forerunner of neurocranial restructuring.

biological rhythms Biological processes occurring or changing at regular intervals, such as hormone release.

biomechanics The study of physical forces acting on, or used by, the body to produce movement.

biopsy A procedure in which a small sample of tissue is removed and analysed for cellular abnormalities.

bloodletting Former medical practice involving removing large quantities of blood, supposedly to prevent or treat disease. It was largely ineffective and often dangerous.

body-mass index (BMI) A mathematical calculation used to assess body fat. It equals the weight in kilograms divided by the height in metres squared (kg/ m2).

body work Any form of therapy intended to improve physical functioning of the body by acting on its physical or energetic properties, for example through massage or manipulation.

bone density The concentration of calcium and other minerals within the bone's mass. A low bone density can be an indicator of osteoporosis.

bone marrow The soft spongy substance located within the cavities of the bones. Blood cells and platelets are produced within the bone marrow.

brain chemistry The study of chemicals in the brain and their effects on brain cells, behaviour and diseases.

bromelain An enzyme found in pineapples and used for its anti-inflammatory properties

bronchodilators The class of drugs that relax the smooth muscle within the walls of the airways thereby causing them to dilate.

Buddhist meditation Forms of meditation used in Buddhism that aim ultimately at spiritual enlightenment.

bursa A fluid-filled sac located between a tendon and a bone that provides lubrication and reduces friction within body parts subject to shearing forces such as the knee, hip, shoulder or elbow.

calcitonin A hormone secreted by the C cells of the thyroid gland. It helps to regulate calcium and phosphorous levels in the bone and blood.

calcium A mineral vital for the formation of bones and teeth within the body and often taken as a dietary supplement.

carcinoma A malignant tumour that originates in the epithelial cells that line the surface of an organ. The majority of cancers can be defined as carcinomas.

cardiopulmonary resuscitation (CPR) A technique of artificial breathing and chest compressions used to circulate oxygen through the body of someone who is unable to breathe on their own and whose heart has stopped beating.

carotenoid supplements Dietary supplements of carotenoids, substances found in yellow or orange plants and converted to Vitamin A within the body.

cartilage Rubbery connective tissue found between bones that allows for the smooth movement of joints and cushions the bone.

catharsis A breakthrough occurring in response to a crisis – an emotional catharsis releases tension by reliving or expressing strong emotions. The term may also be used to mean emptying or cleansing of the bowel.

cauterization The destruction of body tissues through the use of heat, extreme cold, an electrical current or a caustic agent.

cerebrospinal fluid CSF – the watery fluid that circulates within and around the brain and spinal cord.

chakras In Eastern philosophies, seven centres of concentrated life energy running from the base of the spine to the crown of the head.

chanting Repetitive and rhythmic speaking or singing of words or sounds.

chemotherapy A treatment for cancer that involves medications that destroy tumour cells.

cholesterol (HDL, LDL) A fatty substance made by the body or found in food that is derived from animal substances. Cholesterol travels through the blood as either a high density lipoprotein (HDL) or a low density lipoprotein (LDL). HDL aids in the transportation of cholesterol to the liver and out of the bloodstream. On the other hand, LDL transports cholesterol to the body. It is believed that elevated amounts of cholesterol increase the risk of developing clogged arteries or heart disease.

chondroitin A major component of cartilage, composed of a chain of sugars usually attached to proteins. It may be taken as a supplement to ease arthritis, often in combination with glucosamine.

chromosome A structure within the nucleus of most cells that contains genetic information or DNA. Chromosomes are found in pairs. A normal human has 46 chromosomes, 23 from each parent.

chronic Recurring or lasting a long time (the opposite of 'acute'), often used to describe a medical condition.

Circadian rhythms Biological rhythms occurring or changing on a cycle of about 24 hours, such as sleep-wake cycles or body temperature fluctuations.

circulation The flow of fluid around a system, such as blood in the heart and blood vessels (blood circulation)

claudication A recurrent cramping pain in the legs brought on by exercise and due to inadequate blood flow to the leg muscles – intermittent claudication.

clinical trial A research study used to evaluate the effects of a drug, treatment or medical device on a group of human subjects.

coagulate The formation of blood clots.

coenzyme Q$_{10}$ A substance located within most body tissues and within some food sources. It is processed by the body to produce cellular energy and has been found to have antioxidant properties.

cognitive flexibility The ability to adapt mental responses to changing situations and circumstances.

collagen The main component of connective tissue. It provides strength, support and elasticity to many parts of the body such as the skin, bones, tendons and ligaments.

colonic irrigation Flushing out the lower bowel with warm water to cleanse impurities. It uses more water, and is generally introduced higher up into the colon, than with an enema.

complementary therapy Any therapeutic system not encompassed by orthodox medicine but designed to work alongside it.

computerized tomography (CT) scan A diagnostic procedure that uses x-rays and computer technology to produce detailed cross-sectional images of the body.

congenital A medical condition that exists at birth. It may be inherited or caused by environmental factors such as an infection.

consultation The interaction between a patient or client and a practitioner.

contrast therapy In hydrotherapy, the use of alternating hot and cold treatments.

conventional treatment Any therapy prescribed or used within orthodox (allopathic) medicine.

convulsion An uncontrollable contraction of muscles that is often violent that occur as a result of disturbances in brain function.

coral calcium Dietary supplements of calcium where the mineral is derived from coral.

cortex The grey outer layer of brain tissue that is filled with nerve cells. The cortex contains the central area for the processing of all information and control.

corticosteroids A class of hormones that produce an anti-inflammatory effect.

cortisol A hormone that is associated with stress reduction and anti-inflammation within the body. Cortisol is produced by the adrenal gland and helps to regulate blood pressure, cardiovascular functioning, and the processing of fats, carbohydrates and proteins.

Cox table A type of examination couch with an opening for the face, so the patient can lie face-downwards to give comfortable access to the spine. It is usually used in chiropractic.

cranial nerve One of the 12 pairs of nerves that originate in the brainstem and serve the parts of the head.

cranial osteopathy Another term for craniosacral therapy.

cranio-occipital technique Another term for craniosacral therapy.

cruciferous vegetables Members of the cabbage family such as cabbage, broccoli, brussel sprouts and cauliflower. They are rich in antioxidants and a good source of dietary fibre.

cupping In Traditional Chinese Medicine, the use of suction from a heated receptacle applied to the skin in order to stimulate an acupoint.

cybernetics The study of communication and control processes in both biological and artificial systems.

cyst A fluid-filled sac.

cystoscopy A diagnostic procedure in which the bladder and urethra are examined. A thin, flexible viewing device, called a cystoscope, is inserted into the urethra during this procedure.

decoctions A herbal extract prepared by boiling or simmering. It is stronger than a tea or infusion.

decongestant A type of medication that reduces congestion in the respiratory system.

dehydration A state in which the body lacks sufficient amounts of fluids. It is often caused by severe sweating, diarrhoea or vomiting.

detoxification/detoxify To rid the body of a toxic substance, such as alcohol, drugs or poisons.

dharana In yoga, the use of fixed concentration on an object in order to still the mind.

diastolic A measurement of the amount of pressure within the walls of the blood vessels during the period when the heart is at rest and the ventricles are refilling.

dietary supplement Any addition to the normal diet, such as a vitamin, mineral, amino acid, herb or botanical taken by mouth.

dilating Widening or opening up of an aperture, cavity or tube, such as the pupils or blood vessels.

diuretic A substance that causes urination to occur more frequently than usual.

DNA Deoxyribonucleic acid (DNA) is a substance contained within the nucleus of most cells that transports genetic information. DNA is a double-stranded helical molecule that provides the cells with the instructions for growth, development and function.

dopamine A chemical substance that transmits signals between nerve cells within the brain. It regulates mood states, movement and balance.

doshas In Ayurveda, the three constitutional elements making up different body types and personalities: vata, pitta or kapha.

double-blind A type of research study in which the participants are randomly assigned to treatment or placebo groups and neither the patients nor doctors have knowledge of/are aware of the group to which a patient belongs.

dynamic relaxation A state of physical relaxation combined with mental concentration, characteristic of practices such as meditation and sophrology.

echinacea A herb often used to boost the immune system to treat colds and other infections.

electric shock therapy Also called electroconvulsive therapy or ECT, a means of inducing an artificial seizure by passing an electric current through the brain, a controversial treatment sometimes used in conventional psychiatry to manage depression.

electrocardiogram (ECG) A diagnostic procedure in which the electrical current produced by the contractions of the heart muscles are measured and analysed to detect damage. It is often used in diagnosing heart conditions.

electroencephalograph (EEG) A medical device used to measure the electrical activity in the brain. It is used to assess brain damage.

electrolyte A chemical compound that allows for the transportation of ions, charged substances, between the positive and negative portions of a cell.

electronic reactions of Abrams (ERA) The name originally applied to individuals' responses in the diagnostic procedure later developed as radionics.

elimination diet The exclusion of certain foods from the diet, usually in the attempt to pinpoint the cause of an allergy or reaction.

endocrine Used to describe the type of gland that secretes hormones directly into the bloodstream (rather than through a duct). Examples include the thyroid, adrenals and ovaries.

endocrinologist A doctor who specializes in endocrine gland disorders.

endorphins Morphine-like chemicals produced in the body that act as internal painkillers and mood enhancers.

endoscope A viewing device that is shaped as a thin flexible tube. It is inserted within an incision and allows the doctor to see the interior of any part of the body.

enema The procedure of introducing water or other fluids into the rectum to provoke a bowel movement. It can also be used to administer medication or a contrast agent, such as barium, to enable viewing of the lower bowel in conventional medical diagnosis (barium enema).

energy field The subtle energy representing the life force said to flow through and surround a person's physical body in various forms of energy medicine.

enzyme A protein produced by the body to speed up a chemical reaction – a biological catalyst.

epinephrine A hormone produced by the adrenal gland that increases the heart beat rate and blood pressure. It is released in response to stress and is a part of the fight-or-flight response.

ergonomics The science of designing furniture, equipment and environmental conditions around the physical and psychological needs of the person, to enhance comfort, well-being and productivity.

essential oil A volatile chemical that gives a plant its characteristic scent. When distilled or expressed it may be used in aromatherapy, perfumery, cosmetics and flavourings.

eurythmy A type of rhythmic movement intended to promote inner harmony. It is used in anthroposophic medicine to help various physical and psychological disorders.

evening primrose oil The oil extracted from the evening primrose herb, containing a high proportion of the fatty acid gamma linolenic acid (GLA), which has anti-inflammatory properties

extracts Parts of a whole, solutions of component materials, for example of plants or animal tissues.

extrasensory perception (ESP) The purported ability to sense information by intuitive capabilities beyond the reach of the normal five senses – a paranormal phenomenon also known as 'sixth sense'.

fallopian tube A part of the female reproductive system that is the passageway connecting the uterus to the ovaries. Both the egg and sperm are transported through this area and the majority of conceptions occur within the fallopian tubes.

flaxseed The seeds of the flax plant, from which linseed oil may be extracted. They are rich in omega-3 fatty acids, polyunsaturated oils with various health-giving properties.

folic acid One of the B vitamins, found in foods such as liver, yeast and green leafy vegetables. Deficiency causes a type of anaemia.

folk medicine Traditional healing practices often handed down by word of mouth.

follicle-stimulating hormone (FSH) An important hormone in the female reproductive system. FSH is released from the pituitary gland. It regulates the release of eggs and the secretion of oestrogen from the ovaries.

fracture A break in a bone or cartilage.

free radicals (in the body) Highly reactive chemicals that form in the body during oxidation and may damage cells, provoke disease or accelerate ageing.

galactorrhoea A condition in which breast milk is released from the nipple although a woman is not breastfeeding and has not recently given birth. It may also occur in men.

galvanic skin response A fall in the measured electrical resistance of the skin, often signalling anxiety or emotional reaction.

gangrene A condition in which body tissue begins to decay as a result of decreased blood flow or infection. This tissue usually turns black and emits a foul odour.

genetic Characteristics or conditions that are inherited.

ginkgo biloba A herbal medicine derived from the nuts of a Chinese tree and used especially for its antioxidant and brain-boosting effects.

ginseng A North American herb used to improve mental and physical function.

glucosamine A component of connective tissues such as cartilage. It can be extracted from sea creatures and taken as a supplement to ease osteoarthritis, often along with chondroitin.

glucose A type of sugar compound in the blood that is derived from carbohydrate food sources. It is processed by the body to provide energy.

gluten A protein found in wheat, rye, barley and oats that provides elasticity to dough. Gluten holds in gas bubbles produced by yeast thus allowing the bread to rise.

glycaemic index A measurement which reflects on the ability of a food item to raise blood sugar. It illustrates how quickly glucose is processed from carbohydrates and absorbed into the bloodstream. White bread, with a GI of 100, is the benchmark for comparison within this calculation.

growth hormone A hormone produced by the pituitary gland that regulates the growth of the body. The amount of this hormone remains high during childhood and adolescence but begins to decline approximately after age 20.

guru The Sanskrit word for teacher, often used to mean a spiritual leader or master.

hearing aid A device that helps a person with hearing loss to hear. It works by amplifying sound waves.

heart rate variability (HRV) The beat-to-beat variation in heart rate that enables the body to adapt to changing conditions. High HRV is associated with good health, while reductions are seen in various disease states. Heart coherence aims to optimize HRV through biofeedback techniques.

herbalism The use of medicines derived from plants.

histamine A chemical substance produced by the body during an allergic reaction. It causes runny nose, sneezing and itching to develop.

holistic In medicine, assessing and treating the person as a whole (rather than just looking at individual symptoms).

homeopathy A system of medicine in which small doses of naturally occurring substances and medicines are used to stimulate healing and the body's own defence mechanisms.

hypothalamus A tiny organ located in the centre of the cranium that regulates the release of hormones, body temperature, sleep patterns, sexual behaviour, thirst and appetite.

hysterectomy A surgical procedure in which the uterus and sometimes the cervix, ovaries and fallopian tubes are removed.

idiopathic A medical condition that occurs without a known cause or explanation.

immunization A process in which the immune system is stimulated to provide protection from future encounters with an infectious agent. This can be achieved through the use of a vaccine, antibody or toxoid.

immunoglobulin A class of proteins, also known as antibodies, that are produced by the body's immune system in response to foreign substances.

immunotherapy Medical treatments which involve stimulating the immune system to destroy foreign substances and tumour cells. It is also known as biological therapy.

impotence Also known as erectile dysfunction, this is the inability to achieve or maintain an erection.

insulin A hormone produced by the pancreas that regulates the amount of sugar in the blood.

intravenous A term used to describe the injection of medications or other fluids directly into the vein.

iron supplements Dietary supplements containing iron, a vital component of blood, deficiency of which leads to anaemia. They may be given as tablets, drops or by injection

intrauterine device (IUD) A contraceptive device that is inserted into the uterus and prevents a fertilized egg from implanting into the walls of the uterus. It is T-shaped and made from flexible plastic or metal material. Some IUDs release hormones that inhibit ovulation from occurring as well.

Japanese Zen A branch of Buddhism that emphasizes meditation and enlightenment.

jaundice Yellowing of the skin due to build up of bile pigment in the blood. It occurs in various diseases.

karma The inevitable results of a person's actions, according to spiritual laws of cause and effect common to Hindu and Buddhist philosophy. Good or bad deeds have appropriate consequences, either in this life or the next.

kava A shrub or the beverage or herbal preparation made from it. It is used to treat anxiety, though is banned in many countries due to safety concerns.

Kegel exercises An exercise routine to strengthen the vaginal and pelvic muscles to aid continence or enhance sexual enjoyment. It is often used by women in preparation for or recovery from childbirth.

ketone A chemical compound produced by the body that is produced as a result of the breakdown of fat for energy.

kundalini In yoga, the female energy believed to lie coiled in the chakra at the base of the spine.

Lamaze technique A type of childbirth preparation using relaxation and breathing techniques, and emphasizing that birth is a normal and natural process.

laparoscopy A surgical procedure used to visualize the ovaries as well as inside the pelvic cavity, fallopian tubes and uterus. A thin flexible viewing tube is inserted into an incision below the navel.

laser-assisted in situ keratomileusis (LASIK) A medical procedure in which the cornea is treated with a laser to correct vision problems such as nearsightedness, farsightedness and astigmatism.

laxative A substance that promotes bowel movements

and relieves constipation.

leukocyte Also known as a white blood cell, these are an important component of the immune system. This class of cells includes monocytes, lymphocytes, neutrophils, granulocytes, basophils and eosinophils. They each work to destroy foreign substances within the blood.

leutinizing hormone (LH) An important hormone that plays a key role in reproduction. LH stimulates the growth and maturation of eggs in females and sperm in males. In addition, it regulates the secretion of progesterone in females and testosterone in males.

ligament A band of fibrous tissue that connects a bone to either another bone or cartilage. It provides the joint with strength and support.

live fruit (unprocessed) Fresh, raw fruit that has not been cooked or processed and retains its optimum nutritional content.

lumbar Relating to the lower part of the back, below the chest or thorax, particularly the five lumbar vertebrae.

lumpectomy The surgical removal of a tumour and surrounding tissue from the breast.

lymph node A series of bean-sized outgrowths on lymphatic vessels that act as filters for lymphatic fluid. Also called lymph glands.

lymphatic fluids The fluid that circulates within the lymphatic system, a series of vessels with its own circulation that forms a vital part of the body's immune system.

lymphoedema Accumulation of lymphatic fluid in the tissues, causing swelling.

magnesium A mineral important in nerve, muscle and bone function and sometimes taken as a dietary supplement.

magnetic resonance imaging (MRI) A diagnostic procedure that uses radio waves and a powerful magnet to produce two dimensional images of organs or other tissues within the body.

malignancy A cancerous tumour capable of spreading within the body.

malnutrition A condition in which the body lacks a sufficient amount of proper nutrition.

malocclusion Faulty alignment of the upper and lower teeth, resulting in an impaired bite.

mammogram A diagnostic procedure that uses x-rays to detect tumours within breast tissue.

manipulons Sequences of movements in the Feldenkrais technique.

mantra A specific word or sound repeated internally or chanted aloud to focus and clear the mind during meditation.

mastectomy A surgical procedure to remove all or portions of a breast.

melatonin A hormone naturally produced by the pineal gland in the brain to regulate sleep-wake cycles and circadian rhythms. Synthetic forms may be taken as supplements.

meridian system Interconnected channels running along the body through which flow life-energy or Qi in Oriental philosophy and Traditional Chinese Medicine. Acupoints – concentrated foci of energy – are located on the meridians.

metabolic disorders Diseases due to faulty biochemical reactions within the body's metabolic processes – those involved in breaking down food ingredients and building up body components from them. Many such disorders are inherited.

metabolism The sum total of chemical processes occurring in the body, especially the breakdown of foodstuffs and the use of nutrient components in producing energy and maintaining body tissues.

metastasize A state in which cancer cells have moved from their organ of origin and have invaded surrounding tissues.

microbe A tiny organism. This definition includes bacteria, viruses, fungi or protozoa.

microorganisms Living creatures too small to be seen with the naked eye, such as bacteria, viruses and algae.

mindfulness-based stress reduction (MBSR) Techniques involving relaxation, meditation and focused attention, designed to increase awareness of everyday living, enhance inner resources and reduce stress.

mineral supplement A dietary supplement containing a mineral, a naturally occurring substance required for bodily function, such as calcium or magnesium.

motor skills Co-ordinated use of the body's skeletal muscles to achieve purposeful movement, such as walking (a gross motor skill) or writing (a fine motor skill).

moxibustion Stimulation of an acupoint by burning a herb, moxa, on or near it.

mucus A thick, slippery, and stretchy fluid that is secreted by the membranes that line the nose, throat, mouth, gastrointestinal tract and vagina. It helps to lubricate these body parts and to trap foreign substances before they are able to enter the body. The mucus produced by the vagina helps sperm travel to the uterus.

muscle dysfunction Weakness or impaired function of muscles.

muscle spasm Involuntary contractions of the muscles which can be triggered by different types of stress.

musculoskeletal Concerning the bones, muscles, joints and other tissues associated with the skeleton.

myokinetics Massage of muscles and associated tissues in order to release tension, as practised in Aston-Patterning.

n.n-diethyl-metatoluamide (DEET) A substance commonly found in insect repellent. It can be applied to the skin or clothing.

narcotic A class of drugs that are easily addictive. They provide pain relief, can cause drowsiness, as well as alter a patient's behaviour.

nasal douching Ayurvedic practice of irrigating the nose with saline (salt water) in order to cleanse the sinuses and relieve symptoms of sinusitis.

nasoscope Also known as a rhinoscope, this is a thin viewing tube that is inserted into the nose allowing it to be examined.

negative asymmetry In Aston-Patterning, an imbalance between the two sides of the body that inhibits effective movement (contrast adaptive asymmetry).

nerve conduction The transmission of impulses down nerves to control body functions or convey sensations.

neurologic A condition that involves the nervous system – the brain, spinal cord and nerves.

neurons One of the types of cells found in the nervous system. These cells are electrically active and transmit signals to regulate behaviour and body functions.

neurotransmitters Chemical messengers released by nerve cells (neurons) to transmit impulses to other nerves or to muscles.

nitrate A chemical compound that is produced as a result of the decay of plant, animal and human waste.

nonsteroidal A term used to describe substances that do not contain steroids.

nonsteroidal anti-inflammatory drugs (NSAIDS) A class of medications that provide pain relief, reduce temperatures and ease inflammation. Examples include aspirin and ibuprofen.

norepinephrine A substance that serves as both a hormone and a neurotransmitter. It plays a key role in concentration, alertness, motivation, aggression, and the fight-or-flight response.

oestrogen The female sex hormone, produced mainly in the ovaries.

omega-3 fatty acids A component of certain fish tissues and vegetables.

ophthalmologist A type of doctor who specializes in the heath of the eye and vision.

opiate A substance that is a derivative of opium or produces an opium-like effect in the body. It works as an analgesic, causing drowsiness, reducing pain and dulling the senses.

optic nerve A bundle of nerve fibres that connect the brain to the retina. It is responsible for converting visual signals from the retina into images allowing for sight.

optometrist A doctor who cares for the eyes. An optometrist specializes in vision problems and is able to determine which eye glasses or contact lenses would best serve a person.

oral cancers A type of cancer that is found in the mouth, on the lips, or in the upper section of the throat.

organ A part of the body composed of several different tissues and specialized for a particular function, for example the heart or liver.

orthodontic A specialty area of dentistry that focuses on tooth placement irregularities or jaw proportion.

orthopaedic A term used to describe conditions or treatments related to the bones, muscles or joints.

osteopaths Practitioners of osteopathy.

osteosarcoma A type of bone cancer that begins in the tissues of growing bones and easily metastasizes.

outpatient surgery A surgical procedure that is performed and does not require an overnight stay in the hospital.

ovum The mature egg released by the ovary during ovulation.

oximeter A device that monitors the amount of oxygen in the body. It can be worn on the finger or earlobe over a period of time, even while a patient sleeps.

oxygenation Describing the amount of oxygen present or the process of providing oxygen, used especially of blood.

pacemaker A small medical device that is placed under the skin and connected to the heart. It measures the heart rhythm and regulates the heartbeat if it is too fast or too slow.

palliation Treatment aimed at relieving symptoms rather than curing their cause.

palpation (of the skin) Examination of the body surface using pressure with the hands to feel for underlying structures.

palpitations Irregular heartbeats that can be felt has fluttering or pounding within the chest.

paraldehyde A liquid substance that is used as a sedative.

paralysis A state in which a body part is unable to move as a result of a loss in muscle function.

parasite An organism that needs to live on a host to survive. A parasite grows, feeds and lives on or inside its host.

pelvic examination A diagnostic procedure in which the doctor examines the vagina, cervix, uterus, ovaries and rectum of a woman.

peptic ulcer An open sore located in the lining of the stomach, oesophagus or small intestine. It is usually caused by stomach acids, certain medications or a bacterial infection.

pericardium A membrane sac that surrounds the heart. It is filled with fluid that helps to lubricate the heart during pumping.

periodontitis An advanced form of gum disease. The tissues surrounding the gums are inflamed and the structure surrounding the teeth and jaw bone loosens causing the teeth to eventually fall out.

peritoneum The large membrane that covers the wall of the abdomen. It is composed of an outer and an inner membrane that is enclosed in men and connected to the fallopian tubes in women. It provides moisture to the abdominal organs and prevents friction as they glide past one another.

phlebotomy A medical process in which blood is released from a vein.

phlegm Mucus formed in the respiratory tract. In Tibetan medicine, one of the three 'humours', along with wind and bile, said to regulate body functions and energy balance.

phobias Extreme and irrational fears of objects or situations that most people regard as harmless.

photosensitivity A condition in which a person suffers from a skin reaction when exposed to sunlight. Swelling, acne, hives and burns are common – developed as a reaction to sun exposure for those with photosensitivity.

phototherapy Using light in the treatment of disease.

phytochemicals Chemical constituents of plants that have effects on health other than their nutrient value. Many are believed to protect against disease, including cancer.

phyto-oestrogens A type of phytochemical with oestrogen-like effects.

pituitary gland A small gland joined to the hypothalamus at the base of the brain. It produces many of the hormones used by the body.

placebo An inert substance or procedure with no specific therapeutic properties. Placebo tablets that appear identical to active drugs are often given for comparison in clinical trials of new drugs, so that patient expectations do not bias the assessment.

placenta A blood-rich organ formed during pregnancy that provides oxygen and food to the developing foetus. In addition, it filters out waste products produced by the foetus during gestation.

platelet A type of blood cell that is responsible for clotting. They are small and disk shaped.

pleura The membrane that surrounds the lungs. It is filled with a fluid that moistens the lungs as they fill and empty with air.

pneumonia A condition in which the lungs become inflamed. It can be caused by a bacterial, viral, or fungal infection.

polyp A small growth that develops on the surface of a mucous membrane.

polysaturated fatty acids A compound that is found in certain foods such as fish, walnuts, corn, sunflower seeds, soybeans, cottonseed and safflower oil. Diets high in this substance promote healthy cholesterol levels.

polyunsaturated oils Fatty acids containing two or more double bonds. They are found in oils from certain vegetables and fish.

poultice Warm, wet padding made of cloth or plant material applied to the skin to soothe aches and pains or draw out infection. It may contain drugs or herbs.

prakriti In Ayurveda, the individual's unique profile of doshas or biological forces, the combination representing the person's constitution.

pranayama The breathing techniques of yoga that enable an individual to control prana, or life force.

premalignant A term used to describe cells that may become cancerous.

pressure points Specific sites on the body that produce a reaction when touched. In Oriental medicine, the term is often applied to points on the meridian system.

probiotics Microorganisms that have beneficial effects within the body. They are found naturally in the gut and may be taken as a dietary supplement.

progesterone A female sex hormone that helps to regulate the menstrual cycle and maintain pregnancy. It is secreted by the ovaries and prepares the lining of the uterus to receive a fertilized egg or to shed during menstruation.

prolactin A hormone that is secreted by the pituitary gland. It regulates breast development and milk production in lactating women.

prosthesis An artificial device that replaces a missing body part such as an arm or a leg.

pseudohaematuria A condition in which the urine becomes red as a result of the consumption of certain foods or medications.

psychodynamic A term used to describe the interplay of mind, personality and psyche.

psychosis A mental condition in which one cannot

distinguish between what is real and imaginary. It is characterized by hallucinations and delusions.

psychosocial The combination of psychological and social influences, which often interact.

psychostimulant Prescription medication used to treat children, adolescents and adults with symptoms of hyperactivity, impulsivity and inattention, often related to Attention-Deficit Hyperactivity Disorder (ADHD).

psychotherapy The treatment of emotional problems by discussion with a professional or counsellor, sometimes within groups. There are many varieties.

puberty A phase of sexual development when a child becomes physiologically capable of reproduction. During this period children experience physical and hormonal changes associated with rapid growth.

pulse rate The number of heart beats in a set time, usually one minute, measured by the pulsation of arteries close to the skin, for example at the wrist or in the neck.

pus A whitish-yellow fluid that consists of white blood cells, cellular debris and necrotic tissue, usually found at a site of infected tissue.

qi The Chinese term used to describe the life force or vital energy of the body, pronounced 'chee'.

qigong An ancient Chinese healing exercise programme combining movement, breathing control and meditation, with the aim of stimulating the flow of qi.

radiation therapy The use of penetrating beams of high-energy rays to destroy cancer cells and slow their multiplication.

rapid eye movement (REM) sleep Period of sleep distinguished by rapid saccadic movements of the eyes, that is often associated with dreaming. REM sleep usually accounts for 20 percent of sleep.

rash A change in the texture and coloration on the skin surface. Usually marked by red or skin-coloured bumps and blotches.

recommended daily allowance (RDA) The amount of an essential nutrient regarded as sufficient to meet the needs of most healthy people when taken daily from food, as set by the Food Standards Agency in the UK and the Food and Nutrition Board in the USA.

rehabilitation The restoration of health or function after an injury or illness.

rei The Japanese word for 'universal spirit' from which the term 'reiki' is partially derived.

Rescue Remedy The combination of five Bach flower remedies intended to alleviate shock after physical or emotional trauma.

restricted environmental stimulation technique

(REST) A therapeutic form of sensory deprivation in which external sensory input, such as sight, touch and hearing, is minimized. It is used to induce deep relaxation.

rhinoscope A medical instrument with an angled mirror used to examine the nasal passage.

riboflavin The chemical name of Vitamin B2, a water-soluble vitamin vital for health, growth and reproduction.

sacral Relating to the sacrum, the five fused vertebrae forming the lower end of the spine at the level of the hip and pelvis (below the lumbar spine).

sacro-occipital Relates to the sacro-occipital technique, a form of craniosacral therapy or chiropractic based on the premise that cerebrospinal fluid circulates driven by a sacral pump from the base of the spine (sacrum) to the occiput (head).

sacrum The five fused vertebrae forming the lower end of the spine at the level of the hip and pelvis (below the lumbar spine).

salivary glands Consists of three pairs of glands within the oral cavity that releases saliva through ducts throughout the mouth.

SAM-e (s-adenosylmethionine) A natural-forming chemical compound made of methlonine and adenosine triphosphate, found in the body. Available as a non-prescription dietary supplement, which is sometimes used to treat depression and osteoarthritis.

saturated fats Fats that are solid at room temperature, mainly derived from animal sources.

scab A dry crust covering a skin wound.

sedative A drug that eases irritability, agitation and aids sleep.

selective serotonin reuptake inhibitors (SSRIs) Antidepressants prescribed to treat depression, anxiety and some personality disorders.

selenium A trace mineral that protects cell membranes from damage and possibly reduces the risk of cancer.

self-help Any type of intervention that a person or group attempts to create improvements in life, most often applied to emotional and psychological measures.

serotonin Also known as 5-hydroxytryptamine or 5-HT, a chemical found widely in the body and in the brain, where it acts as a neurotransmitter. Low levels have been linked with depression.

sitz bath A shallow tub to be filled with warm water as a hip bath, intended to soothe conditions such as haemorrhoids while leaving the legs and body dry.

skin graft A patch of skin removed from one section of the body and transplanted to another section to repair damaged skin or to create skin cells where they no longer exist. Grafts can also be taken from a donor.

slitlamp Microscope used to examine the anterior structures of the eye.

soul response In Anthroposophic medicine, an individual's inner response to external stimuli such a sound.

spasm Brief involuntary muscle contractions that are focal to one area and often painful.

spermicide A chemical usually consisting of nonoxynol-9 that is used to kill sperm during sexual relations.

sphenoid One of the bones of the skull, forming part of its base at the side of the head and behind the nose.

spinal cord A column of nerve tissue made of 31 pairs of spinal nerves responsible for relaying nerve impulses sent from the brain.

spinal manipulation The main treatment mode of chiropractic. It involves correction of misalignments in the spine by pressure with the hands.

spirometer Device used to test the air capacity of a person's lungs.

splint Mechanism used to hold a part of the body firm and motionless while healing occurs.

sputum A mucus-like secretion created in the lungs and bronchi and commonly coughed up.

St John's wort A herbal medicine that has proved both effective and safe in treating mild to moderate depression.

stem cell Unspecialized cell that can be used to replace cells that are damaged or lost.

sterilize To rid all microorganisms and germs.

steroid A natural fat-soluble substance found in the body.

sterols A group of natural lipids found in animals and plants. Chemically, a steroid alcohol. One example is cholesterol.

stimulant A chemical that causes temporary heightened physiological and organic activity.

stress reduction Any technique that lessens the perceived effects of stress on an individual and thus reduces anxiety, tension, negative behaviours and symptoms such as headache or fatigue.

subluxations An incomplete or partial dislocation of a joint.

succussed Shaken – used especially to describe the preparation of homeopathic remedies.

supplements Extras or additions, particularly substances taken in addition to the diet.

sutures Stitches used to hold wounds together after injury or surgery. Also the fibrous joints between the plates of the skull that allow for expansion during normal growth to adulthood, after which they fuse.

sympathetic nervous system The part of the autonomic nervous system, usually outside conscious control, responsible for 'fight or flight' reactions – such as increased heart rate in response to threat. It is balanced by the parasympathetic system, which does the opposite.

synbiotics The combination of probiotics (beneficial bacteria) with prebiotics, the undigestible carbohydrates that nourish them in the intestines. The combination is said to have a greater therapeutic effect.

systolic Arterial pressure when the heart is contracting. The numerator in a blood pressure measurement.

T-cell A white blood cell that is key to the proper functioning of the immune system.

tai chi A series of flowing exercises often recommended in Traditional Chinese Medicine.

tartar Hardened plaque which results from the build-up of food and bacteria around teeth.

tendon Tough bundles of collagen fibres that attach the ends of muscles to the bones they move.

tension headache A headache brought on by stress and anxiety, often linked with muscle contraction in the neck, scalp and face.

testosterone Male sex hormone produced in the testes.

Thai massage A form that involves both massage and acupressure – gentle pressure on acupoints to harmonize the flow of qi or life energy.

thalassaemia A hereditary form of anaemia due to an abnormality in the haemoglobin molecule that carries oxygen in the blood.

three excreta Faeces, urine and perspiration, routinely assessed in Tibetan medicine for their potential contribution to health and disease.

three humours According to Tibetan medicine, wind, bile and phlegm: the principles of energy, the balance of which controls a person's constitution.

Tibetan sutras A collection of sacred scripts important in Tibetan Buddhism.

tic An uncontrollable recurring spasm of the face, arms, and legs.

tinctures A plant extract prepared by soaking a herb in alcohol.

topical steroids Corticosteroid drugs applied to the skin in cream or ointment form, to relieve inflammation in various skin conditions.

toxic/toxins Anything having a poisonous or harmful effect may be described as toxic. Technically, a toxin is a poison produced by a living organism, such as bacterial toxins; however the word is often used to describe any poisonous substance.

toxoplasmosis Parasitic infection of tissue which can result in brain damage and blindness.

Trager approach A form of massage or manipulation that also involves exercise and relaxation techniques, designed to integrate mind and body.

trans-fatty acids Fats produced especially during food processing by hydrogenation of vegetable oils. Although unsaturated, trans fats behave more like saturated fats, and may be even more harmful to health.

transcranial magnetic stimulation A form of magnet therapy involving an external magnet applied on or near the skull to induce electromagnetic fields within the brain.

trauma Any physical or mental wound caused by an external force.

trycyclic antidepressant Antidepressant drug that allows for the reabsorbtion of neurotransmitters in the central nervous system.

tuina A type of massage used in Traditional Chinese Medicine that involves pressure on acupoints.

ultrasound Sound waves are used to bounce off tissue to create an image of an examined area.

ultraviolet rays Light rays with very short wave lengths, outside the visible spectrum so they cannot be seen with the human eye. They form part of the radiation from the sun responsible for warmth and suntanning.

urologist Doctor who specializes in diseases of the urogenital tract.

vedas The four sacred scriptures of Hinduism.

vena cava Vein that carries expended blood to the right atrium of the heart.

vertebrae The 33 bones comprising the backbone and protecting the spinal cord.

vipassana A type of Buddhist mindfulness meditation using present moment awareness to achieve insight and enlightenment.

virus Microorganism that relies on living cells to multiply. Viral illnesses can be unique in their formation and hard to treat.

visualization The use of mental imagery, often to achieve psychological goals such as enhanced performance, creativity or problem-solving.

vitamins (B_{12}, A, B_6, C) Substances found in foods and essential in tiny amounts for healthy functioning. Vitamin B_{12} is important to healthy nerve cell activity. Vitamin A maintains the skin, eyes and teeth. Vitamin B_6 helps to produce antibodies and red blood cells. Vitamin

C is an antioxidant important in healing wounds.

vitiligo A skin disease causing patchy depigmentation of the skin.

x chromosome Sex chromosome found in males and females. Females usually have two of these chromosomes.

y chromosome Male sex chromosome which appear predominantly in males.

yang In traditional Chinese philosophy, one of the pair of fundamental forces forming the universe. Yang represents male, contraction, active, hot, hard and positive.

yin In traditional Chinese philosophy, one of the pair of fundamental forces forming the universe. Yin represents female, expansion, cold, soft and negative.

yoga sutras Ancient Hindu scripts on yoga philosophy and practice.

yogi A master or teacher of yoga.

Zen A school of Buddhism teaching enlightenment especially through meditation.

zinc A metallic element required in small quantities for healthy body functioning.

RESOURCES

Additional Reading

Becker, Robert O. and Selden, Gary. *The Body Electric: Electromagnetism and the Foundation of Life*, Harper Paperbacks, 1998

Blumer, Ronald H. *The New Medicine: Companion Book to the Public Television Series*, Middlemarch Films, 2006

Borysenko, Joan. *A Woman's Book of Life: The Biology, Psychology, and Spirituality of the Feminine Life Cycle*, Riverhead, 1998

Brantley, Jeffrey, et al. *Five Good Minutes: 100 Morning Practices To Help You Stay Calm and Focused All Day Long*, New Harbinger Publications, 2005

Brantley, Jeffrey. *Calming Your Anxious Mind: How Mindfulness and Compassion Can Free You of Anxiety, Fear, and Panic*, New Harbinger Publications, 2003

Bratman, Steven and Kroll, David. *Natural Health Bible*, Prima Lifestyle, 1999

Brill, Peggy W., et al. *The Core Program: Fifteen Minutes a Day that Can Change Your Life*, Bantam, 2003

Carson, Richard D. *Taming Your Gremlin: A Guide to Enjoying Yourself*, HarperCollins, 1990

Dell, Diana L. and Svec, Carol. *The PMDD Phenomenon: Breakthrough Treatments for Premenstrual Dysphoric Disorder (PMDD) and Extreme Premenstrual Syndrome (PMS)*, McGraw Hill, 2002

Domar, Alice D. and Dreher, Henry. *Healing Mind, Healthy Woman: Using the Mind-Body Connection to Manage Stress and Take Control of Your Life*, Delta, 1997

Domar, Alice D. and Lesch, Alice Kelly. *Conquering Infertility: Dr. Alice Domar's Mind/Body Guide to Enhancing Fertility and Coping With Infertility*, Penguin, 2004

Dossey, Larry. *Healing Words: The Power of Prayer and the Practice of Medicine*, Harper San Francisco, 1997

Ernst, Edzard. *Desktop Guide to Complementary and Alternative Medicine*, C.V.Mosby, 2006

Forrest, Steven. *The Inner Sky: How to Make Wiser Choices for a More Fulfilling Life*, Astro Communications Services, 1999

Gaudet, Tracy. *Body, Soul and Baby: A Doctor's Guide to the Complete Experience of Pregnancy; From Preconception to Postpartum*, Bantam, 2007

Gaudet, Tracy and Spencer, Paula. *Consciously Female: How to Listen to Your Body and Your Soul for a Lifetime of Healthier Living*, Bantam, 2004

Geffen, Jeremy. *The Journey Through Cancer*, Three Rivers Press, 2001

Graedon, Joe and Graedon, Teresa. *The People's Pharmacy Guide to Home and Herbal Remedies*, St. Martin's Paperbacks, 2002

Hanh, Thich Nhat. *Being Peace*, Parallax Press, 2005

Holstein, Lana L. *How to Have Magnificent Sex: The 7 Dimensions of a Vital Sexual Connection*, Harmony, 2001

Horrigan, Bonnie J. *Voices of Integrative Medicine: Conversations and Encounters*, Churchill Livingstone, 2003

Hottinger, Greg. *The Best Natural Foods on the Market Today: A Yuppie's Guide to Hippie Food, Volume 1*, Huckleberry Mountain Press, 2004

Huddleston, Peggy. *Prepare for Surgery, Heal Faster: A Guide of Mind-Body Techniques,* Angel River Press, 2002

Hudson, Tori. *Women's Encyclopedia of Natural Medicine: Alternative Therapies and Integrative Medicine*, McGraw Hill, 1999

Judelson, Debrea R. and Dell, Diana L. *The Women's Complete Wellness Book (American Medical Women's Association)*, St Martin's Press, 2000

Kabat-Zinn, Jon. *Full Catastrophe Living*, Delta, 1990

Kabat-Zinn, Jon. *Wherever You Go, There You Are: Mindfulness Meditation in Everyday Life*, Hyperion, 2005

Kaptchuk, Ted J. *The Web that Has No Weaver: Understanding Chinese Medicine*, Congdon and Weed, 1983

Kliger, Benjamin and Lee, Roberta. *Integrative Medicine: Principles of Practice*, McGraw-Hill Professional, 2004

Koenig, Harold G. *The Healing Power of Faith: How Belief and Prayer Can Help You Triumph Over Disease*, Simon & Schuster, 2001

Krucoff, Carol and Krucoff, Mitchell. *Healing Moves: How to Cure, Relieve, and Prevent Common Ailments with Exercise*, Writers' Collective, 2004

Legato, Marianne J. *Eve's Rib: The New Science of Gender-Specific Medicine and How it Can Save Your Life*, Harmony, 2002

Lerner, Michael. *Choices in Healing: Integrating The Best of Conventional and Complementary Approaches To Cancer*, The MIT Press, 1996

Levine, Stephen. *Healing into Life and Death,* Anchor, 1989

Moyers, Bill. *Healing and the Mind*, Main Street Books, 1995

Myss, Caroline. *Anatomy of the Spirit: The Seven Stages of Power and Healing*, Three Rivers Press, 1997

Nelson, Miriam E. *Strong Women Stay Young*, Bantam, 2000

Northrup, Christiane. *The Wisdom of Menopause: Creating Physical and Emotional Health and Healing During The Change*, Bantam, 2003

Northrup, Christiane. *Women's Bodies, Women's Wisdom: Creating Physical and Emotional Health and Healing*, Bantam, 2002

Ornish, Dean. *Dr. Dean Ornish's Program for Reversing Heart Disease: The Only System Scientifically Proven to Reverse Heart Disease Without Drugs or Surgery*, Ballantine Books, 2007, revised edition

Payne, Niravi B. and Richardson, Brenda Lane. *The Whole Person Fertility Program: A Revolutionary Mind-Body Process to Help You Conceive*, Three Rivers Press, 1998

Pelletier, Kenneth. *The Best Alternative Medicine*, Fireside, 2002

Rakel, David. *Integrative Medicine*, W.B.Saunders, 2002

Remen, Rachel Naomi. *Kitchen Table Wisdom*, Riverhead Books, 1997

Richardson, Cheryl. *Take Time for Your Life: A Personal Coach's Seven-Step Program for Creating the Life You Want*, Broadway, 1999

Rossman, Martin L. *Healing Yourself: A Step-by-Step Program for Better Health Through Imagery*, Awareness Press, 1987

Santorelli, Saki. *Heal Thy Self: Lessons on Mindfulness in Medicine*, Harmony, 2000

Schultz, V. Hansel, R. Blumenthal M., and Tyler, V.E. *Rational Phytotherapy: A Reference Guide for Physicians and Pharmacists*, Springer, 2004

Servan-Schreiber, David. *Healing Without Freud or Prozac*, Rodale Books, 2004

Siegel, Bernie S. *Love, Medicine, and Miracles: Lessons Learned About Self-Healing From A Surgeon's Experience With Exceptional Patients*, Harper Paperbacks, 1990

Stewart, Elizabeth G. and Spencer, Paula. *V Book: A Doctor's Guide to Complete Vulvovaginal Health*, Bantam, 2002

Tarrant, John. *The Light Inside the Dark: Zen, Soul, and the Spiritual Life*, Harper Paperbacks, 1999

Weed, Susan S. *Menopausal Years The Wise Woman Way: Alternative Approaches for Women 30–90*, Ash Tree Publishing, 2001

Weil, Andrew. *Eating Well For Optimum Health: The Essential Guide to Bringing Health and Pleasure Back to Eating*, Collins, 2001

Weil, Andrew. *Health and Healing*, Houghton Mifflin, 2004

Weil, Andrew. *Healthy Aging: A Lifelong Guide to Your Physical and Spiritual Well-being*, Knopf, 2005

Willett, Walter C., and Skerrett, P.J. *Eat, Drink, and Be Healthy: The Harvard Medical School Guide to Healthy Eating*, Free Press, 2005

Williams, Redford, M.D. and Williams, Virginia, PhD. *Anger Kills: Seventeen Strategies for Controlling the Hostility That Can Harm Your Health*, HarperTorch, 1998

Williams, Redford, M.D. and Williams, Virginia, PhD. *In Control: No More Snapping at Your Family, Sulking at Work, Steaming in the Grocery Line, Seething in Meetings, Stuffing Your Frustration*, Rodale Books, 2006

Williams, Virginia, PhD and Williams, Redford, M.D. *Lifeskills: 8 Simple Ways to Build Stronger Relationships, Communicate More Clearly, and Improve Your Health*, Three Rivers Press, 1999

Wilson, Paul. *The Calm Technique: Meditation without Magic or Mysticism*, Barnes & Noble Books, 1999

Internet Resources

ACUPUNCTURE
www.acupuncture.com
www.medicalacupuncture.org
www.aaom.org
www.nccaom.org

CANCER
www.bhma.info
www.breastcancer.org
www.cancer.gov/occam
www.cancersource.com
www.cancer.duke.edu
www.nci.nih.gov

COUNSELLING AND COMMUNICATION
www.aamft.org
www.bacp.co.uk
www.gottman.com
www.ifta-familytherapy.org
www.relate.org.uk

DUKE UNIVERSITY SITES
www.dcim.org
www.dukehealth.org

E-MEDICINE CONSUMER HEALTH
www.emedicinehealth.com
www.netdoctor.co.uk
www.nhsdirect.nhs.uk

EYE MOVEMENT DESENSITIZATION AND REPROCESSING (EMDR)
www.emdria.org
www.emdr.com
www.emdr-europe.net

HEALTH AND WELLNESS
www.cochrane.org
www.instincttoheal.org

HEART COHERENCE
www.heartmath.com
www.theheartofhealth.com
www.futurehealth.org

HERBAL MEDICINES
www.herbalgram.org
www.herbalmedicine.org.uk
www.herbs.org

HOLISTIC MEDICINE
www.bhma.org
www.holisticmedicine.org
www.holisticonline.com

INTEGRATIVE MEDICINE
www.mdanderson.org/departments/CIMER
www.nccam.nih.gov
www.integrativemedicine.upmc.com

MASSAGE
www.amtamassage.org
www.ncbtmb.com

MENOPAUSE
www.menpoause.org
www.menopausematters.co.uk
www.menopause-online.com

NATURAL STANDARD COLLABORATION
www.naturalstandard.com

NUTRITION
www.consumerlab.com
www.dietary-supplements.info.nih.gov
www.isodisnatura.net/
www.fda.gov/opacom/hpnews.html

YOGA
www.himalayaninstitute.org
www.kripalu.org
www.yogadirectory.com

Boldface page references indicate photographs and illustrations.

Picture Credits